ANNALS OF THE NEW YORK ACADEMY OF SCIENCES
Volume 911

THE PARAHIPPOCAMPAL REGION

IMPLICATIONS FOR NEUROLOGICAL AND PSYCHIATRIC DISEASES

Edited by Helen E. Scharfman, Menno P. Witter, and Robert Schwarcz

The New York Academy of Sciences
New York, New York
2000

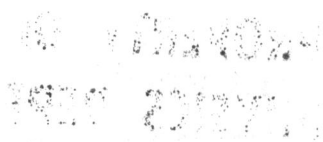

Library of Congress Cataloging-in-Publication Data

The parahippocampal region : implications for neurological and psychiatric diseases / edited by Helen E. Scharfman, Menno P. Witter, and Robert Schwarcz.
    p. ; cm. — (Annals of the New York Academy of Sciences, ISSN 0077-8923 ; v. 911)
    Includes bibliographical references and indexes.
    ISBN 1-57331-263-0 (cloth : alk. paper) . — ISBN 1-57331-264-9 (pbk. : alk. paper)
    1. Hippocampus (Brain)—Physiology. 2. Hippocampus (Brain)—Pathophysiology. I. Scharfman, Helen E. II. Witter, Menno P. III. Schwarcz, Robert. IV. Series.

    Q11 .N5 vol. 911
    [QP383.25]
    500 s—dc21
    [612.8'25]

                           00-036153

GYAT / BMP
Printed in the United States of America
ISBN 1-57331-263-0 (cloth)
ISBN 1-57331-264-9 (paper)
ISSN 0077-8923

ANNALS OF THE NEW YORK ACADEMY OF SCIENCES

Volume 911
June 2000

THE PARAHIPPOCAMPAL REGION

IMPLICATIONS FOR NEUROLOGICAL AND PSYCHIATRIC DISEASES[a]

Editors and Conference Organizers
HELEN E. SCHARFMAN, MENNO P. WITTER, AND ROBERT SCHWARCZ

CONTENTS

[a]This volume is the result of a conference entitled **The Hippocampal Region: Basic Science and Clinical Implications,** held by the New York Academy of Sciences on September 23–26, 1999, in Baltimore, Maryland.

Financial assistance was received from:

Major Funder
• NATIONAL INSTITUTES OF HEALTH

Supporters
• ASTRA ARCUS AB
• JANSSEN PHARMACEUTICA

Contributors
• ALA INSTRUMENTS
• ASTRA ZENECA
• FINE SCIENCE TOOLS INC.
• GLAXO WELLCOME
• GUILFORD PHARMACEUTICALS, INC.
• MERZ & CO. GMBH
• MICROBRIGHTFIELD
• PHARMACIA & UPJOHN COMPANY
• SHIRE RICHWOOD INC.
• SUTTER INSTRUMENT COMPANY

Preface

Several structures in the temporal lobe play a critical role in learning and memory, emotions, and other complex behavioral processes. These include the hippocampus, the most frequently studied part of the temporal lobe, the juxtaposed parahippocampal region, and the amygdala. During the last decade, it has become increasingly clear that pathological changes in the parahippocampal region occur during the early stages of several catastrophic neurological and psychiatric diseases, such as Alzheimer's disease, schizophrenia, and epilepsy. Thus, it is quite likely that parahippocampal neuropathology contributes to dysfunction in these and perhaps other brain disorders. Notably, pathology in these brain structures may be a critical element of several of these diseases, independent of the state of the hippocampus itself.

This volume contains the proceedings of a New York Academy of Sciences conference entitled The Parahippocampal Region: Basic Science and Clinical Implications, which was held in Baltimore, Maryland in September 1999. The idea for the meeting originated from the need to integrate basic and clinical information about the parahippocampal region, as described and interpreted by the experts in the field. The major goal of the two-and-one-half-day symposium was to provide a comprehensive, contemporary review of this brain region and its circuitry, and to stimulate interdisciplinary research including anatomical, biochemical, physiological, behavioral, and pathological studies. It is our hope that the proceedings will provide the reader with the necessary information to further explore the structure and function of the parahippocampal region.

A recurring issue concerning research in this field has been the lack of a universal terminology and a precise definition of the "parahippocampal region." Therefore, an impromptu discussion at the meeting sought a consensus definition for this and associated terms that would ideally apply to multiple species. The outcome of these discussions, which were subsequently consolidated and edited by several meeting participants and additional experts, is briefly summarized here.

Why "parahippocampal region"? Arguments to group a number of brain structures together, and to propose a single term for them, could be based on a variety of considerations. We grouped together several cortical regions that form part of the cortex adjacent to and enwrapping the macroscopically defined "hippocampus." In order to refer to these areas as a unit, we chose the term parahippocampal region, which is defined below. *Region* implies the spatial proximity of the constituents, and functional neutrality. This contrasts with a *system*, which may contain remote but functionally connected components. The term *parahippocampus* implies too much structural homogeneity, and *parahippocampal gyrus* was avoided because it refers to a macroscopically identifiable entity of the primate brain, which is not present in most nonprimate mammals. *Parahippocampal cortex* has become generally accepted in the primate literature to designate the more caudal portions of the parahippocampal gyrus (areas TF and TH, as originally described in the rhesus monkey by von Bonin and Bailey[1]).

Consistent with this nomenclature is the use of the term *hippocampal formation*, which includes the dentate gyrus, areas CA1–3 and the subiculum. In contrast to previous proposals, the entorhinal cortex is not considered part of the hippocampal formation (cf. Amaral and Witter[2]). The term *hippocampal region,* used by many authors—in particular in reference to rodents—as a shorthand for dentate gyrus, CA-fields, subiculum, pre- and parasubiculum, and entorhinal cortex, will not be used (cf. Witter *et al.*[3]). We will also avoid the designation *rhinal cortex* (cf. Murray[4]) because it cannot be equally applied to both primate and nonprimate species. As originally proposed, the rhinal cortex comprises the entorhinal and perirhinal cortices, two areas positioned around the rhinal sulcus in the primate brain. This is in contrast to the more posterior *parahippocampal cortex,* which does have a topological relation to the collateral sulcus, but not to the rhinal sulcus. Unfortunately, as argued by Burwell *et al.*[5] and described further by Witter *et al.* (this volume), the most likely homologue for the primate parahippocampal cortex in nonprimate mammals is formed by the postrhinal cortex, which does have a topological relation to the rhinal sulcus.

Definition of the parahippocampal region. On the basis of its unique laminar organization and connectivity, the parahippocampal region is defined as the pre- and parasubiculum, the entorhinal and perirhinal cortices, as well as the postrhinal (in nonprimate mammalians) or parahippocampal cortex (in primates including human). It is likely that each of these individual components of the parahippocampal region makes unique contributions to the overall cortico-hippocampal interplay.

Laminar organization. Already in the earliest cytoarchitectonic descriptions of the mammalian cortex, two major types of cortex were discussed, that is, a three-layered cortex, called allocortex, and a six-layered cortex, generally called neocortex or isocortex. Moreover, most authors suggested that transitional zones exist between the three-layered and six-layered cortical areas. These transitional zones generally have been referred to as periallocortex and proisocortex (cf. Stephan[6]). The structures included here in the hippocampal formation form a continuum of three-layered cortex (Fig. 1), that is, cortex consisting of a molecular layer, a cell layer, and a polymorph or fiber layer. This holds true for the dentate gyrus, fields CA3, CA2, and CA1, and the subiculum. The border of the subiculum and the presubiculum is characterized by a sudden emergence of a more superficially positioned cortical sheet. This increase in number of layers indicates the border of the hippocampal formation with the parahippocampal region. The parahippocampal region thus comprises cortical areas that form the transition from allocortex into neocortex. In the periallocortex, the additional cortical sheet is strictly separated from the deeper continuation of the subicular sheet by a cell-free zone, generally termed lamina dissecans. This striking organization, which is present in all mammalian species, prompted Rose[7] to designate this cortical region as the schizocortex. Although this term is no longer in use, it describes very well the characteristic cytoarchitectonic features of the pre- and parasubiculum and the entorhinal cortex. At the border between the entorhinal and perirhinal or postrhinal/parahippocampal cortex, the lamina dissecans disappears, giving way to a more homogeneously layered cortex, the proisocortex, that resembles the six-layered neocortex. However, in contrast to the adjacent neocortex, the perirhinal and postrhinal/parahippocampal cortices do not feature a marked inner granular cell layer IV (Fig. 1).

Connectivity. As illustrated in Figure 2, the components of the parahippocampal region show unique connectivity. Each individual area of the parahippocampal region projects directly to one or more of the subfields of the hippocampal formation, and in turn receives a direct afferent input from area CA1 and/or the subiculum. The most prominent cortical input of the entorhinal cortex is collectively supplied by the perirhi-

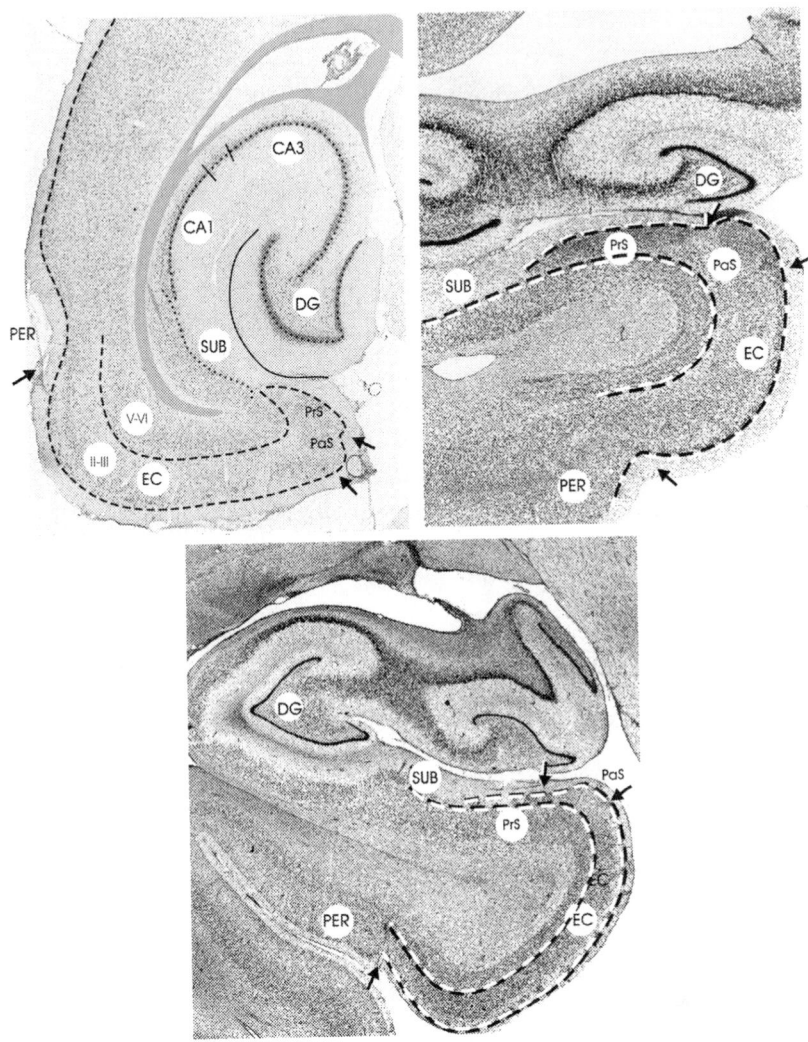

FIGURE 1. Nissl-stained section through rat (*top left*), monkey (*top right*), and human (*bottom*) parahippocampal/hippocampal regions. Note the increase in number of cortical laminae at the border between the subiculum (SUB) and the presubiculum (PrS), indicating the border, according to the criteria outlined here, between the hippocampal formation and the parahippocampal region. Also note the marked cell-free zone in pre- and parasubiculum and entorhinal cortex, known as the lamina dissecans. This characteristic cell-free zone ends at the border of the entorhinal cortex (EC) with the perirhinal cortex (PER).

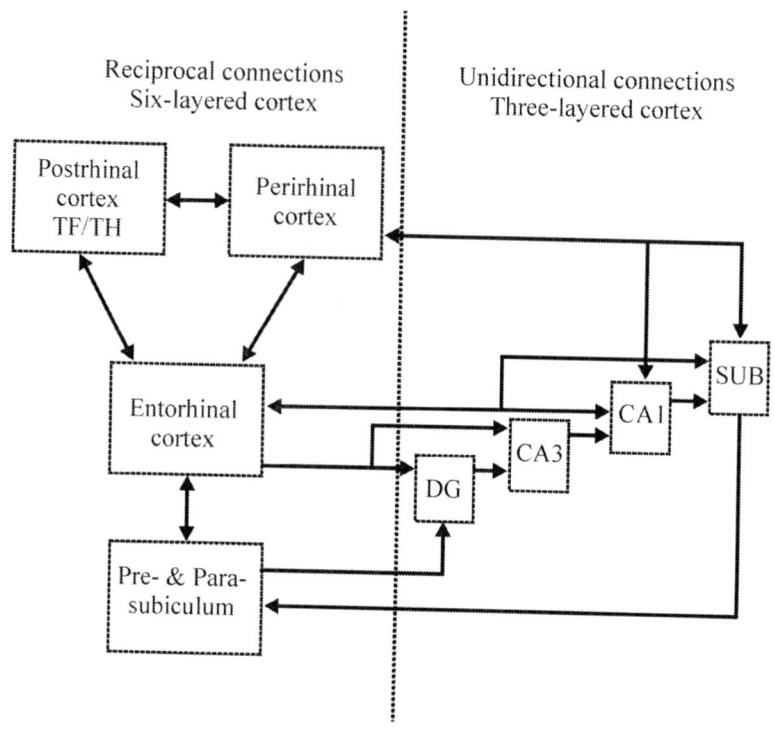

FIGURE 2. Summary of the two main criteria used to define the parahippocampal region (*left*) and the hippocampal formation (*right*). The hippocampal formation is characterized mainly by unidirectional connections between three-layered allocortical regions. The parahippocampal cortex is defined as those six-layered cortical areas which (i) are reciprocally connected to (parts of) the hippocampal formation and (ii) are reciprocally interconnected. *Abbreviations*: DG, dentate gyrus; CA3 and CA1, parts of the Ammon's horn or Cornu Ammonis; SUB, subiculum.

nal and postrhinal/parahippocampal cortices, and a major part of entorhinal output is distributed to these same parahippocampal regions. Moreover, a prominent reciprocal connectivity exists between the entorhinal cortex and the pre- and parasubiculum.[2,8,9]

—HELEN E. SCHARFMAN
—MENNO P. WITTER
—ROBERT SCHWARCZ

REFERENCES

1. VON BONIN, G. & P. BAILEY. 1947. The Neocortex of *Macaca mulatta*. University of Illinois Press. Urbana, IL.
2. AMARAL, D.G. & M.P. WITTER. 1995. The hippocampal formation. *In* The Rat Nervous System, 2nd ed. G. Paxinos, Ed.: 443–493. Academic Press Inc. London.

3. WITTER, M.P. *et al.* 1986. Connections of the parahippocampal cortex in the cat. V. Intrinsic connections with comments on its input/output connectivity in relation to the hippocampus. J. Comp. Neurol. **252:** 78–94.
4. MURRAY, E.A. 1996. What have ablation studies told us about the neural substrates of stimulus memory? Semin. Neurosci. **8:** 13–22.
5. BURWELL, R.D. *et al.* 1995. Perirhinal and postrhinal cortices of the rat: a review of the neuroanatomical literature and comparison with findings from the monkey brain. Hippocampus **5:** 390–408.
6. STEPHAN, H. 1975. Allocortex. *In* Handbuch der Mikroskopischen Anatomie des Menschen IV-9. W. Borgman, Ed.: 1–998. Springer-Verlag. Berlin.
7. ROSE, M. 1927. Der Allocortex bei Tier und Mensch. J. Psychologie Neurologie **34:** 1–111.
8. SUZUKI, W.A. & D.G. AMARAL. 1994. Topographic organization of the reciprocal connections between the monkey entorhinal and the perirhinal and parahippocampal cortices. J. Neurosci. **14:** 1856–1877.
9. BURWELL, R.D. & D.G. AMARAL. 1998. Perirhinal and postrhinal cortices of the rat: interconnectivity and connections with the entorhinal cortex. J. Comp. Neurol. **391:** 293–321.

Anatomical Organization of the Parahippocampal-Hippocampal Network

MENNO P. WITTER,[a] FLORIS G. WOUTERLOOD, PIETERKE A. NABER,[b] AND THEO VAN HAEFTEN

Graduate School Neurosciences Amsterdam, Research Institute Neurosciences, Vrije Universiteit, Department of Anatomy, Amsterdam, The Netherlands

ABSTRACT: The anatomical organization of the parahipppocampal-hippocampal network indicates that it consists of different parallel circuits. Considering the topographical distribution of sensory cortical inputs, the hypothesis is that the major parallel circuits carry functionally different information. These functionally different parallel routes reach different portions of the hippocampal network along the longitudinal axis of all fields as well as along the perpendicularly oriented transverse axis of CA1 and the subiculum. In the remaining fields of the hippocampal formation, that is, the dentate gyrus and CA2/CA3, separation along the transverse axis is not present. By contrast, here the functionally different pathways converge onto the same neuronal population. The entorhinal cortex holds a pivotal position among the cortices that make up the parahippocampal region. By way of the networks of the superficial and deep layers, it mediates, respectively, the input and output streams of the hippocampal formation. Moreover, the intrinsic entorhinal network, particularly the interconnections between the deep and superficial layers, may mediate the comparison of hippocampal input and output signals. As such, the entorhinal cortex may form part of a novelty detection network. In addition, the organization of the entorhinal-hippocampal network may facilitate the holding of information. Finally, the terminal organization of the presubicular input to the medial entorhinal cortex indicates that the interactions between the deep and superficial entorhinal layers may be influenced by this input.

INTRODUCTION

Nomenclature and Overview

The parahippocampal region is comprised of a number of different cortical domains. Although no generally accepted definition is yet available, there is agreement that at least the entorhinal and perirhinal cortices should be included. A third region, which is positioned posterior to these two areas, is also generally included. In primates, this region is referred to as the parahippocampal cortex or areas TF and TH according to the description of Von Bonin and Bailey.[1] In the rat[2,3] and cat[4] this re-

[a]Address for correspondence: M.P. Witter, Ph.D, Department of Anatomy, Vrije Universiteit, van der Boechorststraat 7, 1081 BT Amsterdam, The Netherlands. Tel.: 31-20-4448048; fax: 31-20-4448054.
e-mail: MP.Witter.Anat@med.vu.nl
[b]Currently at the Netherlands Institute for Brain Research, Amsterdam, The Netherlands.

1

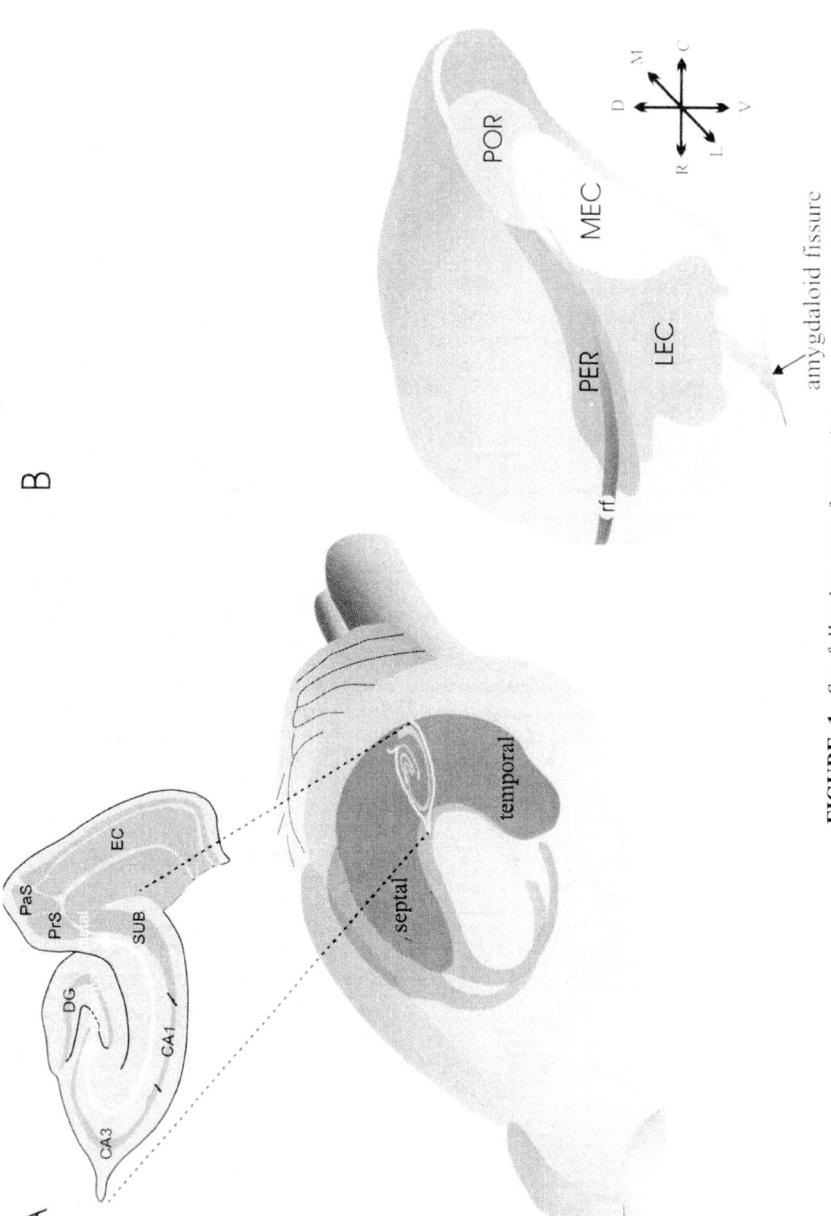

FIGURE 1. *See following page for caption.*

gion is referred to as the postrhinal cortex (FIGS. 1 and 2). (For further discussion concerning nomenclature, the reader is referred to the foreword of this volume).

Functional descriptions of the parahippocampal region should be founded on its neuronal and connectional architecture. Moreover, the precise reciprocal connections between the parahippocampal region and, on the one hand, the hippocampal formation and, on the other, large portions of the association cortex, should also be taken into account. A striking organizational feature of the parahippocampal region is the pivotal position of the entorhinal cortex (EC). This field receives most of its cortical inputs from the perirhinal and postrhinal (TF/TH) cortices and, in turn, gives rise to most of the cortical input to the dentate gyrus, the fields of the Ammon's horn (CA1–CA3), and the subiculum. Moreover, hippocampal output originating in CA1 and the subiculum is relayed back to the entorhinal cortex, from where it may be distributed predominantly to the perirhinal and postrhinal (TF/TH) cortices. One of the most intriguing questions currently facing us is whether the different areas within the parahippocampal region have different functional roles, and if so, what these roles are. One prerequisite for answering this question is a detailed understanding of both the extrinsic and intrinsic connections of each of these regions and of the connections between them. The aim of the present chapter is to summarize some of the fundamental concepts underlying parahippocampal-hippocampal connectivity. For an overview of the organization of the connectivity between the different cortical areas that make up the parahippocampal region, the reader is referred to the contribution by Burwell (this volume).

Historical Account of Parahippocampal-Hippocampal Connections

From the influential work of Ramón y Cajal,[5] it became known that EC gives rise to an extremely dense projection into the macroscopic structure called the hippocampus. More recently, investigators have produced more detailed descriptions of the connectivity between the different hippocampal fields, resulting in what is now well known as the "trisynaptic circuit." As illustrated in FIGURE 3, this circuit includes the *"perforant pathway"* projection to the dentate gyrus, the subsequent *"mossy fiber"* projection to field CA3, and finally the *"Schaffer collaterals"* targeting neurons in CA1. Over time, projections from CA1 to the subiculum were added, as were connections leading from CA1 and the subiculum, by way of the fornix, towards the hypothalamus and mammillary complex (not illustrated). It was only with the publication of the seminal papers by Van Hoesen and colleagues[6–8] in 1975 that

---

FIGURE 1. Three-dimensional drawings indicating where the hippocampus and parahippocampal cortices in the rat brain are situated. (**A**) Drawing of a rat brain seen from a lateral frontal view with, on the inside, the C-shaped hippocampus. The septo-temporal orientation of the hippocampus is indicated. Section taken from the hippocampus (*upper left*) illustrates the subfields of the hippocampus and the orientation of the transverse axis, running from proximal (close to DG) to distal (close to EC). (**B**) Drawing of the left hemisphere of the rat brain seen from a caudal-lateral point of view, with indicated the positions of the lateral (LEC) and medial (MEC) parts of the entorhinal cortex, perirhinal (PER) and postrhinal (POR) cortices. Abbreviations: C, caudal; CA, cornu ammonis; D, dorsal; DG, dentate gyrus; EC, entorhinal cortex; L, lateral; LEC, lateral entorhinal cortex; M, medial; MEC, medial entorhinal cortex; PaS. Parasubiculum; PER, perirhinal cortex; PrS, presubiculum; POR, postrhinal cortex; R, rostral; SUB, subiculum; V, ventral; rf, rhinal fissure.

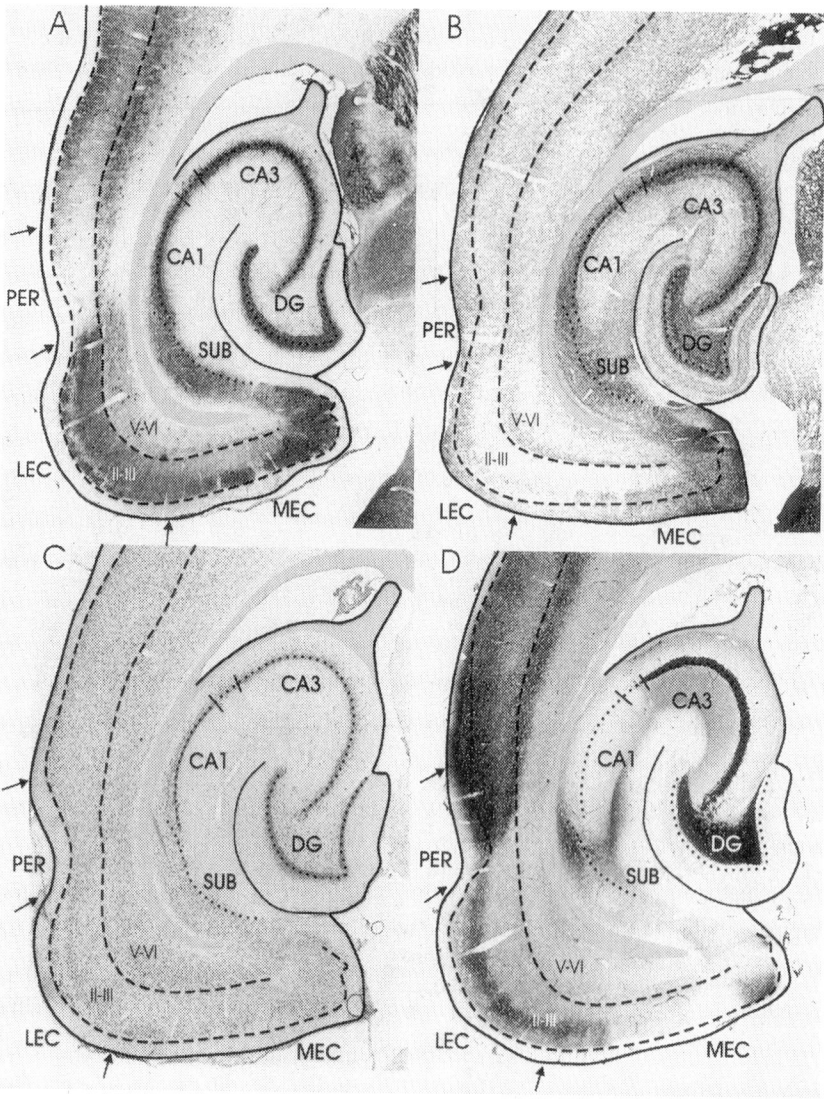

FIGURE 2. Photomicrographs of horizontal (**1**), sagittal (**2**), and coronal (**3**) sections of the rat brain. Adjacent sections are stained for the calcium-binding protein Parvalbumin (Parv; **A**), acetylcholine-esterase (AChE; **B**), Nissl (**C**), and heavy metals by Timm's method (**D**). The boundaries of the perirhinal (PER) and postrhinal (POR) cortices, medial (MEC) and lateral (LEC) entorhinal subdivisions, and parasubiculum (PaS), are demarcated by *arrows*. In the hippocampus the borders between CA1, CA3, and SUB are indicated with *slashes*. In the Parv-stained material, the cytoarchitectonic borders between POR and MEC/PaS and between PER and LEC are characterized by light staining in PER and POR, while MEC/PaS and LEC are darkly stained. In the AChE-stained material the border between PaS

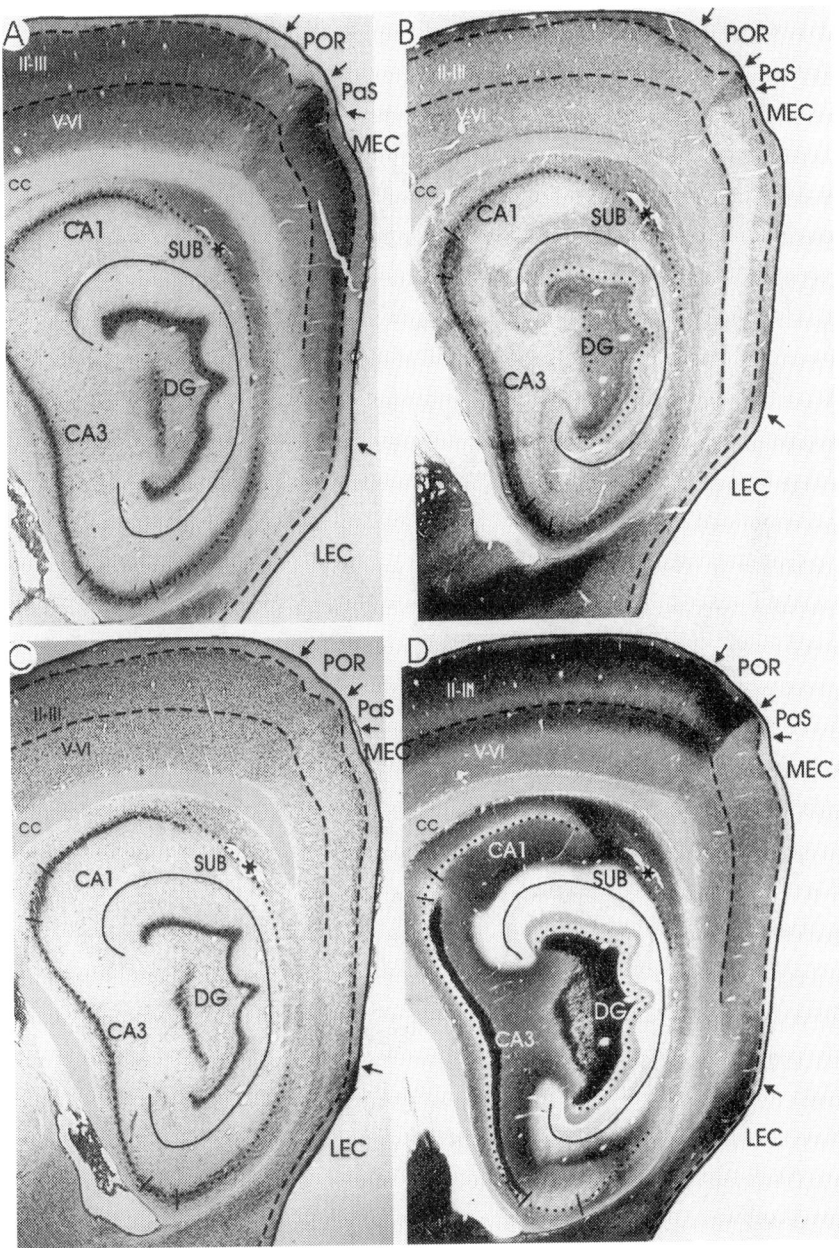

and POR is clear by a dark staining in PaS and only light staining in POR. In contrast, POR is heavily stained in Timm's stained material, while PaS/MEC are only lightly stained. Similar to the latter border, in Timm's material the border between PER/LEC can be recognised on a light staining in LEC, whereas PER is heavily stained. Scale bar: 500 μm. *Asterisks*

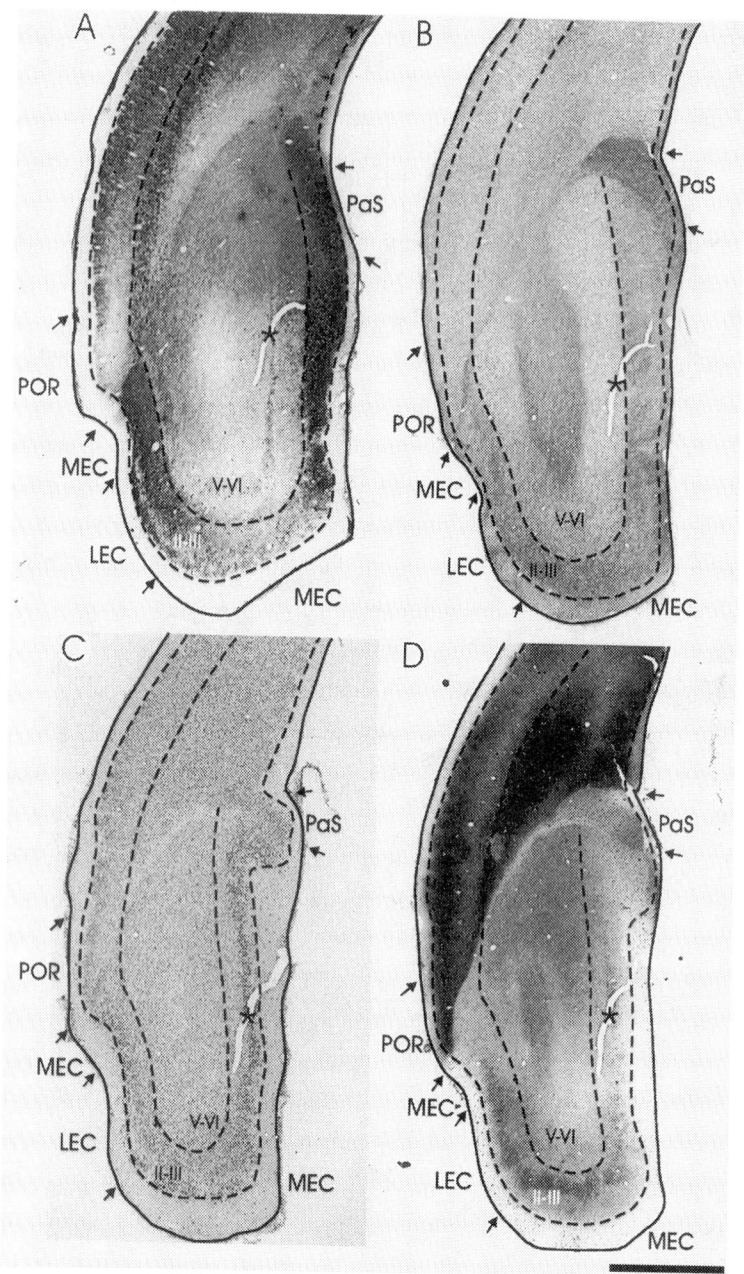

indicate corresponding marks. Abbreviations: CA, cornu ammonis; DG, dentate gyrus; LEC, lateral entorhinal cortex; MEC, medial entorhinal cortex; PaS, parasubiculum; PER, perirhinal cortex; POR, postrhinal cortex; SUB, subiculum; cc, corpus callosum; II-III, superficial cortical layers; V-VI, deep cortical layers.

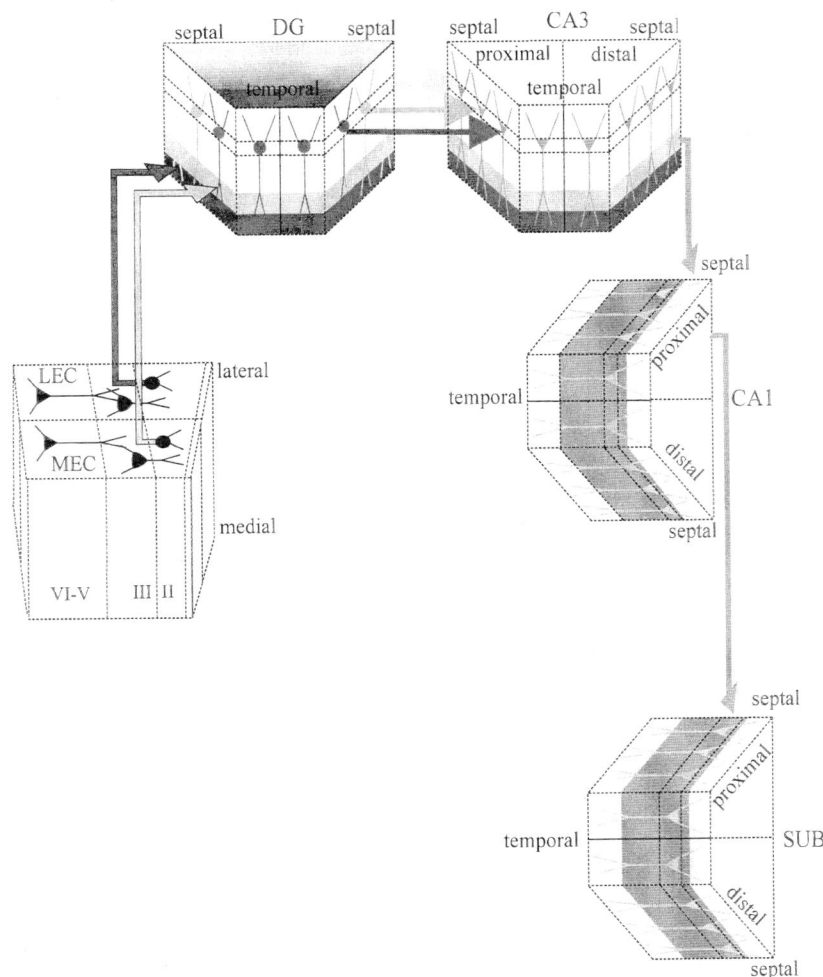

FIGURE 3. Schematic representation of the so-called "Trisynaptic Circuit," comprising the unidirectional connections from the entorhinal cortex-to-the dentate gyrus-to-CA3-to-CA1. Two additional pathways have been indicated in this figure: (i) the projections from CA1 to the subiculum and (ii) the projection form layer II neurons of the entorhinal cortex to CA3. Indicated are the entorhinal cortex with its lateral (LEC) and medial (MEC) subdivisions, the dentate gyrus (DG), hippocampal fields CA3 and CA1, and the subiculum. In each of the fields, the major to-pological characteristics are indicated: in case of the entorhinal cortex, the deep and superficial cell layers are indicated as well as the lateral-to-medial axis; for DG, the different layers as well as the septal-to-temporal axis are represented; for the remaining fields, in addition to the different layers, we indicated the septal-to-temporal (longitudinal) axis as well as the proximal-to-distal (transverse) axis. With respect to the included connections, it is illustrated that the perforant path-way, connecting the entorhinal cortex to DG, orginates from neurons in layer II; moreover, it con-sists of two components, originating in LEC and MEC, and terminating in the outer and middle molecular layer, respectively. Also indicated is the restricted "lamellar" origin and terminal dis-tribution of the mossy fiber projection along the septal-to-temporal axis. This figure forms the template for the expanded versions represented in FIGURES 4 and 6.

researchers started to focus on the connections from CA1 and the subiculum back to the EC. Interestingly, around the same time it was rediscovered that the EC projects not only to the dentate gyrus, but also to fields CA3 and CA1.[9,10] Rediscovered is the appropriate phrase, because in the original Golgi descriptions of Cajal, these fiber systems were already notable and they were actually described. It took another 10 years before the projections from the EC to CA1 were confirmed with the use of electronmicroscopy[11,12] and electrophysiology.[13-15] Moreover, the topographical organization of this projection to CA1 was described in much detail together with that of an additional projection to the subiculum.[16-18] Finally, another projection was added recently to the already complicated picture, namely, a projection to CA1 and the subiculum, originating in the perirhinal and postrhinal cortices[19-21] (see also Naber *et al.*, this volume).

PROJECTIONS FROM THE ENTORHINAL CORTEX TO THE HIPPOCAMPAL FORMATION

The Perforant Pathway Has a Layer II and a Layer III Component

The organization of the perforant pathway has been analyzed in most detail in the rat; however, some facets of its organization have also been well described in the cat and the monkey. The perforant pathway was originally described by Ramón y Cajal[5] as a collection of fibers, leaving the EC and perforating the underlying white matter and adjacent layers of the subiculum, on their way to the molecular layer of the subiculum. From here, Cajal described fibers crossing the hippocampal fissure into the molecular layer of the dentate gyrus. He also described fibers coursing parallel to the hippocampal fissure in the molecular layer of the subiculum and fields CA1 and CA3. This complex set of projections, together constituting the perforant pathway, originates from layers II and III of the EC, so that neurons in layer II project to the dentate gyrus (DG) and CA3, whereas layer III cells project to CA1 and the subiculum.[10,22] However, intracellular tracing studies in the rat provide evidence that layer II cells also send a few collaterals to the subiculum.[23,24]

At this point, further refinement of the organization of the perforant pathway should be introduced, related to the origin of the pathway in two cytoarchitectonically defined subdivisions of the EC. Traditionally, these subdivisions have been called the lateral (LEC) and the medial entorhinal cortex (MEC), respectively. It is most relevant to point out that the terms lateral and medial entorhinal area do not relate in a simple manner to the actual position of these areas on the surface of the hemisphere. FIGURE 1B illustrates that in the rat, and this is more or less true in the guinea pig, cat, monkey, and human as well, the largest portion of the LEC occupies the rostrolateral part of the EC, whereas the MEC occupies the remaining caudomedial portion of the EC. More recently proposed nomenclatures stress the rostro-caudal relations between the different subdivisions.[25-29] The lateral and medial perforant pathways, as these two components of the perforant pathway are generally referred to, have a similar distribution along the longitudinal axis of the hippocampus; by contrast, they show a different distribution along the transverse and radial axes (FIG. 4). Whereas layer II cells of the LEC send their axons to the outer one third of the molecular layer/stratum lacunosum-moleculare of DG and CA3, the pro-

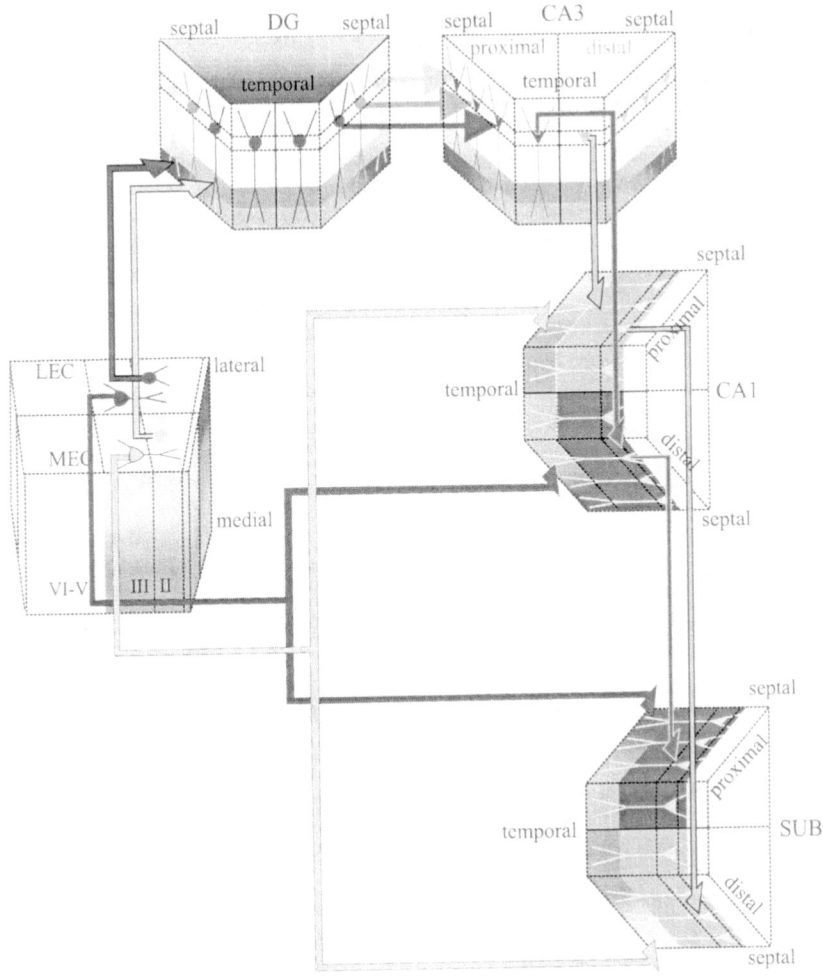

FIGURE 4. Expanded version of FIGURE 3, including the origin and distribution of the layer III component of the perforant pathway. The origin and distribution of the lateral and medial components of this projection to CA1 and the subiculum are shown: LEC projects to the distal portion of CA1 and the proximal portion of the subiculum, whereas the MEC projection targets the remaining proximal portion of CA1 and the distal portion of the subiculum. Note that the perforant path terminates throughout the width of the molecular layer in both fields. The second feature added to this figure is the marked septotemporal topology of both the layer II and layer III components of the perforant pathway: lateral parts of LEC and MEC project to septal portions of all hippocampal fields, and more medial portions of both entorhinal fields distribute projections to increasingly more temporal portions of the hippocampal formation. Finally, the organization of the CA1 to subiculum projection system is illustrated: the proximal half of CA1 projects to the distal half of the subiculum (*light grey arrow*) and the distal half of CA1 projects to the adjacent proximal half of the subiculum (*dark grey arrow*).

jection originating in layer II of the MEC terminates in the middle one third of these layers. Both pathways, originating from cells in layer II in the LEC and MEC, likely influence the same cells in DG and CA3.[30] This is in contrast to the pathway originating from the neurons in layer III of the LEC and MEC. These layer III fibers terminate in the stratum lacunosum-moleculare of area CA1 and the molecular layer of the subiculum, so that they project each to a restricted transverse portion of both hippocampal fields. Fibers from the LEC terminate specifically in the distal part of the CA1 and the proximal part of the subiculum (therefore around the border of CA1/subiculum). By contrast, fibers from the MEC terminate in the proximal part of CA1 and the distal part of the subiculum (FIG. 4). In the cat, the organization of the layer II and III components of the perforant pathway is remarkably similar to that in the rat.[31–33] In the monkey, the different radial distribution of the lateral and medial components of the layer II projection is not as clearcut, whereas organization of the layer III projection is comparable to that in the rat.[4,22] In summary, the organization of the perforant pathway thus indicates that different hippocampal fields show different ways of information processing. The DG and CA3/CA2 can be viewed as being diffusely activated by all parts of the EC along the full transverse axis of a particular septotemporal level but with a selectivity along the dendrites of the cells at the innervated level. By contrast, the CA1/subiculum system appears to receive a much more topologically selective input from the EC, so that inputs from the LEC are kept separate from those arising from the MEC. Although species differences are apparent, the differential organization of the two components of the perforant pathway appears to hold true in all species.

The Perforant Pathway Is Topographically Organized

The perforant pathway shows a topographical organization along the longitudinal axis of the hippocampal formation, so that a lateral-to-medial gradient in the EC corresponds to a septal-to-temporal gradient in the hippocampal formation (FIG. 4). This particular topography was initially reported in the cat regarding the layer II projections to the DG and CA3[31] and subsequently reported in the rat and monkey. We now know that the same topological rules underlie the organization of the layer III projections to CA1 and subiculum.[16,34–38] Although species differences are apparent, the essential organization is strikingly constant in that within the EC three rostrocaudally oriented strips should be differentiated: a laterally situated strip that projects to the septal (in rat and cat) or caudal (in monkey) hippocampus; an intermediate strip that projects mainly to intermediate portions of the hippocampus; and finally, the most medially situated strip that issues fibers targeting the most temporal (in rat and cat) or most rostral (in monkey) portion of the hippocampus. It is critical to point out that each of these three longitudinally oriented strips of EC comprises portions of both the LEC and the MEC. This implies that at all longitudinal levels of the hippocampus, each field receives inputs belonging to the functionally different components of the perforant pathway originating in the LEC and the MEC, respectively. The major point of this organization is that on the basis of its afferents, the EC can be divided into at least three longitudinal zones, which project to different parts along the hippocampal longitudinal axis. The dorsolateral part of the LEC and the caudal part of the MEC, which receive major inputs from the adjacent perirhinal and postrhinal (TF/TH) cortices, respectively, project predominantly to the septal hippocampal formation (cau-

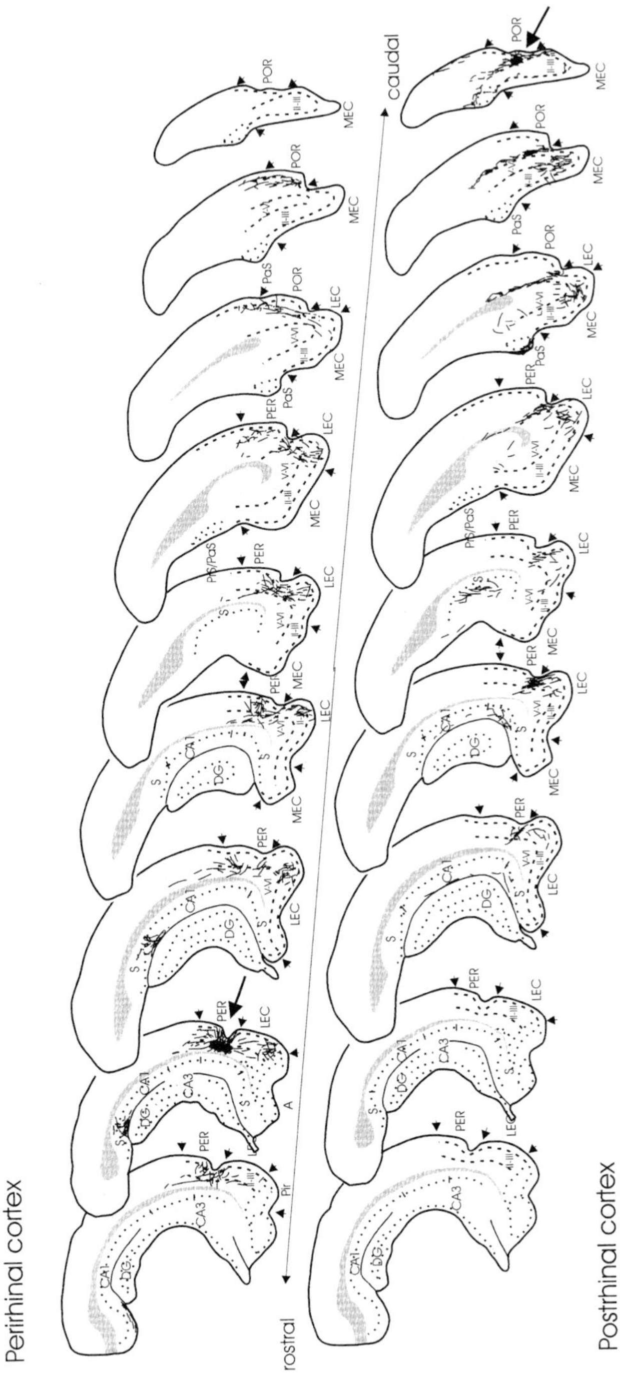

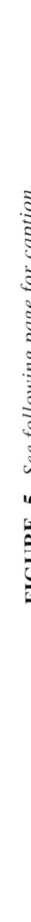

FIGURE 5. *See following page for caption.*

dal hippocampal formation in the monkey). The medial parts of the EC, which receive prominent inputs from the limbic and periamygdaloid cortices, project more temporally (rostrally in the monkey) in the hippocampal formation. The intermediate zone of the EC projects to the intermediate parts of the hippocampal fields.[39–42]

Interestingly, anatomical observations in the rat indicate that also the entorhinal intrinsic connectivity is preferentially organized according to these three longitudinal strips. A strong interconnection exists between parts of a particular longitudinal strip, including strong interconnections between the portions of the LEC and the MEC, which belong to the same strip. Connections from any part of the EC towards more laterally or more medially positioned portions are sparse and only invade the immediately adjacent portion of the neighboring longitudinal strip. This organization implies that parts of the EC that innervate the same longitudinal level of the hippocampus are strongly interconnected, whereas portions of the EC that project to different longitudinal hippocampal levels are interconnected only sparsely or not at all.[16,43] The available anatomical evidence in the cat[42] and monkey[41] indicates a similar topological preference with respect to the intrinsic connections. However, in these species the rostrocaudal extent of these connections is somewhat more restricted, so that in essence the more caudal portions of the MEC may not be connected to the more rostral portions of the LEC.

PROJECTIONS FROM THE PERIRHINAL AND POSTRHINAL CORTICES TO THE HIPPOCAMPAL FORMATION

Earlier anatomical studies indicated that the perirhinal cortex gives rise to a projection to certain fields in the hippocampal formation.[44,45] We recently reanalyzed this projection and extended our study to include the projections from the postrhinal cortex. Both anatomical and electrophysiological data indicate that neurons in the superficial layers of the perirhinal and postrhinal cortices give rise to a projection to the molecular layer of CA1 and the subiculum (FIG. 5). However, similar to what was described above for inputs arising from the LEC and the MEC, we noted that the perirhinal and postrhinal projections target different portions along the transverse

---

FIGURE 5. Distribution of labeled fibers in the hippocampus and EC after anterograde tracer injections in the perirhinal cortex (PER) and the postrhinal cortex (POR). The top series of coronal sections, from rostral to caudal, show the observed terminal labelling in area CA1, the subiculum, and EC after an injection of biotin-conjugated dextran-amine (BDA) in the perirhinal cortex (*large arrow*). In the corresponding bottom series of coronal sections, the terminal fibers in area CA1, the subiculum, and EC, originating in the postrhinal cortex are shown. When the two series are compared, it can be seen that the fibers labeled from either injection terminate in different areas in the subiculum, such that fibers originating in the perirhinal cortex terminate in the proximal subiculum whereas fibers originating in the postrhinal cortex terminate in more distal parts of the subiculum. The terminal labelling in EC differs as well, such that the perirhinal cortex projects preferentially to parts of LEC, in contrast to the postrhinal projection, that mainly targets parts of MEC. Abbreviations: A, amygdala; CA, cornu ammonis; DG, dentate gyrus; LEC, lateral entorhinal cortex; MEC, medial entorhinal cortex, PaS, parasubiculum; PER, perirhinal cortex; Pir, piriform cortex; POR, postrhinal cortex; PrS, presubiculum; S, subiculum; II-III, superficial cortical layers; V-VI, deep cortical layers.

axis of CA1 and the subiculum. Input from the perirhinal cortex terminates predominantly in the most distal part of CA1 and the directly adjacent narrow proximal portion of the subiculum. In contrast, the postrhinal fibers predominantly target the most proximal part of CA1 and the most distal portion of the subiculum. In the rat, projections from the postrhinal cortex are much stronger to the subiculum than to CA1, whereas for those of the perirhinal cortex a more evenly dense distribution to CA1 and the subiculum is apparent. Detailed studies are needed before a more definitive description can be provided, but it is of interest that in the monkey, both the perirhinal and the parahippocampal cortices also project to CA1 and the subiculum; in this species, however, both projections distribute exclusively to the border region between CA1 and the subiculum.[46]

The projections from the perirhinal and the postrhinal cortices have been electrophysiologically analyzed as well. In particular, the projections from the perirhinal cortex to the hippocampal formation have been studied in some detail by different groups. Although there is general agreement concerning the perirhinal projections to the subiculum (for more details see Naber *et al.*, this volume), the perirhinal projection to CA1 is somewhat more controversial in that three groups using current source density analysis in the rat following stimulation of the perirhinal cortex reported contrasting findings. It is most likely that these conflicting results are due to the complicated and restricted topology of this projection (to be discussed). Also, a projection from the perirhinal cortex to the dentate gyrus has been described.[47] On the basis of detailed anatomical and electrophysiological findings, we recently argued that no such projection exists and that the activation in the dentate gyrus following perirhinal stimulation is due to a relay in the adjacent dorsolateral part of the EC.[21,48] Regarding the projection from the postrhinal cortex, we recently provided confirmatory electrophysiological evidence for a projection to the distal parts of the subiculum[49] (see also Naber *et al.*, this volume).

Origin and Distribution of Perirhinal and Postrhinal Projections to CA1 and the Subiculum

With the use of retrograde tracing, we only recently began to study in more detail the distribution of the projections from the perirhinal and postrhinal cortices along the longitudinal axis of the subiculum. We observed that the distribution of this projection along the longitudinal axis of the subiculum depends on the rostrocaudal site of origin in the perirhinal cortex, so that more rostral parts project to more septal levels of CA1/subiculum and more caudal parts predominantly distribute fibers to more temporal levels of CA1/subiculum. With respect to the projection originating from the postrhinal cortex a similar topology was noted, so that the most rostral portion of the postrhinal cortex, bordering the perirhinal cortex, projects to more septal parts of the subiculum, and increasingly more caudomedial parts of the postrhinal cortex distribute a projection to more temporal portions of the distal subiculum (Ammerlaan and Witter, unpublished observations). In all our retrograde tracing studies, we consistently observed that these projections originate predominantly from layers II and III of the perirhinal and postrhinal cortices. As expected, we also observed labeling of neurons in layer III of the LEC and MEC, respectively. Interestingly, comparison of the distribution of the retrogradely labeled neurons indicated a major difference between the entorhinal projections on the one hand and the perirhinal/

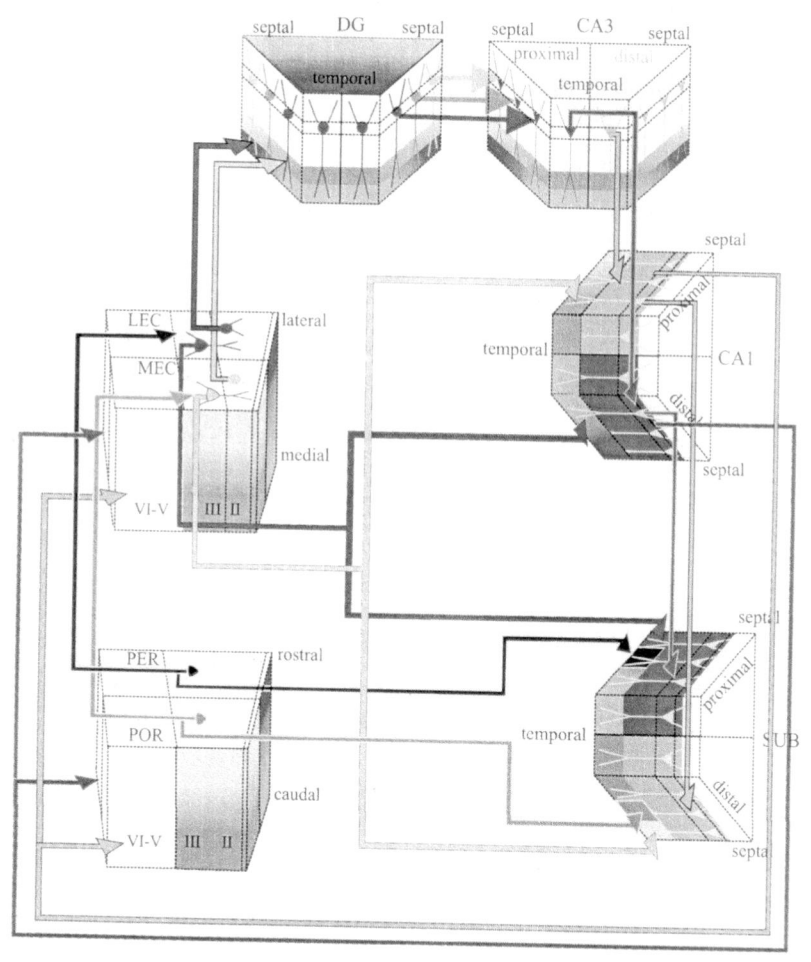

FIGURE 6. Expanded version of FIGURE 4, including projections from the perirhinal (PER) and postrhinal (POR) cortices to CA1 and the subiculum. Note that the perirhinal projection targets areas in CA1 and subiculum, which do overlap with the terminal distribution of the LEC projection; however, the distribution of the perirhinal projection along both the longitudinal and the transverse axes is more restricted than that of the LEC projection. A similar organizational relation exists between the postrhinal and MEC projections. Additional connections included in this figure comprise the projections from the perirhinal and postrhinal cortex to the entorhinal cortex, as well as the projections from CA1 and the subiculum back to the entorhinal, perirhinal and postrhinal cortices. Indicated are the strict reciprocal features of these projections with the incoming ones from the various parahippocampal cortices.

postrhinal projections on the other. It appears that the origin of subicular projections in the perirhinal and postrhinal cortices is much more restricted than the origin of subicular projections in the EC. Moreover, based on anterograde tracing data, we conclude that the distribution of the projections originating from the perirhinal/postrhinal cortices along the longitudinal and transverse axes of the subiculum is much more restricted than the entorhinal-subiculum projection. Whereas a restricted part of the EC gives rise to a projection along approximately 20–25% of the longitudinal axis, the perirhinal/postrhinal projections reach less than 10%. Regarding the distribution along the transverse axis, a similar difference is apparent. Fibers originating in the LEC target the proximal half of the transverse extent of the subiculum, whereas projections from the perirhinal cortex innervate less than one third of the area innervated by the corresponding perforant pathway component from the LEC. Similarly, the projections from the MEC distribute along the entire distal half of the subiculum and those from the postrhinal cortex only reach the most distal one third of this region. It thus appears that the projections from the perirhinal and postrhinal cortices to the subiculum are much more "focal" than are those originating in the EC with respect to both origin and terminal distribution (FIG. 6).

CA1 AND SUBICULUM: INTERCONNECTIONS AND ORIGIN OF RETURN PROJECTIONS TO THE PARAHIPPOCAMPAL REGION

In view of the transverse topology of the projections from the parahippocampal region to CA1 and the subiculum, it is of interest that the projections of CA1 to the subiculum exhibit a strikingly similar transverse organization.[50–52] Two major organizational features have become apparent. (1) The CA1-to-subiculum projection shows extensive longitudinal divergence, so that fibers from one particular point of origin distribute over approximately one third of the long extent of the subiculum. This longitudinal spread is thus comparable to that of the perforant pathway. (2) Projections from the proximal part of CA1 terminate in the distal part of the subiculum. Conversely, projections from the distal part of CA1 predominantly reach the proximal part of the subiculum; projections from the center of CA1 reach the center of the subiculum. Intracellular fills of CA1 neurons have yielded comparable results and furthermore showed that the axon of any one particular neuron distributes along approximately one third of the transverse extent of the subiculum.[51,52] An additional feature of the termination of the CA1-subiculum projection is that it extends throughout the stratum pyramidale and moleculare of the subiculum. The CA1-to-subiculum projections thus not only appear able to influence the proximal dendrites of the subicular pyramidal cells, but also influence the cell at the level of the soma and possibly the basal dendritic domain. In other words, in this respect the subicular connectivity forms a hardwired column or "channel."

Projections from the hippocampal formation to the EC originate in CA1 and the subiculum. With regards to the laminar termination of these projections, it was reported earlier in the rat that most fibers terminate deep to the lamina dissecans, in layer V of the EC over its full transverse extent.[53–55] However, we and others have shown that in all species studied, this projection also distributes to the superficial layers, mainly to layer

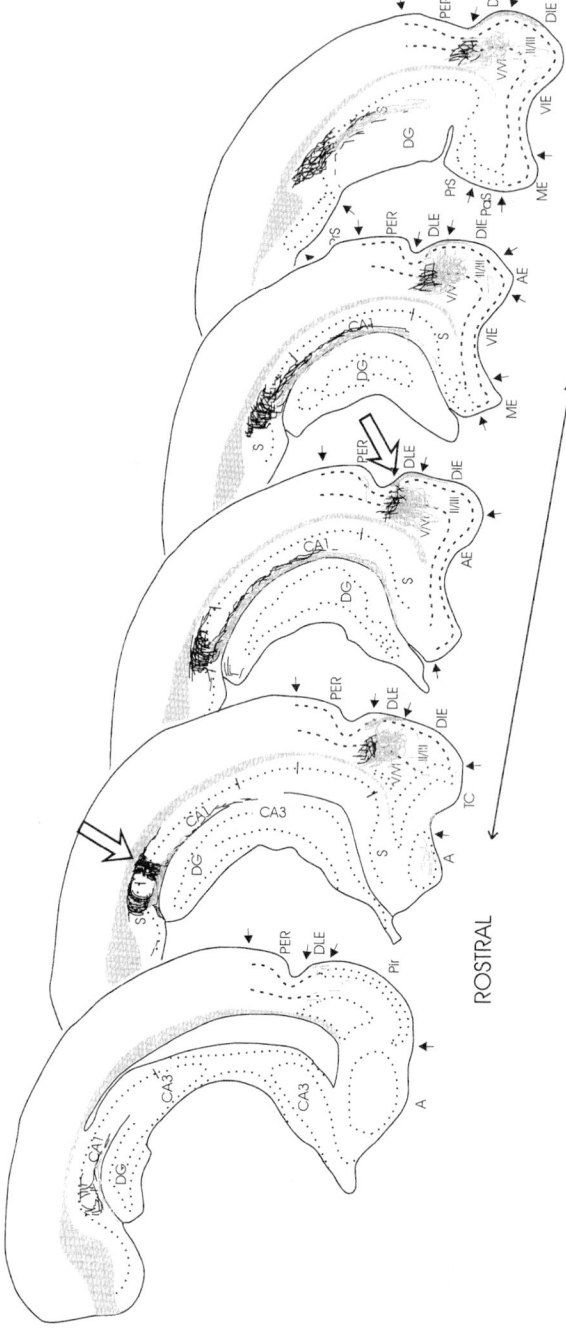

FIGURE 7. Distribution of labeled fibers in the hippocampus and entorhinal cortex after combined anterograde tracer injections in the dorsolateral part of EC (DLE) and in the distal part of hippocampal subfield CA1. Line drawings of coronal sections, from rostal to caudal, indicating the observed terminal labeling in area CA1 and the subiculum (*grey fibers*) after an injection of biotin-conjugated dextran-amine (BDA) in DLE (*open arrow*), and the terminal labelling in the subiculum and EC (*black fibers*) after an injection of Phaseolus vulgaris-leucoagglutinin (Pha-L) in area CA1 (*open arrow*). The terminal fibres originating in DLE overlap with the injection site in CA1 and vice-versa, that is, the terminal labeling of CA1-fibers overlaps with the injection site in DLE. Moreover, the fibers originating from both injections terminate in the same area in the subiculum, close to the border with area CA1. Abbreviations: A, amygdala; CA, cornu ammonis; DG, dentate gyrus; DLE, DIE, VIE, ME, AE, TC, subdivisions of EC see 25; EC, entorhinal cortex; PaS, parasubiculum; PER, perirhinal cortex; Pir, piriform cortex; PrS, presubiculum; S, subiculum (Reproduced from Naber *et al.*,[59] with permission).

III of the EC.[33,56,57] The projections from CA1 and the subiculum originate from the entire longitudinal extent of the hippocampal formation, and in rat, cat, and monkey, this projection shows a topographical distribution along the long axis, similar to that of the perforant pathway.[53–55] Also with respect to the topography along the transverse axis of the CA1 and the subiculum, the projections to the EC are organized similar to the perforant pathway. The proximal part of the subiculum and the adjacent distal part of CA1 project preferentially to the LEC, whereas the distal part of the subiculum and the proximal part of CA1 project preferentially to the MEC. In other words, this output system is in register with the organization of perforant pathway fibers terminating in these two hippocampal subfields.[58] It should be emphasized that the organization along the transverse axis does not interfere in any way with the described topography of these connections along the septotemporal axis. In summary, at septal levels, the distal CA1 and proximal subiculum project to lateral parts of the LEC, whereas the proximal CA1 and distal subiculum distribute fibers to laterocaudal parts of the MEC. At temporal levels, the distal CA1 and proximal subiculum project to medial parts of the LEC, whereas the proximal CA1 and distal subiculum project to rostromedial parts of the MEC.

Based on this information we considered whether the transverse portions in CA1 and the subiculum, as defined on the basis of the intrinsic hippocampal circuitry, overlap with the parts that are characterized on the basis of the restricted distribution of the perforant pathway. In a series of anterograde double-labeling experiments, we analyzed whether projections of the EC target neurons in CA1 and the subiculum that, on the one hand, are interconnected and, on the other hand, give rise to return projections to the EC, so that they terminate deep to the origin of the EC-to-CA1/subiculum projections (FIGS. 7 and 8). Both for the lateral and medial subdivision of the EC, the projections to CA1/subiculum as well as the projections from CA1 to the subiculum and to the EC are rather divergent. Interestingly, we did only rarely observe evidence for the presence of "closed loops," that is, cells in layer III of EC which give rise to projections to interconnected neurons in CA1 and the subiculum, while the targeted CA1 neurons, in turn, project back to the deep layers of the originating part of the EC.[59] We conclude that although fibers originating from a restricted part of the EC distribute extensively along the longitudinal axis of CA1 and the subiculum, only restricted portions of the latter two areas receiving that same entorhinal input are interconnected. Moreover, only a small percentage of the CA1 neurons that project to the correspondingly innervated subicular neurons give rise to projections that return to the deep layers of the originating part of the EC. The present findings are taken to indicate that the EC-hippocampal circuitry functionally comprises many parallel closed loops.

INTRINSIC ORGANIZATION OF THE ENTORHINAL CORTEX

The EC, like the presubiculum and parasubiculum, is characterized by the presence of a marked cell-sparse layer, or lamina dissecans, which results in a more or less clearcut separation of superficial layers I, II, and III from deeper positioned layers V and VI. The neuronal composition of the EC is mainly known on the basis of the seminal Golgi-based description by Lorente de Nó.[60] More recently, important information has been added, based on immunocytochemical and electrophysiological studies.[4,61–65] It is beyond the scope of this chapter to give a detailed description

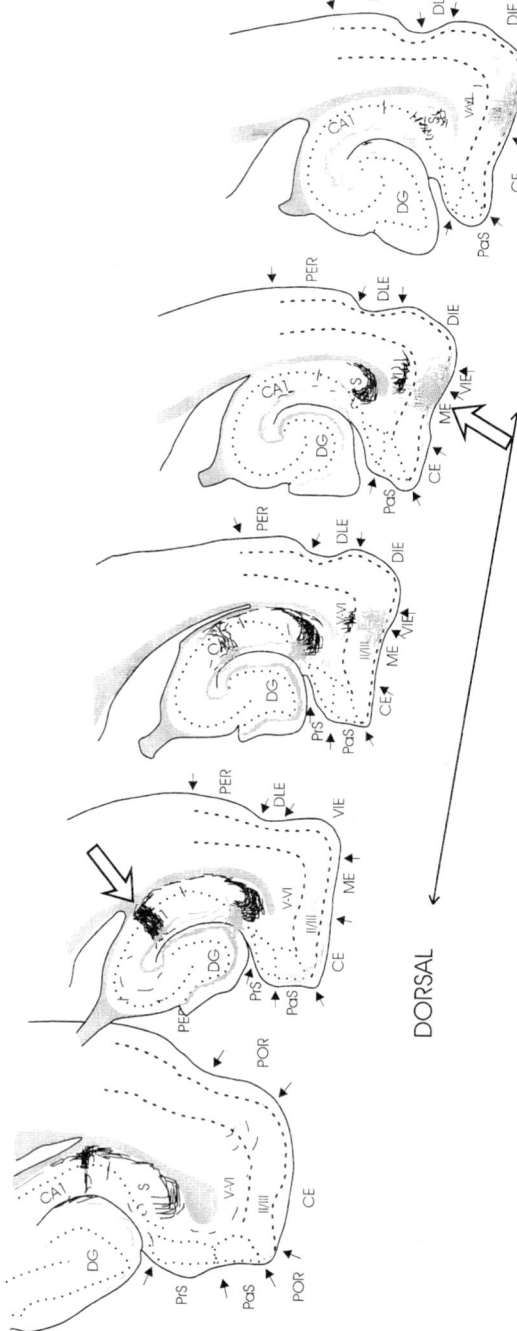

FIGURE 8. Distribution of labeled fibers in the hippocampus and entorhinal cortex after combined anterograde tracer injections in the medial part of the entorhinal cortex (ME) and the proximal part of hippocampal subfield CA1. Line drawings of horizontal sections, from dorsal to ventral, indicating the observed terminal labeling in area CA1 and the subiculum (grey fibers) after an injection of Phaseolus vulgaris-leucoagglutinin (Pha-L) in ME (open arrow), and the terminal labeling in the subiculum and the entorhinal cortex (black fibers) after an injection of biotin-conjugated dextran-amine (BDA) in area CA1 (open arrow). The terminal fibers originating in ME overlap with the injection site in CA1 and the terminal distribution of CA1-fibers overlaps with the injection site in ME. Moreover, the fibers labeled from both injections terminate in the same area in the subiculum, close to the border with the presubiculum. Abbreviations: A, amygdala; CA, cornu ammonis; DG, dentate gyrus; DLE, DIE, VIE, ME, CE, AE, TC, subdivisions of EC (see ref. 25); EC, entorhinal cortex; PaS, parasubiculum; PER, perirhinal cortex; Pir, piriform cortex; POR, postrhinal cortex; PrS, presubiculum; S, subiculum; II-III, superficial cortical layers; V-VI, deep cortical layers. (Reproduced from Naber et al.,[59] with permission).

of all cellular components that make up the entorhinal network. In contrast, we will summarize some recent findings concerning the laminar organization, which may bear to the way we envisage the functional organization of the EC.

The generally accepted model describes that inputs to EC target neurons in superficial layers I–III. According to this traditional scheme, neurons in the deep layers receive the major output from the hippocampal fields CA1 and the subiculum and convey this to neighboring cortical areas of the parahippocampal region and subcortical structures such as the basal ganglia, claustrum, and thalamus. Although this overall scheme has the advantage of being simple, in reality though, it forms a gross oversimplification of the network as we know it today. For example, as described above, hippocampal output also reaches the superficial layers of the EC. Moreover, cortical inputs have been described that either reach both superficial and deep layers or selectively innervate only the deep layers of the EC. In recent anterograde tracing studies in the rat concerning inputs originating from the anterior and posterior cingulate cortex, we, as well as others, noted that inputs from these regions most prominently innervate the deep layers, with only a minor component distributing to the superficial layers.[66,67] Similar observations have been reported in the cat as well.[39] Another, even more striking example that this separation into input and output layers is no longer tenable is the recent observation that inputs from the presubiculum, which are known to distribute selectively to layers I and III of the MEC, also target dendrites of layer V pyramidal cells.[68] Yet another example concerns the origin of the projections to the olfactory bulb and the prefrontal and perirhinal cortices in the rat. In a recent tracing study, it was reported that these entorhinal efferents to large extents originate from cells in superficial layers II and III.[25] Although not specifically tested experimentally, in view of the number of cells that give rise to these entorhinal efferent projections, it is most likely that these cells in layers II and III also give rise to the perforant pathway projection.

FUNCTIONAL RELEVANCE OF THE ORGANIZATIONAL PRINCIPLES OF THE PARAHIPPOCAMPAL-HIPPOCAMPAL NETWORK

In this chapter we have elaborated on the pathways mediated by the perirhinal/ LEC- versus the postrhinal/MEC-hippocampal loops. These pathways most likely mediate the processing of different types of sensory information;[3,41,69,70] see also the chapters by Burwell and Naber *et al.*, this volume. In addition, we have described pathways that are mediated by different lateral-to-medial bands in the EC in relation to different septal (posterior)-to-temporal (anterior) portions along the hippocampal longitudinal axis. The laterally originating pathway will provide for sensory inputs, mediated by either the perirhinal or the postrhinal parallel pathways (see above), reaching the septal (posterior) hippocampal formation. In contrast, the medially originating pathway most likely is involved in the transfer of motivational signals/ reflections of the intrinsic state of the organism to more temporal (anterior) portions of the hippocampal formation.[16,71] In view of the precise reciprocity of these pathways, suggesting the presence of closed loops, we suggest that the parahippocampal-hippocampal network is comprised of a number of functionally different parallel input-output pathways. This complicated three-dimensional matrix, in combination with the recent insights that the entorhinal intrinsic network also subserves functional interactions between the deep and superficial layers,[72-74] led to the following conclusion. The entorhinal network is more than an incidental combination of an input and an output station mediating corticohippocampal interplay. In contrast, it is uniquely situated to monitor, "online," what hippocampal processing does to a particular input. In view of the described specificity and selectivity of the various parallel loops, EC may detect the difference between an incoming stimulus with the net outcome of hippocampal processing of a closely related stimulus that entered earlier in time. The entorhinal circuit generates a new input signal which, by way of the superficial layers, may be transferred back to the hippocampus, to serve, for example, short-term maintenance of information by way of reverberation.[72] In addition, the notion that these same superficial layers also give rise to a projection to the prefrontal cortex makes it feasible that the outcome of the online monitoring process will be transferred to parts of the prefrontal cortex that potentially play a role in the generation of adaptive behavioral responses. Alternatively, the deep layers of the EC may mediate the flow of hippocampal output to the neocortex.[75] Finally, we propose that entorhinal function, be it monitoring, short-term maintenance, or generation of a hippocampal output signal to adjacent temporal association cortex, may depend on the activity of a rather specific set of cortical afferents, such as those from the presubiculum. We have shown that inputs from the presubiculum may interact with neurons in both the superficial and the deep layers of the MEC. It is tempting to speculate that the finding of this superficial and deep termination of presubicular inputs relates to a rather unique feature of this input: presubicular inputs distribute equally dense to both the ipsilateral and the contralateral MEC. In case the proposed relation between neuronal targets and bilateral innervation of the MEC is indeed present and functionally relevant, the prediction would be that a similar neuronal distribution would hold true for the inputs that originate from the infralimbic cortex, because this projection distributes bilaterally to the LEC at almost equal densities (Jones and Witter, unpublished observations).

ACKNOWLEDGMENT

The research reported in this paper was supported by grants 903-47-008 and 903-47-051 of the Netherlands Organization for Scientific Research (NWO).

REFERENCES

1. VON BONIN, G. & P. BAILEY. 1947. The Neocortex of *Macaca mulatta*. University of Illinois Press. Urbana, IL.
2. BURWELL, R.D., M.P. WITTER & D.G. AMARAL. 1995. Perirhinal and postrhinal cortices of the rat: a review of the neuroanatomical literature and comparison with findings from the monkey brain. Hippocampus **5:** 390–408.
3. NABER, P.A., M. CABALLERO-BLEDA, B. JORRITSMA-BYHAM & M.P. WITTER. 1997. Parallel input to the hippocampal memory system through peri- and postrhinal cortices. NeuroReport **8:** 2617–2621.
4. WITTER, M.P., H.J. GROENEWEGEN, F.H. LOPES DA SILVA & A.H.M. LOHMAN. 1989. Functional organization of the extrinsic and intrinsic circuitry of the parahippocampal region. Prog. Neurobiol. **33:**161–254.

5. RAMÓN Y CAJAL, S. 1911. Histologie du Système Nerveux de l'Homme et des Vertebrés. Maloine, Paris.
6. VAN HOESEN, G.W. & D.N. PANDYA. 1975. Some connections of the entorhinal (area 28) and perirhinal (area 35) cortices of the rhesus monkey. I. Temporal lobe afferents. Brain Res. **95:** 1–24.
7. VAN HOESEN, G.W., D.N. PANDYA & N. BUTTERS. 1975. Some connections of the entorhinal (area 28) and perirhinal (area 35) cortices of the rhesus monkey. II. Frontal lobe afferents. Brain Res. **95:** 25–38.
8. VAN HOESEN, G.W. & D.N. PANDYA. 1975. Some connections of the entorhinal (area 28) and perirhinal (area 35) cortices of the rhesus monkey. III. Efferent connections. Brain Res. **95:** 39–59.
9. STEWARD, O. 1976. Topographic organization of the projections from the entorhinal area to the hippocampal formation in the rat. J. Comp. Neurol. **167:** 285–314.
10. STEWARD, O. & S.A. SCOVILLE. 1976. Cells of origin of entorhinal cortical afferents to the hippocampus and fascia dentata of the rat. J. Comp. Neurol. **169:** 347–370.
11. DESMOND, N.C., C.A. SCOTT, J.A. JANE, JR. & W.B. LEVY. 1994. Ultrastructural identification of entorhinal cortical synapses in CA1 stratum lacunosum-moleculare of the rat. Hippocampus **4:** 594–600.
12. WITTER, M.P. B. JORRITSMA-BYHAM & F.G. WOUTERLOOD. 1992. Perforant pathway projection to the Ammon's horn and the subiculum in the rat. An electron micrsocopical PHA-L study. Soc. Neurosci. Abstr. **18:** 323.
13. LEUNG, L.S. 1995. Stimulation of perforant path evoked field and intracellular potentials in hippocampal CA1 area. Hippocampus **5:** 129–136.
14. PARÉ, D. & R. LLINAS. 1995. Intracellular study of direct entorhinal inputs to field CA1 in the isolated guinea pig brain in vitro. Hippocampus **5:** 115–119.
15. YECKEL, M.Y. & T.W. BERGER. 1995. Monosynaptic excitation of hippocampal CA1 pyramidal cells by afferents from the entorhinal cortex. Hippocampus **5:** 108–114.
16. WITTER, M.P. 1989. Connectivity of the rat hippocampus. *In* The Hippocampus-New Vistas; Neurology and Neurobiology, Vol. X. V. Chan-Palay & Y. Ben-Ari, Eds.: 67–82. Alan Liss Inc. New York.
17. WITTER, M.P. 1993. Organization of the entorhinal-hippocampal system: a review of current anatomical data. Hippocampus **3:** 33–44.
18. WITTER, M.P., A.W. GRIFFIOEN, B. JORRITSMA-BYHAM & J.L.M. KRIJNEN. 1988. Entorhinal projections to the hippocampal CA1 region in the rat: an underestimated pathway. Neurosci. Lett. **85:** 193–198.
19. CANNING, K.J. & L.S. LEUNG. 1997. Lateral-entorhinal, perirhinal and amygdalaentorhinal transition projections to hippocampal CA1 and dentate gyrus in the rat: a current source density study. Hippocampus **7:** 643–655.
20. LIU, P. & D.K. BILKEY. 1997. Current source density analysis of the potential evoked in hippocampus by perforant cortex stimulation. Hippocampus **7:** 389–396.
21. NABER, P.A., M.P. WITTER & F.H. LOPES DA SILVA. 1999. Perirhinal cortex input to the hippocampal formation in the rat: evidence for parallel pathways, both direct and indirect. A combined physiological and anatomical study. Eur. J. Neurosci. **11:** 4119–4133.
22. WITTER, M.P. & D.G. AMARAL. 1991. Entorhinal cortex of the monkey. V. Projections to the dentate gyrus, hippocampus, and subicular complex. J. Comp. Neurol. **307:** 437–459.
23. LINGENHOHL, K. & D.M. FINCH. 1991. Morphological characterization of rat entorhinal neurons in vivo: soma-dendritic structure and axonal domains. Exp. Brain Res. **84:** 57–74.
24. TAMAMAKI, N. & Y. NOJYO. 1993. Projection of the entorhinal layer II neurons in the rat as revealed by intracellular pressure-injection of neurobiotin. Hippocampus **3:** 471–480.
25. INSAUSTI, R., M.T. HERRERO & M.P. WITTER. 1997. Entorhinal cortex of the rat: cytoarchitectonic subdivisions and the origin and distribution of cortical efferents. Hippocampus **7:** 146–183.
26. WITTER, M.P. & P. ROOM. 1985. Connections of the parahippocampal cortex. A neuroanatomical tracing study in the cat.: 15–36. Thesis Vrije Universiteit.
27. AMARAL, D.G., R. INSAUSTI & W.M. COWAN. 1987. The entorhinal cortex of the monkey. I. Cytoarchitectonic organization. J. Comp. Neurol. **264:** 326–355.

28. AMARAL, D.G. & R. INSAUSTI. 1990. Hippocampal formation. *In* The Human Nervous System. G. Paxinos, Ed.: 711–756. Academic Press. New York.
29. INSAUSTI, R., T. TUNÓN, T. SOBREVIELA *et al.* 1995. The human entorhinal cortex: a cytoarchitectonic analysis. J. Comp. Neurol. **355:** 171–198.
30. MCNAUGHTON, B.L. & C.A. BARNES. 1977. Physiological identification and analysis of dentate granule cell responses to stimulation of the medial and lateral perforant pathways in the rat. J. Comp. Neurol. **175:** 439–454.
31. WITTER, M.P. & H.J. GROENEWEGEN. 1984. Laminar origin and septotemporal distribution of entorhinal and perirhinal projections to the hippocampus in the cat. J. Comp. Neurol. **224:** 371–385.
32. VAN GROEN, T. & F.H. LOPES DA SILVA. 1986. The organization of the reciprocal connections between the subiculum and the entorhinal cortex in the cat. II. An electrophysiological study. J. Comp. Neurol. **251:** 111–120.
33. VAN GROEN, T., F.J. VAN HAREN, M.P. WITTER & H.J. GROENEWEGEN. 1986. The organization of the reciprocal connections between the subiculum and the entorhinal cortex in the cat. I. A neuroanatomical tracing study. J. Comp. Neurol. **250:** 485–497.
34. RUTH, R.E., T.J. COLLIER & A. ROUTTENBERG. 1982. Topography between the entorhinal cortex and the dentate septotemporal axis in rats. I. Medial and intermediate entorhinal projecting cells. J. Comp. Neurol. **209:** 69–78.
35. RUTH, R.E., T.J. COLLIER & A. ROUTTENBERG. 1988. Topographical relationship between the entorhinal cortex and the septotemporal axis of the dentate gyrus in rats. II. Cells projecting from lateral entorhinal subdivisions. J. Comp. Neurol. **270:** 506–516.
36. WITTER, M.P. G.W. VAN HOESEN & D.G. AMARAL. 1989. Topographical organization of the entorhinal projection to the dentate gyrus of the monkey. J. Neurosci. **9:** 216–228.
37. DOLORFO, C.L. & D.G. AMARAL. 1998. Entorhinal cortex of the rat: topographic organization of the cells of origin of the perforant path projection to the dentate gyrus. J. Comp. Neurol. **398:** 25–48.
38. AMARAL, D.G. & M.P. WITTER. 1989. The three-dimensional organization of the hippocampal formation: a review of anatomical data. Neuroscience **31:** 571–591.
39. ROOM, P. & H.J. GROENEWEGEN. 1986. Connections of the parahippocampal cortex. I. Cortical afferents. J. Comp. Neurol. **251:** 415–450.
40. BURWEL, R.D. & D.G. AMARAL. 1998. Perirhinal and postrhinal cortices of the rat: interconnectivity and connections with the entorhinal cortex. J. Comp. Neurol. **391:** 293–321.
41. SUZUKI, W.A. & D.G. AMARAL. 1994. Topographic organization of the reciprocal connections between the monkey entorhinal and the perirhinal and parahippocampal cortices. J. Neurosci **14:** 1856–1877.
42. WITTER, M.P., P. ROOM, H.J. GROENEWEGEN & A.H.M. LOHMAN. 1986. Connections of the parahippocampal cortex in the cat. V. Intrinsic connections; comments on input/output connections with the hippocampus. J. Comp. Neurol. **252:** 78–94.
43. DOLORFO, C.L. & D.G. AMARAL. 1998. Entorhinal cortex of the rat: organization of intrinsic connections. J. Comp. Neurol. **398:** 49–82.
44. KOSEL, K.C, G.W. VAN HOESEN & D.L. ROSENE. 1983. A direct projection from the perirhinal cortex (area 35) to the subiculum in the rat. Brain Res. **269:** 347–351.
45. MCINTYRE, D.C., M.E. KELLY & W.A. STAINES. 1996. Efferent projections of the anterior perirhinal cortex in the rat. J. Comp. Neurol. **369:** 302–318.
46. SUZUKI, W.A. & D.G. AMARAL. 1990. Cortical inputs to the CA1 field of the monkey hippocampus originate from the perirhinal and parahippocampal cortex but not from area TE. Neurosci. Lett. **115:** 43–48.
47. LIU, P. & D.K. BILKEY. 1996. Direct connections between perirhinal cortex and hippocampus is a major constituent of the lateral perforant path. Hippocampus **6:** 125–134.
48. WITTER, M.P., P.A. NABER & F.H. LOPES DA SILVA. 1999. Perirhinal cortex does not project to the dentate gyrus (letter to the editor). Hippocampus **9:** 605–606.
49. NABER, P.A., M.P. WITTER & F.H. LOPES DA SILVA. 2000. Evidence for a direct projection from postrhinal cortex to subiculum in the rat. Hippocampus. In press.

50. TAMAMAKI, N., K. ABE & Y. NOJYO. 1987. Columnar organization in the subiculum formed by axon branches originating from single CA1 pyramidal neurons in the rat hippocampus. Brain Res. **412:** 156–160.
51. TAMAMAKI, N. & Y. NOJYO. 1990. Disposition of the slab-like modules formed by axon branches originating from single CA1 pyramidal neurons in the rat hippocampus. J. Comp. Neurol. **291:** 509–519.
52. AMARAL, D.G., C. DOLORFO & P. ALVAREZ-ROYO. 1991. Organization of CA1 projections to the subiculum: a PHA-L analysis in the rat. Hippocampus **1:** 415–435.
53. SWANSON, L.W. & W.M. COWAN. 1977. An autoradiographic study of the organization of the efferent connections of the hippocampal formation in the rat. J. Comp. Neurol. **172:** 49–84.
54. KÖHLER, C. 1985 Intrinsic projections of the retrohippocampal region in the rat brain. I. The subicular complex. J. Comp. Neurol. **236:** 504–522.
55. VAN GROEN, T. & J.M. WYSS. 1990. Extrinsic projections from area CA1 of the rat hippocampus: olfactory, cortical, subcortical, and bilateral hippocampal formation. J. Comp. Neurol. **302:** 515–528.
56. VAN HAEFTEN, T., B. JORRITSMA-BYHAM & M.P. WITTER. 1995. Quantitative morphological analysis of subicular terminals in the rat entorhinal cortex. Hippocampus **5:** 452–459.
57. SAUNDERS, R.C. & D.L. ROSENE. 1988. A comparison of the efferents of the amygdala and the hippocampal formation in the rhesus monkey. I. Convergence in the entorhinal, prorhinal, and perirhinal cortices. J. Comp. Neurol. **271:** 153–184.
58. TAMAMAKI, N. & Y. NOJYO. 1995. Preservation of topography in the connections between the subiculum, field CA1, and the entorhinal cortex in rats. J. Comp. Neurol. **353:** 379–390.
59. NABER, P.A., F.H. LOPES DA SILVA & M.P. WITTER. 2000. Reciprocal connections between the entorhinal cortex and hippocampal fields CA1 and the subiculum are in register with the projections from CA1 to the subiculum. Hippocampus. In press.
60. LORENTE DE NÓ, R. 1933. Studies on the structure of the cerebral cortex. I. The area entorhinalis. J. Psychol. Neurol. **45:** 381–438.
61. WOUTERLOOD, F.G., W. HÄRTIG, G. BRÜCKNER & M.P. WITTER. 1995. Parvalbumine-immunoreactive neurons in the entorhinal cortex of the rat: localization, morphology, connectivity and ultrastructure. J. Neurocytol. **24:** 135–153.
62. SCHMIDT, S., E. BRAAK & H. BRAAK. 1993. Parvalbumine-immunoreactive structures of the adult human entorhinal and transentorhinal region. Hippocampus **3:** 459–470.
63. Tunón, T., R. Insausti, I. Ferrer *et al.* 1993. Parvalbumine and calbindin D-28K in the human entorhinal cortex. Brain Res. **589:** 24–32.
64. KLINK, R. & A. ALONSO. 1997. Morphological characteristics of layer II projection neurons in the rat medial entorhinal cortex. Hippocampus **7:** 571–583.
65. VAN DER LINDEN, S. & F.H. LOPES DA SILVA. 1998. Comparison of the electrophysiology and morphology of layers III and II neurons of the rat medial entorhinal cortex in vitro. Eur. J. Neurosci. **10:** 1479–1489.
66. WYSS, J.M. & T. VAN GROEN. 1992. Connections between the retrosplenial cortex and the hippocampal formation in the rat: a review. Hippocampus **2:** 1–13.
67. JONES, B.F. & M.P. WITTER. 1999. Cingulate cortex projections to the (para)hippocampal area in the rat: an anatomical tracing study. Soc Neurosci. Abstr. **25:** 891.
68. VAN HAEFTEN, T, F.G. WOUTERLOOD & M.P. WITTER. 2000. Presubicular input to the dendrites of layer V entorhinal neurons in the rat. Ann. N.Y. Acad. Sci. **22:** this volume.
69. BURWELL, R.D. & D.G. AMARAL. 1998. Cortical afferents of the perirhinal, postrhinal and entorhinal cortices of the rat. J. Comp. Neurol. **398:** 179–205.
70. SUZUKI, W.A. & D.G. AMARAL. 1994. The perirhinal and parahippocampal cortices of the Macaque monkey: Cortical afferents. J. Comp. Neurol. **350:** 497–533.
71. WITTER, M.P. 1986. A survey of the anatomy of the hippocampal formation, with emphasis on the septotemporal organization of its intrinsic and extrinsic connections. Adv. Exp. Med. Biol. **203:** 67–82.
72. IIJIMA, T., M.P. WITTER, M. ICHIKAWA *et al.* 1996. Entorhinal-hippocampal interactions revealed by real-time imaging. Science **272:** 1176–1179.

73. DICKSON, C.T. & A. ALONSO. 1997. Muscarinic induction of synchronous population activity in the entorhinal cortex. J. Neurosci. **17:** 6729–6744.
74. STEWART, M. 1999. Columnar activity supports propagation of population burst in slices of rat entorhinal cortex. Brain Res. **830:** 274–284.
75. BUZSÁKI , G. 1996. The hippocampo-neocortical dialogue. Cerebr. Cortex **6:** 81–92.

The Parahippocampal Region: Corticocortical Connectivity

REBECCA D. BURWELL[a]

Department of Psychology, Brown University, Providence, Rhode Island 02912, USA

ABSTRACT: The parahippocampal region, as defined in this review, comprises the cortical regions that surround the rodent hippocampus including the perirhinal, postrhinal, and entorhinal cortices. The comparable regions in the primate brain are the perirhinal, parahippocampal, and entorhinal cortices. The perirhinal and postrhinal/parahippocampal cortices provide the major polysensory input to the hippocampus through their entorhinal connections and are the recipients of differing combinations of sensory information. The differences in the perirhinal and postrhinal cortical afferentation have important functional implications, in part, because these two regions project with different terminal patterns to the entorhinal cortex. The perirhinal cortex projects preferentially to the lateral entorhinal area (LEA), and the postrhinal cortex projects preferentially to the medial entorhinal area (MEA) and the caudal portion of LEA. Although the perirhinal and postrhinal cortices provide the major cortical input to the entorhinal cortex, the entorhinal cortex itself receives some direct cortical input. An examination of the cortical afferentation of the entorhinal cortex reveals an interesting principle of connectivity among these regions; the composition of the direct neocortical input to the LEA is more similar to that of the perirhinal cortex, and the composition of the direct neocortical input to the MEA is more similar to that of the postrhinal cortex. Thus, polymodal associational input to the LEA and the MEA exhibits some segregation and is organized in parallel. The organization of intrinsic connections for each of the parahippocampal regions also contributes to the segregation of information into parallel pathways.

INTRODUCTION

The parahippocampal region comprises a group of cytoarchitectonically and connectionally distinct cortical regions. While these regions are easily discriminable, what joins them is that together they account for the large majority of the cortical input to the hippocampus. In this chapter, I briefly review the fundamental neuroanatomical features of the perirhinal, postrhinal, and entorhinal cortices, the cortical afferentation of these regions, and the organization of the interconnections among these regions in the rat brain. Along the way comparisons will be made with what is known about the mouse, monkey, and human brains.

Studies in the human, monkey and rat now suggest that the parahippocampal regions contribute substantially to some memory processes.[1–5] The suspected role of these regions in normal memory function initiated a flurry of neuroanatomical stud-

[a]Address for correspondence: Rebecca D. Burwell, Ph.D., Department of Psychology, Brown University, Providence, RI 02912. Tel.: (401) 863-9208; fax: (401) 863-1300.
e-mail: Rebecca_Burwell@Brown.edu

ies conducted primarily in the monkey and the rat.[6–17] For some years now we have known that the the majority of the cortical input to the hippocampus is funneled through the association cortices that surround the hippocampus. Neuroanatomical approaches show that the individual areas within the parahippocampal region differ in their structural and connectional organization, suggesting that they are not merely conduits of information for the hippocampus, but that they have different functions with regard to memory. This notion of differential contributions is supported by differences among them in cortical and subcortical afferentation, patterns of intrinsic connectivity, and patterns of interconnectivity.

The large majority of research on hippocampal and parahippocampal function has been conducted in rat and monkey models. Consequentially, an important question is the extent of neuroanatomical and functional homology with similar regions in the human brain. The recent increase in the use of mutant mice to study hippocampal function also raises questions of how the parahippocampal regions in the mouse compare with the comparable regions in the rat, monkey and human brains. Although considerable information is now available about the structure and function of parahippocampal regions in the rat and monkey brains, the data on the these regions are lacking for the mouse and human brains. It will be important to document cross-species differences in these regions to promote the usefulness of animal models of human memory.

NOMENCLATURE

In the rodent brain, there is a prominent sulcus, the rhinal sulcus, that arises at the joining of the olfactory bulb and frontal pole and extends almost to the caudal pole of the brain (FIG. 1). The caudal extension of the rhinal sulcus in most rats is barely evident as no more than a shallow indentation. The cortical regions that surround the caudal portion of the rhinal sulcus in the rat brain include the perirhinal, postrhinal, and entorhinal regions. In the primate brain, the three comparable regions are the perirhinal, parahippocampal, and entorhinal cortices. Although still identifiable, the rhinal sulcus is substantially more limited in extent in the monkey and is even less prominent in the human brain (FIG. 2). In the primate brain, then, only the perirhinal and entorhinal (rhinal cortices) are contiguous with the rhinal fissure. In both the rodent and the primate brains, the three regions can be described as surrounding the hippocampus; thus, the term "parahippocampal region" is especially useful in a comparative framework. Nevertheless, care must be taken not to equate the term with "parahippocampal cortex" or "parahippocampal gyrus" in the primate brain.

In the rat, the perirhinal cortex consists of areas 35 and 36 (reviewed in Ref. 3). The postrhinal cortex has not been subdivided at this writing. In the monkey, the perirhinal cortex consists of areas 35 and 36, and area 36 is further partitioned into five subdivisions. The monkey parahippocampal cortex consists of areas TH and TF, each comprising two subdivisions.[16] Although the data on the mouse and human are sufficiently limited as to preclude a confident application of a consistent nomenclature across species, indications are that the regions that surround the hippocampus can at least be divided into three comparable regions: perirhinal, postrhinal, and entorhinal for the mouse (FIG. 1A); perirhinal, parahippocampal, and entorhinal for the human (FIG. 2B).

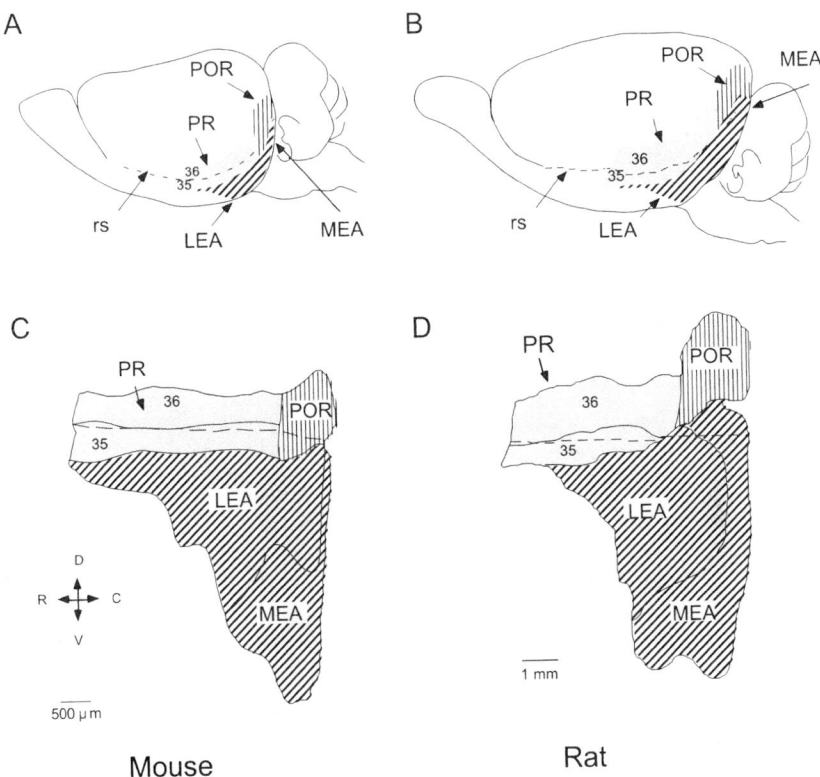

FIGURE 1. A lateral surface view of the mouse brain (**A**) and the rat brain (**B**; adapted from Burwell *et al.*[3]). Unfolded two-dimensional surface maps of the mouse (**C**) and the rat (**D**) entorhinal, perirhinal and postrhinal cortices. Perirhinal cortex (PR, areas 35 and 36) is shown in gray, postrhinal cortex (POR) in vertical stripes, and the entorhinal cortex (EC) in diagonal stripes. LEA, lateral entorhinal area; MEA, medial entorhinal area.

The perirhinal cortex exhibits substantial cross-species similarity in cytoarchitectonic features in the rat and monkey brains (see below), but the postrhinal and parahippocampal regions share few apparent structural or cytoarchitectonic similarities. Thus, in defining these areas in the rat brain, Burwell and colleagues[3,18] called the region postrhinal cortex, a name already found in the rodent literature,[19] rather than employing terminology in use for the primate brain. Subsequent connectional studies indicated that the rat postrhinal and monkey parahippocampal regions exhibit striking connectional similarities,[9,15] which provided the basis for hypothesizing functional homology between the two regions.

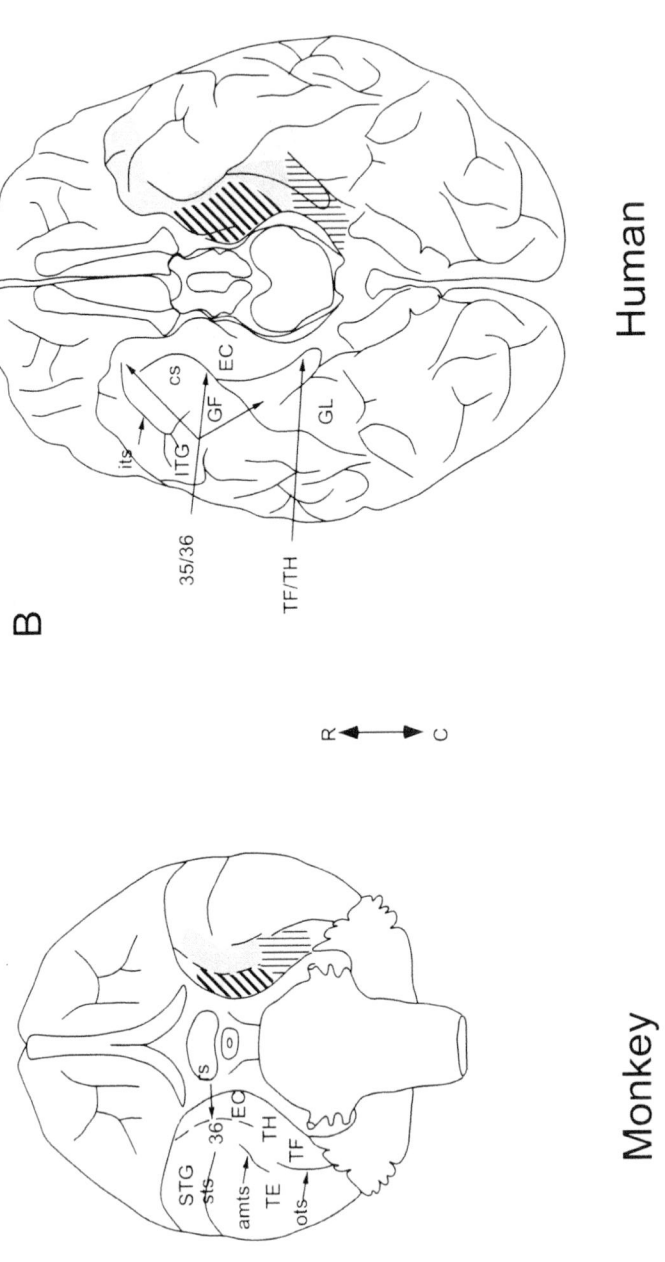

FIGURE 2. Ventral surface views of the monkey brain (**A**; adapted from Suzuki & Amaral[16]) and the human brain (**B**; adapted from Insausti, Tuñón, *et al.*[46]) showing borders of the entorhinal (EC), perirhinal (PR), and parahippocampal (PH) cortices as described in this chapter. amts, anterior middle temporal sulcus; Audv, auditory association cortex; cs, collateral sulcus; GF, fusiform gyrus; GL, lingual gyrus; ITG, inferotemporal gyrus; its, inferotemporal sulcus; ls, lateral sulcus; ots, occipitotemporal sulcus; PaSub, parasubiculum; rs, rhinal sulcus; STG, superior temporal gyrus; area TE of von Bonin and Bailey (1947); and Visl, visual association cortex.

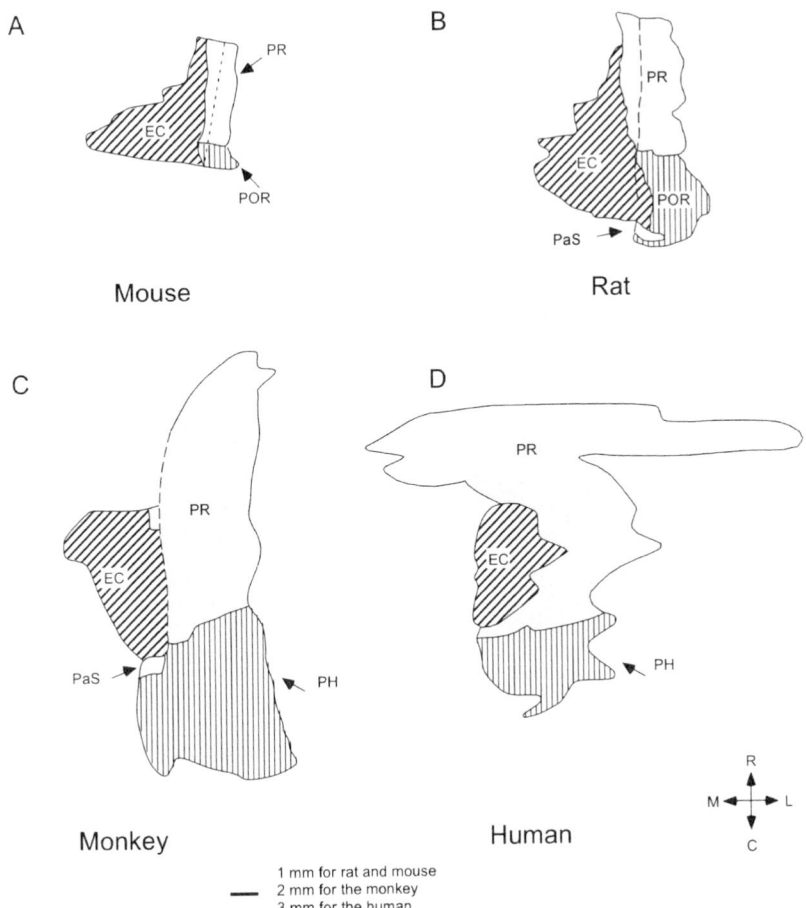

FIGURE 3. Representative unfolded two-dimensional maps. For comparison, unfolded maps for all four species are shown here. Either layer IV or a line between layers III and V was unfolded in the mouse (**A**) and rat (**B**), layer IV was unfolded in the monkey (**C**), and the outer margin of layer V was unfolded in the human (**D**). Again, perirhinal cortex (areas 35 and 36) is shown in gray, parahippocampal (PH) and postrhinal (POR) cortices in vertical stripes, and the entorhinal cortex (EC) in diagonal stripes. PaSub, parasubiculum.

STRUCTURE AND CYTOARCHITECTONIC FEATURES

Unfolded maps of layer IV of the parahippocampal region of four species (FIG. 3, note the differences in scale) provide the basis for some interesting comparisons. Allowing for differences in size and shape, the spatial relationships among the sub-areas are similar in the mouse, rat, monkey, and human brains. Although there are obvious differences in absolute size, the perirhinal cortex accounts for about 5% of the total cortical surface area, at least for the rat and monkey.[3,20] Thus, it has been

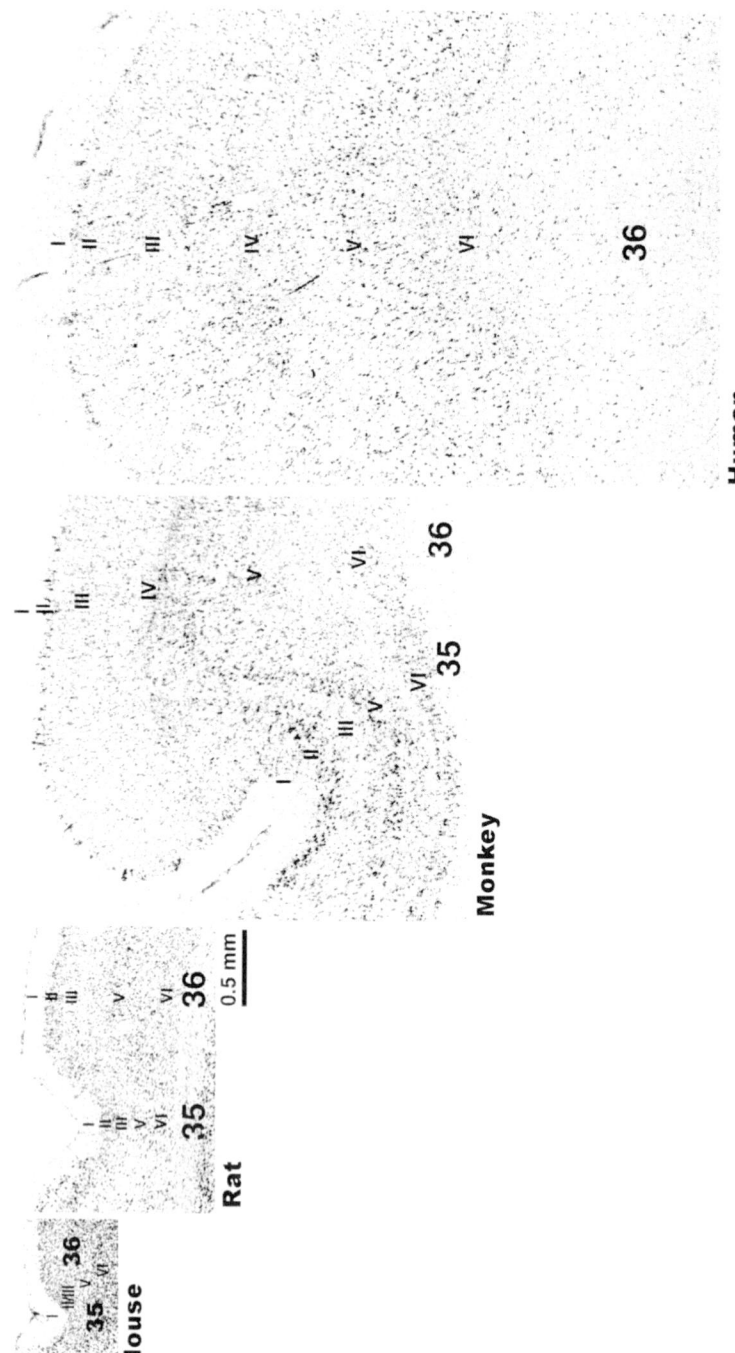

FIGURE 4. Photomicrographs of Nissl-stained coronal sections through perirhinal cortex (areas 35 and 36) of the mouse (**A**), rat (**B**), the macaque monkey (**C**), and the human (**D**). The laminar pattern is indicated by Roman numerals. Note that the characteristic patchy layer II is apparent in all four species.

TABLE 1. Cortical surface area (sq mm)

Region	Mouse	Rat	Monkey	Human
Perirhinal cortex	1.50	9	93	422
Parahippocampal or postrhinal cortex	0.36	5	78	89
Entorhinal cortex	3.50	12	41	81

SOURCE: Burwell et al.[45] for areas for rat, monkey, and human; Burwell, unpublished observations, for areas for the mouse.

suggested that the perirhinal cortex may scale up relative to cortical surface area. It is noteworthy that the relative sizes of the other cortices vary across the four species (TABLE 1). For example, the size of the entorhinal cortex appears to scale down exponentially with increase in cortical surface area, suggesting that the area might be less important as one goes up the evolutionary scale.

In addition to cortical surface area, another cross-species difference is apparent in cortical thickness. FIGURE 4 shows the perirhinal cortex of the mouse, the rat, the macaque monkey, and the human brains in coronal section in the same scale. This cortex is substantially thicker in primate brains as compared with the rodent models. Additionally, the laminar characteristics of the cortex are much more prominent in the primate brains as compared to either rodent model. Yet, as we shall see, closer comparisons indicate that there are similarities in the general organizational principles of the perirhinal and parahippocampal/postrhinal cortices across species as well as some signature characteristics that are common across species.

All reports of the cytoarchitecture of area 35 of the rat perirhinal cortex indicate that the region is agranular.[3,21,22] Recent investigations further conclude that it is distinguished by a prominent layer V characterized by large, darkly staining pyramidal cells.[3] Area 36 is easily distinguished cytoarchitectonically from area 35 because it is granular. Additionally, area 36 has a distinctive layer II characterized by patches of spherical and pyramidal cells. In the ventral subdivision, only a weak layer IV is present such that the granule cells are intermixed with the cells forming layers III and V. This granular layer is more distinct at progressively more dorsally situated portions of area 36.

The available cytoarchitectonic information on the perirhinal and postrhinal cortices in the rat indicates that there are similarities with the monkey. The macaque monkey area 35 is agranular and homogeneous in its cytoarchitectonic characteristics as is true for the rat.[4,15,23,24] Layer V is populated by large, darkly staining, densely packed cells. As in the rat, these cells form an arc around the fundus of the rhinal sulcus. In contrast to area 35, area 36 shows substantial cytoarchitectonic regional variation. In general, it becomes more densely cellular, more columnar, and more distinctly laminated as one moves either laterally or caudally.[15] Unlike area 35, area 36 has a distinct layer IV, although it tends to be very weakly populated in the medial and rostral portions of the area. In the monkey as in the rat, the most distinctive feature of area 36 is the patchy layer II, which is composed of islands of darkly stained cells that form an irregular border with layer I, especially at rostral levels. In fact, this characteristic patchiness of area 36 layer II is easily identified across species in the mouse, rat, monkey, and human (FIG. 4).

The postrhinal cortex in the rat is not clearly differentiated from the perirhinal cortex on cytoarchitectonic grounds. This may be in part because of the way in which postrhinal cortex wraps obliquely around the caudal pole of the rat brain. This spatial arrangement makes it impossible to clearly observe the organization of laminar and cellular characteristics without dissecting out the region and flattening it. Thus, in most planes of the section, the border between the rat perirhinal and postrhinal cortices is difficult to ascertain. In coronal sections, the rostrally adjacent perirhinal cortex can be distinguished from the postrhinal cortex by the presence of ectopic layer II cells in the postrhinal ventral division. These outpouchings of cells into layer I give layer II a distinctively irregular appearance. In general, the postrhinal cortex is more highly laminated than perirhinal cortex, the cells are smaller and more homogeneously packed, and the cortex exhibits a weak granular layer. In the caudal half of the region, the lamination is obscured by the plane of sectioning.

In the monkey, the parahippocampal cortex comprising areas TH and TF is easily distinguished from the neighboring perirhinal region. The rostral portion of area TH is agranular and bilaminate in appearance due to the merging of layers II/III and layers V/VI. The caudal subdivision of area TH is more laminar in appearance and contains a meager internal granular layer. In contrast, area TF is more highly granular with large pyramidal cells populating a layer V that merges with layer VI.

CORTICAL AFFERENTATION

The perirhinal and postrhinal cortices of the rat receive widespread and entirely different neocortical input from unimodal and polymodal associational areas. Although earlier studies provided the initial information about perirhinal afferentation,[19,25–28] our recent more quantitative study based on new borders confirmed and extended the earlier findings (FIG. 5).[9] Perirhinal cortex receives a substantial olfactory input from piriform cortex (FIG. 5, upper left), which terminates almost exclusively in area 35. All other cortical input terminates preferentially in dorsal area 36 and is distributed across all remaining sensory modalities. The postrhinal cortex, in contrast, receives strong input from visual and visuospatial association cortex, somewhat less input from auditory association regions, and only weak input from the remaining modalities.

Our recent examination of the polymodal associational input to the perirhinal and postrhinal cortices (FIG. 5, lower)[9] confirmed, in a more quantitative manner, earlier reports of substantial associational input to perirhinal cortex.[19,28–31] Again, the two regions receive very different complements of cortical associational input. Projections from ventral temporal association cortices to the perirhinal cortex have been well-documented,[19,31,32] and we now know that the postrhinal cortex also receives ventral temporal input. The location of the origins of that input, however, differs for the two regions. The perirhinal cortex is interconnected with the full rostrocaudal extent of ventral temporal association cortex (Te_V as defined by Swanson), whereas the postrhinal cortex is interconnected preferentially with the caudal portion of the region. Our earlier observations indicate that rostral Te_V receives more input from somatosensory regions, mid-rostrocaudal portions from auditory regions, and the caudal portion from visual regions.[9] Thus, the organization of perirhinal and postrhi-

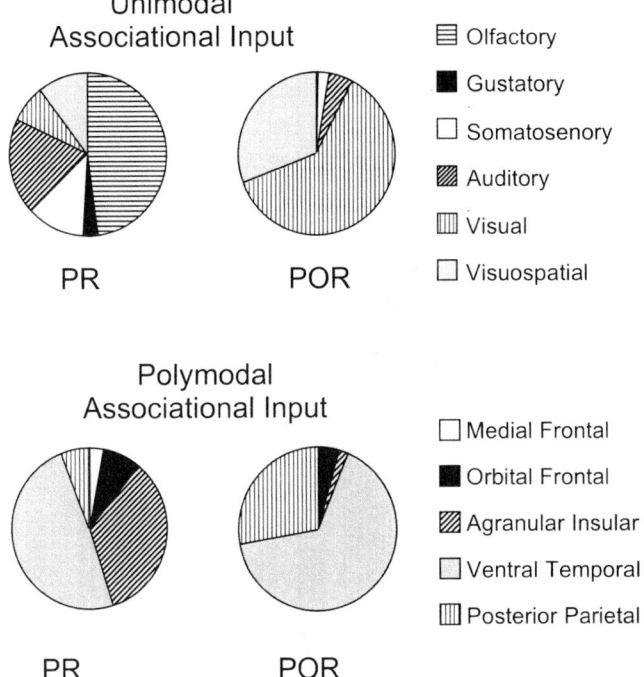

FIGURE 5. Pie charts showing the proportion of unimodal associational input to the perirhinal cortex (PR, *upper left*) and the postrhinal cortex (POR, *upper right*). Pie charts showing the proportion of polymodal associational input to the perirhinal cortex (PR, *lower left*), and the postrhinal cortex (POR, *lower right*). Ventral temporal cortex here represents a band of cortex that lies along the dorsal borders of the perirhinal and postrhinal cortices. The perirhinal cortex receives input from more rostral portions of this region, whereas the postrhinal cortex receives input from more caudal portions of this region.

nal input from ventral temporal areas further upholds the principle that the perirhinal cortex receives input from all sensory modalities, whereas postrhinal cortex is preferentially innervated by visual and visuospatial regions.

Although the perirhinal and postrhinal cortices receive substantially more input from higher-order polymodal associational regions, the entorhinal cortex does itself receive some extra-peri-postrhinal associational input (FIG. 6). Interestingly, the direct associational input to the lateral entorhinal area (LEA) is more similar to that of the perirhinal cortex in that it arises predominantly in anterior associational regions such as medial frontal cortex. The medial entorhinal area (MEA), in contrast, receives direct associational input more similar to that of the postrhinal cortex in that it arises predominantly in posterior associational regions such as retrosplenial cortex.

The perirhinal and parahippocampal cortices of the macaque monkey are also distinguished by their cortical input.[15,24,33,34] Suzuki and Amaral[15] provided evidence that unimodal associational inputs arise from somatosensory, auditory, and visual as-

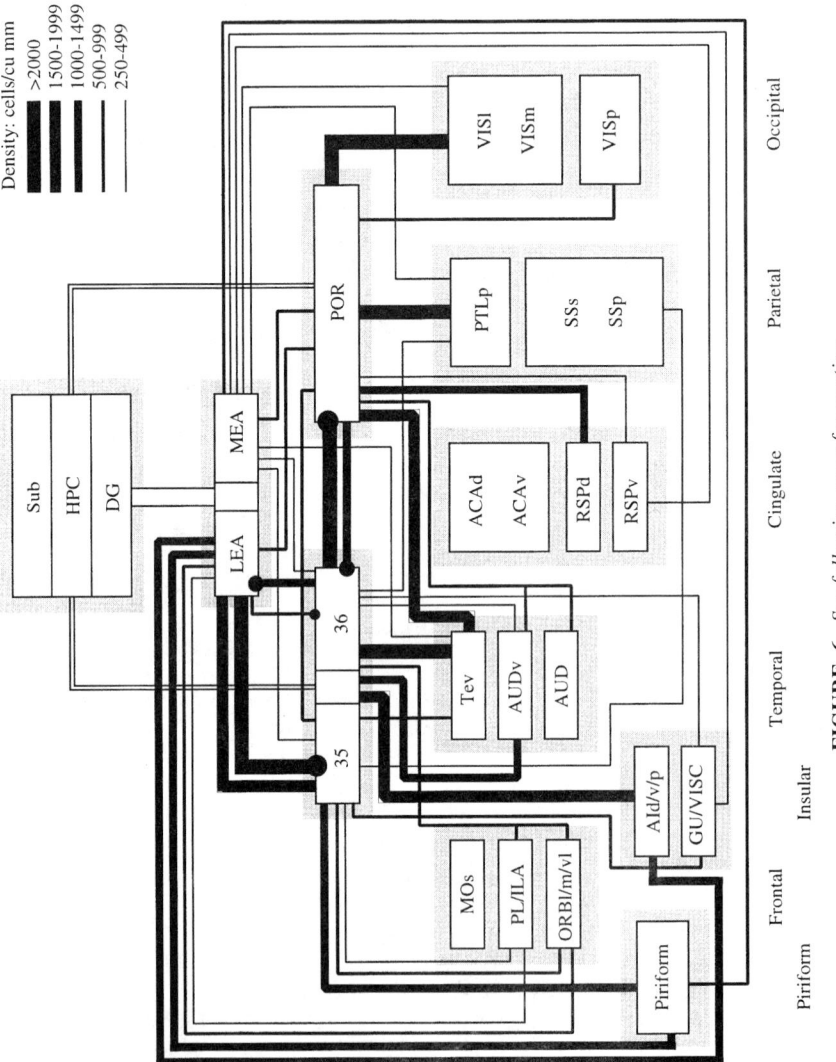

FIGURE 6. See following page for caption.

sociation cortices. Different from the rat, the majority of the input to both of these cortices is from visual areas although not the same visual regions. Visual object information derived from projections originating in area TE predominantly reaches the perirhinal cortex, whereas visuospatial information, arising from posterior parietal cortex and area V4, is more heavily directed to the parahippocampal cortex. Cortices identified with somatosensory processing, primarily the granular and dysgranular insular cortices, project both to perirhinal and parahippocampal cortices. Unlike the rat in which auditory association cortex projects to both perirhinal and postrhinal cortices, in the monkey only the parahippocampal cortex receives input from auditory associational regions. The monkey perirhinal and parahippocampal cortices receive polysensory information from ventrolateral and orbital cortices, cingulate and retrosplenial cortices, posterior parietal cortex, and the polymodal region of the dorsal bank of the superior temporal sulcus.[15] All of these cortices project to parahippocampal cortex, but the predominant polymodal associational input to perirhinal cortex arises from the parahippocampal cortex and the superior temporal sulcus. Interestingly, in both the rat and the monkey, the parahippocampal/postrhinal cortex projects heavily to the perirhinal cortex, whereas the reciprocal projection is relatively meager.

INTRINSIC CONNECTIONS

We previously identified a number of principles of intrinsic connectivity in the parahippocampal region.[7] Area 36 of the perirhinal cortex has extensive intrinsic connections such that any location is connected to the entire subregion (FIG. 7A). The projections are heaviest to the locations closest to the origin and attenuate as the distance from the origin increases. Although projections to a focus in area 36 originate about equally from regions located rostrally and caudally to the focus, there is a prominent dorsal to ventral gradient. This dorsal to ventral polarity is also reflected in connections between areas 35 and 36. Continuing the dorsal to ventral polarity of projections, area 36 projects heavily to area 35, but area 35 returns a weaker projection to area 36. In general, the ventrally directed projections terminate at the same rostrocaudal level at which they originate. The area 36 projection to area 35 resembles a lateral pathway according to criteria described by Felleman and Van Essen;[20] that is, the cells in superficial and deep layers terminate in all layers. In contrast, the

---

FIGURE 6. A diagram representing the pattern and strength of the cortical connectivity of the hippocampal formation [dentate gyrus (DG), hippocampus proper (HPC), subicular complex (sub), and entorhinal cortex (EC)], the perirhinal cortex (PR, areas 35 and 36), and the parahippocampal (PH, areas TF and TH) or postrhinal cortices (POR) for the rat. The thickness of the *solid lines* represents the relative strength of the remaining cortical input to the respective areas based on densities of labeled neurons. *Open lines* reflect connections that are known, but were not quantified in the referenced study. ACA, anterior cingulate cortex; AId, v, and p, dorsal, ventral, and agranular insular cortices; Aud, primary auditory cortex; AUDv, auditory association cortex; GU, gustatory granular insular cortex; MOp and MOs, primary and secondary motor areas; Pir, piriform cortex; RSP, retrosplenial cortex; SSp and SSs, primary and supplementary somatosensory areas; VISC, visceral granular insular cortex; VISl and m, visual association cortex; VISp, primary visual cortex.

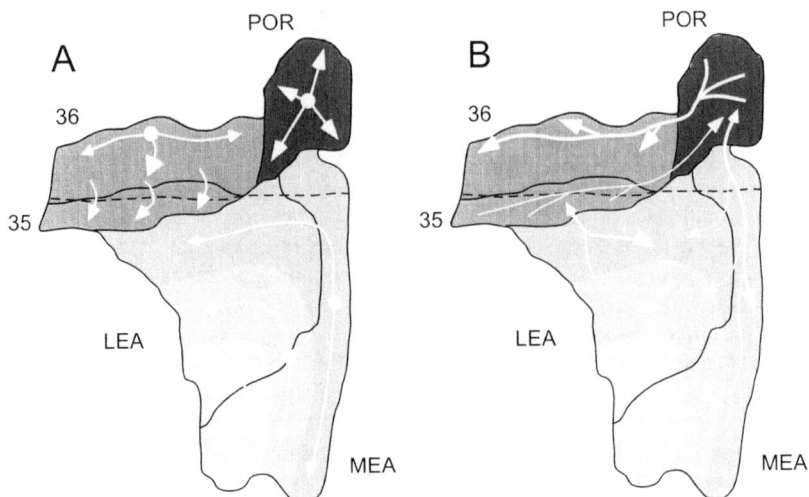

FIGURE 7. Unfolded maps of the parahippocampal areas in the rat showing the patterns of intrinsic connections (*left*) and the patterns of interconnections (*right*). The postrhinal cortex (POR) is shown in dark grey, the perirhinal cortex (PR) in middle grey, and the entorhinal cortex (EC) in three shades of light grey. The shades of light grey for the entorhinal cortex are progressively lighter to represent the lateral to medially located dentate-gyrus projecting bands. See text for details.

return projection exhibits characteristics of a feedback pathway in that the projection exhibits a bilaminate origin in area 35 and a bilaminate termination in area 36.

Unlike area 36 and area 35, the intrinsic connections of POR exhibit no polarity. Although they show no topography of terminations, the associational projections within POR are extensive. Thus, any focus within the region gives rise to strong intrinsic projections to the entire region (FIG. 7A). Indeed, this characteristic of the intrinsic connections of the postrhinal cortex was useful in defining its borders.[7] The laminar pattern of the postrhinal associational connections in the postrhinal cortex is similar to that found in area 36 in that they originate in layers II, V, and VI and terminate in layers I and V/VI.

The entorhinal cortex exhibits an unusual organization of interconnections that does not respect cytoarchitectonically defined subfields. There are three lateral to medially located, nonoverlapping domains or bands, each of which contains portions of LEA and MEA (FIG. 7A). The associational projections terminate preferentially within the band of origin.[23,37–39] The intrinsic entorhinal connections arise in layers II and III and the deep layers, but terminate preferentially in superficial layers.[39] Thus, it appears that the entorhinal cells of origin of the perforant pathway receive associational input from both deep and superficial layers. Each band projects to a different septotemporal level of the dentate gyrus, hippocampus, and subiculum.[14,23,35,36] More specifically, a caudolaterally situated band of entorhinal cortex projects to the septal half of the dentate gyrus; an intermediate band projects to the third quarter; and a medially situated band project to the fourth septotemporal border.

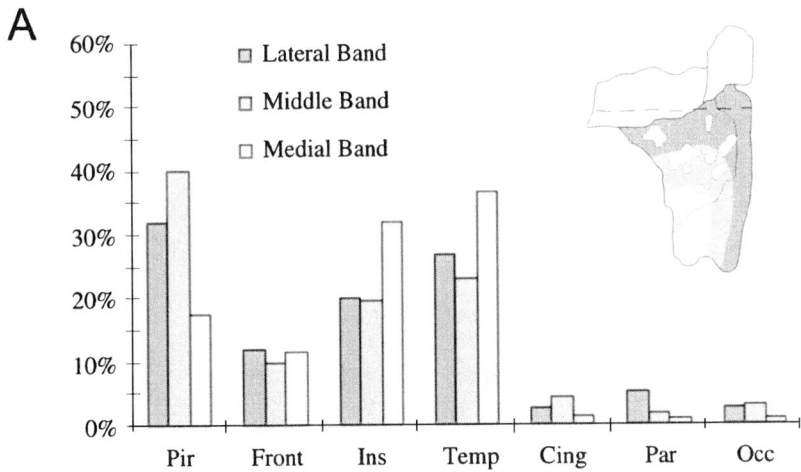

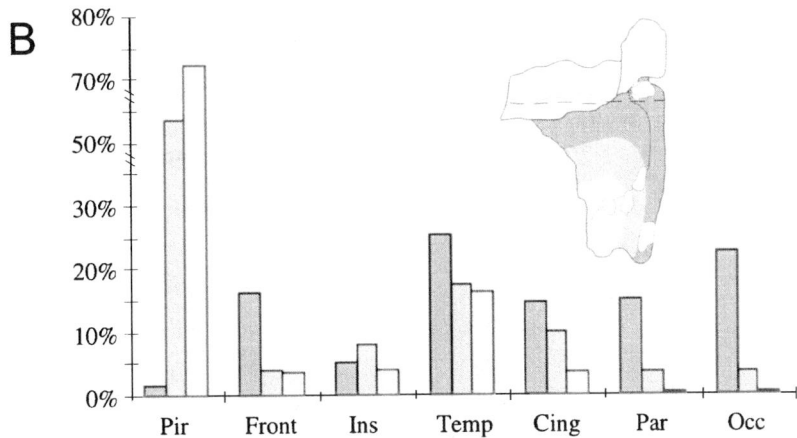

FIGURE 8. The results of a reanalysis of data from Burwell and Amaral[7] to show the organization of direct associational input to the entorhinal cortex according to its lateral to medially situated dentate-gyrus projecting bands. LEA, lateral entorhinal area; MEA, medial entorhinal area; perirhinal cortex areas 35 and 36; postrhinal cortex, POR.

The organization of entorhinal cortex into dentate-projecting bands appears also to reflect differences in cortical afferentation. Although the entorhinal cortex receives the majority of cortical input via the perirhinal and postrhinal cortices, it also receives some direct cortical input. We reanalyzed cortical afferent input to the entorhinal cortex[7] according to the medial to laterally situated bands and made some interesting discoveries. FIGURE 8 shows percentage of total input per band from different cortical regions for the LEA (panel A) and the MEA (panel B). Cortical input appears to be ordered according to band, especially for the MEA. The lateral band, which would innervate septal levels of the dentate gyrus, receives the largest portion of polymodal association input that might be considered visuospatial in nature. In contrast, the middle and medial bands, which innervate more temporal levels of the dentate gyrus, receive the bulk of their input from olfactory regions. In fact, the MEA portion of the medial band is almost exclusively innervated by olfactory regions and thus shows some similarities in location and connectivity to the olfactory field of the monkey entorhinal cortex (EO).[40] It should be noted, however, that EO in the monkey is defined by olfactory bulb input and is considered to belong to the LEA.

INTERCONNECTIVITY

We now know that in the rat, as in the monkey, widespread cortical input reaches the hippocampal formation via the perirhinal and postrhinal cortices and their connections with the entorhinal cortex.[6,7,17,19] Thus, it is important to know how these two regions are interconnected in order to discern the influence each region has over hippocampal processing. The postrhinal cortex projects strongly to dorsal levels of the perirhinal cortex (Fig. 7B).[7] Accordingly, postrhinal input to the perirhinal cortex is likely to influence other cortical inputs that also terminate in dorsal levels of area 36. The reciprocal projection—that from perirhinal cortex to the postrhinal cortex—is noticeably weaker and arises primarily from area 35.

The perirhinal and postrhinal cortices give rise to robust projections to the entorhinal cortex, which are stronger to the lateral band (Fig. 7B). Perirhinal cortex projects more strongly to the LEA and exhibits a topography such that rostral perirhinal cortex projects more strongly to rostral LEA, and caudal perirhinal cortex projects more strongly to caudal LEA. Postrhinal cortex projects preferentially to the MEA although it also projects to caudal LEA. Projections from the postrhinal cortex innervate all three DG-projecting bands of the entorhinal cortex, although the labeling in the lateral band is heavier. As in the monkey, the entorhinal cortex also gives rise to a return projection to the perirhinal and postrhinal cortices.[7,19,37,38] Moreover, the topography of the return projection is similar. The rostral entorhinal cortex (LEA) projects preferentially to the perirhinal cortex, whereas the caudal entorhinal cortex (caudal LEA and MEA) projects both to perirhinal and postrhinal cortices.

The topography of the entorhinal interconnections among the perirhinal, parahippocampal, and entorhinal cortices in the monkey was extensively described by Suzuki and Amaral.[16] Similar to the rat, the monkey parahippocampal cortex projects strongly to the perirhinal cortex, but the reciprocal projection is substantially weaker. Another similarity with the rat is that the perirhinal cortex projects most heavily to the rostrolateral two-thirds of the entorhinal cortex, and the parahippocampal cortex projects most heavily to the caudal two-thirds.

CONCLUSION

The intrinsic connections and interconnections of the parahippocampal areas are complex, but orderly in their arrangement. To summarize, the perirhinal and postrhinal receive different combinations of unimodal and polymodal sensory input. The

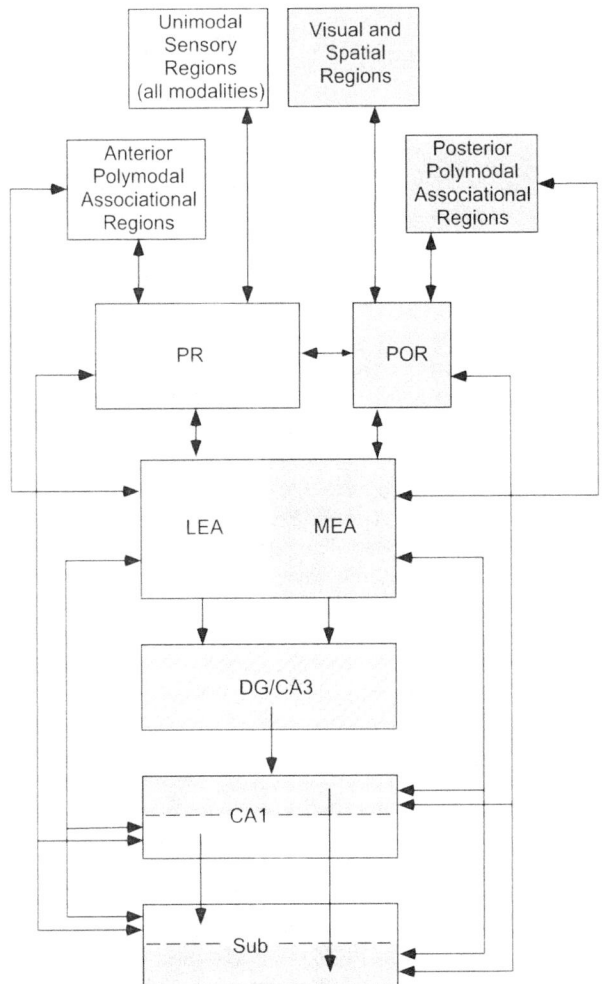

FIGURE 9. Schematic of corticohippocampal circuitry that shows the multiple parallel pathways by which unimodal and polymodal associational input reaches the hippocampal formation. Information appears to be somewhat segregated into a PR-LEA associated pathway (*light grey*), which is influenced by anterior associational regions such as the medial and orbital frontal cortices, and a POR-MEA associated pathway (*dark grey*), which is influenced by posterior associational regions such as the retrosplenial cortex. Several principles of connectivity are illustrated in the schematic. First, the polymodal associational input to PR vs. POR is similar to the direct polymodal associational input to the LEA and MEA, respectively. Second, PR and LEA project with similar terminal patterns to the CA1 field of the hippocampus and the subiculum; likewise POR and MEA terminate similarly in the CA1 and the subiculum. Third, there is convergence of infomation both in the dentate gyrus (DG) and CA3 field of the hippocampus, and in the intrinsic connections of the entorhinal cortex (see Fig. 7).

perirhinal cortex receives input from all modalites with the olfactory input terminating primarily in area 35 and all others terminating preferentially in dorsal area 36. The postrhinal cortex is heavily innervated by visual and visuospatial regions. In terms of polymodal input, the perirhinal cortex tends to receive polymodal associational input from more anterior regions, whereas the postrhinal cortex is more closely interconnected with posterior polymodal associational regions. The exception is that perirhinal cortex does receive a strong input from the postrhinal cortex which also terminates in dorsal area 36. The perirhinal and postrhinal cortices project to different portions of the entorhinal cortex, maintaining some segregation of information flow. The flow of information is organized both according to cytoarchitectonic subdivisions (LEA and MEA) and according to the dentate-projection bands. Perirhinal cortex projects preferentially to LEA and postrhinal cortex projects preferentially to MEA and caudal LEA. The medial to laterally situated entorhinal bands are important in that they provide for both integration of information (within bands) and segregation of information (across bands), providing the circuitry for parallel pathways through the hippocampal formation. There is now evidence that a similar organization exists in the mouse entorhinal cortex[41] and the monkey entorhinal cortex.[42] Thus, this feature of entorhinal connectivity appears to be conserved across species.

In conclusion, the perirhinal and postrhinal cortices in the rodent and primate brains are connected with both the full range of unimodal and polymodal associational cortices and with multiple fields of the hippocampal formation.[7,9,10,14–16] The organization of cortical afferentation, intrinsic connections, and interconnectivity suggests that there may be two parallel corticohippocampal-processing streams (FIG. 9).

In neuroscientific research the parahippocampal region has been most consistently implicated in memory functions. Based on functional neuroanatomical grounds, however, it is reasonable to hypothesize an additional function for these regions in attention. The processing stream associated with the perirhinal cortex and anterior associational systems (FIG. 9, light grey) includes prefrontal areas thought to contribute to attention and working memory. It is also interconnected with subcortical reward systems.[44] Based on the neuroanatomy, this stream might be involved in focused attentional processing of behaviorally relevant stimuli. In contrast, the processing stream more closely associated with the postrhinal cortex and posterior associational systems (FIG. 9, dark grey) has robust connections with regions involved with visuospatial orienting, for example, the posterior parietal cortex and the lateral posterior nucleus of the thalamus. Thus, this processing stream is uniquely situated to contribute to attentional orienting toward spatially relevant stimuli. Continued investigation of these regions is necessary in order to fully understand their contributions to cognitive functions.

REFERENCES

1. CORKIN, S., et al. 1997. H.M.'s medial temporal lobe lesion: findings from magnetic resonance imaging. J. Neurosci. **17**(10): 3964–3979.
2. WITTER, M.P. 1993. Organization of the entorhinal-hippocampal system: A review of the current anatomical data. Hippocampus **3**: 33–44.
3. BURWELL, R.D., M.P. WITTER & D.G. AMARAL. 1995. The perirhinal and postrhinal cortices of the rat: A review of the neuroanatomical literature and comparison with findings from the monkey brain. Hippocampus **5**: 390–408.

4. VAN HOESEN, G.W. 1982. The parahippocampal gyrus: new observations regarding its cortical connections in the monkey. TINS **5:** 345–350.
5. EICHENBAUM, H., T. OTTO & N.J. COHEN. 1994. Two functional components of the hippocampal memory system. Behav. Brain Sci. **17:** 449–518.
6. NABER, R. 1999. The hippocampal memory system: Functional analysis of parallel pathways through the subiculum. Vol. dissertation. Ponsen & Looijen B.V. Wageningen, the Netherlands.
7. BURWELL, R.D. & D.G. AMARAL. 1998. The perirhinal and postrhinal cortices of the rat: interconnectivity and connections with the entorhinal cortex. J. Comp. Neurol. **391**(3): 293–321.
8. DOLORFO, C.L. & D.G. AMARAL. 1998. Entorhinal cortex of the rat: organization of intrinsic connections. J. Comp. Neurol. **398**(1): 49–82.
9. BURWELL, R.D. & D.G. AMARAL. 1998. Cortical afferents of the perirhinal, postrhinal, and entorhinal cortices. J. Comp. Neurol. **398**(2): 179–205.
10. NABER, P.A., et al. 1997. Parallel input to the hippocampal memory system through peri- and postrhinal cortices. Neuroreport **8**(11): 2617–2621.
11. McDONALD, A.J. & F. MASCAGNI. 1996. Projections of the lateral entorhinal cortex to the amygdala: a *Phaseolus vulgaris* leucoagglutinin study in the rat. Neuroscience **77**(2): 445–459.
12. McINTYRE, D.C., M.E. KELLY & W.A. STAINES. 1996. Efferent projections of the anterior perirhinal cortex in the rat. J. Comp. Neurol. **369**(2): 302–318.
13. AGGLETON, J.P. & M.W. BROWN. 1999. Episodic memory, amnesia, and the hippocampal-anterior thalamic axis. Behav. Brain Sci. **22:** 425–489.
14. DOLORFO, C.L. & D.G. AMARA. 1998. The entorhinal cortex of the rat: topographic organization of the cells of origin of the perforant path projection to the dentate gyrus. J. Comp. Neurol. **398**(1): 25–48.
15. SUZUKI, W.A. & D.G. AMARAL. 1994. The perirhinal and parahippocampal cortices of the Macaque monkey: Cortical afferents. J. Comp. Neurol. **350:** 497–533.
16. SUZUKI, W.A. & D.G. AMARAL. 1994. Topographic organization of the reciprocal connections between the monkey entorhinal cortex and the perirhinal and parahippocampal cortices. J. Neurosci. **14**(3): 1856–1877.
17. WITTER, M.P., G.W. VAN HOESEN & D.G. AMARAL. 1989. Topographical organization of the entorhinal projection to the dentate gyrus of the monkey. J. Neurosci. **9**(1): 216–228.
18. BURWELL, R.D. & D.G. AMARAL. 1995. The issue of parahippocampal cortex in the rat. Soc. Neurosci. Abstr. **21**(2): 1494.
19. DEACON, T.W. et al.1983. Afferent connections of the perirhinal cortex in the rat. J. Comp. Neurol. **220:** 168–190.
20. FELLEMAN, D.J. & D.C. VAN ESSEN. 1991. Distributed hierarchical processing in the primate cerebral cortex. Cereb. Cortex **1:** 1–47.
21. KREIG, W.J.S. 1946. Connections of the cerebral cortex. I. The albino rat. B. Structure of the cortical areas. J. Comp. Neurol. **84:** 277–323.
22. TURNER, B.H. & J. ZIMMER. 1984. The architecture and some of the interconnections of the rat's amygdala and lateral periallocortex. J. Comp. Neurol. **227:** 540–557.
23. WITTER, M.P. et al. 1989. Functional organization of the extrinsic and intrinsic circuitry of the parahippocampal region. Prog. Neurobiol. **33:** 161–253.
24. JONES, E.G. & T.P.S. POWELL. 1970. An anatomical study of converging sensory pathways within the cerebral cortex of the monkey. Brain **93:** 793–820.
25. VAUDANO, E., C.R. LEGG & M. GLICKSTEIN. 1990. Afferent and efferent connections of temporal association cortex in the rat: a horseradish peroxidase study. Eur. J. Neurosci. **3:** 317–330.
26. PAPERNA, T. & R. MALACH. 1991. Patterns of sensory intermodality relationships in the cerebral cortex of the rat. J. Comp. Neurol. **308:** 432–456.
27. LUSKIN, M.B. & J.L. PRICE. 1983. The topographic organization of associational fibers of the olfactory system in the rat, including centrifugal fibers to the olfactory bulb. J. Comp. Neurol. **216:** 264–291.
28. GULDIN, W.O. & H.J. MARKOWITSCH. 1983. Cortical and thalamic afferent connections of the insular and adjacent cortex of the rat. J. Comp. Neurol. **215:** 135–153.

29. BECKSTEAD, R.M. 1979. An autoradiographic examination of corticocortical and sub-cortical projections of the mediodorsal-projection (prefrontal) cortex in the rat. J. Comp. Neurol. **184:** 43–62.

30. TAKAGISHI, M. & T. CHIBA. 1991. Efferent projections of the infralimbic (area 25) region of the medial prefrontal cortex in the rat: an anterograde tracer PHA-L study. Brain Res. **566:** 26–39.

31. MASCAGNI, F., A.J. MCDONALD & J.R. COLEMAN. 1993. Corticoamygdaloid and cortic-ocortical projections of the rat temporal cortex: a *Phaseolus vulgaris* leucoagglutinin study. Neuroscience **57**(3): 697–715.

32. ROMANSKI, L.M. & J.E. LEDOUX. 1993. Information cascade from primary auditory cortex to the amygdala: corticocortical and corticoamygdaloid projections of tempo-ral cortex in the rat. Cereb. Cortex **3**(6): 515–532.

33. VAN HOESEN, G.W. & D.N. PANDYA. 1975. Some connections of the entorhinal (area 28) and perirhinal (area 35) cortices of the rhesus monkey. I. Temporal lobe affer-ents. Brain Res. **95:** 1–24.

34. VAN HOESEN, G.W. & D.N. PANDYA. 1975. Some connections of the entorhinal (area 28) and perirhinal (area 35) cortices of the rhesus monkey. II. Frontal lobe afferents. Brain Res. **95:** 25–38.

35. RUTH, R.E., T.J. COLLIER & A. ROUTTENBERG. 1982. Topography between the entorhi-nal cortex and the dentate septotemporal axis in rats. I. Medial and intermediate entorhinal projecting cells. J. Comp. Neurol. **209:** 69–78.

36. RUTH, R.E., T.J. COLLIER & A. ROUTTENBERG. 1988. Topography between the entorhi-nal cortex and the dentate septotemporal axis in rats. II. Cells projecting from lateral entorhinal subdivisions. J. Comp. Neurol. **270:** 506–516.

37. KOHLER, C. 1988. Intrinsic connections of the retrohippocampal region in the rat brain. II. The medial entorhinal area. J. Comp. Neurol. **246:** 149–169.

38. KOHLER, C. 1988. Intrinsic connections of the retrohippocampal region in the rat brain: III. The lateral entorhinal area. J. Comp. Neurol. **271:** 208–228.

39. DOLORFO, C.L. & D.G. AMARAL. 1994. Information processing in the entorhinal cortex of the rat: a neuroanatomical study of entorhinal intrinsic connections. Soc. Neuro-sci. Abstr. **20**(1): 350.

40. AMARAL, D.G., R. INSAUSTI & W.M. COWAN. 1987. The entorhinal cortex of the mon-key: I. Cytoarchitectonic organization. J. Comp. Neurol. **264:** 326–355.

41. VAN GROEN, T., J. KADISH & P.J. RIEKKINEN. 1998. The projections from the entorhinal cortex to the hippocampus in the mouse. Soc. Neurosci. Abstr. **24**(1): 677.

42. CHROBAK, J.J. & D.G. AMARAL. 1997. Organization of associational connections in the monkey entorhinal cortex. Soc. Neurosci. Abstr. **23**(1): 903.

43. SUZUKI, W.A. & D.G. AMARAL. 1990. Cortical inputs to the CA1 field of the monkey hippocampus originate from the perirhinal and parahippocampal cortex but not from area TE. Neurosci. Lett. **115:** 43–48.

44. MCDONALD, A.J. 1998. Cortical pathways to the mammalian amygdala. Prog. Neuro-biol. **55:** 257–332.

45. BURWELL, R.D., W.A. SUZUKI, *et al.* 1996. Some observations on the perirhinal and parahippocampal cortices in the rat, monkey, and human brains. *In* Perception, Mem-ory, and Emotion: Frontier in Neuroscience. T. Ono, Ed. Elsevier. New York.

46. INSAUSTI, R., T. TUÑÓN, *et al.* 1995. The human entorhinal cortex: a cytoarchitectonic analysis. J. Comp. Neurol. **355:** 171–198.

Development of the Entorhino-Hippocampal Projection: Guidance by Cajal-Retzius Cell Axons

KATJA CERANIK, SHANTING ZHAO, AND MICHAEL FROTSCHER[a]

ABSTRACT: The entorhinal cortex gives rise to a massive projection to the hippocampus and fascia dentata. In the rat, this projection forms early in development with first entorhinal axons reaching the hippocampus around embryonic day (E) 17. From the very beginning, the entorhinal axons recognize their appropriate termination zones in the hippocampus proper and fascia dentata, i.e., stratum lacunosum-moleculare and the outer molecular layer of the dentate. This is remarkable, because at the time of entorhinal fiber ingrowth, the definitive target cells of entorhinal axons, pyramidal cells and granule cells, are not yet fully developed, and the majority of their distal dendritic tips have not yet reached these layers. This raises the question as to the cellular and molecular signals guiding the entorhinal axons to and keeping them in their target layers. Here we hypothesize that early generated Cajal-Retzius (CR) cells located in stratum lacunosum-moleculare and the outer molecular layer of the dentate, and in particular their axons projecting to the entorhinal cortex, provide a template that is used by the entorhinal axons to find their target layers in the hippocampus.

INTRODUCTION

A characteristic feature of hippocampal organization is the segregated termination of afferent fibers in distinct layers. In the dentate gyrus, for instance, fibers from the entorhinal cortex populate the outer molecular layer, whereas commissural/associational (CA) fibers innervate the inner molecular layer. The entorhinal fibers accordingly establish synapses with the distal dendrites of the granule cells, whereas the CA fibers impinge on proximal dendritic portions. The functional consequences of this segregated termination of dentate afferents as well as the factors governing its development are unknown.

Previous studies have suggested that the sequential ingrowth of hippocampal afferents determines their position on the target cells' dendritic arbors.[1] According to this hypothesis, early formed projections such as the entorhino-hippocampal projection impinge on distal dendrites, whereas projections generated later on in development contact dendritic portions closer to the cell body. This explanation appeared plausible, since commissural fibers, which invade the hippocampus after the afferents from the entorhinal cortex, generally contact proximal dendrites close to the cell body.[2] A good example in favor of this hypothesis is the termination of the mossy

[a]Address for correspondence: Michael Frotscher, Institute of Anatomy, University of Freiburg, P.O. Box 111, D-79001 Freiburg, Germany. Tel.: +49 761 203-5056; fax: +49 761 203-5054.
e-mail: frotsch@uni-freiburg.de

fibers. These axons of the late-generated dentate granule cells terminate very close to the cell bodies of CA3 pyramidal neurons by establishing characteristic synapses with the large *excrescences* originating from proximal dendrites.

We previously tested this temporal hypothesis of fiber lamination in the hippocampus by confronting a hippocampal slice culture first with commissural afferents and then with entorhinal fibers, thereby reversing the normal sequence of fiber ingrowth in a triplet culture paradigm.[20] Despite the reversal of fiber ingrowth, both entorhinal and commissural axons recognized their proper target layers, suggesting that the lamination of these fiber systems may not be due to their sequential ingrowth but may rather be determined by local cellular and molecular signals.

In our search for these signals, we have next focused on Cajal-Retzius (CR) cells located in stratum lacunosum-moleculare of the hippocampus proper and the outer molecular layer of the dentate. CR cells are early generated transient neurons that are present at the time of ingrowth of entorhinal axons into exactly these layers. Moreover, entorhinal axons were found to establish transient synapses with CR cells.[13] Here we describe the projection of CR cells by using intracellular recording and labeling techniques. Hippocampal CR cells give rise to a projection to the entorhinal cortex, which may be used as a template by the later outgrowing entorhinal axons to find their appropriate target layers in the hippocampus and fascia dentata.

MATERIALS AND METHODS

In the present study we used acute brain slices containing the entorhinal cortex and hippocampus and slice cultures of these regions in order to record from hippocampal CR cells and trace their axonal projections following intracellular biocytin filling. Briefly, 4- to 10-day-old Wistar rats were decapitated, and transverse sections of the hippocampal formation (300–400 μm) were cut and used for experiments in acute slices. Cultures were obtained from brains of P0–P1 rat pups. Sections (400 μm) were placed onto moistened Millipore membranes, which were transferred to 6-well plates filled with 1 ml of medium each. Sections were then incubated for 6 to 10 days. Details concerning slice culture preparation, the medium, and recording conditions have been described elsewhere.[5,6]

Putative CR cells in the dentate outer molecular layer (OML) and stratum lacunosum-moleculare (SLM) of the hippocampus proper were visualized using infrared differential interference contrast (IR-DIC) video microscopy,[37] recorded, and biocytin-filled (whole-cell configuration of the patch-clamp technique with 1 to 5 mg/ml biocytin in the patch pipette).

During recording at $34 \pm 2°C$ the membrane potential was set to -70 mV. The resting membrane potential (RMP) was measured after obtaining the whole-cell configuration. The input resistance (R_N) was calculated according to Ohm's law from averages of -20 pA-current injections (1 s duration) in the current-clamp configuration and the resulting voltage deflection at the end of the pulse. Half-duration[28] of single action potentials (APs) was determined from the first spike in response to a slightly suprathreshold current injection. AP amplitude was measured from baseline ($V_h = -70$ mV) to the peak voltage deflection. AP threshold was measured as the voltage deflection from baseline to the onset of the steep rising phase of the AP. Sag ratio was determined using averages of the voltage deflections following -80 pA hy-

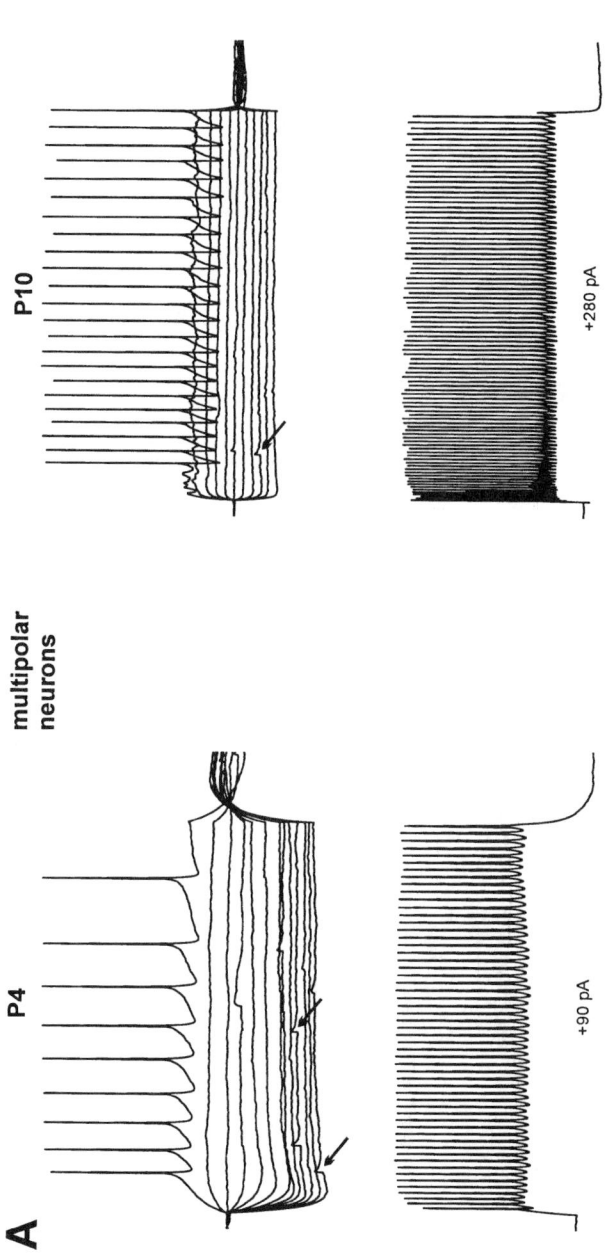

FIGURE 1. Discharge properties of presumed CR cells in the OML of young postnatal rats. (**A**) *Upper traces:* voltage responses of multipolar neurons to hyper- and depolarizing current injections (1 s) recorded at P4 (*left*) and P10 (*right*). In the P4 neuron, current injections ranged from −100 pA to +20 pA in steps of 10 pA. In the P10 neuron, current injections ranged from −100 pA to +100 pA in steps of 20 pA. Note that both neurons express only little or no sag and show spontaneous postsynaptic potentials (*arrows*). *Lower traces:* to large depolarizing current injections, both the P4 and the P10 multipolar neurons responded with a high frequency train of brief action potentials with little adaptation and large amplitudes.

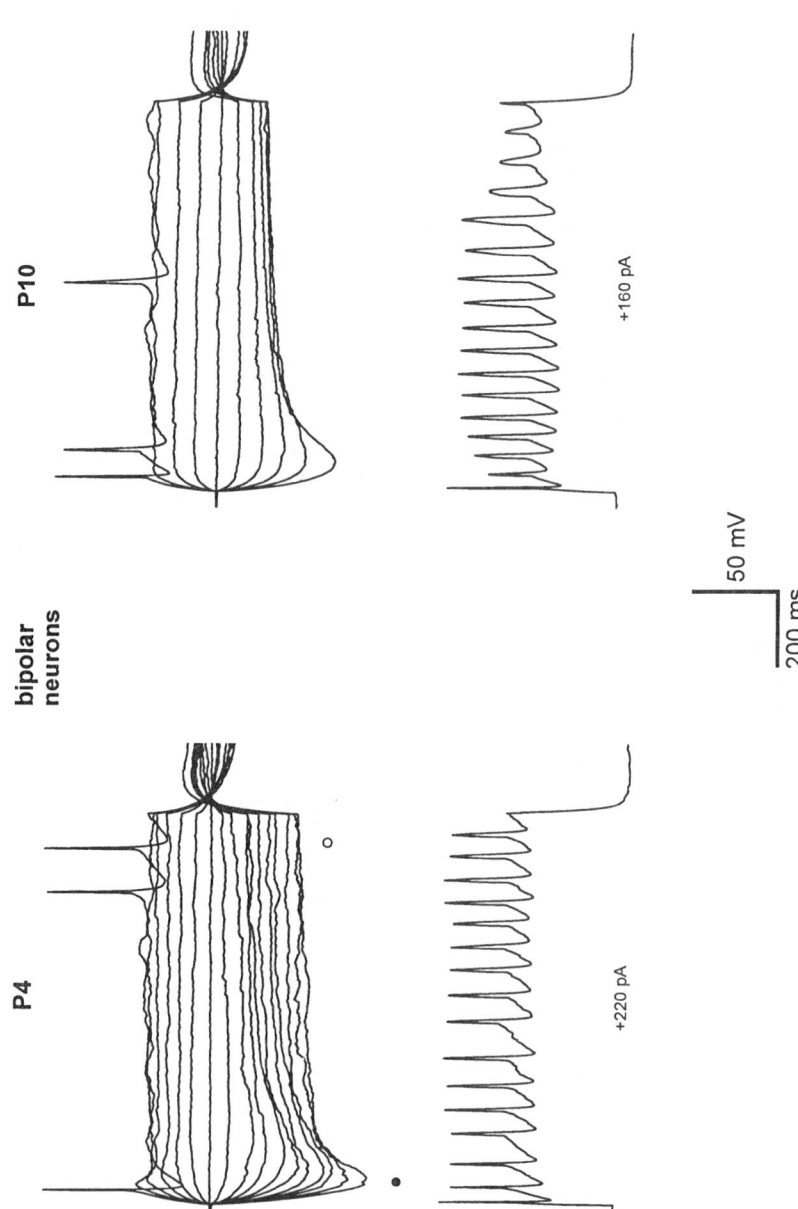

FIGURE 1. (B) *See following page for caption.*

perpolarizing current pulses (1 s duration) and calculated as the steady state voltage at the end of the pulse (open circle in FIG. 1B) divided by the peak voltage deflection during the pulse (filled circle in FIG. 1B). Values are given as mean ± SEM. Student's *t*-test was used.

The slices were immersion-fixed in a phosphate-buffered aldehyde solution containing 1% paraformaldehyde and 2.5% glutaraldehyde in 0.1 M phosphate buffer (PB; pH 7.4) for 12 hours at 4°C. Slices were further processed by a diaminobenzidine (DAB) reaction, postfixed in osmium tetroxide, dehydrated, and embedded as described.[5,6] Some acute slices and cultures were briefly frozen in liquid nitrogen and thawed in 0.1 M PB in order to increase the penetration of the reagents.

RESULTS

Patch-clamp Recordings from Presumed CR Cells

Neurons recorded in the OML and SLM were very heterogeneous in their physiological properties. Although they were not different in their resting membrane potentials (multipolar neurons: -53.6 ± 1.6 mV, $n = 18$; bipolar neurons: -54.0 ± 1.6 mV, $n = 22$; $p > 0.1$), they showed marked differences regarding their discharge patterns. One group consisting of multipolar, fusiform, or pyramidal-like neurons displayed relatively high frequency trains of APs with little or no adaptation (FIG. 1A, right). By P10, 3 of 5 neurons had already developed firing patterns similar to those of GABAergic interneurons,[17] i.e., short duration of APs and a marked afterhyperpolarization following a spike (FIG. 1A, compare neurons from P4 and P10). In contrast, the second group of neurons consisting of bipolar, horizontally oriented cells, fired low frequency trains of APs (FIG. 1B), some with marked adaptation and broadening of the AP. This property remained developmentally unchanged (FIG. 1B, compare neurons from P4 and P10). Passive and active membrane properties of both neuronal groups differed significantly (R_N of multipolar neurons was 373 ± 54 MΩ, of bipolar neurons 612 ± 42 MΩ, $p < 0.01$; AP half-duration of multipolar neurons was 0.8 ± 0.1 ms, of bipolar neurons 2.8 ± 0.3 ms, $p < 0.001$; AP amplitude of multipolar neurons was 104.5 ± 2 mV, of bipolar neurons 81.7 ± 2.9 mV, $p < 0.001$, and the firing threshold of multipolar neurons was -36.2 ± 1.1 mV, of bipolar neurons -28.1 ± 1.2 mV, $p < 0.001$). A very prominent feature of bipolar neurons was the expression of a hyperpolarization-activated current ("sag" or h-current, see FIG. 1B) that was significantly ($p < 0.001$) more pronounced in bipolar neurons (sag ratio: 0.6 ± 0.03) compared to multipolar neurons displaying no or only little

---

FIGURE 1. (B) Voltage responses to hyper- and depolarizing current injections (1 s) of bipolar neurons recorded at P4 (*left*) and P10 (*right*). In the P4 neuron, current injections ranged from −100 pA to +60 pA in steps of 10 pA. To large depolarizing current injections, the P4 bipolar neuron responded with a low frequency train of action potentials of increasing width. In the P10 bipolar neuron, current injections ranged from −100 pA to +80 pA in steps of 20 pA. This neuron responded to a larger depolarizing pulse with a low frequency train of action potentials. The width of the action potentials increased and their amplitude decreased. *Filled* and *open circle* represent the peak and the steady state voltage deflection, respectively, that were used for sag ratio determination.

sag (sag ratio: 0.9 ± 0.02). Spontaneous synaptic potentials were frequently observed in multipolar neurons (FIG. 1A, arrows). To summarize, in 5 of 6 physiological parameters shown, the two neuronal groups differed significantly. Taken together with the differences in morphology (see below), these data point to the existence of two distinct groups of putative CR cells.

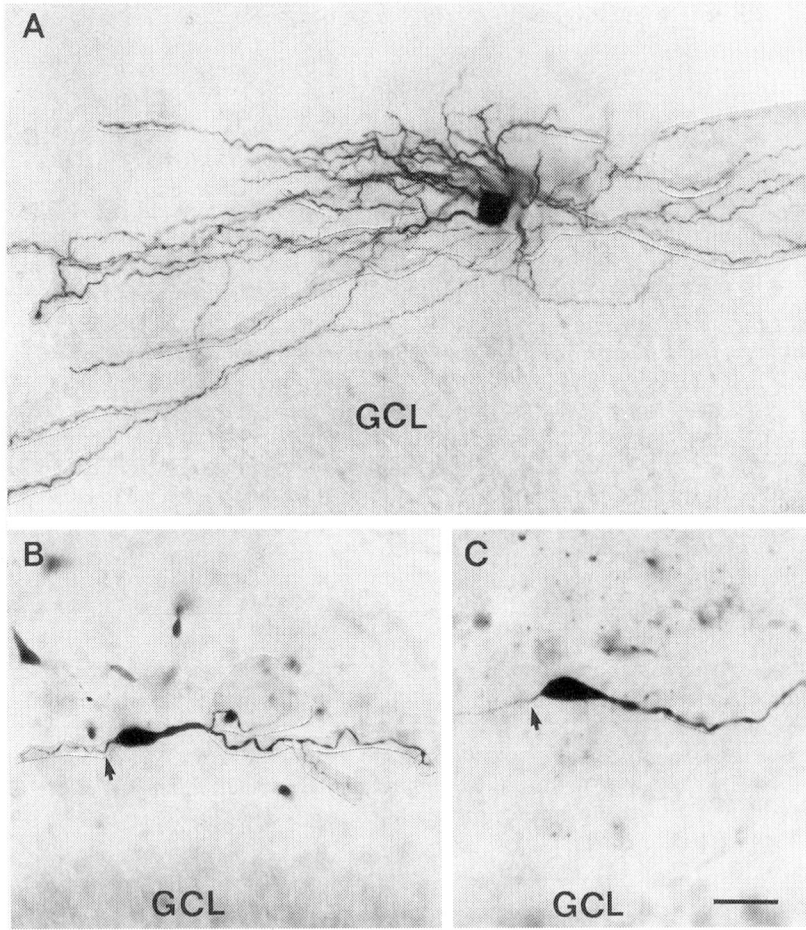

FIGURE 2. Biocytin-filled presumed Cajal-Retzius cells in the outer molecular layer of the fascia dentata. (**A**) Multipolar type of CR cell with a complex dendritic arbor in a slice culture incubated for 7 days. Note that most dendrites are in one plane due to the flattening of the culture. GCL, granule cell layer. (**B,C**) Two typical bipolar CR cells in the outer molecular layer of the dentate in acute slices (B: P6; C: P9). From the two opposing poles of the ovoid cell body, one thick main dendrite and the axon (*arrows*) originate. Scale bar (A–C): 25 μm.

Morphological Characteristics of CR Cells

Following recording, the slices and cultures were fixed and embedded, and the biocytin-stained cells were photographed. FIGURES 2A–C are photomontages illustrating the two different types of CR cell all of them located in the OML. While the cell in FIGURE 2A is multipolar, the two cells in FIGURE 2B and C represent typical bipolar neurons with one thick horizontal dendrite and the axon originating from the opposing pole of the cell body. The neuron in FIGURE 2A is from an entorhino-hippocampal coculture incubated for 7 days, whereas the two bipolar cells are from acute slice preparations. The fusiform, pyramidal-like or multipolar cells, giving rise to 2–5 smooth, sometimes sparsely spiny dendrites, generally had a more complex dendritic arbor than the bipolar neurons. However, the more complete appearance of distal dendritic branches of the cultured neuron (FIG. 2A) may be due to flattening of the cell during incubation. Thus, relatively more dendritic branches are visible in one plane of the section. The main dendrite of the bipolar cells parallels the hippocampal fissure and frequently shows long spine-like appendages.

The axons of both types of CR cell give rise to collaterals branching in the OML and SLM, respectively. Many axonal processes crossed the hippocampal fissure and invaded the subiculum. Some collaterals could be traced as far as to the entorhinal cortex. We have reason to assume that these collaterals to the entorhinal cortex are underestimated in our sample. First, in acute slices we regularly observed cutoff profiles in the subiculum indicating a more extended projection of the cell. It should be pointed out that the axons of hippocampal CR cells have to descend to reach the entorhinal cortex and are thus transected by slice preparation. Interestingly enough, the number of CR cells whose axon could be traced to the entorhinal cortex was larger in entorhino-hippocampal complex cultures than in acute slices of entorhinal cortex/hippocampus. We conclude that some of the transected CR cell axons have regenerated and reentered their normal target region, the entorhinal cortex, under these *in vitro* conditions. We have recently confirmed this projection of hippocampal CR cells to the entorhinal cortex by retrograde tracing *in vivo* with Fast-Blue and in fixed tissue with the carbocyanine dye DiI.[6]

DISCUSSION

In the present study an attempt was made to analyze the physiological and morphological characteristics of hippocampal CR cells. Like their counterparts in the neocortex, hippocampal CR cells are located in the marginal zone that in the hippocampus is represented by the layers adjoining the hippocampal fissure, i.e., the OML and SLM. We found that the neurons in the OML and SLM do not form a homogeneous class with respect to both their physiological and morphological characteristics. In spite of their morphological and physiological variability, we tentatively regard them as Cajal-Retzius cells, because virtually all neurons in the OML and SLM with morphological and physiological characteristics described in the present report were found to express the glycoprotein Reelin,[6] a marker of CR cells.[8,9,13,16,23,31] Since the OML and SLM are cell-poor layers in the adult rodent brain, it is conceivable that these physiologically and morphologically diverse neurons represent subforms of the transient CR cells which undergo degeneration within the first postnatal weeks.[12,14] However, some of the neurons in the OML do not disappear during later development. We accordingly described these cells as a separate type of hippocampal interneuron.[5]

Following a brief discussion of the physiological properties of CR cells, we will speculate about their role in the pathfinding and layer-specific termination of entorhinal fibers.

Physiological Properties of Presumed CR Cells

As has been shown in numerous other studies, the morphological and physiological maturation of neurons mutually influence each other.[25,29,34,39] During anatomical differentiation, the addition of new membrane area associated with an increase in the size of the soma and the elaboration of dendritic arborization takes place. This is paralleled by an increase in the membrane surface area and an increased density of ionic channels in the membrane. It was shown that the density of sodium channels, rather than their kinetics, changes during development.[24] These changes could account for the fast spiking pattern, shorter APs with larger amplitudes, and lower input resistance (R_N) of the multipolar group of neurons compared to the bipolar neurons. The bipolar CR cells, in contrast, display a relatively simple morphology with only one or two dendrites resulting in a smaller membrane surface area and lower density of ionic channels. This may be the reason for their significantly higher R_N, their broader and smaller APs, and their low firing frequencies. It may, however, also be possible that bipolar CR cells express different types of ionic channels. For instance, bipolar cells show a pronounced sag in contrast to multipolar neurons that display only little or no sag. The sag or h-current is activated by hyperpolarization beyond approximately −50 to −70 mV, is carried by Na^+ and K^+ ions, and slowly depolarizes the cell towards resting potential values.[26] The functional significance of the sag is not clear, but it seems possible that in cells with high AP threshold, like the bipolar CR cells, the sag counterbalances any sustained hyperpolarizing influence that inhibits discharge initiation.[39]

In contrast to multipolar neurons, bipolar CR cells showed almost no spontaneous synaptic potentials, which is in agreement with previous studies.[30,38] Derer and Derer[14,15] reported a few symmetric, supposedly GABAergic synapses on Cajal-Retzius cells. The high R_N of bipolar cells is likely to contribute to an increased degree of excitability. Small membrane conductance fluctuations are able to produce large voltage responses in neurons with high input resistances. Thus, the high R_N may compensate for the relative immaturity of synaptic inputs in newborn animals.

In this report as well as in our recent study[6] we provide evidence for an axonal projection of hippocampal CR cells to the entorhinal cortex. We hypothesize that outgrowing entorhinal axons use CR cell axons as a scaffold on their way to their appropriate termination zones, the OML and SLM (see below). CR cells seem to be GABAergic,[32,39] but see del Rio.[11] Early in development, GABA acts as an excitatory neurotransmitter that depolarizes postsynaptic cells.[7] This depolarization may be associated with an increase in the internal Ca^{2+} concentration, possibly triggering gene expression and promoting neuronal differentiation.[35,36] Thus, hippocampal CR cells may serve an inductive function in the development of the entorhino-hippocampal projection.

Role of CR Cells in the Pathfinding of Entorhinal Fibers

The early generation of CR cells as well as their degeneration soon after birth suggest a role of these neurons in developmental processes. In fact, the glycoprotein reelin, synthesized and secreted by CR cells,[8,9,23,31] appears to be crucially involved in the formation of cortical layers.[18,19,27,33] In the natural mutant *reeler* lacking reelin, there are severe malformations of the neocortex, hippocampus, and cerebellum.[3,4,33]

We have focused on Cajal-Retzius cells in our search for the cellular and molecular factors governing the layer-specific termination of entorhinal afferents to the hippocampus and fascia dentata. Hippocampal CR cells are located in the SLM and OML, both well-known termination zones of entorhinal fibers. Unlike the definitive postsynaptic partners of entorhinal fibers, the distal dendrites of pyramidal cells and granule cells, early generated CR cells are present at the time of entorhinal fiber ingrowth during development. We hypothesized that hippocampal CR cells serve as transient targets for the early ingrowing fibers from the entorhinal cortex, keeping them in their proper termination zones. This assumption was confirmed, at least in part, by our finding of synaptic contacts between entorhinal fibers and CR cells.[6,13] Moreover, elimination of CR cells by excitotoxic lesion in slice culture prevented cocultured entorhinal fibers from finding their appropriate target layers. Initially, we

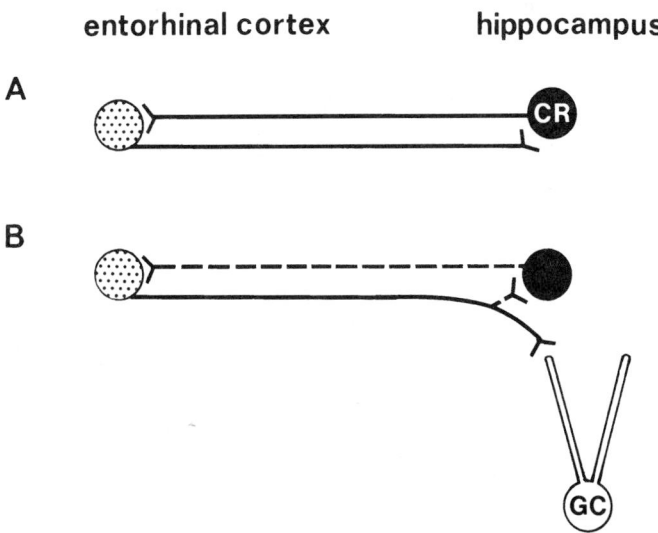

FIGURE 3. Hypothetical role of Cajal-Retzius cells in the pathfinding of entorhinal axons. Axons of neurons in the entorhinal cortex are guided to the hippocampus by the axons of early generated hippocampal Cajal-Retzius (CR) cells. The entorhinal fibers are kept in the outer molecular layer and stratum lacunosum-moleculare by synaptic contacts with CR cells until the distal dendritic tips of pyramidal cells and granule cells (GC) are available for synaptic contact. When these definitive synapses with pyramidal and granule cells are established in the early postnatal period, the majority of CR cells undergo degeneration and their contacts with entorhinal fibers are lost.

assumed that reelin would be involved in this process. However, antibody blockade of reelin with the CR-50 antibody[31] did not interfere with the normal pathfinding of entorhinal axons in entorhino-hippocampal cocultures.[13] Similarly, anterograde tracing of entorhinal axons in reeler mutant mice revealed an essentially normal entorhino-hippocampal projection.[10,19] We accordingly had to assume a reelin-independent guidance function of CR cells, because not the blockade or absence of reelin, but the selective elimination of Cajal-Retzius cells interfered with the pathfinding of entorhinal axons.

The results of the present experiments and those of our recent retrograde tracing studies[6] may provide a clue to the presumed guidance role of CR cells for entorhinal fibers. It is a well established concept that early generated pioneer neurons form a scaffold for later outgrowing projections. For instance, subplate neurons, early generated neurons like Cajal-Retzius cells, project to the thalamus, thereby guiding later outgrowing thalamo-cortical fibers.[21,22] The majority of CR cells in the SLM and OML project heavily to the subiculum with some collaterals reaching the entorhinal cortex. This is exactly the route later outgrowing entorhinal fibers have to take on their way to the hippocampus and fascia dentata, however, in opposite direction. We accordingly hypothesize that the early generated projection of hippocampal CR cells to the entorhinal cortex provides a template for entorhino-hippocampal fibers, very much in analogy to the guidance role of subplate cells in the formation of thalamo-cortical projections (FIG. 3). This hypothesis is compatible with the altered pathfinding of entorhinal axons following CR cell elimination.[13]

ACKNOWLEDGMENTS

The authors thank Drs. J.R.P. Geiger and B. Heimrich for their helpful comments and M. Winter for her help with the figures. This work was supported by the Deutsche Forschungsgemeinschaft (SFB 505, TP A3, A8, and Leibniz Program).

REFERENCES

1. BAYER, S.A. & J. ALTMAN. 1987. Directions in neurogenetic gradients and patterns of anatomical connections in the telencephalon. Prog. Neurobiol. **29:** 57–106.
2. BLACKSTAD, T.W. 1956. Commissural connections of the hippocampal region of the rat, with special reference to their mode of termination. J. Comp. Neurol. **105:** 417–537.
3. CAVINESS, V.S., Jr. & P. RAKIC. 1978. Mechanisms of cortical development: a view from mutations in mice. Annu. Rev. Neurosci. **1:** 297–326.
4. CAVINESS, V.S., Jr. et al. 1988. The reeler malformation: implication for neocortical histogenesis. Cereb. Cortex **7:** 59–89.
5. CERANIK, K. et al. 1997. A novel type of GABAergic interneuron connecting the input and the output regions of the hippocampus. J. Neurosci. **17:** 5380–5394.
6. CERANIK, K. et al. 1999. Hippocampal Cajal-Retzius cells project to the entorhinal cortex: retrograde tracing and intracellular labelling studies. Eur. J. Neurosci. **11:** 4278–4290.
7. CHERUBINI, E. et al. 1991. GABA: an excitatory transmitter in early postnatal life. Trends Neurosci. **14:** 515–519.
8. D'ARCANGELO, G. et al. 1995. A protein related to extracellular matrix proteins deleted in the mouse mutant reeler. Nature **374:** 719–723.
9. D'ARCANGELO, G. et al. 1997. Reelin is a secreted glycoprotein recognized by the CR-50 monoclonal antibody. J. Neurosci. **17:** 23–31.

10. DELLER, T. *et al.* 1999. Different primary target cells are important for fiber lamination in the fascia dentata: a lesson from reeler mutant mice. Exp. Neurol. **156:** 239–253.
11. DEL RIO, J.A. *et al.* 1995. Glutamate-like immunoreactivity and fate of Cajal-Retzius cells in the murine cortex as identified with calretinin antibody. Cereb. Cortex **1:** 13–21.
12. DEL RIO, J.A. *et al.* 1996. Differential survival of Cajal-Retzius cells in organotypic cultures of hippocampus and neocortex. J. Neurosci. **16:** 6896–6907.
13. DEL RIO, J.A. *et al.* 1997. A role for Cajal-Retzius cells and reelin in the development of hippocampal connections. Nature **385:** 70–74.
14. DERER, P. & M. DERER. 1990. Cajal-Retzius cell ontogenesis and death in mouse brain visualized with horseradish peroxidase and electron microscopy. Neuroscience **36:** 839–856.
15. DERER, P. & M. DERER. 1992. Development and fate of Cajal-Retzius cells *in vivo* and *in vitro. In* Development of the Central Nervous System in Vertebrates. S.C. Sharma & A.M. Goffinet, Eds.: 113–129. Plenum. New York.
16. DRAKEW, A. *et al.* 1998. Developmental distribution of a reeler gene-related antigen in the rat hippocampal formation visualized by CR-50 immunocytochemistry. Neuroscience **82:** 1079–1086.
17. FREUND, T.F. & G. BUZSÁKI. 1996. Interneurons of the hippocampus. Hippocampus **6:** 345–470.
18. FROTSCHER, M. 1997. Dual role of Cajal-Retzius cells and reelin in cortical development. Cell Tissue Res. **290:** 315–322.
19. FROTSCHER, M. 1998. Cajal-Retzius cells, reelin and the formation of layers. Curr. Opin. Neurobiol. **8:** 570–575.
20. FROTSCHER, M. & B. HEIMRICH. 1993. Formation of layer-specific fiber projections to the hippocampus *in vitro.* Proc. Natl. Acad. Sci. USA **90:** 10400–10403.
21. GHOSH, A. & C.J. SHATZ. 1993. A role for subplate neurons in the patterning of connections from thalamus to neocortex. Development **117:** 1031–1047.
22. GHOSH, A. *et al.* 1990. Requirement for subplate neurons in the formation of thalamocortical connections. Nature **347:** 179–181.
23. HIROTSUNE, S. *et al.* 1995. The reeler gene encodes a protein with an EGF-like motif expressed by pioneer neurons. Nat. Genet. **10:** 77–83.
24. HUGUENARD, J.R. *et al.* 1988. Developmental changes in Na^+ conductances in rat neocortical neurons: appearance of a slowly inactivating component. J. Neurophysiol. **59:** 778–795.
25. KANDLER, K. & E. FRIAUF. 1995. Development of electrical membrane properties and discharge characteristics of superior olivary complex neurons in fetal and postnatal rats. Eur. J. Neurosci. **7:** 1773–1790.
26. LÜTHI, A. & D.A. MCCORMICK. 1998. H-current: properties of a neuronal and network pacemaker. Neuron **21:** 9–12.
27. MARIN-PADILLA, M. 1998. Cajal-Retzius cells and the development of the neocortex. Trends Neurosci. **21:** 64–71.
28. MCCORMICK, D.A. *et al.* 1985. Comparative electrophysiology of pyramidal and sparsely spiny stellate neurons of the neocortex. J. Neurophysiol. **54:** 782–806.
29. MCCORMICK, D.A. & D.A. PRINCE. 1987. Post-natal development of electrophysiological properties of rat cerebral cortical pyramidal neurones. J. Physiol. **393:** 743–762.
30. MIENVILLE, J.-M. 1998. Persistent depolarizing action of GABA in rat Cajal-Retzius cells. J. Physiol. **512**(Pt. 3): 809–817.
31. OGAWA, M. *et al.* 1995. The reeler gene-associated antigen on Cajal-Retzius neurons is a crucial molecule for laminar organization of cortical neurons. Neuron **14:** 899–912.
32. PESOLD, C. *et al.* 1998. Reelin is preferentially expressed in neurons synthesizing gamma-aminobutyric acid in cortex and hippocampus of adult rats. Proc. Natl. Acad. Sci. USA **95:** 3221–3226.
33. RAKIC, P. & V.S. CAVINESS, JR. 1995. Cortical development: view from neurological mutants two decades later. Neuron **14:** 1101–1104.
34. SPIGELMAN, I. *et al.* 1992. Patch-clamp study of postnatal development of CA1 neurons in rat hippocampal slices: membrane excitability and K^+ currents. J. Neurophysiol. **68:** 55–69.
35. SPITZER, N.C. *et al.* 1993. Calcium dependence of differentiation of GABA immunoreactivity in spinal neurons. J. Comp. Neurol. **337:** 168–175.

36. SPITZER, N.C. *et al.* 1995. Spontaneous calcium transients regulate neuronal plasticity in developing neurons. J. Neurobiol. **26:** 316–324.
37. STUART, G.J. *et al.* 1993. Patch-clamp recordings from the soma and dendrites of neurons in brain slices using infrared video microscopy. Pflügers Arch. **423:** 511–518.
38. VON HAEBLER, D. *et al.* 1993. Properties of horizontal cells transiently appearing in the rat dentate gyrus during ontogenesis. Exp. Brain Res. **94:** 33–42.
39. ZHOU, F. & J.J. HABLITZ. 1996. Postnatal development of membrane properties of layer I neurons in rat neocortex. J. Neurosci. **16:** 1131–1139.

Physiology of the Entorhinal and Perirhinal Projections to the Hippocampus Studied by Current Source Density Analysis

KEVIN J. CANNING, KUN WU, PASCAL PELOQUIN, FABIAN KLOOSTERMAN, AND L. STAN LEUNG[a]

Department of Physiology and Clinical Neurological Sciences, University of Western Ontario, London, Ontario, Canada N6A 5A5

ABSTRACT: Evoked field potentials and current-source-density analysis were used to study the olfactory, entorhinal, and perirhinal projections to the hippocampus. In urethane-anesthetized rats, various structures were electrically stimulated, and evoked potentials were mapped using glass micropipettes or multichannel silicon probes. Stimulation of the olfactory bulb, lateral olfactory tract, piriform cortex, amygdala-entorhinal transition, lateral entorhinal cortex, or lateral perforant path (LPP) evoked an outer molecular layer sink (inferred distal dendritic excitation) in the dentate gyrus, with progressively decreasing onset latency. Medial perforant path (MPP) stimulation evoked a middle molecular layer sink (mid-dendritic excitation) in the dentate gyrus. LPP and MPP were also inferred to monosynaptically excite the distal dendrites of CA3, often resulting in a population spike in CA3. CA3 spiking, in turn, was often followed by excitation at the inner molecular layer of the dentate gyrus. LPP and MPP evoked distal dendritic sinks but no population spikes in CA1. Stimulation of the perirhinal cortex activated a sink in the subiculum/CA1 border without activating the dentate gyrus. In addition, reverberatory activity through a hippocampal-entorhinal-hippocampal pathway may be activated by MPP or CA3 stimulation. It is suggested that the parallel projections of the entorhinal and perirhinal inputs to the distal dendrites of hippocampal principal neurons enhance local and distributed processing as characterized by CA3 to dentate gyrus feedback, and hippocampal-entorhinal reverberation.

INTRODUCTION

In all mammals studied, including rat, cat, monkey, and human, the hippocampus receives its major input from the entorhinal cortex.[1–3] Ramón y Cajal[4] first showed that perforant fibers from the spheno-occipital cortex (entorhinal cortex) perforate the subiculum en route to the dentate gyrus (DG), CA3, and the stratum lacunosum-moleculare of CA1. It is known that the medial entorhinal cortex (MEC) projects to the middle molecular layer of the DG via the medial perforant path (MPP). The lateral entorhinal cortex (LEC) projects to the outer molecular layer of the DG via the

[a]Address for correspondence: Dr. L. Stan Leung, Department of Clinical Neurological Sciences, University Campus, London Health Sciences Centre, The University of Western Ontario, London, Ontario, Canada N6A 5A5. Tel.: (519) 663-3733; fax: (519) 661-3827.
e-mail: sleung@julian.uwo.ca

lateral perforant path (LPP).[5–9] In addition, anatomical evidence suggests that MEC and LEC project respectively to proximal and distal layers of the molecular layer of CA3.[9–11] Recent anatomical evidence also substantiates an entorhinal projection to the stratum lacunosum-moleculare of CA1[10,12,13] and a restricted perirhinal cortex (PRh) input to the CA1/subiculum border.[14–18]

Studies on the physiological projection from the perirhinal and entorhinal cortex to the hippocampus have been less systematic. Most of the studies have focused on the perforant path projection to the DG starting with the classic studies of Andersen[19] and Lomo.[20] Yeckel and Berger[11] and Gloor et al.[21,22] concluded that, in the rabbit and the cat, respectively, the perforant path excited CA3 and CA1. The dearth of physiological information on the entorhinal/ perirhinal projections to the hippocampus provides the rationale of our studies.

Our approach was to study the functional inputs the hippocampus receives from the entorhinal/perirhinal cortices in urethane-anesthetized rats using current source density (CSD). CSD analysis removes the effect of volume conduction and reveals the local synaptic activation.[23,24] With careful application of CSD analysis, the synaptic activation of CA1 or CA3 can be separated from that of the DG, and the amplitude and time course of the dendritic synaptic currents can be localized to particular layers. Other than a few studies that will be reviewed below, CSD analysis has not been extensively used in the study of cortico-hippocampal afferents. The use of the *in vivo* preparation emphasizes the holistic and system processing of the hippocampus. The long connections among neurons, such as those between the hippocampus and the entorhinal cortex and those between inhibitory interneurons and principal cells, are preserved. From one view, CSD analysis is a study of anatomy of the functioning synapses. From another view, it reveals systems physiology and neural interactions in the hippocampal-rhinal cortex, which may determine complex behavioral and cognitive functions.

METHODS

The general procedures have been reported elsewhere[25–28] and will only be briefly stated here. Male hooded rats were anesthetized with 1.2 g/kg i.p. urethane and placed in a stereotaxic apparatus, with rectal temperature maintained at 37°C. The location of the stimulating electrode was placed at approximately: (1) MPP at P8.0, L4.0–4.4 (with respect to bregma[29]), and 3.0–3.6 mm deep below the skull surface (D); (2) CA3 at P2–3.2, L3.2–3.5, and D3.4–3.8; (3) LPP at P8.0, L6.0–6.4, and D3.0–5.0; (4) LEC at P8.0, L6.0, and D3.0–5.0; (5) amygdala-entorhinal transition (TR) at P5.8–6.3, L5.0–7.0, and D7.0–9.0; (6) PRh at P5.0–6.3, L4.0–7.0, D~6.0, and sometimes angled 5° away from the midline; (7) piriform cortex (PC) at A2.2–P2.8, L4.0–6.0, and D7.0–9.0; (8) lateral olfactory tract (LOT) at A3.7, L3.5, and D~6.8; (9) olfactory bulb (OB) at A6.7, L1.2–2.0, and D3.0–6.0; or (10) contralateral hippocampus at P4.5, L3.0–3.5, and D3.0. Photo-isolated constant current pulses of 0.15–0.2 ms duration were delivered cathodally to one stimulating electrode at <0.15 Hz repetition rate, with a screw in the frontal skull serving as the anode. Paired-pulse stimulation of 20–500 ms interpulse intervals was often used, in order to assess paired-pulse facilitation or depression. Extracellular potentials were recorded either by (1) a glass micropipette filled with 2 M sodium acetate and 4% pon-

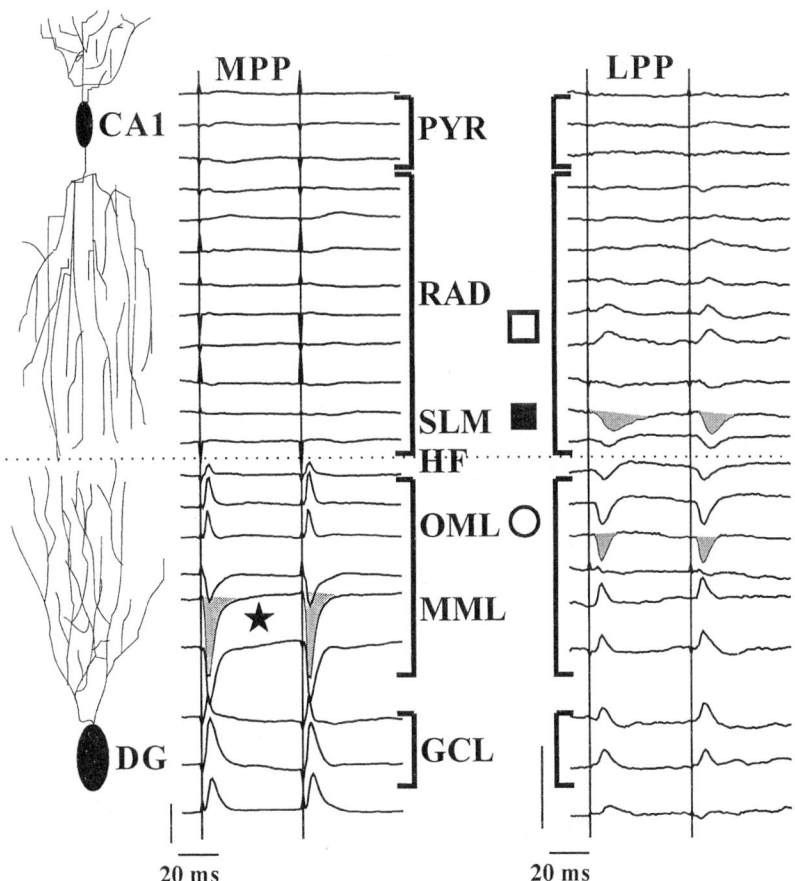

FIGURE 1. Schematic diagram of a granule cell in the dentate gyrus (DG) and a pyramidal cell in CA1 (*at left*) and the CSD traces acquired using a roving microelectrode, at 50-mm intervals. The maximum sinks are *shaded*. Paired pulses of 50-ms interpulse interval were delivered to the medial perforant path (MPP) or lateral perforant path (LPP). MPP stimulation evoked a sink in the middle molecular layer of the dentate gyrus (*star*) but little activity in CA1. LPP simulation evoked a sink in the outer molecular layer of the DG (*open circle*) and in the distal apical dendrites of CA1 (*closed square*); a source (*open square*) is observed at the CA1 proximal dendrites. This figure is constructed from the data used in Canning and Leung,[26] and the recording track was in CA1 near the subiculum, at the approximate level of P5.2 and L3.4 of Paxinos and Watson.[29] *Abbreviations*: Pyramidal cell layer (Pyr), stratum radiatum (RAD), stratum lacunosum-moleculare (SLM), hippocampal fissure (HF), dentate gyrus (DG), outer molecular layer (OML), middle molecular layer (MML), and granule cell layer (GCL). *Calibration*: 500 mV/mm^2, 20 ms with sink shown downwards. The *vertical lines* represent the times of stimuli which were 80 and 30 μA for MPP and LPP, respectively.

tamine sky blue (4–12 MΩ) stepped by a Burleigh inchworm at 1 micron resolution, or (2) a 16-channel silicon probe of 50 or 100 micron interval separation on a vertical shank[30] kindly provided by the Center for Neural Communication Technology, University of Michigan. Recordings were primarily acquired from CA1 and the DG at P3.2–4.5, L2.0–3.0, from CA3 at P3.2, L3.5, and angled 5–10° towards the midline, or from the subiculum near CA1 at P5.6–6.3, L4.0–6.2, and angled from 0–30° towards the midline. The recording and stimulation sites were verified by observing lesions and dye spots in the thionin-stained brain sections.

One-dimensional (depth z) CSDs were calculated from the laminar profile of average evoked potentials using the formula:

$$CSD(z) = \left[\frac{[2 \times \phi(z) - \phi(z + N\Delta z) - \phi(z - N\Delta z)]}{(N \times \Delta z)^2} \right] \sigma_z$$

where $CSD(z)$ is the current-source-density at depth z, in arbitrary units (mV/mm^2), $\Phi(z)$ is the average evoked potential at depth z, Δz is the depth interval (50 or 100 microns), σ_z is the conductivity in the z-direction, assumed constant $N = 2$ or 1.

RESULTS

Functional Synapses in the Dentate Gyrus are Organized in Layers

The layered structure of the afferent excitation of the DG is readily revealed using CSDs following stimulation of various structures. Following a low-intensity MPP stimulus pulse, the evoked potential was negative at the molecular layer and reversed to a positive wave at the granule cell layer; this was the population excitatory postsynaptic potential (EPSP) in the DG.[20] CSD analysis revealed a short-latency sink at the middle molecular layer (MML), surrounded by sources at the granule cell layer and the outer molecular layer (OML) (FIGS. 1 and 2). LPP stimulation evoked a short-latency sink at the OML, accompanied by an extended source at both the MML and the granule cell layer (FIG. 1). The sink following MPP or LPP activation is inferred to correspond to the inward current at the excitatory synapse. The MPP-evoked sink was abolished by intraventricular injection of glutamate receptor antagonist 6-cyano-7-nitroquinoxaline-2,3-dione and not by gamma-aminobutyric acid receptor type A ($GABA_A$) antagonist bicuculline.[27] Thus, MPP and LPP activated excitatory synapses at different parts of the dendritic tree, as expected from the neuroanatomical evidence (see Introduction).

Stimulation of the olfactory bulb (OB), lateral olfactory tract (LOT), piriform cortex (PC), amygdala-entorhinal transition area (TR), or lateral entorhinal cortex (LEC) activated an OML sink in the dentate gyrus with progressively decreasing latency (FIG. 3). However, OB, LOT, PC, TR, and LEC stimulation all gave a spatial sink-source profile similar to LPP stimulation (FIG. 2).[26,31]

Occasionally, LPP stimulation evoked a sink in the OML that was more proximal on the dendrites than that evoked by stimulation of OB, LOT, or PC (FIG. 2). We believe that stimulation of LPP may activate perforant path axons that are normally not derived from the part of the LEC that receives olfactory inputs, perhaps including

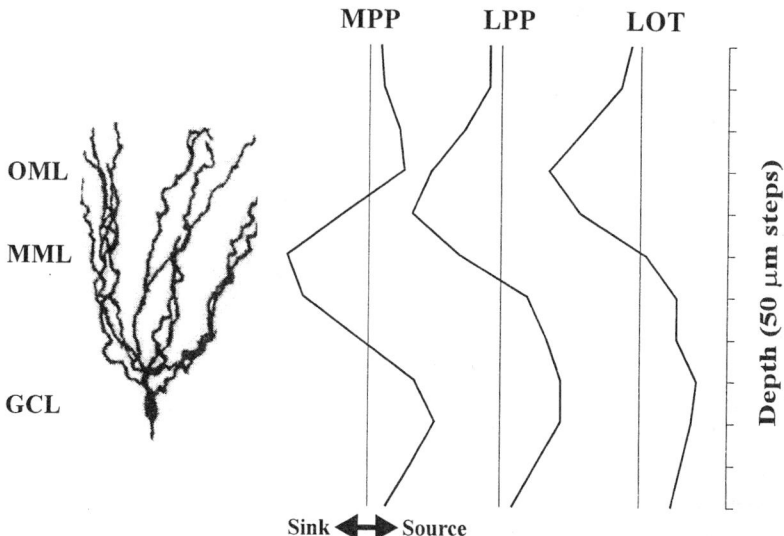

FIGURE 2. Schematic diagram of a granule cell in the dentate gyrus (*at left*) and the depth profiles of current source density after medial perforant path (MPP), lateral perforant path (LPP), and lateral olfactory tract (LOT) stimulation. Profiles are shown at times during the rising phase of the evoked response following stimulation of MPP (240 μA, 3.5 ms after stimulus), LPP (48 μA, 6 ms after stimulus), and LOT (450 μA, 21 ms after stimulus). Potential recordings were simultaneously acquired for each afferent at 16 channels of a silicon probe with a 50-μm interelectrode distance and spatial differencing in the CSD formula applied with a 100-μm interval (Rat PBP008). LOT and LPP stimuli evoked a distal dendritic sink, whereas MPP stimulus evoked a middendritic sink accompanied by a distal dendritic source.

some axons derived from MEC. Autoradiographic data showed that the more lateral part of the entorhinal cortex projects to more distal part of the DG molecular layer.[8]

The threshold for evoking a population EPSP was similar following MPP or LPP stimulation. In a recent series of 11 rats in which both MPP and LPP responses were available, the population EPSP threshold and population spike threshold was assessed for the first pulse in a paired-pulse stimulation paradigm. The population EPSP threshold was similar for MPP and LPP, measured at 42 ± 2 μA (0.2 ms pulses). However, the population spike threshold was higher for LPP than MPP stimulation ($p < 0.01$, paired Wilcoxon), measuring 450 ± 6 μA and 123 ± 11 μA for LPP and MPP stimulation, respectively for the same 11 rats. The threshold spike evoked by LPP stimulation was typically on the falling phase of the population EPSP,[33] in contrast to the rising phase of the EPSP for the MPP-evoked spike. Higher threshold and later onset for spiking are consequences of activating distal as compared to proximal dendritic synapses.[34] Paired-pulse facilitation was larger following LPP than MPP stimulation,[26,32] but the largest paired-pulse facilitation was observed for inputs that projected to the LEC (FIG. 3).

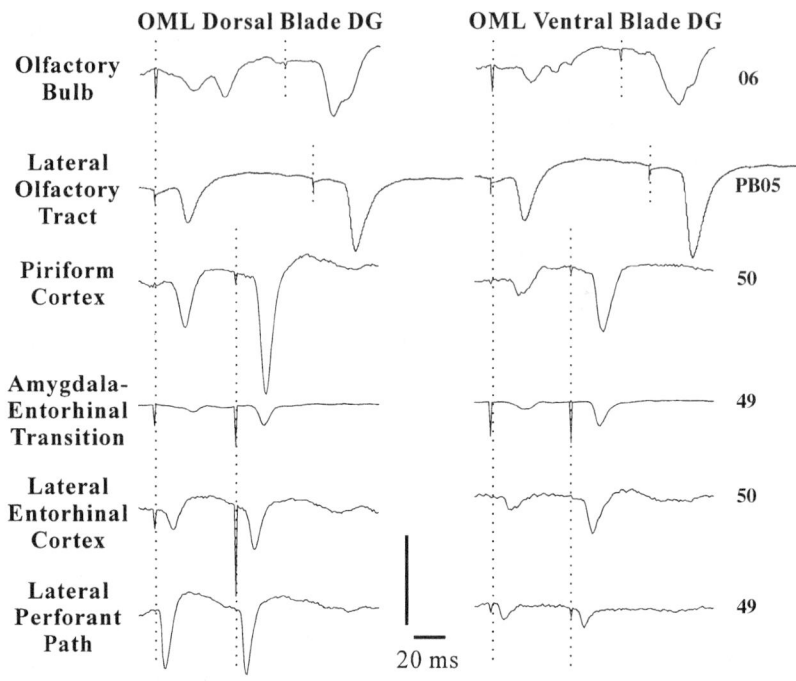

FIGURE 3. CSD transients from the outer molecular layer (OML) (sum of three adjacent 50-mm depths) of the dorsal or ventral blade of the dorsal dentate gyrus following stimulation of the olfactory bulb (OB), lateral olfactory tract (LOT), piriform cortex (PC), amygdala-entorhinal transition (TR), lateral entorhinal cortex (LEC), and lateral perforant path (LPP). The approximate average onset latency for the early sink (excitatory synaptic current) in the OML was 20, 17, 13, 12, 8, and 4 ms following stimulation of the OB, LOT, PC, TR, LEC, or LPP, respectively. There was large paired-pulse facilitation for all stimuli except the LPP stimulus, which showed small paired-pulse facilitation. *Calibration*: 500 mV/mm^2 and 20 ms, and stimulus intensity was 450, 280, 100, 400, 500, and 30 μA, respectively, for the OB, LOT, PC, TR, LEC, and LPP stimuli.

Perforant Path Excitation of CA1 at the Distal Dendrites

Either LPP or MPP stimulation could evoke a distal dendritic sink in CA1 at the stratum lacunosum-moleculare (FIG. 1).[24,26] Anatomical evidence indicated that MPP and LPP project to proximal (CA3 side) and distal (subiculum side) of CA1, respectively. FIGURE 1 shows a recording track through CA1 near the subiculum, which is expected to receive input from the LPP.[12] The CA1 distal dendritic sink was typically evoked at a higher stimulus intensity than the DG sink. The distal dendritic sink in CA1 (located at stratum lacunosum-moleculare (SLM) of FIG. 1 following LPP stimulation) showed more paired-pulse facilitation than that in the DG (located at OML in FIG. 1). The characteristics of paired-pulse facilitation and long-term potentiation[25] suggest that the sink was caused by an excitatory inward current at the distal dendrites. However, no monosynaptic population spike was observed in CA1 following MPP or LPP

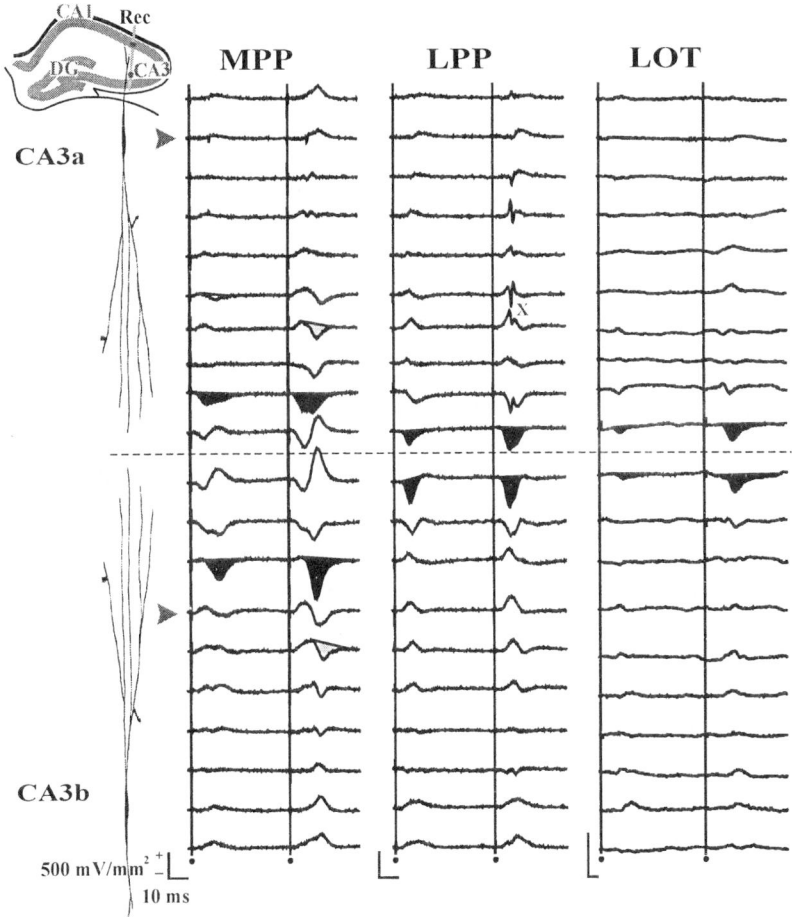

FIGURE 4. CSD time transient profiles recorded in a track passing through CA3a and CA3b (*top left cross section*), following stimulation of the MPP, LPP, and LOT at 200 μA. CA3 pyramidal cells are shown schematically on the *left*. *Black filled areas* indicate the early distal dendritic sink at CA3a and b. Note that the early sink evoked by LPP or LOT stimulation are located more distally (50–100 μm) on the dendrites than the early sink evoked by MPP stimulation. *Shaded areas (light grey)* indicate late (presumably disynaptic) proximal dendritic sink at CA3a and CA3b following MPP, which are less apparent following LPP stimulation. The *arrows* beside the MPP profile indicate dye deposits at the sites of the recording traces. *Dots* under the profiles indicate the stimulus artefacts. The CSDs at "X" under the LPP profile may be artifacts generated by a nonstationary population spike.

stimulation at up to 800 μA. This is in contrast to a previous study in the anesthetized rabbit.[11] The weak excitation provided by the direct input of the entorhinal cortex to the distal dendrites of CA1 in the rat is in accordance with the conclusion of *in vitro* studies.[35,36] Intracellular recordings *in vitro* or *in vivo*[37] also revealed strong feed-forward inhibition that was not clearly detected in the CSD profile.[23,38]

Perforant Path Excitation of CA3 at the Distal Dendrites

MPP stimulation induced an early, presumed monosynaptic sink (of about 2 ms latency) at the stratum lacunosum-moleculare of CA3a and CA3b (FIG. 4).[28] We are not aware of any CSD study of the projection of LPP to CA3. Thus, we undertook the latter project, and the results below have not been reported elsewhere. We found that the maximal sink activated by LPP in CA3a or CA3b was more distal on the dendrites than that activated by MPP (black filled-in areas in FIG. 4). LOT stimulation also activated distal sinks in CA3a or CA3b like LPP stimulation (FIG. 4). In CA3c within the hilus, an early (monosynaptic) sink was only detected in 3 of 12 rats following MPP stimulation,[28] possibly because of the relatively dispersed projection of MPP to the hilus. It is noted that uniform depolarization of all parts of a neuron (or a structure) will give no extracellular currents, i.e., zero CSDs.

The threshold for evoking a population EPSP in CA3 was similar following MPP or LPP stimulation (40 ± 2 μA, *n* = 6), which was also not significantly different from the population EPSP threshold in the DG. MPP stimulation evoked a population spike in CA3a, CA3b, or CA3c in about 60% of the rats (a maximal current of 400 μA was used). LPP stimulation readily evoked CA3a spikes as well but less readily in CA3b and CA3c. The CA3 population spike could clearly be discriminated from the DG population spike by having a slightly higher threshold and later onset latency.[28] Intracellular recordings *in vitro*[39] and *in vivo*[40] also revealed relatively strong excitation of CA3 by the perforant path, which however was weaker than that of the DG. Previous inference of a dendritic excitation of CA3[11,41] was based solely on field potentials without CSD analysis.

A disynaptic/polysynaptic sink in the IML was found in about half of the rats following MPP stimulation. A population spike in CA3c was found to reliably precede the late IML sink by 2–3 ms (data not shown). A similarly late IML sink may occur after LPP stimulation, but this has not been studied systematically. It is inferred that MPP stimulation first activates CA3 pyramidal cells and mossy cells in the hilus,[40] both ipsi- and contralaterally.[42] CA3c pyramidal cells and mossy cells send their axon collaterals to the IML,[43-45] and mossy cells excite DG granule cells and other neurons at the IML.[46] Stimulation of contralateral or ipsilateral CA3 also activated an early IML sink.[27,47] Blockade of GABA$_A$ receptors by bicuculline induced spike bursts arising from the IML sink without affecting the IML sink itself.[27] Thus, the sink at the IML was inferred to correspond to excitatory postsynaptic currents. Similar to anesthetized rats, IML excitation after CA3 stimulation was strong only after GABA$_A$ receptor blockade *in vitro*.[48]

Reverberations of the Hippocampo-Entorhinal Circuit

CA3 stimulation and occasionally MPP stimulation evoked a late wave in the DG at >20 ms latency.[27] The late wave in the DG was found to correspond to a MML sink, and was thus inferred to arise from the MEC and project through the MPP.[27,30]

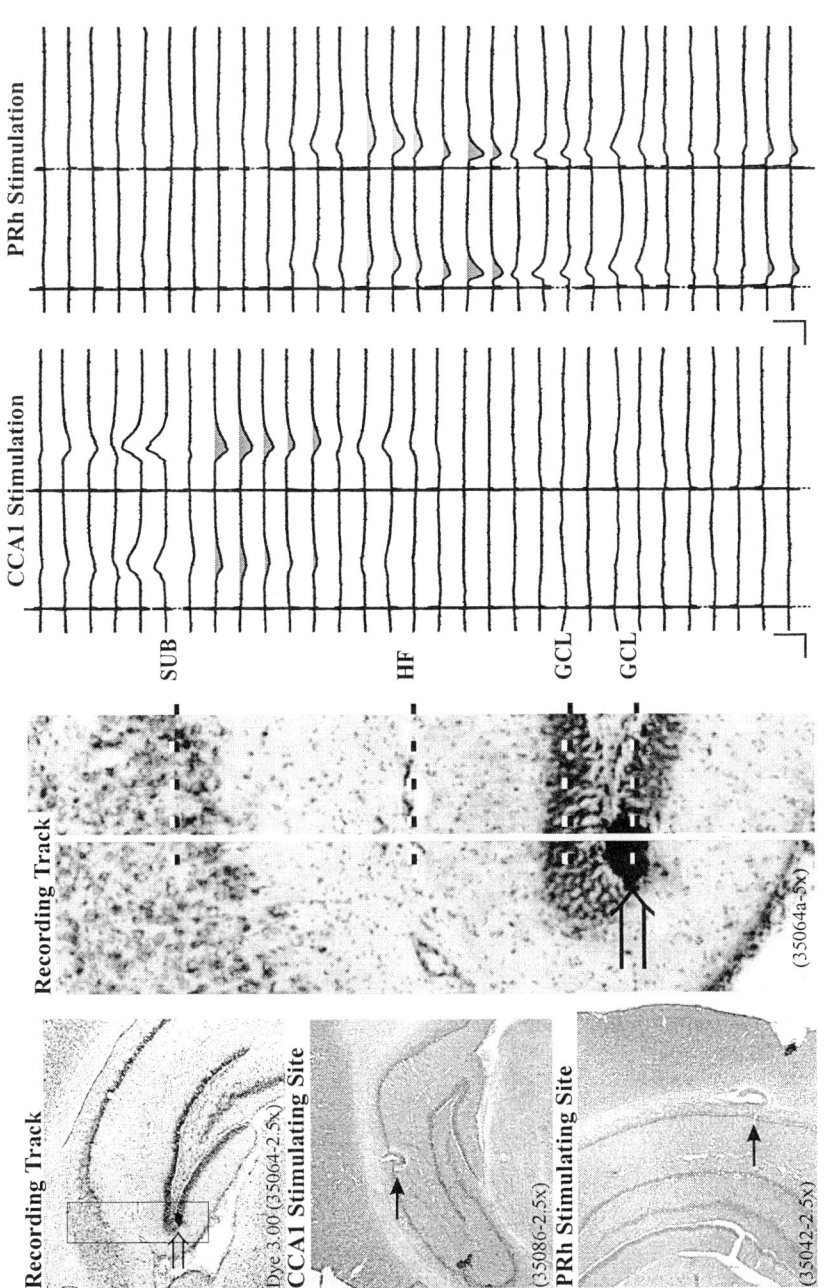

FIGURE 5. *See following page for caption.*

Thus, the late wave represents a reverberation from the hippocampus through the entorhinal cortex, as first proposed by Deadwyler et al.[47] CSD analysis allows for the interpretation that MEC but not LEC is the main structure involved in the entorhinal-hippocampal reverberations following dorsal CA3 stimulation. Lesion of the entorhinal cortex,[47,49] apparently in the MEC,[47] and inactivation of the MPP in the angular bundle[27] abolished the late DG wave. Enhanced entorhinal-hippocampal reverberations may be induced by hippocampal seizure activity.[50,51]

Perirhinal Cortex Input to the Hippocampus

Recently, there has been a great deal of debate concerning the perirhinal cortical input to the hippocampus.[26,52–54] We failed to find a direct PRh projection to the septal part of CA1 using CSD analysis,[26] in contrast to studies by Liu and Bilkey.[53,54] We also inferred that PRh did not project directly to the DG,[26] which was reported by Liu and Bilkey.[53,54] In a subsequent study, presented in abstract form[55] in 1996, we did find that PRh stimulation evoked a substantial dendritic sink near the subiculum-CA1 border at a restricted part (mid-septotemporal level) of the hippocampus. These results are reported as follows.

Stimulation of the deep PRh resulted in an early sink (presumably monosynaptic excitation) at the distal dendritic layers of the DG and the subiculum near CA1 (FIG. 5). The subiculum was inferred from the dispersed cell body layer along the recording track. In the DG, a sink was at both dorsal and ventral blades, accompanied by sources near the granule cell layer. The subiculum sink was near the hippocampal fissure, accompanied by sources near the cell body layer. Subiculum and DG sinks have different characteristics in that the subiculum sink was later than the DG sink and it showed paired-pulse facilitation while the DG sink did not (FIG. 5). We inferred that the DG sink was caused by the spread of stimulus currents to fibers of passage, likely from the LEC, for reasons that have been discussed before.[26] It is possible that axons of the LEC may also contribute to the subiculum sink.

FIGURE 5. CSD traces recorded in a vertical track through the dentate gyrus and the subiculum at its border with CA1 following stimulation of the deep white matter underlying the perirhinal cortex or the contralateral CA1 (CCA1). Photomicrographs of the recording track (*vertical white line*) and stimulus location are shown at the *left* along with a magnified portion of the hippocampus that is lined up with the CSD traces shown at the *right*. The CCA1 stimulus evoked a middendritic sink (*shaded grey*) surrounded by sources located more distally on the dendrites and proximally near the pyramidal cell layer. The deep PRh stimulus evoked a sink in the distal dendrites of the pyramidal cells (*shaded light grey*) as well as the distal dendrites of the dentate gyrus in the outer molecular layer (*shaded grey*). Note that in the subiculum, the distal sink was accompanied by a proximal dendritic source. The recording track passed through the subiculum near CA1 at ~P5.8, the CCA1 stimulus was at ~P4.3, and the PRh stimulus was at ~P6.04–6.30 of Paxinos and Watson.[29] *Abbreviations*: Subiculum pyramidal cell region (SUB), hippocampal fissure (HF), and granule cell layer (GCL). *Calibration*: 500 mV/mm^2 and 10 ms, with sink downwards. *Vertical lines* represent the times of the stimuli that were of 50 and 200 µA intensity for CCA1 and PRh respectively.

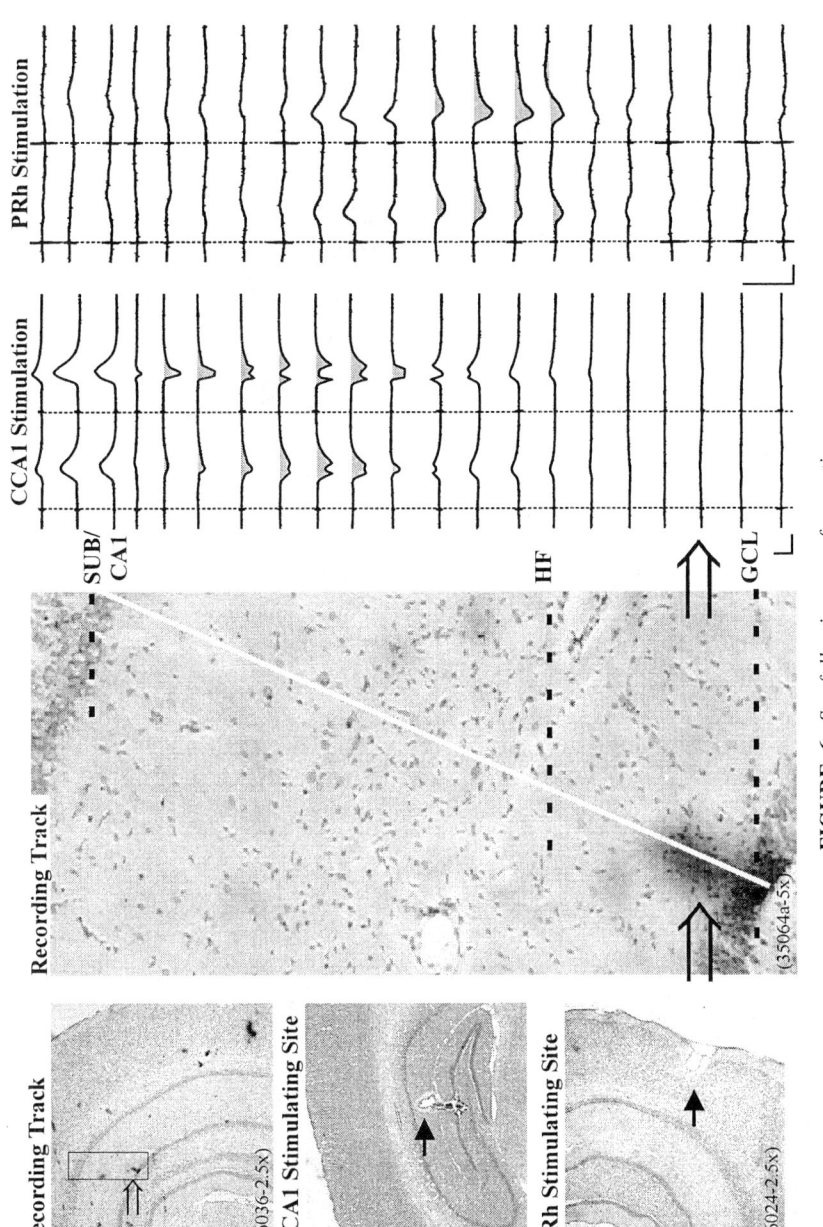

FIGURE 6. *See following page for caption.*

Stimulation of the superficial PRh resulted in an early (presumably monosynaptic) sink in the distal dendrites of subiculum/CA1, without significant DG activation (FIG. 6). A source in the proximal dendritic layers of subiculum/CA1 accompanied the distal dendritic sink. It is unlikely that the LEC contributes to this subiculum/CA1 sink, since the LEC stimulation should activate the DG as well. Distal dendritic excitation following superficial PRh stimulation was only found in recording tracks where pyramidal cell bodies were dispersed and not packed into a single discrete layer. This suggests that the subiculum was activated by PRh stimulation, although activation of CA1 near the subiculum cannot be ruled out. Using higher stimulus intensity, superficial PRh stimuli can also evoke DG activity through spread of stimulus current to fibers from LEC that course near the PRh or through a multisynaptic pathway from PRh to the LEC and then the DG.[17,18,52] When PRh stimulation resulted in multisynaptic activation of the DG, the excitatory sink responses had longer onset latencies and exhibited more paired-pulse facilitation.

SUMMARY AND CONCLUSIONS

Perirhinal Projection to Subiculum/CA1

We found a presumably monosynaptic projection from the PRh to the subiculum/CA1 border at a mid-septotemporal level of the hippocampus. The PRh projection was inferred to excite a sink at the distal dendritic layer of subiculum/CA1 (FIGS. 5 and 6). Stimulation of the superficial layer of PRh activated the subiculum/CA1 without significant activation of the DG (FIG. 6),[52] as would be expected for a perirhinal to subiculum/CA1 pathway[16] and not the LEC to subiculum/CA1 pathway. This result is also consistent with other neuroanatomical data[14,15] and with the CSD study done independently by Naber et al.[18] While Liu and Bilkey[53,54] claimed to find a PRh to CA1 projection using CSD analysis, we disagreed with their conclusion based on their data.[56,57]

FIGURE 6. CSD traces recorded in an angled track through the dentate gyrus and subiculum/CA1 following stimulation of the superficial perirhinal cortex at the rhinal fissure or the contralateral CA1 (CCA1). Format of figure same as that of FIGURE 5. The CCA1 stimulus evoked a mixed radiatum sink (*shaded grey*) that was likely due to stimulation of both the contralateral DG and CA1. There are sources at the distal dendrites and near the pyramidal cell layer. The superficial PRh stimulus evoked a sink in the distal dendrites of the pyramidal cells (*shaded grey*) without any significant activity in the DG. Note that in the subiculum/CA1 there is a source more proximal to the cell body layer that was temporally related to the distal sink. The recording track was at the border between the subiculum and CA1 where the pyramidal cell layer is less compact at (~P6.04–6.30) than in the middle CA1, the CCA1 stimulus was at ~P4.3, and the PRh stimulus was at ~P6.04–6.30 of Paxinos and Watson.[29] *Abbreviations:* Subiculum/CA1 cell layer (SUB/CA1), hippocampal fissure (HF), and granule cell layer (GCL). *Calibration:* 500 mV/mm^2 and 10 ms sink downwards. *Vertical lines* represent the times of stimuli, of 100 and 200 μA intensity for CCA1 and PRh, respectively.

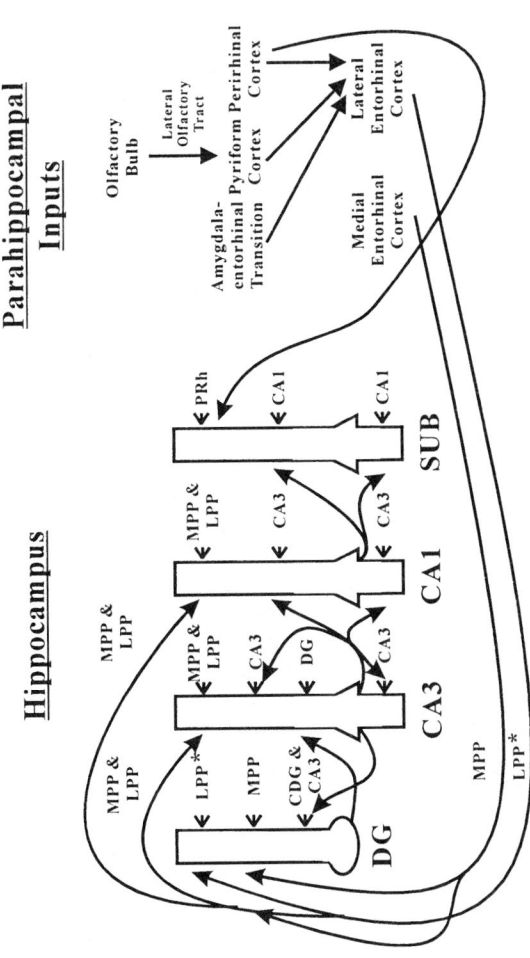

FIGURE 7. Summary of the synaptic connections studied by CSD analysis in the hippocampus. The main projections as well as the location of synapse made by each type of principal cell are shown. Only parahippocampal (entorhinal/perirhinal) inputs to the hippo-campus are included, and the intrinsic connections are included for comparison. *Abbreviations*: subiculum (SUB), dentate gyrus (DG), perirhinal cortex (PRh), medial perforant path (MPP), lateral perforant path (LPP), and contralateral and ipsilateral dentate gyrus (hilus) (CDG).

CSD Analysis Reveals Functional Synapses in Layers

Stimulation of the LPP, MPP, and CA3 evoked a sink at the OML, MML, and IML of the DG, respectively. The presence of excitatory sinks at various locations of the molecular layer of the DG following LPP or MPP stimulation is expected (Introduction). The results confirm the power of the CSD analytic technique in locating the site of synaptic activation in a cortical structure.

Ento- and Perirhinal Projections are Mainly on the Distal Dendrites of Principal Cells in the Hippocampus

Except for the projection to the mid-dendrites of DG granule cells, entorhinal and perirhinal cortices project to the distal dendritic synapses of the principal hippocampal neurons (FIG. 7). In the DG and CA3, these dendritic synapses are sufficiently powerful to generate spikes, as shown by the synchronously firing neurons or the population spike in this study. In the urethane- anesthetized rat, a population spike was not observed in CA1 following MPP or LPP stimulation or in subiculum/CA1 following PRh stimulation, although a distal dendritic sink was found. In contrast to the distal projection of the entorhinal/perirhinal afferents, the major association pathways in the hippocampus, e.g., the mossy fibers to CA3, recurrent fibers of CA3, the Schaffer collaterals to CA1, and association afferents to the subiculum all synapse on the proximal dendrites and strongly excite the target neurons (FIG. 7).

The long physical and electrotonic distance of the distal dendritic synapses from the spike trigger zone (presumably near the soma) suggests the possibility of failure of conduction in the dendrites. Various interneurons inhibit the dendrites through $GABA_A$ or $GABA_B$ receptors,[58] and the apical dendrites may be subjected to rhythmical modulation by synaptic and active conductances oscillating at the theta frequency.[59–62] Inhibition at the dendrites may drastically reduce electrotonic conduction[24,36,37] or active conduction in the dendrites.[63]

Frequency-dependent transmission across the hippocampus has been proposed,[64,65] and it may enhance the effectiveness of distal dendritic synapses. Frequency-dependent transmission partly depends on paired-pulse facilitation (FIG. 3) and frequency potentiation, both of which increase the EPSP amplitude and the likelihood of spiking.[26,66]

Parallel Feedforward Excitation, Feedback, and Reverberation

Based mainly on anatomical evidence, Amaral and Witter[67] criticized the sequential trisynaptic pathway in the hippocampus, involving the entorhinal cortex-DG-CA3-CA1/subiculum. Our studies provide physiological evidence that complement and extend those reviewed by Amaral and Witter[67] and Lopes da Silva et al.[68] In brief, we found evidence that either medial or lateral entorhinal cortex provides parallel monosynaptic excitation of both CA3 and DG, and that CA3c/hilar neurons provide an excitatory feedback of the DG. Other parallel pathways are found in the relatively weak entorhinal to CA1 and perirhinal to subiculum/CA1 projections. We also found evidence of reverberatory hippocampo-entorhinal activity,[69] which may serve to process the entorhinal/perirhinal inputs locally and in a distributed manner among the hippocampo-entorhinal circuits.

39. BERZHANSKAYA, J., N.N. URBAN & G. BARRIONUEVO. 1998. Electrophysiological and pharmacological characterization of the direct perforant path input to hippocampal area CA3. J. Neurophysiol. **79:** 2111–2118.
40. BUCKMASTER, P.S. & P.A. SCHWARTZKROIN. 1995. Interneurons and inhibition in the dentate gyrus of the rat *in vivo*. J. Neurosci. **15**(1)**:** 774–789.
41. BREINDL, A., B.E. DERRICK, S.B. RODRIGUEZ & J.L. MARTINEZ, JR. 1994. Opioid receptor-dependent long-term potentiation at the lateral perforant path-CA3 synapse in rat hippocampus. Brain Res. Bull. **33:** 17–24.
42. GOLARAI, G. & T.P. SUTULA. 1996. Bilateral organization of parallel and serial pathways in the dentate gyrus demonstrated by current-source density analysis in the rat. J. Neurophysiol. **75:** 329–342.
43. GOTTLIEB, D.I. & W.M. COWAN. 1973. Autoradiographic studies of the commissural and ipsilateral association connection of the hippocampus and detentate gyrus of the rat. I. The commissural connections. J. Comp. Neurol. **149:** 393–422.
44. LI, X.G., P. SOMOGYI, A. YLINEN & G. BUZSAKI. 1994. The hippocampal CA3 network: an *in vivo* intracellular labeling study. J. Comp. Neurol. **339:** 181–208.
45. BUCKMASTER, P.S., H.J. WENZEL, D.D. KUNKEL & P.A. SCHWARTZKROIN. 1996. Axon arbors and synaptic connections of hippocampal mossy cells in the rat *in vivo*. J. Comp. Neurol. **366:** 271–292.
46. SCHARFMAN, H.E. 1995. Electrophysiological evidence that dentate hilar mossy cells are excitatory and innervate both granule cells and interneurons. J. Neurophysiol. **74:** 179–194.
47. DEADWYLER, S.A., J.R. WEST, C.W. COTMAN & G. LYNCH. 1975. Physiological studies of the reciprocal connections between the hippocampus and entorhinal cortex. Exp. Neurol. **49:** 35–57.
48. SCHARFMAN, H.E. 1994. EPSPs of dentate gyrus granule cells during epileptiform bursts of dentate hilar "mossy" cells and area CA3 pyramidal cells in disinhibited rat hippocampal slices. J. Neurosci. **14**(10)**:** 6041–6057.
49. BRAGIN, A., J. CSICSVARI, M. PETTOMEN & G. BUZSAKI. 1997. Epileptic afterdischarge in the hippocampal-entorhinal system: current source density and unit studies. Neuroscience **76:** 1187– 1203.
50. PARE, D., M. DECURTIS & R. LLINAS. 1992. Role of the hippocampal-entorhinal loop in temporal lobe epilepsy: extra- and intracellular study in the isolated guinea pig brain *in vitro*. J. Neurosci. **12**(5)**:** 1867–1881.
51. WU, K. & L.S. LEUNG. 1999. Enhancement of multisynaptic transmission through the hippocampo-entorhino-hippocampal loop in partially kindled rats *in vivo*. Soc. Neurosci. Abstr. **25:** 1351.
52. CANNING, K.J. & L.S. LEUNG. 1994. Entorhinal and perirhinal cortical inputs to the hippocampus: a current-source-density study. Soc. Neurosci. Abstr. **20:** 340.
53. LIU, P. & D.K. BILKEY. 1996. Direct connection between perirhinal cortex and hippocampus is a major constituent of the lateral perforant path. Hippocampus **6:** 125–134.
54. LIU, P. & D.K. BILKEY. 1997. Current source density analysis of the potential evoked in hippocampus by perirhinal cortex stimulation. Hippocampus **7:** 389–396.
55. CANNING, K.J. & L.S. LEUNG. 1996. An electrophysiological analysis of the projection from the perirhinal cortex to the subiculum in the rat using current source density. Soc. Neurosci. Abstr. **22:** 903.
56. CANNING, K.J. & L.S. LEUNG. 1999. Current source density analysis does not reveal a direct projection from the perirhinal cortex to septal part of hippocampal CA1 or dentate gyrus. Hippocampus **9:** 599–600.
57. LEUNG, L.S. & K.J. CANNING. 1999. Reply to Liu and Bilkey's reply. Hippocampus **9:** 603–604.
58. FREUND, T.F. & G. BUZSÀKI. 1996. Interneurons of the hippocampus. Hippocampus **6:** 347–470.
59. VANDERWOLF, C.H. & L.-W.S. LEUNG. 1983. Hippocampal rhythmical slow activity: a brief history and the effects of entorhinal lesions and phencyclidine. *In* Neurobiology of the Hippocampus. G. Siefert, Ed.: 275–302. Academic Press. London.
60. LEUNG, L.S. 1984. Model of gradual phase shift of theta rhythm in the rat. J. Neurophysiol. **52:** 1051–1065.

61. BRANKACK, J., M. STEWART & S.E. FOX. 1993. Current source density analysis of the hippocampal theta rhythm: associated sustained potentials and candidate synaptic generators. Brain Res. **615:** 310–327.
62. KAMONDI, A., L. ACSADY, X.J. WANG & G. BUZSAKI. 1998. Theta oscillations in somata and dendrites of hippocampal pyramidal cells *in vivo*: activity-dependent phase-precession of action potentials. Hippocampus **8:** 244–261.
63. TSUBOKAWA, H. & W.N. ROSS. 1996. IPSPs modulate spike backpropagation and associated $[Ca^{2+}]_i$ changes in the dendrites of hippocampal CA1 pyramidal neurons. J. Neurophysiol. **76:** 2896–2906.
64. JONES, R.S.G. 1993. Entorhinal-hippocampal connections: a speculative view of their function. TINS **16**(2): 58–64.
65. YECKEL, M.F. & T.W. BERGER. 1998. Spatial distribution of potentiated synapses in hippocampus: dependence on cellular mechanisms and network properties. J. Neurosci. **18:** 438–450.
66. LEUNG, L.S. & X. FU. 1994. Factors affecting paired-pulse facilitation in hippocampal CA1 neurons *in vitro*. Brain Res. **650:** 75–84.
67. AMARAL, D.G. & M.P. WITTER. 1989. The three-dimensional organization of the hippocampal formation: a review of anatomical data. Neurosci. **31**(3): 571–591.
68. LOPES DA SILVA, F.H., M.P. WITTER, P.H. BOEIJINGA & A.H.M. LOHMAN. 1990. Anatomic organization and physiology of the limbic cortex. Physiol. Rev. **70**(2): 453–511.
69. IIJIMA, T., M.P. WITTER, M. ICHIKAWA, T. TOMINAGA, R. KAJIWARA & G. MATSUMOTO. 1996. Entorhinal-hippocampal interactions revealed by real-time imaging. Science **272:** 1176–1179.

Molecular Effects of the Psychotropic NMDA Receptor Antagonist MK-801 in the Rat Entorhinal Cortex: Increases in AP-1 DNA Binding Activity and Expression of Fos and Jun Family Members

OUTI KONTKANEN,[a] MERJA LAKSO,[a] EIJA KOPONEN,[a] GARRY WONG,[a] AND EERO CASTRÉN[a,b,c]

[a]A.I. Virtanen Institute and [b]Department of Psychiatry, University of Kuopio, P.O. Box 1627, 70211 Kuopio, Finland

ABSTRACT: Noncompetitive NMDA receptor antagonists such as phencyclidine and MK-801 produce psychotropic symptoms that closely resemble schizophrenic psychosis and induce the expression of immediate early genes in limbic cortical areas. We are concentrating on analyzing molecular and physiological effects that these drugs produce in the entorhinal cortex and on the potential connection between these effects and the psychotic symptoms. We show here that MK-801 increases the DNA binding activity of the activator protein-1 (AP-1) complex in the entorhinal cortex. We also observed increased expression of mRNAs for Fos and Jun transcription factor family members c-Fos, FosB, Fra-2, and JunB, as well as Fos family proteins in the entorhinal cortex after MK-801 administration. This suggests that the activated AP-1 complex consists of these transcription factors. Genes regulated by the AP-1 complex in the entorhinal cortex might be involved in the pathophysiology of psychotic behavior and are potential targets for new antipsychotic drugs.

INTRODUCTION

Noncompetitive NMDA receptor antagonists, such as MK-801, phencyclidine (PCP), and ketamine, produce in humans emergence reactions which resemble schizophrenic psychosis and aggravate psychotic symptoms of schizophrenic patients.[1,2] Because PCP produces symptoms that resemble not only the positive but also negative symptoms of schizophrenia, it is generally considered the best experimental model of psychosis.[2] Olney and co-workers demonstrated that PCP and other noncompetitive NMDA receptor antagonists produce reversible neurotoxic effects in neurons in the posterior cingulate and retrosplenial cortices of rat brain.[3–6] These effects are characterized by reversible intracellular vacuolization[3] and induction of mRNAs for c-Fos[7–10] and brain-derived neurotrophic factor (BDNF).[8,11] These excitatory symptoms are observed only in adult rats[12] and are blocked by antipsychotic

[c]Address for correspondence: Eero Castrén, M.D., A.I. Virtanen Institute, University of Kuopio, P.O. Box 1627, 70211 Kuopio, Finland. Tel.: +358-17-162 084; fax: +358-17-163 030. e-mail: eero.castren@uku.fi

drugs.[13,14] This strongly suggests that excitatory effects are linked to the psychotropic side effects of PCP-like drugs. Because the excitatory symptoms are observed only in a relatively small population of neurons, PCP-like drugs could be used as a tool to identify the neuronal populations that may be involved in the psychotic behavior.

We have observed that MK-801 and PCP produce excitatory changes also in the entorhinal cortex (EC).[11,14] In view of the psychotropic effects that PCP and MK-801 produce, the EC is of particular interest because several different lines of evidence link this brain area to schizophrenic psychoses.[15–18] In addition, anatomical and physiological properties of the EC are relatively well understood,[19,20] which facilitates the interpretation of the effects of psychotropic drugs in this brain area. EC is an input and output station for information going to and coming from the hippocampus. It is thought that the EC–hippocampus loop is very important in the processing of sensory information, and defects in its normal function might produce cognitive disturbances.[20]

MK-801 increases c-Fos and BDNF mRNAs in the EC.[11,14] Induction of these genes is confined to a circumscribed neuronal population within the EC: mRNA for c-Fos is increased in neurons in layer III of the medial EC,[14] in the area which has also been termed caudal EC.[19] We have also shown that the induction of c-Fos expression in the EC can be blocked by prior administration of antipsychotic drugs.[14]

In collaboration with U. Heinemann's laboratory, we have investigated the electrophysiological consequences of the excitatory symptoms produced by MK-801 using a preparation that contains both EC and hippocampus in the same slice of rat brain.[21] Neurons in layer II of the EC send their projections to the dentate gyrus, from where the so-called trisynaptic loop through the hippocampus originates. EC layer II neurons are normally strongly inhibited and fire only in response to repetitive stimulations. In contrast, neurons in layer III project to the CA1 area. These projections are readily activated by single stimuli, but respond to a repetitive stimulation by a long-lasting inhibition.[22] In slices from rats treated with MK-801, stimulus-induced field potentials representing excitatory synaptic responses were strongly prolonged in layer III, but not in layer II and layer V of the EC. Furthermore, slow inhibitory postsynaptic potentials and afterhyperpolarizations following trains of action potentials in EC layer III neurons were weakened.[21] These data suggest disturbed information flow between EC and hippocampus, which may produce severe problems in the processing of sensory information and could quite well produce psychotic symptoms.

We hypothesize that PCP-like NMDA receptor antagonists produce similar kinds of disturbances in the EC-hippocampal information flow which occur during psychotic symptoms in schizophrenia. This hypothesis predicts the neuronal circuitry that could be disturbed in psychosis. Analysis of genes regulated by MK-801 in the EC may yield valuable information about the molecular events underlying psychosis. Moreover, physiological responses of the affected neurons in the EC as well as neurons in the hippocampus can be analyzed. This information may allow the generation of more precise experimental models for psychosis, and it could be used in the search for more effective drugs for schizophrenia.

In this paper, we have further characterized the effects of MK-801 in the EC. Fos (c-Fos, FosB, Fra-1, and Fra-2) and Jun (c-Jun, JunB, JunD) family proteins are activated rapidly in brain in response to various stimuli such as injury, growth factors, and drug treatment.[23,24] No prior protein production is needed for their expression; hence, they are called immediate early genes. Fos and Jun members form activator protein-1 (AP-1) complexes consisting of either Jun homodimers or Jun/Fos heterodimers. Binding of the AP-1 complex to a specific DNA sequence, the AP-1/TRE enhancer element regulates transcription of the target genes.[23,24] AP-1 complex binding to DNA typically activates transcription, but depending on the composition of the complex it may also reduce or have no effect on it.[24] Different stimuli may induce different sets of Fos/Jun family genes, thereby influencing the composition of the AP-1 complex, and subsequently the expression of the target genes.

We show that increased c-Fos expression has functional effects, since the DNA binding activity of the AP-1 complex is increased after MK-801 treatment. Furthermore, by analyzing the expression of Fos and Jun family members after MK-801 treatment, we have identified components that contribute to the increased AP-1 binding activity.

MATERIALS AND METHODS

Male Wistar rats (~200 g, National Laboratory Animal Center, University of Kuopio, Kuopio, Finland) were kept under standardized temperature, humidity, and lighting conditions with free access to food and water. All animal experiments were performed in accordance with the guidelines of the Society for Neuroscience and were accepted by the experimental animal ethics committee of the University of Kuopio. For electromobility shift assays (EMSA), rats were treated either with MK-801 (5 mg/kg, Dizocilpine maleate; RBI, Natick, MA) or saline. After 4, 8 or 24 hours, rats were quickly anesthetized with CO_2, decapitated, and the brains were removed for dissection. Both entorhinal cortices and hippocampi were collected, rapidly frozen in isopentane, and stored frozen at $-75°C$ until nuclear proteins were extracted. For *in situ* hybridization, rats were treated with MK-801, and brains were collected after 5 hours and kept in dry ice until completely frozen and stored at $-75°C$. Rats used for immunohistochemistry experiments were treated with MK-801. Four hours later, the animals were anesthetized with pentobarbital and transcardially perfused with 4% paraformaldehyde (PFA) in PBS (phosphate buffered saline, pH 7.4). After removal, the brains were postfixed overnight in 4% PFA/PBS at $+4°C$ and cryoprotected in 20% sucrose in PBS. Brains were stored at $-75°C$ until cut.

For EMSA, the nuclear proteins were extracted from the tissue by homogenization in hypotonic buffer containing 10 mM Hepes (pH 7.9), 1.5 mM $MgCl_2$, 10 mM KCl, 0.2 mM (*p*-amidinophenyl)methanesulfonyl fluoride (PMSF), 1 mM dithiothreitol (DTT), 1 μg/ml leupeptin, and 1 μg/ml aprotinin. The homogenate was centrifuged for 15 min at 4000 rpm at $+4°C$ and resuspended in a mixture of low-salt buffer (20 mM Hepes (pH 7.9), 25% glycerol, 1.5 mM $MgCl_2$, 1.2 mM KCl, 0.2 mM EDTA, 0.2 mM PMSF, 1 mM DTT, 1 μg/ml leupeptin and 1 μg/ml aprotinin) and high-salt buffer (same as low-salt buffer but with 20 mM KCl) in a ratio of 2:1. After 30 min incubation on ice, the homogenate was centrifuged at 13,000 rpm for 30 min at $+4°C$, and the nuclear proteins were collected and stored at $-75°C$.

A double-stranded oligonucleotide, 5′-CGC TTG ATG AGT CAG CCG GAA-3′ (Promega, Madison, WI), containing the AP-1/TRE enhancer element and binding to the AP-1 protein complex, was labeled with $[\gamma\text{-}^{32}P]ATP$ using T4 polynucleotide kinase (Promega). Five micrograms of nuclear protein extract isolated from the EC or hippocampus was combined with labeled AP-1 oligonucleotide in binding buffer containing 10 mM Tris/HCl (pH 7.5), 5% glycerol, 1 mM $MgCl_2$, 50 mM NaCl, and 0.5 mM EDTA. DNA-protein complexes were allowed to form for 15 min on ice and were resolved by 4% polyacrylamide gel electrophoresis at 100 V for 1.5 hours in Tris/glycine buffer, pH 8.5. The gels were then dried and exposed to X-ray films. DNA binding activity was quantitated with MCID^{TM} image analysis software (Imaging Research Inc., St. Catharine, Ontario, Canada). Activities were converted to percent of AP-1 binding in comparison to protein extracts from saline-treated rats. Results are shown as the mean ± SEM.

In situ hybridization was performed on 14 μm sections cut from frozen brains. Sections were postfixed with 4% PFA and hybridized with oligonucleotides that had been labeled with $[\alpha\text{-}^{33}P]dATP$ by terminal deoxynucleotidyl transferase (MBI Fermentas, Vilnius, Lithuania). The antisense oligonucleotides recognizing rat c-Fos, FosB, c-Jun, JunB,[25] Fra-1 (nt 961-986), and Fra-2 (nt 421-456) mRNAs were designed to minimize nonspecific hybridization. Hybridization was performed with 1–3 $\times 10^3$ cpm/μl of labeled probe in buffer containing 50% formamide, 10% dextran sulfate and 4 × SSC at +42°C overnight. After incubation, the sections were dipped into 1 × SSC at room temperature, washed for 30 min at +55°C in 1 × SSC, washed sequentially for 3 min each at room temperature in 1 × SSC, 0.1 × SSC, 70% ethanol, and 94% ethanol. Sections were exposed onto Hyperfilm-βmax films (Amersham, Buckinghamshire, England) for 2–3 weeks and developed in D-19 (Kodak, Rochester, NY).

Immunohistochemistry was performed on free-floating 30 μm thick sections cut with a microtome. Sections were stored in buffer containing 30% ethylene glycol and 25% glycerin in 0.05 M phosphate buffer (PB) (pH 7.4) at +4°C. Prior to immunohistochemistry, the sections were washed first 3 × 10 min in 0.1 M PB (pH 7.4) and then in 0.1 M PBS (pH 7.4). Sections were permeabilized for 30 min at room temperature in buffer containing 1% Triton X-100 and 3% heat-inactivated fetal bovine serum (FBS) in PBS. Anti-Fos antibody (Santa Cruz Biotechnology, Inc., Santa Cruz, CA) recognizing rat c-Fos, FosB, Fra-1, and Fra-2 proteins was used at 1:2000 dilution in 1% Triton X-100/1% FBS/PBS for overnight at +4°C. Immunoreactivity was visualized using an avidin-biotin conjugated secondary antibody (Vectastain, Vector Laboratories, CA) and diaminobenzidine precipitation (Zymed Laboratories, Inc., San Francisco, CA).

RESULTS

AP-1 DNA binding activity was measured in the EC and hippocampus 4, 8 or 24 h after the MK-801 treatment. AP-1 DNA binding was increased by 378 ± 99% ($p <0.05$) in the EC 4 hours after MK-801 treatment (5 mg/kg, $n = 9$) when compared to saline-treated controls ($n = 9$) (FIG. 1A). After 8 hours, this induction in binding activity was reduced to near the levels of saline-treated control tissue, and remained at this level after 24 hours. In contrast, AP-1 DNA binding activity in the hippocampus was not significantly affected by MK-801 treatment at any of the time points investigated (FIG. 1B).

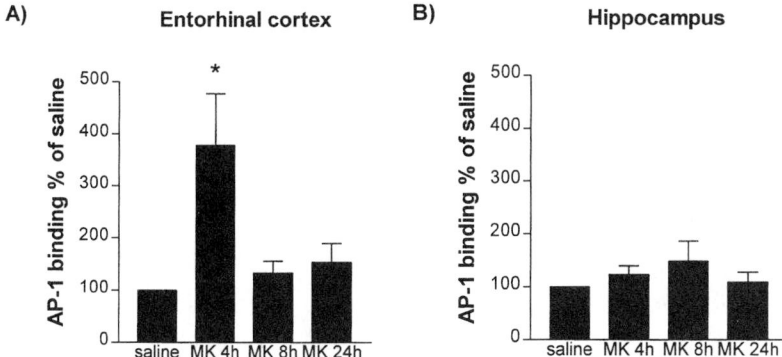

FIGURE 1. Effect of MK-801 treatment (5 mg/kg) on AP-1 complex DNA binding activity shown by electromobility shift assay. (**A**) MK-801 administration increases AP-1 binding in the entorhinal cortex at 4 hours compared to saline-treated control tissue (saline and MK-801 4 h, $n = 9$, MK-801 8 h and 24 h, $n = 5$). (**B**) In the hippocampus, MK-801 treatment does not significantly affect AP-1 binding activity at any time point investigated ($n = 5$ for each time point). Results are shown as mean ± SEM, $* p < 0.05$ (one sample Student's t test).

The composition of the induced AP-1 complex in the EC was investigated using oligoprobes complementary to c-Fos, FosB, Fra-1, Fra-2, c-Jun, and JunB mRNAs. From the Jun family members investigated, the expression of only JunB was positively regulated in the EC (FIG. 2), whereas c-Jun was not affected at the 5-hour time point (data not shown). mRNAs coding for the immediate early genes c-Fos, FosB, and Fra-2 of the Fos family genes were all upregulated 5 hours after MK-801 treatment in the EC, although upregulation of FosB was not as marked as for the other regulated Fos family members (FIG. 2). Expression of Fra-1 was not altered 5 hours after the MK-801 injection (data not shown).

The increased expression of Fos proteins in the EC 4 hours after the MK-801 injection was shown by immunostaining using an antibody recognizing all members of the Fos protein family (FIG. 3). Increased staining was most prominent in layer III, but individual stained nuclei were also observed in layer VI of the mEC.

DISCUSSION

Noncompetitive NMDA receptor antagonists are known to increase c-Fos expression in retrosplenial, cingulate, and entorhinal cortices.[7–10,14] This increase in one of the AP-1 complex components led us to investigate whether MK-801 affects the expression of other Jun/Fos proteins and the functional activity of the AP-1 complex. Here, we showed that a single MK-801 injection increases both the amounts of c-Fos, FosB, Fra-2, and JunB mRNAs and Fos proteins in the rat EC. Moreover, we

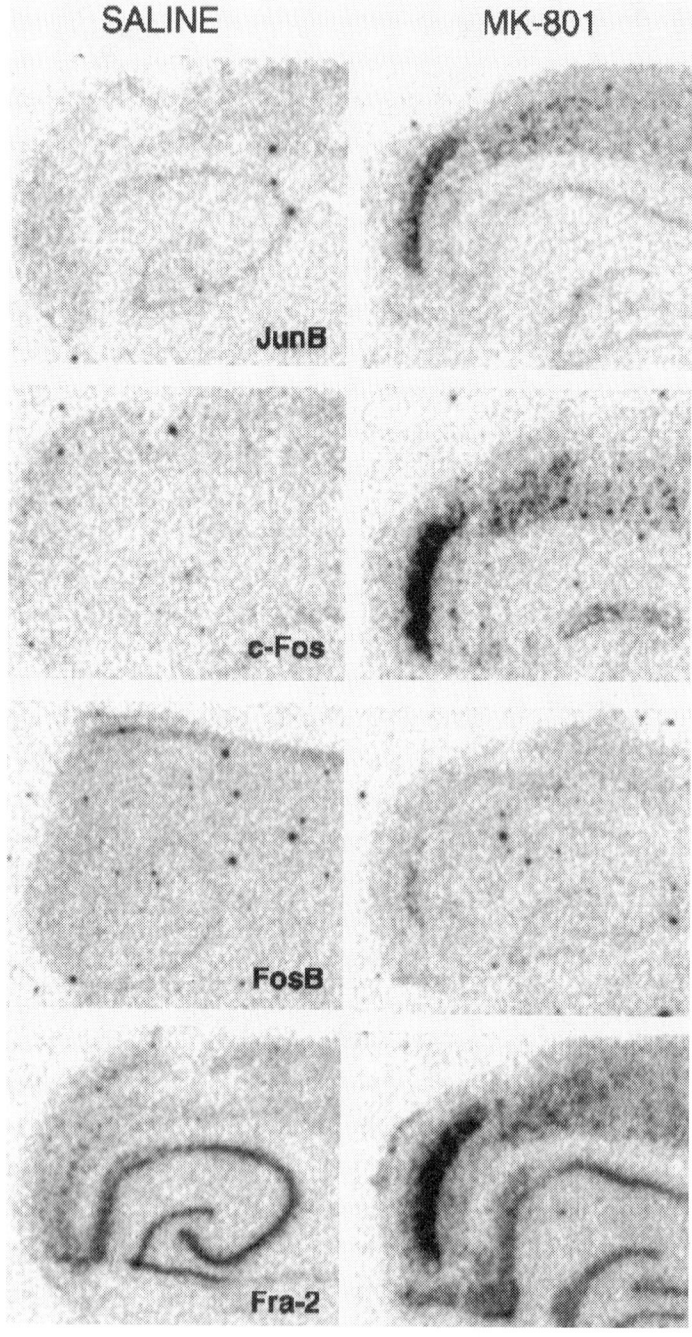

FIGURE 2. *See following page for caption.*

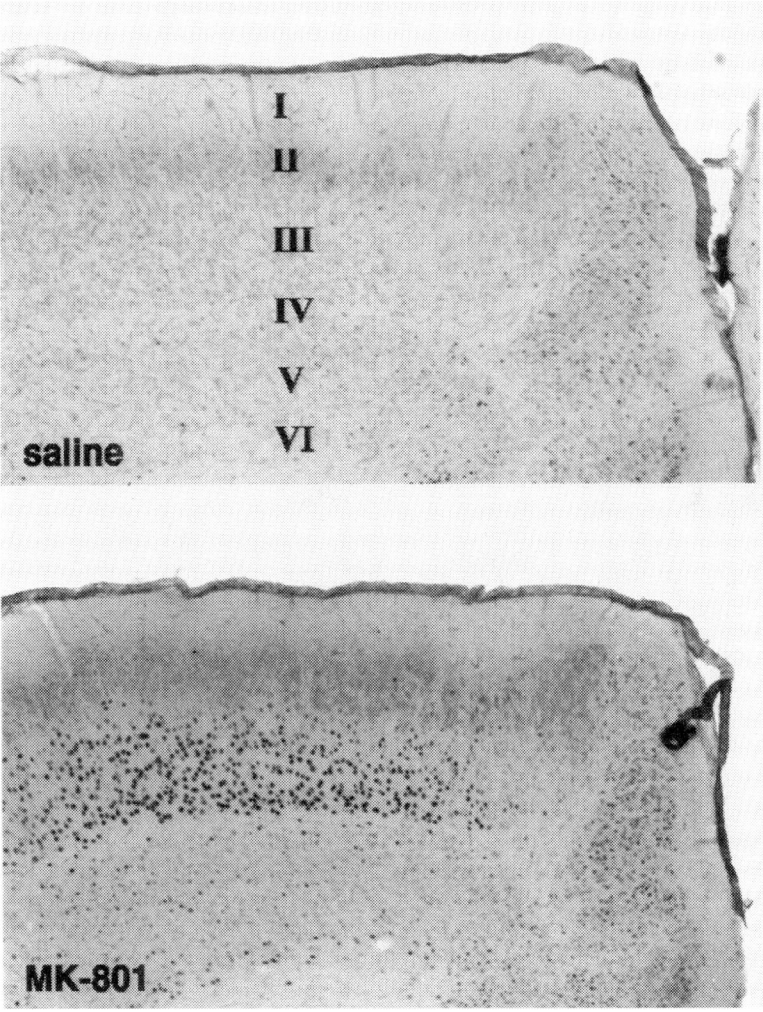

FIGURE 3. Immunohistochemistry showing increased expression of Fos family proteins in rat entorhinal cortex (EC) at 5 hours after MK-801 administration (5 mg/kg). The antibody recognizes all Fos proteins and stains nuclei mainly in layer III of the EC. Layers are indicated by roman numerals. Caudal is up, rostral down.

FIGURE 2. Effects of MK-801 treatment (5 mg/kg) on Jun/Fos family mRNA levels shown in horizontal sections of rat brain by *in situ* hybridization. mRNAs for JunB, c-Fos, FosB, and Fra-2 were increased in rat entorhinal cortex layer III 5 hours after MK-801 administration. Caudal is left, rostral right.

were able to show that DNA binding activity of the AP-1 complex is increased after MK-801 treatment. Of the time points studied, the DNA binding activity of AP-1 in the EC was highest at 4 hours after MK-801 administration, after which the activity declined. Hippocampal DNA binding activity of the AP-1 complex did not respond to MK-801 treatment, consistent with our previous observation that MK-801 does not increase c-Fos mRNA or protein levels in the hippocampus.[14]

We have previously shown that MK-801 treatment increases c-Fos mRNA and protein expression in the EC.[14] It had been reported earlier, by using *in situ* hybridization and immunohistochemical methods, that MK-801 increases c-Fos mRNA and protein levels in the retrosplenial and posterior cingulate cortex.[7–10] In addition to increases in c-Fos protein, an induction of FosB, c-Jun, JunB, and JunD protein levels after MK-801 has been shown in the same areas by immunohistochemical methods.[10] We also observed an increased expression of JunB, c-Fos, and FosB by *in situ* hybridization and enhanced immunoreactivity of Fos proteins by immunohistochemistry after MK-801 administration. Moreover, we could show a dramatic increase in Fra-2 mRNA levels in layer III of mEC at 5 hours after MK-801 administration. However, in contrast to previous reports of MK-801 effects in the retrosplenial cortex,[8,10] we were not able to detect increased c-Jun mRNA levels at 5 hours in the EC. This discrepancy may be due to different brain areas studied or differences in the chosen time intervals.

Our results suggest that the AP-1 complex induced by MK-801 in the EC at 4 hours may be composed of JunB and one of the following Fos family members: c-Fos, FosB or Fra-2. JunB is known to heterodimerize with c-Fos, FosB, and Fra-2, but it also forms homodimers.[24] JunB/c-Fos and JunB/FosB heterodimers increase the DNA binding affinity to target genes. Also, JunB/Fra-2 dimerization has been observed, but the effect of this complex on the transcription of target genes is not clear.[24] FosB mRNA was increased in the EC by MK-801, but based on its relatively weak expression compared to c-Fos and Fra-2 mRNA levels, its contribution to AP-1 complex formation is probably minor at the studied time point. This does not rule out the possibility that FosB may play a more prominent role in the regulation of target gene expression at later time points.

In conclusion, we have shown that the psychotropic agent MK-801 increases the mRNA levels of c-Fos, FosB, Fra-2, and JunB, and the DNA binding activity of the AP-1 complex in layer III of the medial EC in rats. The set of target genes which are regulated by the AP-1 complex in the EC are currently not well established, but these genes may be of great interest because they might be involved in psychotic behavior. Moreover, products of these genes are potential targets for antipsychotic drug development.

ACKNOWLEDGMENTS

We are grateful to Anne Lehtelä and Laila Kukkonen for their excellent technical assistance, Dr. Antero Salminen for help with EMSA assays, and Dr. Jari Koistinaho for oligonucleotide probes. This work was supported by grants from the Academy of Finland, Finnish Technical Development Center (TEKES), Sigrid Juselius Foundation, and Jalmari and Rauha Ahokas Foundation.

REFERENCES

1. KRYSTAL, J.H., L.P. KARPER, J.P. SEIBYL, G.K. FREEMAN, R. DELANEY, J.D. BREMNER, G.R. HENINGER, M.B. BOWERS & D.S. CHARNEY. 1994. Subanesthetic effects of the noncompetitive NMDA antagonist, ketamine, in humans. Psychotomimetic, perceptual, cognitive, and neuroendocrine responses. Arch. Gen. Psychiatry **51**: 199–214.
2. JAVITT, D.C. & S.R. ZUKIN. 1991. Recent advances in the phencyclidine model of schizophrenia. Am. J. Psychiatry **148**: 1301–1308.
3. OLNEY, J.W., J. LABRUYERE & M.T. PRICE. 1989. Pathological changes induced in cerebrocortical neurons by phencyclidine and related drugs. Science **244**: 1360–1362.
4. OLNEY, J.W., J. LABRUYERE, G. WANG, D.F. WOZNIAK, M.T. PRICE & M.A. SESMA. 1991. NMDA antagonist neurotoxicity: mechanism and prevention. Science **254**: 1515–1518.
5. OLNEY, J.W. & N.B. FARBER. 1995. Glutamate receptor dysfunction and schizophrenia. Arch. Gen. Psychiatry **52**: 998–1007.
6. OLNEY, J.W. & N.B. FARBER. 1995. NMDA antagonists as neurotherapeutic drugs, psychotogens, neurotoxins, and research tools for studying schizophrenia. Neuropsychopharmacology **13**: 335–345.
7. DRAGUNOW, M. & R.L.M. FAULL. 1990. MK-801 induces c-fos protein in thalamic and neocortical neurons of rat brain. Neurosci. Lett. **113**: 144–150.
8. HUGHES, P., M. DRAGUNOW, E. BEILHARZ, P. LAWLOR & P. GLUCKMAN. 1993. MK801 induces immediate-early gene proteins and BDNF mRNA in rat cerebrocortical neurones. Neuroreport **4**: 183–186.
9. NÄKKI, R., F.R. SHARP, S.M. SAGAR & J. HONKANIEMI. 1996. Effects of phencyclidine on immediate early gene expression in the brain. J. Neurosci. Res. **45**: 13–27.
10. GASS, P., T. HERDEGEN, R. BRAVOS & M. KIESSLING. 1993. Induction and suppression of immediate early genes in specific rat brain regions by the non-competitive N-methyl-D-aspartate receptor antagonist MK-801. Neuroscience **53**: 749–758.
11. CASTRÉN, E., M.P. BERZAGHI, D. LINDHOLM & H. THOENEN. 1993. Differential effects of MK-801 on the brain-derived neurotrophic factor mRNA levels in different regions of rat brain. Exp. Neurol. **122**: 244–252.
12. FARBER, N.B., D.F. WOZNIAK, M.T. PRICE, J. LABRUYERE, J. HUSS, H. ST. PETER & J.W. OLNEY. 1995. Age-specific neurotoxicity in the rat associated with NMDA receptor blockade: potential relevance to schizophrenia? Biol. Psychiatry **38**: 788–796.
13. FARBER, N.F., M.T. PRICE, J. LABRUYERE, J. NEMNICH, H. ST. PETER, D.F. WOZNIAK & J.W. OLNEY. 1993. Antipsychotic drugs block phencyclidine receptor-mediated neurotoxicity. Biol. Psychiatry **34**: 119–121.
14. VÄISÄNEN, J., A.M. LINDÉN, M. LAKSO, G. WONG, U. HEINEMANN & E. CASTRÉN. 1999. Excitatory actions of NMDA receptor antagonists in rat entorhinal cortex and cultured entorhinal cortical neurons. Neuropsychopharmacology **21**: 137–146.
15. BROWN, R., N. COLTER, J.A.N. CORSELLIS, T.C. CROW, C.D. FRITH, R. JAGOE, E.C. JOHNSTONE & L. MARSH. 1986. Postmortem evidence of structural brain changes in schizophrenia. Arch. Gen. Psychiatry **43**: 36–42.
16. ARNOLD, S.E., B.T. HYMAN, H.G. VAN & A.R. DAMASIO. 1991. Some cytoarchitectural abnormalities of the entorhinal cortex in schizophrenia. Arch. Gen. Psychiatry **48**: 625–632.
17. BOGERTS, B. 1993. Recent advances in the neuropathology of schizophrenia. Schizophrenia Bull. **19**: 431–445.
18. FALKAI, P., B. BOGERTS & M. ROZUMEK. 1988. Limbic pathology in schizophrenia: the entorhinal region—a morphometric study. Biol. Psychiatry **24**: 515–521.
19. AMARAL, D.G. & M.P. WITTER. 1995. Hippocampal formation. *In* The Rat Nervous System. G. Paxinos, Ed: 443–493. Academic Press. Sydney.
20. JONES, R.S.G. 1993. Entorhinal-hippocampal connections: a speculative view of their function. Trends Neurosci. **16**: 58–64.
21. GLOVELI, T., C. ISERHOT, D. SCHMITZ, E. CASTRÉN, J. BEHR & U. HEINEMANN. 1997. Systemic administration of the phencyclidine compound MK-801 affects stimulus-induced field potentials selectively in layer III of rat medial entorhinal cortex. Neurosci. Lett. **221**: 93–96.

22. GLOVELI, T., D. SCHMITZ, R.M. EMPSON & U. HEINEMANN. 1997. Frequency-dependent information flow from the entorhinal cortex to the hippocampus. J. Neurophysiol. **78:** 3444–3449.
23. MORGAN, J.I. & T. CURRAN. 1991. Stimulus-transcription coupling in the nervous system: involvement of the inducible proto-oncogenes fos and jun. Annu. Rev. Neurosci. **14:** 421–451.
24. HERDEGEN, T. & J.D. LEAH. 1998. Inducible and constitutive transcription factors in the mammalian nervous system: control of gene expression by Jun, Fos and Krox, and CREB/ATF proteins. Brain Res. Rev. **28:** 370–490.
25. KOISTINAHO, J., M. PELTO-HUIKKO, S.M. SAGAR, A. DAGERLIND, R. ROIVAINEN & T. HÖKFELT. 1993. Differential expression of immediate early genes in the superior cervical ganglion after nicotine treatment. Neuroscience **56:** 729–739.

Two-Phase Computational Model Training Long-Term Memories in the Entorhinal-Hippocampal Region

ANDRÁS LÖRINCZ[a] AND GYÖRGY BUZSÁKI[b,c]

[a]Department of Information Systems, Eötvös Loránd University, Pázmány Péter sétány 1/D, Budapest, Hungary H-1117

[b]Center for Molecular and Behavioral Neuroscience, Rutgers, The State University of New Jersey, 197 University Avenue, Newark, New Jersey 07102, USA

ABSTRACT: The computational model described here is driven by the hypothesis that a major function of the entorhinal cortex (EC)-hippocampal system is to alter synaptic connections in the neocortex. It is based on the following postulates: (1) The EC compares the difference between neocortical representations (primary input) and feedback information conveyed by the hippocampus (the "reconstructed input"). The difference between the primary input and the reconstructed input (termed "error") initiates plastic changes in the hippocampal networks (error compensation). (2) Comparison of the primary input and reconstructed input requires that these representations are available simultaneously in the EC network. We suggest that compensation of time delays is achieved by predictive structures, such as the CA3 recurrent network and EC-CA1 connections. (3) Alteration of intrahippocampal connections gives rise to a new hippocampal output. The hippocampus generates separated (independent) outputs, which, in turn, train long-term memory traces in the EC (independent components, IC). The ICs of the long-term memory trace are generated in a two-step manner, the operations of which we attribute to the activities of the CA3 (whitening) and CA1 (separation) fields. (4) The different hippocampal fields can perform both nonlinear and linear operations, albeit at different times (theta and sharp phases). We suggest that long-term memory is represented in a distributed and hierarchical reconstruction network, which is under the supervision of the hippocampal output. Several of these model predictions can be tested experimentally.

COMPUTATIONAL ASSUMPTIONS IN THE HIPPOCAMPAL-ENTORHINAL CORTEX SYSTEM

The main goal of this chapter is to discuss how the various subnetworks of the entorhinal-hippocampal system can perform different operations depending on the "state" of the brain. We attempt to describe the entorhinal cortex (EC)-hippocampal system as a collection of structure-function relationships. Our basic assumption is that the major function subserved by the hippocampus is to develop a representation that can rehearse past events—episodes—and can make predictions about ongoing events based on previously learned temporal sequences. From this single principle and theoretical considerations, we assign symbolic (mathematical) functions to each anatomical field of the EC-hippocampal loop. We also derive that an important function of the

[c]e-mail: buzsaki@axon.rutgers.edu

EC-hippocampal system is to modify synaptic connections in those structures that provide inputs to the hippocampal formation. For present purposes, we define long-term memory (LTM) formation as the alteration of synaptic connections in those cortical networks whose activity gave rise to hippocampal input. Ample clinical and experimental evidence is available to support the view that the hippocampal formation is essential for forming certain types of LTM.[87,94,95] The exact definition of the types of memories involving the EC-hippocampal system, however, is still debated.[13,31,73,94]

Our computation speculation takes its origin from a simple anatomical question: why does the hippocampal formation receive two distinct inputs from the EC? As discussed in detail in the chapter by Witter *et al.* (this volume), layer III of the EC provides a direct input to the CA1 and subicular regions. This projection is topographic.[102] In contrast, layer II neurons send their axons to the dentate gyrus (DG) and the CA3 region. The divergence in this pathway is substantial. We postulate that the two EC outputs carry qualitatively different types of information. The architecture of our speculative hippocampal-EC model is characterized as follows. First, the EC-hippocampal formation can be conceived as "novelty"-detecting "reconstruction network."[37,93,111] In the computational jargon, the term "novelty" can be defined as "error," that is, the difference between the expected (top-down) and experienced (bottom-up) neuronal representations. A second assumption is that neocortical representations are funneled to the hippocampus primarily by way of layer III of the EC (primary input). The third assumption is that the main function of layer II EC neurons is to compare neuronal representations between the neocortical (bottom-up) inputs and feedback (top-down) inputs from the hippocampus, that is, to compute and input the "error." The top-down information is conveyed by the hippocampus—EC layer V–layer II projections. The fourth assumption is that a main operation of the hippocampus is to reconstruct (or re-represent) the template of the neocortical input in order to optimize neocortical circuits to represent temporal sequences, that is, events and series of events.

We conjecture that temporal sequences are coded by directed associative connections (directed graphs) between neurons.[70] This functionality is advantageous because pattern completion is not restricted to single inputs but to input series, which improve noise-filtering properties. A directed graph has directed paths. Paths can have branches. Branching corresponds to different outcomes of the similar episodes that have been experienced. Thus, the directed graph will have a tree-like structure. The various episodes can be represented by various tree-like structures, that is, a mixture of trees. The smaller the branching ratio within the tree-like structures and the longer the directed paths, the longer the learned predictions. The mutual information delivered by the computational units (the neurons) and the number of associative connections correlate (e.g., Ref. 68). Consequently, by decreasing the mutual information delivered by computational units the branching ratio is reduced. In short, minimizing mutual information between computational units can optimize the directed graph.

With the foregoing ingredients, the operation of the model hippocampus-EC is this. The neocortical representations (primary input) and EC layer V-transformed hippocampal output (i.e., the reconstructed input) are compared by layer II of the EC. The difference between the primary input and the reconstructed input (termed the reconstruction error) is the novel information that activates the dentate gyrus and CA3 circuits, resulting in alterations of the internal connectivity of the CA3 recurrent matrix (plasticity). If the neocortical input to the EC is not novel (e.g., a rat is

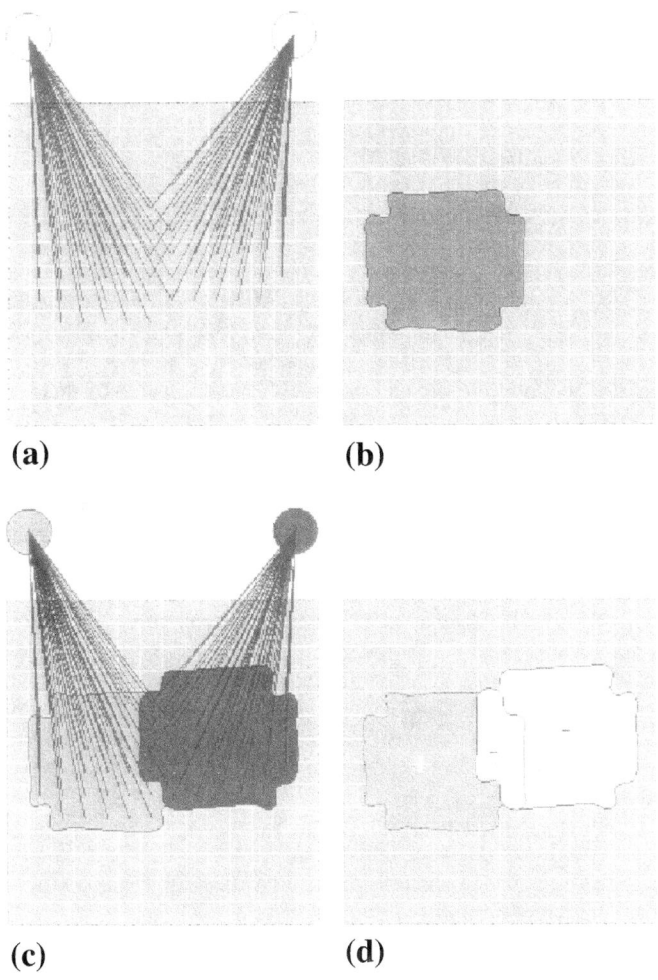

FIGURE 1. Explanation of terms. **(a)** Input layer arranged as a 14 by 14 matrix representing the 196-dimension input vector. Inputs project onto 2 units with overlapping input areas. Lines of different thickness depict synaptic strengths between the input layer and the unit. Thicker lines denote stronger inputs. The absence of a line indicates zero connection strength between the corresponding component of the input and the unit. Zero input is depicted by the background gray level. **(b)** Input to the network (positive values are darker than the background). **(c)** Reconstructed input. Two units are activated by the input. The darker unit receives stronger activation. The units reconstruct their inputs by means of their synaptic memories. The reconstructed inputs are shown superimposed on the 14 by 14 matrix. **(d)** Reconstruction error. Negative values: reconstructed activity is larger than the input activity (lighter regions); background gray: no reconstruction error; positive values: reconstruction error (darker region).

placed into a highly familiar environment), then the output of the hippocampus simply iterates previously stored hippocampal representations to the EC. Novel inputs,
on the other hand, will induce synaptic changes in the circuits of the hippocampus.
Because of the change in the hippocampal output, the EC will be trained until the
difference (error) between the input from the neocortex and the reconstructed input
conveyed by the hippocampal output is eliminated. Error elimination is also con-
strained by novelty-driven learning in the hippocampus. We conjecture that hippocampal synaptic modification gives rise to hippocampal outputs with minimized
mutual information (MMI). One can show that these outputs, referred to as independent components (ICs), can also train synapses in the EC and neocortical circuits to
transfer ICs. Then the circuits of the EC and neocortical regions become optimized
for the learning of temporal sequences. Development of the ICs requires a two-phase
operation, a nonlinear operation phase that tunes the circuits within the hippocampus
and a linear operation phase that tunes EC and neocortical circuits in a supervised
manner.

Comparator networks require that the inputs to be compared (primary and reconstructed inputs in our case) are available simultaneously. However, propagation of
activity within the hippocampus-EC is associated with finite delays, due to relatively
slow conduction velocity of axons, synaptic delays, and EPSP-spike delays. Compensation of time delays can be achieved by means of predictive structures. We assume that the EC-CA1 connections form such predictive structures and can
compensate for the time delays. We also conjecture that the recurrent collateral system of the CA3 field learns temporal sequences and serves as a means to replay the
learned sequences in the absence of EC inputs. This role of the recurrent collateral
system is assisted by a two-phase operation: patterns and pattern series that modify
hippocampal circuits are replayed to tune the EC and neocortical circuits to hold the
same information in an optimized manner. In short, we assume that the hippocampus
is involved in both signal reconstruction and prediction operations. These computational functions require both nonlinear and linear operations. We hypothesize that
the same anatomical circuits can perform both operations, albeit at different times.
We assign nonlinear (leaky) and linear (nonleaky) modes to the theta and sharp wave
physiological states of the hippocampus,[13] respectively. Before discussing the proposed computational model in detail, the mathematical tools needed for model construction are overviewed briefly.

MAIN BUILDING BLOCKS OF THE MODEL

Reconstruction Network

An assumption of our hippocampus-EC model is that it functions as a reconstruc-
tive network. An example of a simple reconstruction network is given in FIGURE 1.
Panel a illustrates the input layer with inputs arranged in a 14 by 14 square matrix
(i.e., the input vector has 196 dimensions) and two computational units in another
layer. The input layer can be considered as a representation of the external space,
e.g., at the level of the entorhinal cortex. The units can be considered as hippocampal
cells; they will be active in a limited region of the external space.[73] No topography
is assumed. The connection vectors of the units are shown by the lines connecting
the units to the input layer. Connection strengths are denoted by the thickness of the

lines. Zero connection strength is indicated by zero thickness. Panel b represents the input to the network. Gray scale value 0.5 corresponds to zero input. Darker and lighter gray values correspond to positive and negative inputs, respectively. Inputs and connection strength values can be arranged in vector form. We note that each element of the connection strength vector corresponds to an element of the input. Thus, in principle, the connection vector could be a particular input. If this particular input is activated, it may give rise to output activities in more than one computational units, that is, memory vectors are not orthogonal. Let us assume that the actual input is exactly equal to the to the connection strength vector of one of the units (panel b) that activates both units (panel c). Connection vectors are not orthogonal and both units are activated (panel c). Weighing their connection vectors with their activities, we can derive the *reconstructed input* (panel c). In the general case, the reconstructed input will not match the input. The difference between the input and the reconstructed input is the *reconstruction error vector* (panel d). The reconstruction error vector can be decreased or eliminated by iteratively *correcting the input* with the reconstruction error vector itself. The corrected input decreases the activity of the unit on the right-hand side (as indicated by the − sign) and increases the activity of the unit on the left-hand side (marked by + sign). Note that at the arrival of the input, no output and thus no reconstruction vector have been developed yet; thus at that time the reconstruction error is equal to the input. Thus, it is satisfactory if only the reconstruction error is fed into the network. We can formalize the iterative method in the following way:

$$a = P^T v \tag{1}$$

$$\Delta v = \alpha\,(x - y) \tag{2}$$

$$y = Qa \tag{3}$$

where x is the *input* vector of the network, y is the *reconstructed input* vector, $x - y$ is the *reconstruction error* vector, Δv is the *actual correction error* vector, α is the gain factor, and P^T is the input-to-output matrix. Superscript ^{T} denotes matrix transposition. Matrix P^T filters the *corrected input* vector v and forms the *internal representation* (or output) vector a. The output-to-input matrix Q weighs the output vector and forms the new reconstructed input and so on.[33,73,80,116] It has been tacitly assumed that matrices P^T and Q are of full rank and matrix $P^T Q$ is positive definite. Note that if the reconstructed input is zero ($y = 0$), the corrected input (v) is proportional to the input (x). Note also, that the correction becomes zero (and the iteration stops) when the input and the reconstructed input are equal. The reconstruction network is represented in FIGURE 2a. This is a recurrent architecture.

The dynamics of the network is shown in a one-dimensional example. Panel c of FIGURE 2 represents two connection strength vectors of 201 dimensions belonging to two computational units (not shown). Components of the connection strength vectors are connected with solid lines and look like smooth functions. The input equals to one of the connection strength vectors. The reconstructed input is shown at times 1, 2, …, 10 (in arbitrary units) in panel d. At early times (e.g., at time 1) the two connection strength vectors are superimposed to form the reconstructed input and the reconstructed input does not resemble the input. At time 10 the reconstructed input is close to the input, the network has almost relaxed. The temporal evolution of the activities of the computational units is shown in panel e. Activities rise sharply at the

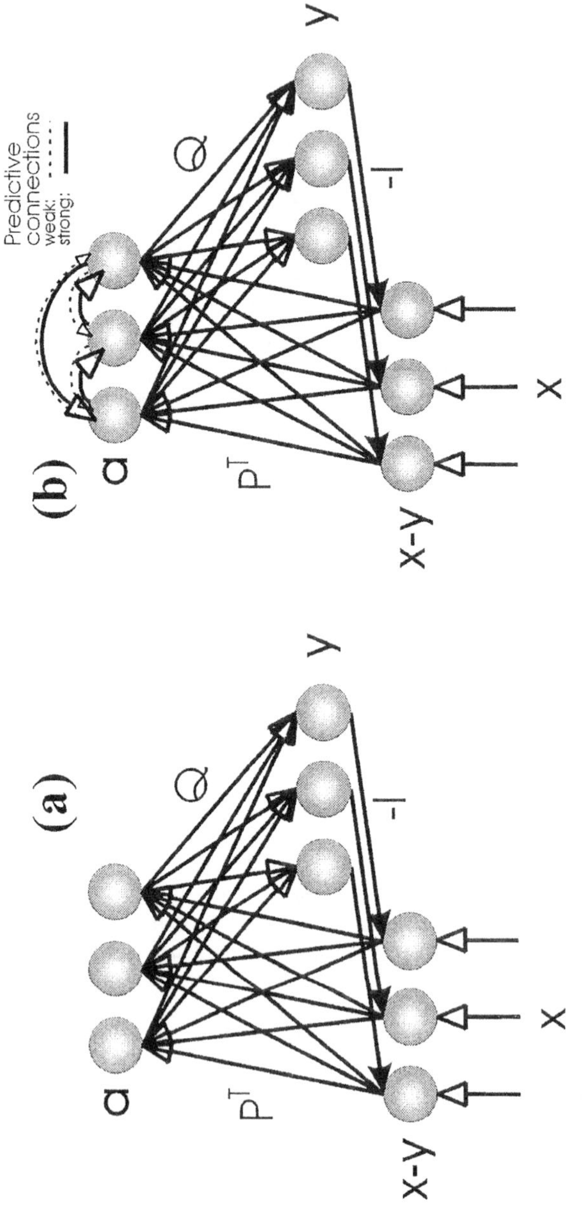

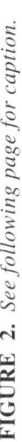

FIGURE 2. *See following page for caption.*

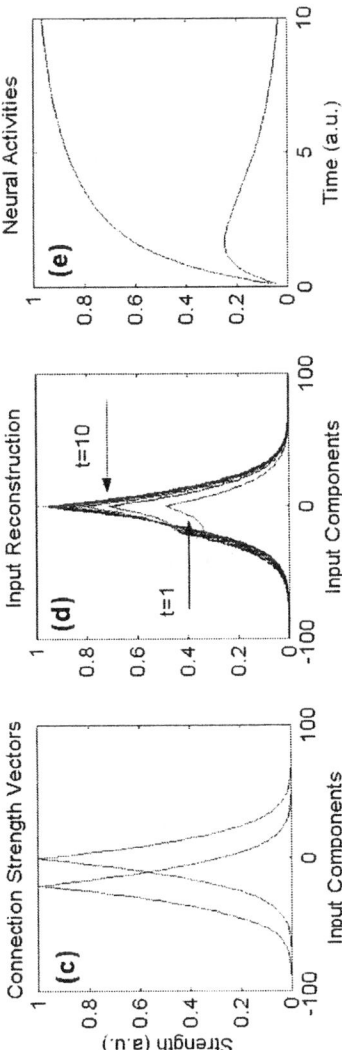

FIGURE 2. Reconstruction network and reconstruction dynamics. (a) Reconstruction network. Input, reconstructed input, and reconstruction error are computed in a dynamic network. The reconstruction error is inputted to the network (matrix P^T). The internal representation (vector a) is used to reconstruct the input by means of matrix Q. The reconstructed input is subtracted from the input to form the reconstruction error. *Open and solid arrows* represent excitatory and inhibitory synapses, respectively. (b) Reconstruction network with predictive connections. (c) Two connection strength vectors of 201 dimensions. Vector components are connected with a *solid line* that looks like a smooth function. The input is equal to one of the connection strength vectors. (d) The reconstructed input is shown at times 1, 2, ..., 10 (in arbitrary units). (e) The temporal evolution of the activities of the computational units. The reconstruction principle acts as competition between units (2 shown here).

start, but the activity of one of the computational units becomes depressed later, whereas the activity of the other unit saturates. The reconstruction dynamics act as competition between units.

Whitening (Decorrelation) and Independent Component Analysis

The information stored as memory in the brain is believed to be coded as discharge patterns of pyramidal neurons. The spatial resolution of the memory trace is that of a single cell and its temporal resolution may be determined by the ensemble firing rate and/or the relationship among spike times (e.g., cells with spatially localized receptive fields—"place cells"—and predictive connections representing temporal relations between place cells). The storage capacity of the network (number of storable and retrievable information) is determined, among other factors, by the number of possible ensemble discharge patterns.[108] The more the patterns differ, the less is the likelihood of false retrieval. We hypothesize that minimization of mutual information (independent component analysis, ICA) is an economic solution for storing memory traces.

ICA assumes that signals derive from independent sources. Consider the two-dimensional example depicted in panel a of FIGURE 3. The figure represents the case when the input vector has two components and there are two computational units. Inputs are distributed evenly within a limited space of rhomboid-like shape. Any input corresponds to a point within this area, and the two inputs to the network are the values of the two projections of the input point onto the two coordinate axes. A layer whitens if (1) it can *transform* the coordinate system, (2) in the new coordinate system the transformed inputs (i.e., the outputs of the layer) are decorrelated, and (3) the standard deviation along the coordinate axes are equal. (The term "white" in this context means that components—consider color, for example—are equal.) Higher order correlation, however, may still exist. For example, if the input gives rise to maximum activity in any of the whitened coordinates in the illustrated example, the value of the other component is granted (i.e., zero). *Separation* is also a coordinate transformation that minimizes information between the components. In case of separation we refer to ICA, or IC transformation, which provides separated or MMI outputs. If the lowest possible value of mutual information (zero) is achieved, *independent components* are developed.

Another aspect of ICA is presented in panel b of FIGURE 3. Here, a *single* matrix, utilizing oblique coordinate axes, represents the IC transformation. MMI outputs can be developed using projections parallel to the oblique ICA axes. A connection can be made here to principal component analysis (PCA). PCA removes second order correlation but does not re-scale the coordinate system. Two inputs (x and x_S) are shown. Consider the case of input x_S. If its component along axis PCA (1) is given, then we can infer that the other component should be close to zero. This is not the case for the MMI outputs denoted by $a_{ICA(1)}$ and $a_{ICA(2)}$. In the ICA coordinate system one component provides no (or minimal) information about the other component. The orthogonal projections of the inputs to the coordinate axes are denoted by a_1 and a_2. Orthogonal projections differ from the oblique projections. The vector sum of the oblique projections *recovers* (reconstructs) the original input, whereas orthogonal projections do not. The reconstruction network can be understood as a system that uses orthogonal projections but computes the oblique projections upon relaxation. The single matrix that represents the oblique coordinate system (IC transformation) will be called IC representation.

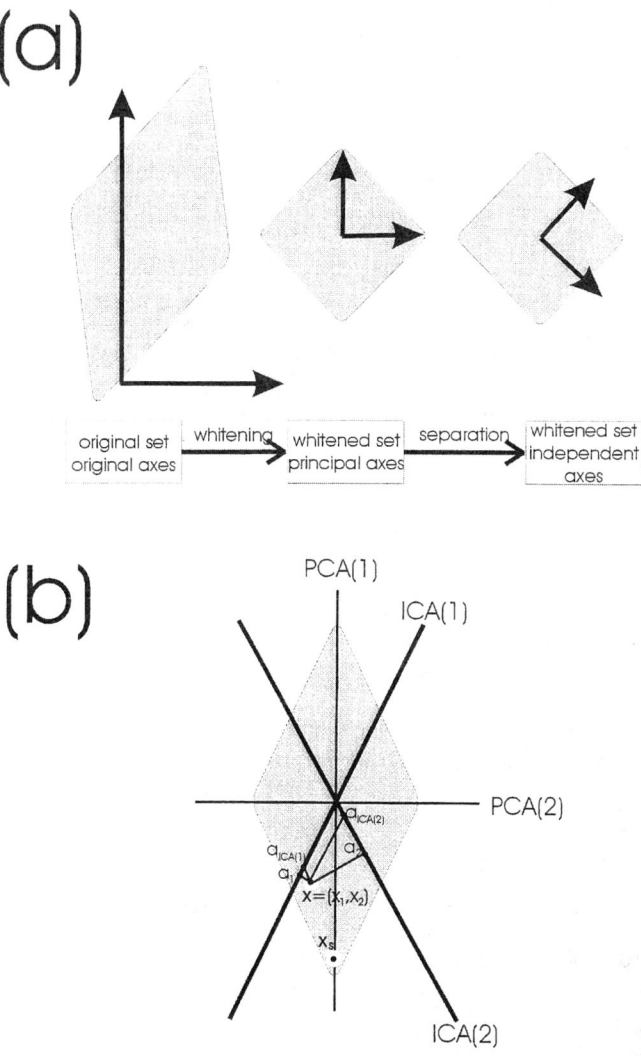

FIGURE 3. Whitening, separation, and independent components. **(a)** Left-hand side: Inputs are distributed evenly within a limited space of rhomboid-like shape. Any input corresponds to a point within the rhomboid. Inputs are given by their projections to the two coordinate axes. Middle: *Whitening* is a transformation that moves, rotates, re-scales the coordinate system, removes second order correlations and provides signals of equal variance. Right-hand side: *Separation* is a coordinate transformation that minimizes information between the components (see text). **(b)** Inputs are distributed evenly within a limited space of rhomboid-like shape. PCA(1) and PCA(2): Axes developed by principal component analysis. ICA(1) and ICA(2): Axes belonging to independent component analysis using single matrix transformation. Inputs: $\mathbf{x}$ and $\mathbf{x}_S$. IC projections to ICA axes: a_1 and a_2. IC components: $a_{ICA(1)}$ and $a_{ICA(2)}$. The vector sum of the IC components recovers (reconstructs) the original input.

Fast and efficient development of MMI outputs requires a two-layer learning scheme, a first layer that whitens and the second layer that separates.[6,46] The tuning (training) of the separation layer requires two-step operation, a linear and a nonlinear (leaky) phase. The separating layer is trained in the nonlinear phase, but the separated outputs are produced in the linear operation mode. Thus, a two-phase operation is required. The outputs of the two-step system can be used to train matrix Q in a supervised manner, because components of the input and the MMI outputs are available. Matrix Q corresponds to the oblique coordinate transformation.

Blind Source Deconvolution

During the development of our model we will face the challenge that reconstruction dynamics corrupt the input distribution and prohibit the development of proper MMI outputs. If, for example, the input rises suddenly from zero to one, then the output will not follow the input change immediately (panel e of FIG. 2). The amplitude distribution of the output signal will be modified by the relaxation. If, for example, the input distribution within the original rhomboid is even, it will be corrupted by the reconstruction network. The phenomenon is called temporal convolution (i.e., introduction of decorrelation in time). Panel e of FIGURE 2 depicts a step function temporally convolved with the exponential decay function of the reconstruction network. We will be forced to assume that one part of the HC (dentate gyrus, DG) counteracts this problem and *deconvolves* the input. Deconvolution means that the original temporal structure is recovered. Consider our step function example. At early times, activities of computational units increase, and we know that previously the input had to be smaller. Thus, we have information about the past. Consequently, different time windows may have mutual information. Using delay lines one can design a learning scheme that removes mutual information between time segments. No information between time segments, however, means that temporal convolution is removed and thus the original signal is recovered.[8,105,106] This is the blind source deconvolution (BSD) method. The architecture that learns to temporally deconvolve is depicted in panel a of FIGURE 4. This type of deconvolving architecture is called the feedback architecture. It has been shown that feedback architectures can be utilized provided that delayed parts are weaker than the direct signal.[52,105] Reconstruction networks represent exponential decays, and thus the condition is satisfied. One can show, using matrix manipulations, that temporal convolutions caused by reconstruction dynamics can be made diagonal using whitening and separation methods. This observation allows us to map the strict requirements of BSD onto the DG.

Tuning (Training) Rules of Synapses[d]

Most computational models follow a "strict" Hebbian tuning rule. According to this rule, a synapse undergoes modification if presynaptic and postsynaptic discharges of the neurons coincide in time. One can describe this rule in matrix form:

$$\Delta P = \beta_1 x a^T \tag{4}$$

---

[d]Tuning rules are not related to the error backpropagation algorithm of multilayer perceptrons, because we restrict ourselves to information available locally. The restriction excludes the propagation of tuning information.

(a)

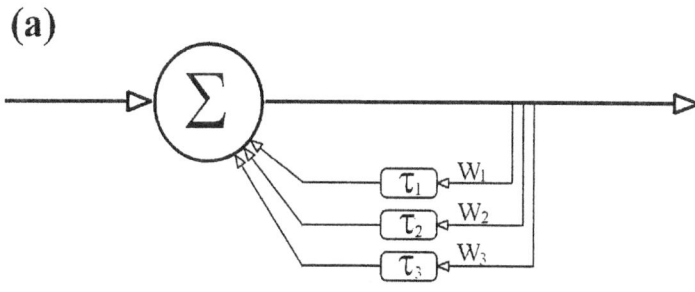

(b)

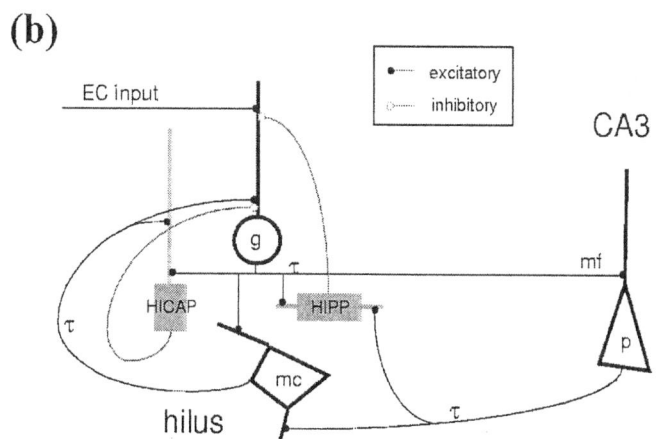

FIGURE 4. Architecture for temporal deconvolution. (**a**) Output x is fed back to a summing stage using different delays (denoted by τ_1, τ_2, and τ_3) and different connection strengths (denoted by w_1, w_2, and w_3). The connection strengths can be optimized by blind source deconvolution. (**b**) The excitatory connections between granule cells (g) and hilar mossy cells (mc) as well as g-CA3 pyramidal cells (p). These synapses, together with feed feed-back connections to g cells form delay lines. Feedback inhibitory neurons innervate specific dendritic segments of the granule cells at the termination zone of the EC and mc afferents. HIPP: hilar interneuron with axonal termination in the perforant path zone; HICAP: hilar interneuron with axon termination in the commissural and association paths. The activity of these interneurons also controls plastic changes (i.e., training) of the mc-g synapses.

where β_1 is the tuning rate, x and a represent the input and the output vectors of the neuronal network of a layer, respectively, and P is the memory matrix that multiplies the input. It has been argued that Hebbian tuning can be established by backpropagating action potentials that may serve as "acknowledgement" signals.[47] The output of the network is a function of the input ($a = g(P^T x)$), where the functional form could be linear or nonlinear. Nonlinearity can arise from feedback inhibition. In hippocampal CA1 pyramidal cells, the spread of backpropagating action potentials may be attenuated by IPSPs.[18] For computational purposes we model the nonlinear function by a saturating tangent hyperbolic function for the CA1 pyramidal cells and the mossy cells. Another nonlinear functional form is assumed for the EC afferent synapses to the granule cells. In this case we assume a function that rises in a supralinear fashion and becomes linear for large signal amplitudes.[76]

According to the tuning rule of Eq. (4) the postsynaptic discharge can be influenced by several factors in recurrent networks. Consider the case of output-to-input matrix Q. From the point of view of synapses of matrix Q the input equals to the output of the network, whereas the output is equal to -1 times the reconstruction vector, y. The matrix, however, is not tuned if the input vector and the reconstruction vector are equal. We assume that tuning is also influenced by the balance between excitatory and inhibitory contributions at the synapse, a more realistic assumption than simple Hebbian rule. Then the learning rule takes the form of the delta-rule

$$\Delta Q = \gamma(x - y)a^T \qquad (5)$$

where γ is the tuning rate and $y = Qa$. This tuning rule will encode the oblique representation of the ICA transformation into matrix Q.[46,75]

In our model, synaptic normalization[1] plays an important role. In the brain, synaptic modification requires a large postsynaptic membrane depolarization of sufficient duration to open Ca^{2+}-permeable N-methyl-D-aspartate (NMDA) channels or voltage-gated Ca^{2+} channels.[11,61] This may be brought about by bursting presynaptic neurons or synchronous firing of several presynaptic fibers.[56] We assume that "effective coincidences" are responsible for another type of learning that gives rise to the development of MMI outputs in the hippocampus. This part of learning depends on the synaptic strength in a complex fashion. During a high frequency afferent input, a stronger synapse will give rise to stronger postsynaptic depolarization and it will become even stronger. The tuning rule therefore should have a term, which is proportional to the strength of the synapse. On the other hand, the magnitude of postsynaptic depolarization may be dampened by the increased discharge of recurrently or feed-forwardly connected interneurons. Consequently, the magnitude of potentiation is inversely related to the activity of inhibitory interneurons impinging upon the postsynaptic principal cell. We thus modify Eq. (5) and write the tuning equation in the form:

$$\Delta P = \beta_1 xa^T + \beta_2(P - Paa^T) \qquad (6)$$

where matrix P denotes feed-forward matrices; β_2 is a positive parameter that depends on the firing rate. We assume that β_2 becomes zero at low firing rates, that is in lossy mode. It can be shown that the new part of the learning rule, $(P - Paa^T)$, normalizes. The first term is P. This linear (strengthening) term dominates for small synaptic strength values. Thus, synaptic vectors cannot diminish provided the tuning rate β_2 is sufficiently large. On the other hand, the other term has a negative sign, it represents the limiting effect on synaptic tuning. Because the number of inhibitory neurons is much smaller than the number of pyramidal cells, we can approximate the cumulated inhibition at synapse P_{ik} as $\Sigma P_{ij}a_j$. The summation is weighted by the elements of the synaptic matrix because, as before, the stronger the synapse the larger the probability that a given synapse contributes to the limiting effect. The limiting effect is also proportional to the postsynaptic activity of the neuron. Then the expression Paa^T follows. This limiting term overrides the strengthening effect when the synaptic weights become large: synaptic vectors cannot grow without limit. The new part of Eq. (6) will be referred to as the statistical part of the tuning rule. Note that the firing rate-dependence of the statistical part of the tuning rule makes the traditional Hebbian part relatively less effective at very high discharge rates. The limit when the traditional part of the learning rule can be neglected corresponds to the whitening equation.[19,51]

Associative connections (matrices) that represent temporal order are assumed to learn correlations between activities and rate changes of activities. The correlations between these quantities can represent temporal relationships. Predictive matrices can connect inputs to outputs, or outputs to outputs. Detailed description of this approach is given by Rao and Ballard.[80]

COMPUTATIONAL MODEL OF THE HIPPOCAMPUS-EC NETWORK

In this section, we attempt to map the aforediscussed mathematical operations onto the structure-function of the hippocampus-EC (FIG. 5). The hippocampus communicates with the perirhinal, parahippocampal and neocortical regions by way of the EC. The main information flow in the EC is from the deep (V–VI) to superficial (II and III) layers. LTM is hypothesized to be stored in the excitatory synapses between the deep and the superficial layers of the EC and in analogous synapses of the neocortex. The EC directly innervates all major hippocampal fields. Layer III of the EC is re-mapped onto the CA1 field and these afferents (input) serve a predictive role (temporal compensation) during theta-associated behaviors. The difference between neocortical information and processed signal in the hippocampus — layer V — layer II loop (i.e., the "reconstructed input") is regarded as "novelty" or "reconstruction error" in the model. This "error" signal drives the DG and the CA3 field. Recurrent collaterals in the CA3 field represent predictive connections and can replay temporal sequences during SPW. Granule cells of the fascia dentata and mossy cells of the hilus form delay lines. These reciprocal excitatory loops of the DG function primarily as a deconvolution network. The EC provides a double input to the CA3 field (perforant path and mossy fiber afferents), and these inputs are decorrelated (whitened) by the CA3 field. The whitened representation undergoes blind source separation in the CA1 field. The resulting MMI outputs are used to train LTM in the EC and the neocortex. The supervised training of the LTM by the hippocampus gives rise to oblique IC representation that requires reconstruction network to develop MMI outputs. Feedforward and feedback inhibitory connections are present in all fields (cf. Freund and Buzsáki[34]). All fields receive subcortical innervation and the activities of these pathways determine the operational modes of the EC-hippocampal region (theta vs. sharp wave phases). Details of the model follow below.

The CA3 Field Performs Whitening (Decorrelation of Inputs)

The CA3 field receives a direct and indirect (by way of the DG) from layer II of the EC.[5,57,101] When activities in the CA3 region are high, the "statistical part" of the tuning rule (Eq. 6) is in effect and that the other part of Eq. (6) can be neglected. As discussed earlier, the statistical part decorrelates (whitens) the EC-conveyed in-

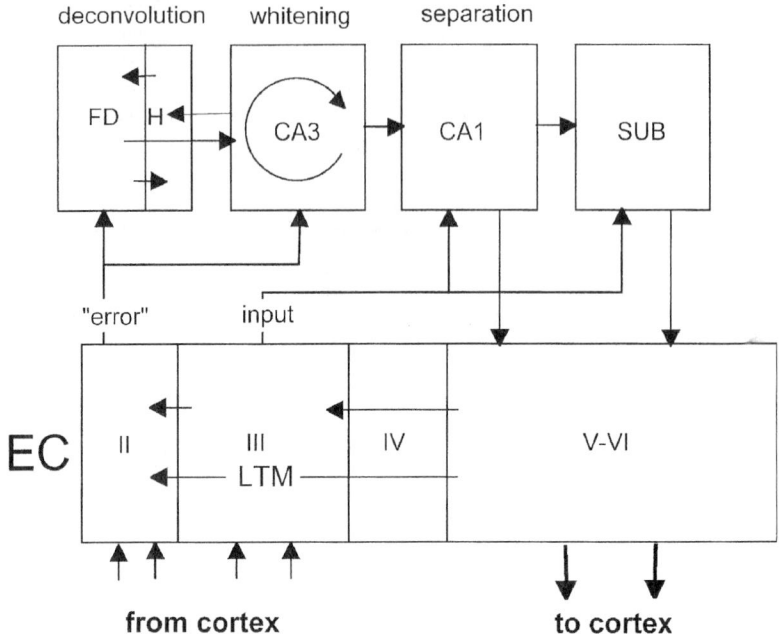

FIGURE 5. Schematic of major fields and connections in the entorhinal cortex (EC)-hippocampal formation and their hypothesized functions in the model. The hippocampus communicates with the perirhinal, parahippocampal and neocortical regions by way of the EC (from cortex; to cortex). The main information flow in the EC is from the deep (V–VI) to superficial (III and II) layers. Long-term memory (LTM) is stored in the excitatory synapses between the deep and the superficial layers of the EC. The EC directly innervates all major hippocampal fields. Layer III of the EC is re-mapped onto the CA1 field. The difference between neocortical information and processed signal in the hippocampus-layer V-layer II loop (the "reconstructed input") is the "reconstruction error". This error signal drives the dentate gyrus and the CA3 field. Granule cells of the fascia dentata (FD) and mossy cells of the hilus (H) form delay lines. These reciprocal excitatory loops of the dentate gyrus (FD and H) function primarily as a deconvolution network. The EC provides the input to the CA3 field (perforant path and mossy fiber synaptic matrices), and this input is decorrelated (whitened) by the CA3 field. The whitened representation undergoes blind source separation in the CA1 field. The resulting independent components are used to train LTM in the EC. All fields receive subcortical innervation and the activities of these pathways determine the operational modes of the EC-hippocampal region (theta vs. sharp wave phases). The anatomical connectivity and certain physiological properties of the subiculum are similar to those of the CA1 region. However, the present model does not specifically deal with this important region (see chapter by Deadwyler et al. on this issue). Some anatomical connections are omitted for simplicity (see chapter by Witter).

formation. The whitening process takes place both during theta and SPW states. In the awake (theta) state inputs from the perforant path and mossy fibers are whitened, whereas during the sleep phase (SPW) whitening process involves signals generated by the recurrent collateral matrix of the CA3 region. Tuning of the recurrent collateral synapses will be discussed below.

The CA1 Field Is a Separation Network

The CA3-CA1 projections (Schaffer collateral synapses) are very divergent. A single CA3 pyramidal cell may innervate as many as 30,000 CA1 neurons.[55] We hypothesize that separation of whitened information takes place in these synapses. Separation requires a two-step (non-linear and linear) operation[6,46,113,114] During theta behaviors, CA1 pyramidal cells discharge sparsely, a feature that we attribute to non-linear leakages. At low population firing rates, the second term of Eq. (6) can be neglected. In the linear (SPW) phase, population firing rate is high (Csicsvari et al.[117]) and the statistical term of Eq. (6) is in effect. Because the CA3 activities are already whitened, the two-step bigradient tuning rule of Wang et al.[113] can be applied for separation. We suggest that the bigradient tuning rule trains the network to provide MMI outputs.

The EC Computes the Reconstruction Error and Represents the Independent Components (ICA)

The EC is both the input stage and the output stage of the autoassociator/autoencoder hippocampal architecture. In addition, the EC provides information about the error of the autoassociation (i.e., the reconstruction error). Layer III represents the neocortical input to the EC. Layer II receives the same input as layer III and it is "upstream" from layer III. In addition, the input is combined with the intracolumnar efferents of layers V–VI of the EC. The intracolumnar connections have both excitatory and feed-forward inhibitory components.[21,28,48,49] On the basis of the anatomical arrangement and the requirements of the mathematical reconstruction network, we suggest that the reconstruction error (the difference between the neocortical input and the reconstructed input) is computed in layer II.

Layers V–VI of the EC are driven by the output of the CA1 field. This projection is topographically organized.[100] We consider the activities in layers V–VI of the EC as efferent copies (neuronal representation) of the CA1 field. However, because of the intrinsic properties of layer V–VI neurons and the internal dynamics of the EC, the neuronal activities in layers V–VI of the EC are different than in the CA1 region. Activities of layers V–VI of the EC represent the *output* of the hippocampus-EC system. The *internal* representation develops the reconstructed input for the EC by means of the layers V–VI to layer II synaptic activities. We refer to these connections as the long-term synaptic memory of the EC. We suggest that the plastic changes, underlying the synaptic memory of the EC, are brought about by the supervised tuning rule[46] of the CA1 outputs and the reconstruction error and serve to generate ICs. The reconstruction error is developed during theta behaviors, whereas the supervisory function of the hippocampus is operative in the linear mode (i.e., during SPW state). Proper tuning can be achieved by using the *sign* of the reconstruction error. In short, we hypothesize that the internal synaptic memory of the EC is modified during the theta-associated behaviors and that the modification represents the sign of the reconstruction error. The modification is consolidated by the SPW activities of the CA1 outputs. We should mention here that the network can perform reconstruction also during nonlinear operation, albeit at a much lower speed.[58,98,99]

The CA1 Region Has a Predictive Function

Afferents from layer III of the EC terminate in a spatially restricted manner on the distal apical dendrites of CA1 pyramidal neurons. Through this pathway, the EC is remapped topographically onto the CA1 field.[102] We suggest that this pathway serves as a predictive structure that counteracts the delays during the theta phase and calculates the correlation between activity rates of CA1 principal cells and EC layer III neurons. The CA3 afferents to the CA1 field transfer activities proportional to the reconstruction error and thus the activity rate of CA1 neurons is proportional to the reconstruction error. Tuning promotes the transfer of EC activities to the CA1 field therefore reconstruction becomes faster. Tuning stops if there is no reconstruction error. Networks of this type have been described by Rao and Ballard.[80] Predictive contribution should be adaptable on-line to compensate for the speed of input changes (e.g., the speed of the animal). Local adaptation rules can be derived using linear approximations.

CA3 Recurrent Collateral Network: Replay of Learned Information during SPW

The CA3 field is active during both theta and SPW states. A major difference between the two behavioral states is that the effectiveness of the recurrent collaterals is reduced in the theta state.[38] We assume that the tuning rule for the recurrent collaterals during the theta behaviors is guided by the activity of the initiating CA3 pyramidal neurons and the change in firing rate of the target CA3 pyramidal neurons. The predictive matrix is now between output nodes, it is not symmetric and represents temporal sequences. During SPW, when extrinsic inputs to the CA3 region are reduced, the recurrent collateral system can "replay" the patterns learned during the theta state. The tuning rule allows for the "distortion" of temporal scale during the short SPW events. As a result, the output pattern sequences of the CA3 are similar in both theta and SPW states.[71,91,115]

The Dentate Gyrus Performs Temporal Deconvolution

Although in the present model the layer V to layer II synapses are assigned as the neuronal substrate of LTM, we onjecture that the SPW-associated bursts train neocortical circuits in a fashion analogous to the training of the EC by the CA1 field[21,65,87,90,94,95] Specifically, we suggest that the outputs of the hippocampus provide the training information for the neocortical hierarchy. Thus, the neocortex may operate in a single (e.g., linear) mode. However, because of the hippocampal supervisory training new constraints emerge for the hippocampus itself. Such training can corrupt predictive networks in neocortical regions and, as a result, temporally convolved inputs may arise from the neocortex. The temporal convolution (decorrelation) needs to be removed. We assign this unique role to the DG. This is a unique function that, according to the model's prediction, should not be replicated in the neocortex. As the neocortex operates as a hierarchical set of linear reconstruction networks, temporal convolution that arise in neocortical networks may be removed by using *component-wise deconvolution* complemented with whitening and separation by the hippocampus (FIG. 4).

Granule cells of the DG number almost one million in the rat.[23,88] Thus, the internal dimension of the DG is larger than its input dimension so that the network can compress information and can form a sparse representation.[64] As shown earlier,[73,76] linear response within active subspaces is possible provided that subspaces are sparse. The model requres that the lossy properties of the granule cells should be different from those of the CA1 pyramidal neurons. Losses in this network should not saturate neuronal responses but, instead, should allow approximately linear response even when the inputs are large.[76] In physiological terms, it predicts that the dynamic firing frequency range of granule cells is larger than that of the pyramidal neurons. We assume that the tuning of synapses targeting granule cell dendrites far from the somata (i.e., termination of entorhinal afferents) will not be limited by the losses and thus these synapses can undergo statistical tuning. Thus, these synapses whiten. Synapses targeting granule cells close to the somata (i.e., termination of mossy cell afferents) are assumed to perform statistical tuning limited by the leaky properties of granule cells. We assume nonlinear saturation in the tuning but not in response properties. Moreover, we assume that the response of mossy cells to granule cell excitation can be shifted in time. The exact time shift may be determined by the gamma frequency population oscillation which is especially prominent in the dentate hilus.[12] Then the mossy fibers with approximately zero (i.e., very short) delays separate, whereas the more delayed mossy cell afferents and/or granule cell-CA3 pyramidal neuron-mossy cell loops deconvolve.[103,106] The convergence-divergence pattern in the model may be described as follows. Sparse representation means that separation and deconvolution involve a small subset of granule cells, corresponding to the small number of granule cell to mossy cell and granule cell to CA3 pyramidal cell connections.[2,4] Mossy cells can serve different granule cell subsets and thus the number of mossy cells may be small (approximately 20,000 in the rat). The divergent mossy cell to the granule cell connections[84,86] whiten in the model. In short, the assumptions of our model for the DG are as follows:

- Granule cells and inhibitory cells form a leaky structure

- Leakages of granule cells are supra-linear for small output activities, become approximately linear in the high output activity region, and give rise to sparse representation

- Sparse sets represent short time statistical properties produced by temporal convolution

- Entorhinal afferents to granule cells are trained by the statistical tuning rule and perform whitening.

- Mossy fiber connections to granule cells (associational afferents) separate and deconvolve.

- Mossy cell – granule cell loops with mossy cells and CA3 pyramidal cells form delay lines with variable delays.

The feedback contribution from the CA3 pyramidal cells to mossy cells is an important property according to our model. The temporally convolved EC input signals reach the CA3 field in a direct fashion and the convolution should be removed. We suggest that the CA3 pyramidal cell – mossy cell – granule cell feedback route[79] can perform this deconvolution task. Computer simulation of the deconvolution in the DG is shown in FIGURE 7.

RELATIONSHIP BETWEEN MODEL AND
HIPPOCAMPUS-EC NETWORK

The overall scenario for how LTM traces (i.e., independent components) are formed in the EC/neocortex by the two-stage operation of our model is as follows:

Theta phase

- EC layer III conveys neocortical representations directly to the CA1 field. This pathway is topographic. Layer II provides reconstruction error to the granule cells and CA3 pyramidal cells. Layers V and VI control the reconstruction process in layer II.

- Granule cells undergo statistical tuning and form sparse representation, operating in leaky mode. Active granule cells overcome leakages and operate in linear mode. Sparse sets represent short time statistical properties produced by temporal convolution. Granule cells and mossy cells learn to remove temporal convolutions. Mossy cells represent a bank of delay lines. Mossy cells with approximately zero delay learn to separate. Mossy cells with longer delays deconvolve.

- Perforant path synaptic matrix to CA3 pyramidal cells form whitened (decorrelated) outputs. CA3 recurrent collaterals predict temporal sequences.

- Schaffer synapses learn to separate whitened information (blind source separation).

- The predictive network activity of the hippocampal fields ensures that the reconstructed output from the CA1 region and the neocortical input are simultaneously present in the EC.

SPW phase

- The major initiator of hippocampal activities is the CA3 pyramidal cells.

- The CA3 recurrent collaterals replay activity sequences acquired during theta phase.

- The CA1 field operates in linear mode and trains the LTM of the EC (encodes independent components into the EC).

A generally accepted view is that the EC and hippocampal formation is one of the critical brain structures for storing of recently acquired information. Several previous theories share the common view that one of the main roles of the hippocampal region is to compare information.[13,29,30,37,97,111,103] The difference between old and novel knowledge can be conceived as an "error" signal which, we suggest, is compensated for by the activities of the hippocampus. Our model differs from early formulations of the "comparator" hypothesis. Sokolov[93] and Vinogradova[111] suggested that the hippocampal formation is both the comparator and novelty detector. In our model, the comparison between new and old is attributed to the EC and the plastic circuits of the hippocampus serve to compensate for the difference (i.e., reconstruction error). A more novel aspect of our model is that once the hippocampus learns to compensate for the error, the altered synaptic structure will continue to generate the same output, provided that the EC-hippocampus receives the same input vectors. In other words, the comparator in the EC requires comparison of the input (from the neocortex) with the reconstructed input (produced by the hippocampal output). Thus even after the input has become familiar (i.e., learned), the activity patterns of the hippocampal formation persist as long as the same input vectors (i.e., the same neocortical inputs) are presented. When new information enters the EC-hippocampus region, the new reconstruction error will modify synaptic connections within the hippocampus. The accuracy and the total number of novelty vectors represented simultaneously in the hippocampus are determined by the finite capacity of the synaptic matrix of the hippocampal neurons. What is learned by the hippocampus (i. e., the reconstruction error) becomes the LTM of the EC/neocortex. Given supervised training of the LTM, it follows that recently learned information is stored first in the hippocampus.

The model features are compatible with the experimental observations. Rat hippocampal "place" cells show long-term stability if the rat is not exposed to a novel environment.[50,104] However, when a rat is exposed to a variety of new environments between tests, place fields in the old environment can deteriorate.[67] The model is also compatible with the view that damage to the hippocampus produces graded amnesia, affecting mostly those recent memories which are predominantly stored in the hippocampus and not yet fully represented in the EC/neocortex.[3,63,95,96]

A second major assumption of the model is that the temporal delays, brought about by the physiological properties of the brain, can be offset by predictive mechanisms. The minimum time lag to be compensated is the reverberation time in the EC-hippocampal loop (15–25 ms in the rat[26]). This epoch corresponds to roughly one gamma oscillation cycle.[12] Although the exact physiological mechanisms responsible for prediction are not known at the moment, several potential mechanisms have been postulated.[17,43,45,60,74,92] Furthermore, several computation models have used time advanced prediction for learned events.[36,53,65,66,85]

We have conjectured that the hippocampus performs blind source separation and trains the EC and neocortical regions to hold the independent components. We also conjecture that neocortex also uses reconstruction network algorithms. Because the neocortical information becomes temporarily correlated (convolved) during tuning, a deconvolution architecture is postulated between neocortical inputs and hippocampal pyramidal cell fields. We hypothesized that the delay lines, formed by the granule cell-mossy cell loops of the DG can perform component-wise deconvolution. To date, we cannot provide any physiological support for the existence of this conjectured operation.

PREDICTIONS OF THE HIPPOCAMPUS-EC MODEL

Perhaps the most important and critical prediction of our model is the differential roles attributed to the EC outputs from layers II and III. Our assumption is that increased activity in layer II represents the reconstruction "error" between the neocortical input and its reconstructed representation by the hippocampus. In turn, the "error" signal is the main driving force to the granule cells and CA3 pyramidal cells, an input necessary for the induction of synaptic plasticity in the CA3 recurrent collateral system. The model suggests that elimination of EC layer II neurons will prevent modification of the intrahippocampal circuits by the neocortical inputs and results in the preseveration of previously trained patterns. Removal of the EC has been shown to eliminate most activity of the DG and increased population bursts in the CA3 region.[12] As an indirect support of this prediction, colchicin-induced damage to the DG did not change the place field characteristics of pyramidal neurons but altered the animal's ability to learn new spatial information.[66]

Selective elimination of the layer III input would deprive the hippocampus from its abilitiy to predict (temporally advance information). This should result in an instability and large variability of place fields of CA1 pyramidal cells. Another testable prediction is the absence of the theta-phase precession pyramidal cells[74] after layer III damage, a phenomenon implied in prediction of future places.[92] In addition, the hippocampus-assisted memory will be lost because the comparator role of the EC will be impaired. Relatively selective degeneration of layer II neurons occurs in Alzheimer's disease and in the senescence rat.[110] In support of the model's prediction, Barnes et al.[7] reported unstable place fields of pyramidal cells and impaired spatial navigation in aged rats. However, it is not known whether this deficit is due to the selective degeneration of layer II cells or simply part of a more general neuronal impairment. Selective, layer-specific toxin lesion of the EC will help examine these model predictions more critically.[32]

Testing the assumption that LTM traces represent the neuronal analogues of ICs will require simultaneous sampling of numerous neurons in several hippocampus-EC regions. Similarly, the hypothesized role of the DG in deconvolving the neocortical information will require multisite multiple unit recordings. However, once the data sets are gathered, the mathematical tools are available for testing these hypotheses.

RELATIONS TO OTHER MODELS

Some of the model's features share similarities with previous models of the hippocampus and other cortical structures. Over the last few years, Levy,[53] Tsodyks et al.,[109] and Zhang et al.[118] have constructed predictive models of hippocampal circuits. Carpenter and Grossberg[20] developed resonating models to match inputs to "top-down expectations." The idea that the same basic architecture can be used in different operational modes has been exploited by Buzsáki,[15] Hinton et al.,[39] Hasselmo et al.,[38] Shen and McNaughton,[89] Bibbig,[10] Neal and Dayan,[72] and Menschik and Finkel.[69] Our model is closely related to generative networks[40,41,82] including the dynamical sparse representation network introduced by Olshausen and Field.[75] Another part of our model concerns Kalman filters that have been proposed for the modeling of the visual cortex.[80] Blind source deconvolution (BSD) and blind source separation (BSS) methods are intimately related to the information maximizing principles.[6,8,19,24,44,46,113] Several previous modeling efforts considered the CA3 field with its extensive recurrent collaterals as a critical region of the hippocampus.[35,38,54,56,62,64,70,77,81,107,108,112] Although many of these models are similar in spirit to our model, the architecture presented here is an attempt to provide a coherent view of the EC-hippocampal loop. Importantly, each of the hippocampal fields and EC layers is assigned to perform distinct roles. Each network as well as their interactions contributes uniquely to the overall performance of the hippocampus-EC architecture.

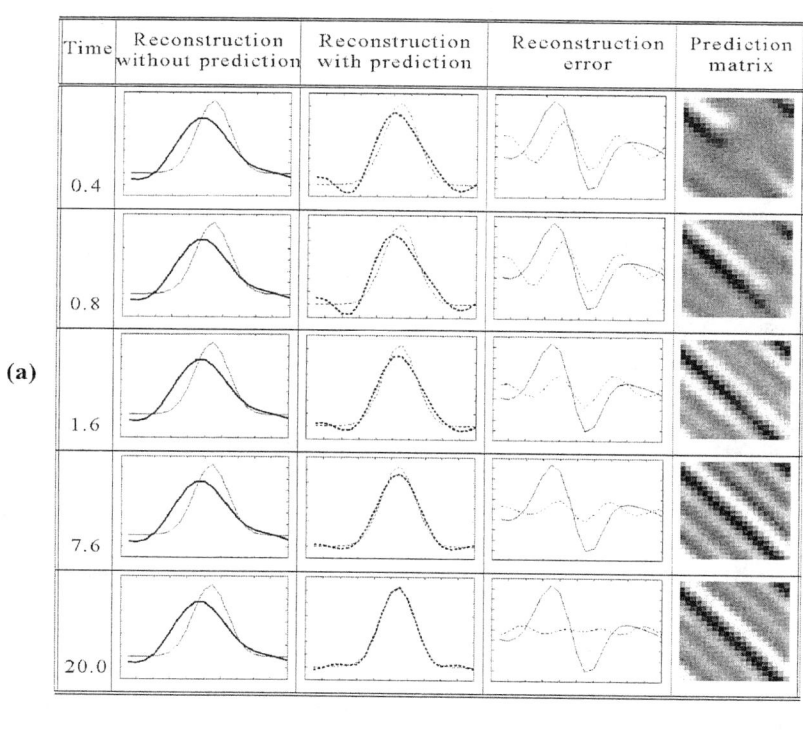

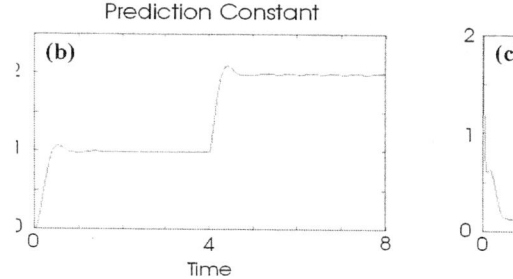

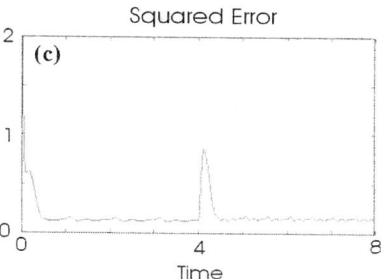

FIGURE 6. Properties of predictive matrix T. **(a)** The first (Time) column gives the actual time for Gaussian excitation to move around a circle. 20 time units correspond to 20 round-trip time. Bold lines: reconstructed inputs. Thin solid lines: inputs and reconstruction errors without prediction. Thin dashed lines: inputs and reconstructed error with prediction. Note that training the prediction matrix in a single run decreases the reconstruction error. (Reconstruction error is not to scale.) Predictive matrix elements (depicted in gray scale) are shown in the right-hand column at different stages of the training. Matrix elements were initialized by zeros and are depicted in matrix form. The strength of an element is illustrated in gray scale in the right-hand column at different stages of training. The farther a matrix element is from the diagonal the further apart are the receptive fields of the corresponding computational units and the larger is the time span of prediction. Gray level 0.5 corresponds to zero connection strength, darker (lighter) gray levels represent positive (negative) con-

COMPUTER SIMULATIONS

Effect of Predictive Matrix on Reconstruction Dynamics

The simulations described here can be viewed as a model when the rat is moving along a circular platform. Simulations were performed on a one-dimensional ring. The ring was constructed by considering a finite input interval ([0.0, 1.0]) and setting points 0.0 and 1.0 identical. The ring was discretized by 20 input units – this corresponds to 20, topographically organized cells. Input units sampled the excitations at equidistant discrete points around the ring. The network consisted of 20 computational units. That is, the system was a "square network": it had the same input and output dimensions. Matrices P and Q of the reconstruction network were set equal and were prewired. Connection strengths to each memory vector were sampled values of Gaussian functions of variance of 0.1 centered at different grid points: the computational units were "place cells." No topography for the place cell layer was assumed. The centers of connection strength vectors were placed equidistantly on the grid. It was assumed that a "previous processing stage" provided local excitations in the form of Gaussian functions. The Gaussian function had a variance of 0.1. The values of the Gaussian function at discretization points at a given time instant were considered as the components of the input vector at that time. The excitatory input was moved around the ring — representing the moving rat. The motion had unit speed and the Gaussian excitation circled once per unit time. The predictive matrix connected output units (output-to-output prediction) and full connectivity was assumed. The architecture is depicted in panel b of FIGURE 2. Initial predictive connection strengths were set to zero. Panel a of FIGURE 6 depicts the evolution of the predictive matrix and its effect on the reconstruction error. The time of the simulation was 20 time units and thus the Gaussian excitation (the rat) moved 20 times around the circle. Reconstruction dynamics was utilized. The second and the third rows of the third column illustrate that reconstruction error can be improved considerably in a "single session," that is, by making a single presentation of the input along the circle. Analogous simulations, using images, have been presented in the literature.[80]

The prediction matrix becomes asymmetric during tuning. The largest absolute values appear along the diagonal and in the lower left and upper right corners. These connections bridge those "place cells" which have receptive fields close to each other. (Note that we have a ring and connections between points 1 and 20 and points 20 and 1 are represented in the upper right and lower left corners of the matrix). In between, predictive connection strengths are closer to zero (gray). The strengths of predictive connections represent spatial closeness. The connectivity of the predictive structure represents the episode: the motion of the rat on the circle.

---

nection strengths. (**b**) Adaptive prediction. The reconstruction architecture with prediction was inputted with a Gaussian that started to move. First, speed was set to the speed that the predictive matrix was trained for. The speed was doubled at 4.0 time units. The initial value of the prediction constant, v_a, was zero and it was allowed to adapt. Prediction constant is shown as a function of time. (**c**) Reconstruction error as a function of time. Note that the error increased only transiently after the speed change.

The speed of motion along the circle may change. The value of the predictive gain constant can be adapted. The adaptation properties are shown in panels b and c of FIGURE 6. The two fast transients of the figure correspond to the start of the motion and to the time instant when motion speed was doubled. After the initial change, the transient substantially reduced.

Deconvolution in the DG

The goal of these simulations was to demonstrate the concept that *component-wise deconvolution* is satisfactory to deconvolve outputs of reconstruction networks. We used a three-layer structure made of input layer, granule cell layer and mossy cell layer. The architecture received convolved and then mixed inputs made of two independent series of random integer values and using two different temporal convolutions. We assume that these inputs are mixed. The case corresponds to the output of a two-unit reconstruction network with "mistuned" predictive matrices. This input enters the network and excites granule cells through the input-to-granule cell matrix (the EC afferents). The output of the granule cells enters a loop and excites a bank of delay neurons (the mossy cells). Delays can be approximately zero and non-zero. In physiological reality they may be considered as short and long delays in the granule cell-mossy cell loops determined by excitatory and inhibitory influences. Granule cell-to-mossy cell connections perform whitening. Both components of the bigradient learning were utilized simultaneously for mossy cell-to-granule cell connections, irrespective of the delays. The main restriction imposed by our model is component-wise deconvolution: every delay line targets that computational unit which gave the input to the delay line. The bank of delay lines with non-zero delays had 20 units for both granule cells that is $2 \times 20 = 40$ for the full network. In case of the general deconvolution architecture, the number should be $2 \times 2 \times 80$. This number grows fast with the number of granule cells. Delay lines with zero delay were exceptions: separation requires full connectivity. This meant that we had 4 zero delay mossy cells. This number of zero delay mossy cells scales with the square of the granule cell number within sparse subsets. The sparser the representation the less the number of separating mossy cells can be. In the computations, all synapses were tuned simultaneously.

We have used a never repeating spike series in the course of learning. Learning is demonstrated by the fact that the convolved and never repeating function became deconvolved as tuning proceeded. One of the two outputs of the network is shown in FIGURE 7 by the dashed lines. Different time windows represent different absolute times during the course of learning. Thus, the inputs are different for the different panels of the figure. One of the original signal, novel to the network, was made of positive and negative going "events" placed at random time intervals. This artificial signal was chosen to demonstrate the principle of component-wise deconvolution. Deconvolution of temporally convolved and mixed spikes is demanding yet the trained network was able to deconvolve *any temporal signal* that underwent the same temporal convolution and mixing. Panel a depicts the output signal before tuning, panels b, c, and d show the output signal of the first layer at different stages of tuning. It can be seen that convolved features became sharper and the correlation between the solid and the dashed lines is improved progressively. The tuned network provides approximately separated signals and deconvolved sharp features. Note that the archi-

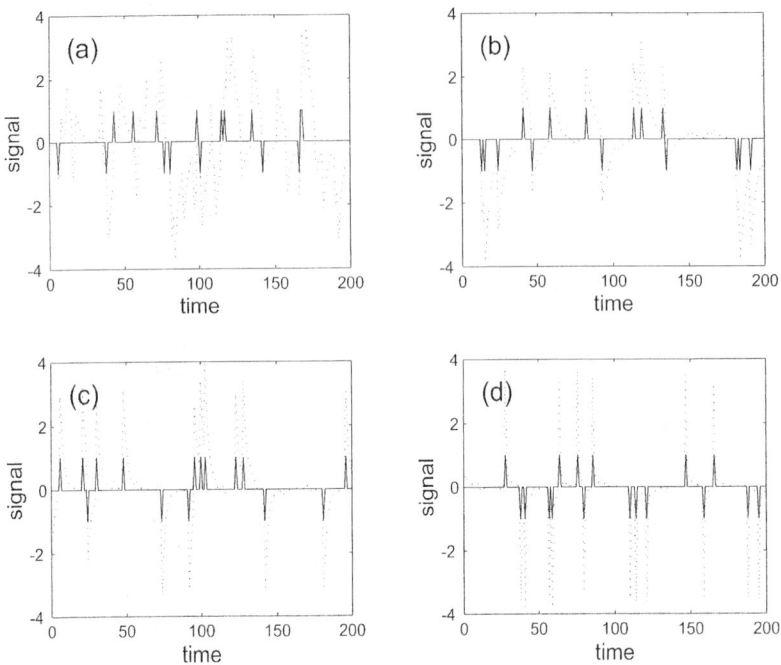

FIGURE 7. Deconvolution of the output of a reconstruction network. **(a)** *Solid line:* one of the two original signals, a random time series of three integer values; zeros, and plus ones and minus ones. Points of the time series are connected for the sake of visualization. Dotted line: one of the two output signals of the network created by temporally convolving and then mixing the two signals. **(b, c,** and **d)** Evolution of the output signal during concurrent whitening, separation and deconvolution. Solid lines: one of the two original signals; dotted lines: one of the output signals. Time is given in arbitrary units.

tecture deconvolves *and* separates within sparse subsets, but the full signal represented by the set of the sparse subsets will not be separated. The task of signal separation is assigned to the CA3 and CA1 fields in the full model.

ACKNOWLEDGMENTS

Helpful discussions with Peter Aszalós, László Balázs, M. E. Hasselmo, Darrell Henze, Gyula Kovács, B. W. Levy, and Csaba Szepesvári are gratefully acknowledged. Numerical simulations on predictive reconstruction networks conducted by Lehel Csató and Zoltán Gábor are also acknowledged. This work was supported by OTKA (T14566, T17100), the National Institutes of Health (NS34994, MH54671), and the US-Hungarian Joint Fund (No. 519).

REFERENCES

1. ABBOTT, L.F. & S. SONG. 1999. Temporally asymmetric Hebbian learning, spike timing and neuronal response variability. *In* Neural Information Processing Systems 11. M.S. Kearns, S.A. Solla & D.A. Cohn, Eds.: 69-75. MIT Press. Cambridge, MA.

2. ACSÁDY, L., A. KAMONDI, A. SÍK, T.F. FREUND & G. BUZSÁKI. 1998. GABAergic cells ar the major postsynaptic targets of mossy fibers in the rat hippocampus. J. Neurosci. **18:** 3386–3403.

3. ACKLEY, D.H., G.E. HINTON & T.J. SEJNOWSKI. 1985. A learning algorithm for Boltzman machines. Cognit. Sci. **9:** 147–169.

4. AMARAL, D.G. 1978. A Golgi study of cell types in the hilar region of the hippocampus in the rat. J. Comp. Neurol. **182:** 851–914.

5. AMARAL, D.G. & M.P. WITTER. 1989. The three-dimensional organization of the hippocampal formation: A review of anatomical data. Neuroscience **31:** 571–591.

6. AMARI, S.L., A. CICHOCKI & H.H. YANG. 1996. A new learning algorithm for blind signal separation. *In* Advances in Neural Information Processing Systems 8. D. Touretzky, M. Mozer & M. Hasselmo, Eds.: 757–763. MIT Press. Cambridge, MA.

7. BARNES, C.A., M.S. SUSTER, J. SHEN & B.L. MCNAUGHTON. 1997. Multistability of cognitive maps in the hippocampus of old rats. Nature **388:** 272–275.

8. BELL, A.J. & T.J. SEJNOWSKI. 1995. An information maximization approach to blind separation and blind deconvolution. Neural Comput. **7:** 1129-1159.

9. BI, G. & M. POO. 1999. Activity-induced synaptic modifications in hippocampal culture: dependence on spike timing, synaptic strength and cell type. J. Neurophysiol. In press.

10. BIBBIG, A. 1997. Physiologically realistic learning rule for active learning and unlearning during hippocampal sharp waves. Soc. Neurosci. Abstr. **23:** 508.

11. BLISS, T.V.P. & G.L. COLLINGRIDGE. 1993. A synaptic model of memory: long-term potebtiation in the hippocampus. Nature **361:** 31–39.

12. BRAGIN, A., G. JANDO, Z. NADASDY, J. HETKE, K. WISE & G. BUZSAKI. 1995. Gamma (40–100 Hz) oscillation in the hippocampus of the behaving rat. J. Neurosci. **15:** 47–60.

13. BURGESS, N. & J. O'KEEFE. 1996. Neuronal computation underlying the firing of place cells and their role in navigation. Hippocampus **7:** 1–15.

14. BUZSÁKI, G. 1984. Feed-forward inhibition in the hippocampal formation. Prog. Neurobiol. **22:** 131–153.

15. BUZSÁKI, G. 1989. A two-stage model of memory trace formation: a role for "noisy" brain states. Neuroscience **31:** 551–570.

16. BUZSÁKI, G. 1996. The hippocampal-neocortical dialogue. Cereb. Cortex **6:** 81–92.

17. BUZSÁKI, G. & J.J. CHROBAK. 1995. Temporal structure in spatially organized neuronal ensembles: a role for interneuronal networks. Curr. Opin. Neurobiol. **5:** 504–510.

18. BUZSÁKI, G., M. PETTONEN, Z. NÁDASDY & A. BRAGIN. 1996. Pattern and inhibition-dependent invasion of pyramidal cell dendrites by fast spikes in the hippocampus in vivo. Proc. Natl. Acad. Sci. USA **93:** 9921–9925.

19. CARDOSO, J.F. & B. LAHELD. 1996. Equivalent adaptive source separation. IEEE Trans. Signal Proc. **44:** 3017–3030.

20. CARPENTER, G.A. & S. GROSSBERG. 1993. Normal and amnesic learning, recognition and memory by a neural model of cortico-hippocampal interactions. Trends Neurosci. **16:** 131–137.

21. CHROBAK, J.J. & G. BUZSÁKI. 1994. Selective activation of deep layer (V-VI) retrohippocampal cortical neurons during hippocampal sharp waves in the behaving rat. J. Neurosci. **14:** 6160–6170.

22. CHROBAK, J.J. & G. BUZSÁKI. 1996. High-frequency oscillations in the output networks of the hippocampal-entorhinal axis of the freely moving rat. J. Neurosci. **16:** 3056–3066.

23. CLAIBORNE, B.J., D.G. AMARAL & W.M. COWAN. 1986. A light and electron microscopic analysis of the mossy fibers of the rat dentate gyrus. J. Comp. Neurol. **246:** 435–458.

24. COMON, P. 1994. Independent component analysis, a new concept? Signal Processing **36:** 287–314.

25. CORMEN, T.H., C.E. LEISERSON & R.R. RIVEST. 1990. Introduction to algorithms. MIT Press. Cambridge, MA.

26. DEADWYLER, S.A., J.R. WEST, C.W. COTMAN & G. LYNCH. 1975. Physiological studies of the reciprocal connections between the hippocampus and entorhinal cortex. Exp. Neurol. **49:** 35–57.
27. DEBANNE, D., B.H. GAHWILER & S.M. THOMPSON. 1998. Long-term synaptic plasticity between pairs of individual CA3 pyramidal cells in rat hippocampal slices. J. Physiol. **507:** 237–247.
28. DICKSON, C.T. & A. ALONSO. 1997. Muscarinic induction of synchronous population activity in the entorhinal cortex. J. Neurosci. **17:** 6729–6744.
29. EICHENBAUM, H., T. OTTO & N.J. COHEN. 1992. The hippocampus—what does it do? Behav. Neural Biol. **57:** 2–36.
30. EICHENBAUM, H., T. OTTO & N.J. COHEN. 1994. Two functional components of the hippocampal memory system. Behav. Brain Sci. **17:** 449–472.
31. EICHENBAUM, H., P. DUDCHENKO, E. WOOD, M. SHAPIRO & H. TANILA. 1999. The hippocampus, memory, and place cells: is it spatial memory or a memory space? Neuron **23:** 209–226.
32. EID, T., F. DU & R. SCHWARCZ.1995. Differential neuronal vulnerability to amino-oxyacetate and quinolinate in the rat parahippocampal region. Neuroscience **68:** 645–656.
33. FOMIN, T., J. KÖRMENDY-RÁCZ & A. LÖRINCZ.1997. Towards a unified model of cortical computation I: data compression and reconstruction architecture using dynamic feedback. Neural Network World **7:** 121–135.
34. FREUND, T.F. & G. BUZSÁKI. 1996. Interneurons of the hippocampus. Hippocampus **6:** 345–470.
35. GLUCK, M.A. 1996. Computational models of hippocampal function in memory. Hippocampus **6:** 565–762.
36. GLUCK, M.A. & C.E. MYERS. 1993. Hippocampal mediation of stimulus representation: a computational theory. Hippocampus **3:** 491–516.
37. GRASTYAN, E., K. LISSAK, I. MADARASZ & H. DONHOFFER. 1959. The hippocampal electrical activity during the development of conditioned reflexes. Electroencephal. Clin. Neurophysiol. **11:** 409–430.
38. HASSELMO, M.E., B.P. WYBLE & G.V. WALLENSTEIN. 1996. Encoding and retrieval of episodic memories: role of cholinergic and GABAergic modulation in the hippocampus. Hippocampus **6:** 693–708.
39. HINTON, G.E., P. DAYAN, B.J. FREY & R.M. NEAL. 1995. The "wake-sleep" algorithm for unsupervised neural networks. Science **268:** 1158–1161.
40. HINTON, G.E. & Z. GHAHRAMANI. 1997. Generative models for discovering sparse distributed representations. Proc. Trans. R. Soc. B **352:** 1177–1190.
41. HINTON, G.E. & T.J. SEJNOWSKI. 1983. Optimal perceptual inference. Proc. IEEE Computer Soc. Conf. on Vision and Pattern Recognition.: 448–453.Washington, D.C.
42. HOFFMAN, K. & R. KUNZE. 1971. Linear Algebra, 2nd Ed. Prentice-Hall. Englewood Cliffs, NJ.
43. HOPFIELD, J.J. 1995. Pattern recognition computation using action potential timing for simulus representation. Nature **376:** 33–36.
44. JUTTEN, C. & J. HERAULT. 1991. Blind separation of sources. Part I: An adaptive algorithm based on neuromimetic architecture. Signal Processing **24:** 1–10.
45. KAMONDI, A., L. ACSÁDY & G. BUZSÁKI. 1998. Dendritic spikes are enhanced by cooperative network activity in the intact hippocampus. J. Neurosci. **18:** 3919–3928.
46. KARHUNEN, J., E. OJA, L. WANG, R. VIGARIO & J. JOUTSENSALO. 1997. A class of neural networks for independent component analysis. IEEE Trans. Neural Networks **8:** 486–504.
47. KOCH, C. 1997. Computation and the single neuron. Nature **385:** 207–210.
48. KÖHLER, C. 1985a. Intrinsic projections of the retrohippocampal region in the rat brain. I. The subicular complex. J. Comp. Neurol. **236:** 504–522.
49. KÖHLER, C. 1985b. Intrinsic projections of the retrohippocampal region in the rat brain. II. The medial entorhinal area. J. Comp. Neurol. **246:** 149–169.
50. KUBIE, J.L. & R.U. MULLER. 1991. Multiple representations in the hippocampus. Hippocampus **1:** 240–242.
51. LAHELD, B. & J.-F. CARDOSO. 1994. Adaptive source separation with uniform performance. *In* Signal Processing VII: Theories and Applications. Proceedings of EUSIPCO-94. M. Holt, Ed.: 183–186. EURASIP. Lausanne, Switzerland.

52. LEE, T.W., A.J. BELL & R.H. LAMBERT. 1997. Blind separation of convolved and delayed sources. *In* Advances in Neural Information Processing Systems 9. M.I. Jordan, M.J. Kearns & S.A. Solla, Eds. MIT Press **9:** 758–764.
53. LEVY, B.W. 1996. A sequence predicting CA3 is a flexible associator that learns and uses context to solve hippocampal-like tasks. Hippocampus **6:** 579–590.
54. LEVY, B.W., C. COLBERT & N. DESMOND. 1989. Elemental adaptive processes of neurons and synapses. *In* Neuroscience and Connectionist Theory. M. Gluck & D. Rummelhart, Eds.: 187–236. Erlbaum Associates. Hillsdale, NJ.
55. LI, X.-G., P. SOMOGYI, A. YLINEN & G. BUZSÁKI. 1994. The hippocampal CA3 network: an in vivo intracellular labeling study. J. Comp. Neurol. **339:** 181–208.
56. LISMAN, J.E. & M.A.P. IDIART. 1995. A mechanism for storing 7±2 short-term memories in oscillatory subcycles. Science **267:** 1512–1514.
57. LOPES DA SILVA, F.H., M.P. WITTER, P.H. BOEIJINGA & A.H.M. LOHMAN. 1990. Anatomic organization and physiology of the limbic cortex. Physiol. Rev. **70:** 453–511.
58. LÖRINCZ, A. 1997. Static and dynamic state feedback control model of basal ganglia-thalamocortical loops. Int. J. Neural Systems **8:** 339–358.
59. LÖRINCZ, A. 1998. Forming independent components via temporal locking of reconstruction architectures: a functional model of the hippocampus. Biol. Cybernet. **79:** 263–275.
60. LYTTON, W.W. & T.J. SEJNOWSKI. 1991. Simulations of cortical pyramidal neurons synchronized by inhibitory interneurons. J. Neurophysiol. **66:** 1059–1079.
61. MARKRAM, H., J. LUBKE, M. FROTSCHER & B. SAKMANN. 1997. Regulation of synaptic efficacy by coincidence of postsynaptic APs and EPSPs. Science **275:** 213–215.
62. MARR, D. 1971. Simply memory: a theory of archicortex. Philos. Trans. R. Soc. [Biol.] **262:** 23–81.
63. MCCLELLAND, J.L., B.L. MCNAUGHTON & R.C. O'REILLY. 1995. Why are there complimentary learning systems in the hippocampus and neocortex: Insights from the successes and failures of connectionistic models of learning and memory. Psychol. Rev. **102:** 419–457.
64. MCNAUGHTON, B.L. & R.G.M. MORRIS. 1987. Hippocampal synaptic enhancement and information storage within a distributed memory system. Trends Neurosci. **10:** 408–415.
65. MCNAUGHTON, B.L., B. LEONARD & L. CHEN. 1989a. Cortical-hippocampal interactions and cognitive mapping: a hypothesis based on reintegration of parietal and inferotemporal pathways for visual processing. Psychobiology **17:** 230–235.
66. MCNAUGHTON, B.L., C.A. BARNES, J. MELTZER & R.J. SUTHERLAND. 1989b. Hippocampal granule cells are necessary for normal spatial learning but not for spatially-selective pyramidal cell discharge. Exp. Brain Res **76:** 485–496.
67. MCNAUGHTON, B.L., C.A. BARNES, J.L. GERRARD, K. GOTHARD, M.W. JUNG, J.J. KNIERIM, H. KUDRIMOTI, Y. QIN, W.E. SKAGGS, M. SUSTER & K.L. WEAVER. 1996. Deciphering the hippocampal polyglot: the hippocampus as a path integration system. J. Exp. Biol. **199:** 173–185.
68. MEILA, M. 1999. Mixture of trees. PhD thesis. MIT. Cambridge, MA.
69. MENSCHIK, E.D. & L.H. FINKEL. 1998. Neuromodulatory control of hippocampal function: towards a model of Alzheimer's disease. Artif. Intelligence Med. In press.
70. MULLER, R.U., M. STEAD & J. PACH. 1996. The hippocampus as a cognitive graph. J. Gen. Physiol. **107:** 663–694.
71. NADASDY, Z., H. HIRASE, A. CZURKO, J. CSICSVARI & G. BUZSAKI. 1999. Replay and compression of recurring spike sequences in the hippocampus. J. Neurosci. **19:** 9497–9507.
72. NEAL, R.M. & P. DAYAN. 1997. Factor analysis using delta-rule wake-sleep learning. Neural Comput. **9:** 1781–1803.
73. O'KEEFE, J. & J. NADEL. 1978. The Hippocampus As a Cognitive Map. Clarendon Press. Oxford.
74. O'KEEFE, J. & M. RECCE. 1993. Phase relationship between hippocampal place units and the EEG theta rhythm. Hippocampus **3:** 317–330.
75. OLSHAUSEN, B.A. & D.J. FIELD. 1996. Emergence of simple-cell receptive field properties by learning a sparse code for natural images. Nature **381:** 607–609.
76. OLSHAUSEN, B.A. & D.J. FIELD. 1997. Sparse coding with an overcomplete basis set: a strategy employed by V1? Vision Res. **37:** 3311–3325.

77. O'REILLY, R.C. & J.L. MCCLELLAND. 1994. Hippocampal conjunctive encoding, storage, and recall: avoiding a trade-off. Hippocampus **4:** 661–682.
78. PAVLOV, I.P. 1927. Conditioned reflexes. Oxford University Press. Oxford.
79. PENTTONEN, M., A. KAMONDI, A. SIK, L. ACSÁDY & G. BUZSÁKI. 1997. Feed-forward and feed-back activation of the dentate gyrus *in vivo*: dentate EEG spikes and sharp wave bursts. Hippocampus **7:** 437–450.
80. RAO, R.P.N. & D.H. BALLARD. 1997. Dynamic model of visual recognition predicts neural response properties in the visual cortex. Neural Comput. **9:** 721–763.
81. ROLLS, E.T. 1996. A theory of hippocampal function in memory. Hippocampus **6:** 601–620.
82. ROWEIS, A. & Z. GHAHRAMANI. 1999. A unifying review of linear Gaussian models. Neural Comput. **11:** 305–345.
83. RUMELHART, D.E., G.E. HINTON & J.L. MCCLELLAND. 1986. A general framework for parallel distributed processing. *In* Parallel Distributed Processing: Explorations in the Microstructure of Cognition. D.E. Rumelhart & J.L. McClelland, Eds. Vol. 1.: 45–76. MIT Press. Cambridge, MA.
84. SCHARFMAN, H.E. 1995. Electrophysiological evidence that dentate hilar mossy cells are excitatory and innervate both granule cells and interneurons. J. Neurophysiol. **74:** 179–194.
85. SCHMAJUK, N.A. & J.J. DICARLO. 1992. Stimulus configuration, classical conditioning, and hippocampal function. Psychol. Rev. **99:** 268–305.
86. SCHWARTZKROIN, P.A. 1994. Role of the hippocampus in epilepsy. Hippocampus **3:** 239–242.
87. SCOVILLE, W.B. & B. MILNER. 1957. Loss of recent memory after bilateral hippocampal lesions. J. Neurol. Neurosurg. Psychiatry **20:** 11–21.
88. SERESS, L. 1992. Morphological variability and developmental aspects of monkey and human granule cells: differences between the rodent and primate dentate gyrus. Epilepsy Res. Suppl. **7:** 3–28.
89. SHEN, B. & B.L. MCNAUGHTON. 1996. Modeling the spontaneous reactivation of experience-specific hippocampal cell assembles during sleep. Hippocampus **6:** 685–692.
90. SIAPAS, A.G. & M.A. WILSON. 1998. Coordinated interactions between hippocampal ripples and cortical spindles during slow-wave sleep. Neuron **21:** 1123–1128.
91. SKAGGS, W.E. & B.L. MCNAUGHTON. 1996. Replay of neuronal firing sequences in rat hippocampus during sleep following spatial experience. Science **271:** 1870–1873.
92. SKAGGS, W.E., B.L. MCNAUGHTON, M.A. WILSON & C.A. BARNES. 1996. Theta phase precession in neuronal populations and the compression of temporal sequences. Hippocampus **6:** 149–172.
93. SOKOLOV, E.N. 1963. Perception and the Conditioned Reflex. Pergamon Press. London.
94. SQUIRE, L.R. 1992a. Declarative and nondeclarative memory: multiple brain systems supporting learning and memory. J. Cognit. Neurosci. **4:** 232–243.
95. SQUIRE, L.R. 1992b. Memory and hippocampus: a synthesis of findings with rats, monkeys and humans. Psychol. Rev. **99:** 195–231.
96. SQUIRE, L.R., A.P. SHIMAMURA & D.G. AMARAL. 1989. Memory and the hippocampus. *In* Neural Models of Plasticity: Experimental and Theoretical Approaches. J.H. Byrne & W.O. Berry, Eds.: 208–239. Academic Press. New York.
97. SUTHERLAND, R.W. & J.W. RUDY. 1989. Configural association theory: the role of the hippocampal formation in learning, memory and amnesia. Psychobiology **17:** 129–144.
98. SZEPESVÁRI, C., S. CIMMER & A. LÖRINCZ. 1997. Dynamic state feedback neurocontroller for compensatory control. Neural Networks **10:** 1691–1708.
99. SZEPESVÁRI, C. & A. LÖRINCZ. 1997. Approximate inverse-dynamics based robust control using static and dynamic feedback. *In* Applications in Neural Adaptive Control Technology. J. Kalkkuhl, K.J. Hunt, R. Zbikowski & A. Dzielniski, Eds.: 151–179. World Scientific. Singapore.
100. TAMAMAKI, N. & Y. NOJYO. 1990. Disposition of the slab-like modules formed by axon branches originating from single CA1 pyramidal neurons in the rat hippocampus. J. Comp. Neurol. **291:** 509–519.

101. TAMAMAKI, N. & Y. NOJYO. 1993. Projection of the entorhinal layer-II neurons in the rat as revealed by intracellular pressure-injection of neurobiotin. Hippocampus **3:** 471–480.
102. TAMAMAKI, N. & Y. NOJYO. 1995. Preservation of topography in the connections between the subiculum, field CA1, and the entorhinal cortex in rats. J. Comp. Neurol. **353:** 379–390.
103. TEYLER, T.J. & P. DISCENNA. 1986. The hippocampal memory indexing theory. Behav. Neurosci. **100:** 147–154.
104. THOMPSON, L.T. & P.J. BEST. 1990. Long-term stability of the place-field activity of single units recorded from the dorsal hippocampus of freely behaving rats. Brain Res. **509:** 299–308.
105. TORKKOLA, K. 1996a. Blind separation of delayed sources based on information maximization. *In* Proceedings of the IEEE International Conference on Acoustics. Speech and Signal Processing, May 7–10, 1996.: 3510–3513. IEEE Press. Atlanta, GA.
106. TORKKOLA, K. 1996b. Blind separation of convolved sources based on information maximization. *In* IEEE Workshop on Neural Networks for Signal Processing, Kyoto, Japan.: 423–432. IEEE Press. USA.
107. TRAUB, R.D. & R. MILES. 1991. Neuronal Networks of the Hippocampus. Cambridge University Press. Cambridge, UK.
108. TREVES, A. & E. ROLLS. 1994. Computational analysis of the role of the hippocampus in memory. Hippocampus **4:** 374–391.
109. TSODYKS, M.V., W.E. SKAGGS, T.J. SEJNOWSKI & B.L. MCNAUGHTON. 1996. Population dynamics and theta rhythm phase precession of hippocampal place cell firing: a spiking neuron model. Hippocampus **6:** 271–280.
110. VAN HOESEN, G.W., J.C. AUGUSTINACK & S.J. REDMAN. 1999. Ventromedial temporal lobe pathology in dementia, brain trauma, and schizophrenia. Ann. N.Y. Acad. Sci. **877:** 575–594.
111. VINOGRADOVA, O.S. 1975. Registration of information and the limbic system. *In* Short-Term Changes in the Neural Activity and Behavior. G. Horn & R.A. Hinde, Eds.: 95–148. Cambridge University Press. Cambridge, UK.
112. WALLENSTEIN, G.V. & M.E. HASSELMO. 1997. GABAergic modulation of hippocampal population activity: sequence learning, place field development, and the phase precession effect. J. Neurophysiol. **78:** 393–408.
113. WANG, L., J. KARHUNEN & E. OJA. 1995. A bigradient optimization approach for robust PCA, MCA, and source separation. Proceedings of the IEEE ICNN, Perth, Australia: 1684–1689. IEEE Publishing. USA.
114. WANG, L. & J. KARHUNEN. 1996. A unified neural bigradient algorithm for robust PCA and MCA. Int. J. Neural Systems **7:** 53–67.
115. WILSON, M.A. & B.L. MCNAUGHTON. 1994. Reactivation of hippocampal ensemble memories during sleep. Science **265:** 676–679.
116. WITTMEYER. 1936 Ueber die Loesung von linearen Gleichungssystemen durch Iteration. Z. Angew. Mat. Mech. **16:** 301–310.
117. CSICSVARI, J., H. HIRASE, A. CZURKO, A MAMIYA & G. BUZSAKI. 1999. Oscillatory coupling of hippocampal pyramidal cels and interneurons in the behaving rat. J. Neurosci. **19:** 274–287.
118. ZHANG, K., I. GINSBURG, G.L. MCNAUGHTON & T.J. SEJNOWSKI. 1988. Interpreting neuronal population activity by reconstruction: unified framework with application to hippocampal place cells. J. Neurophysiol. **79:** 1017–1044.

Properties of Entorhinal Cortex Projection Cells to the Hippocampal Formation

U. HEINEMANN, D. SCHMITZ,[a] C. EDER, AND T. GLOVELI[b]

Institute of Physiology at the Charité, Department of Neurophysiology,
Humboldt University, 10117 Berlin, Germany

ABSTRACT: There are multiple connections from the entorhinal cortex (EC) to the hippocampus that carry the information from the EC to the hippocampus. Layer II cells of the medial EC innervating the dentate gyrus (DG)–molecular layer possess K^+-outward currents and inward rectifier currents that are potentially modulated by changes in intracellular second messengers. Layer II cells responded to synaptic stimulation with a rather flat input-output curve, and much stronger stimuli are required to generate action potentials in these neurons than in EC layer III cells. During repetitive stimulation at frequencies of 10 Hz and more, EC layer II cells respond with increased likelihood to generate action potentials. Two different NMDA conductances can be demonstrated in these neurons. A slow, less Mg, less voltage-dependent component is responsible for the transient depolarization between the fast and slow IPSP. A second group of neurons also projects to the DG. These are either pyramidal or nonpyramidal cells in the deep layers of the EC. At least part of these neurons also possess rhythmogenic properties. In contrast to layer II cells, layer III neurons have a steep input-output curve and show during repetitive synaptic activation a tendency to repolarize and to display long-lasting inhibitions dependent on $GABA_B$-, atropine-, and naloxone-sensitive components. As a consequence, they are readily activated during low frequency stimulation, but project only a few action potentials to area CA1 initially during higher (more than 10 Hz) frequency synaptic stimulation.

The rhinal cortex, which in the rat comprises the entorhinal, perirhinal, and postrhinal cortices,[1] is a crucial structure for some forms of memory.[2–4] The perirhinal and postrhinal cortices serve as major input sources to the entorhinal cortex (EC), in addition to well-established inputs from olfactory areas.[1] The perirhinal and postrhinal cortices receive functionally different types of information. While the perirhinal cortex is the major recipient of projections from somatosensory, auditory, and olfactory areas,[5] the postrhinal cortex is characterized by inputs from visually related areas.[5] These two cortical areas project preferentially to different portions of the EC. The perirhinal cortex preferentially projects to the lateral EC, whereas the postrhinal cortex mainly innervates the medial EC.[6,7] Since the lateral and medial EC are differ-

[a]Present address: Department of Cellular and Molecular Pharmacology, University of California at San Francisco, 513 Parnassus, San Francisco, CA 94141-0450.

[b]Author for correspondence: Tengis Gloveli, Institute of Physiology at the Charité, Department of Neurophysiology, Humboldt University, Tucholskystrasse 2, 10117 Berlin, Germany. Tel.: +49-30-2802-6651; fax: +49-30-2802-6669.

e-mail: tengis.gloveli@charite.de

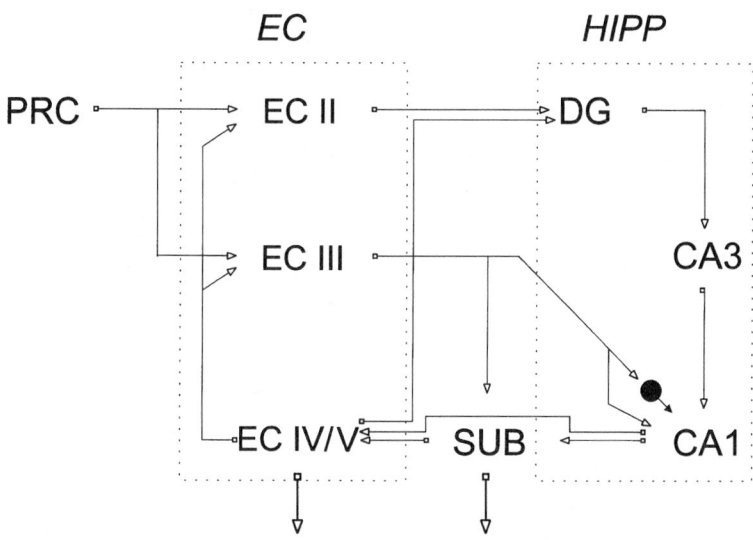

FIGURE 1. Schematic drawing of the entorhinal cortex–hippocampal connections. Note a trisynaptic input from layer II of the medial entorhinal cortex to area CA1 of the hippocampus, and monosynaptic inputs from layer II and IV/V to the dentate gyrus. Layer III neurons project to the pyramidal cells of area CA1 either directly or via the inhibitory interneurons. PRC: perirhinal cortex; EC: entorhinal cortex; ECII, ECIII, ECIV/V: entorhinal cortex layers II, III, and IV/V, respectively; HIPP: hippocampus; DG: dentate gyrus; CA1 and CA3: hippocampal areas CA1 and CA3, respectively; SUB: subiculum.

entially connected with the hippocampus, the functionally different types of information might be processed in parallel in the hippocampal memory system.[6]

The six-layered EC occupies a key position in the limbic system because it functions as a relay station between the hippocampus and isocortical brain structures. The EC provides major input to the hippocampal formation through two pathways. The stellate cells of layer II give rise to projections that distribute to the dentate gyrus (DG) and CA3.[8–10] A second prominent pathway originates from pyramidal cells of layer III and terminates on neurons in CA1 and subiculum (FIG. 1).[1,11,12] Layer III projection cells terminated mostly on the interneurons of CA1 as revealed by anatomical and physiological studies[13] (FIG. 1). In addition to these major entorhino-dentate projections, arising from the superficial layers of the EC, the anatomical data demonstrate that a small number of deep layer (IV–VI) neurons of the EC also project to the DG and hippocampus.[14] Recently, Deller and coworkers[15] using anterograde tracing demonstrate a previously unknown projection originating from the deep layers (IV–VI) of the medial EC (mEC) to the rat DG and terminating in the outer and inner molecular layer, granular cell layer, and hilus of the DG. The hippocampal output originating from area CA1 and subiculum projects back to the deep layers (IV–VI) of the EC (FIG. 1),[16–20] which in turn are reciprocally connected with multimodal association areas.[1,21] This hippocampal-cortical backward projection via the subiculum and the EC can account for the mechanism by which information processed by hippocampus can be transferred to permanent storage sites in the neocortex. Thus, it has been assumed that the parahippocampal regions, including the EC, maintain information in an intermediate store before transferring information into a long-term store.[22] The EC makes important, albeit distinct, contributions to spatial memory storage and retrieval in rats.[23] In addition, a possible functional dissociation between parahippocampal cortex and hippocampal formation has been proposed recently by Gabrieli and coworkers,[24] who reported preferential activation of the parahippocampal cortex during encoding and activation of the hippocampal formation during retrieval of information.

The EC also has gathered much attention because of its critical role in various neurological and psychiatric disorders. A characteristic of patients with Alzheimer's disease is their profound anterograde amnesia in early stages of the disease,[25] which is thought to be related to the early occurring pathological alteration in the EC.[26] This structure plays important roles also for the induction and/or maintenance of epilepsy and schizophrenia. In the phencyclidine model of schizophrenia, open channel block of NMDA receptor channels leads to a selective functional and structural affection of layer III neurons of the EC.[27–29] A critical interaction between different transmitters like GABA, acetylcholine, dopamine, and glutamate has been made responsible for the dysfunction and subsequent structural loss of neurons in this model.[30–32] The EC is also a key structure for seizure generation in temporal lobe epilepsy.[33,34] One reason for this might be the reciprocal synaptic connectivity between deep and superficial layers of the EC, which leads to massive excitation, largely driven via NMDA receptors.[33,35]

The EC has complex intrinsic and network properties that contribute to signal processing.[36,37] In the hippocampal-entorhinal network, the theta rhythm occurs during exploratory behavior and rapid eye movement sleep and represents a period when hippocampal circuits receive rhythmic input from neurons within the superficial layers of the EC.[38,39] In contrast, during sharp waves, which occur during consummatory behaviors and slow-wave sleep, the output neurons of the hippocampus and EC participate in organized population burst.[40,41] In addition, a gamma oscillation (40–100 Hz) was recently described that occurs within the superficial layers of the EC in association with entorhinal theta waves during exploratory behavior and rapid eye movement sleep.[42] The theta-gamma frequency synchronization of neuronal activity within the EC and hippocampus may provide a basis for effective communication among these neuronal populations.[42]

This information suggests that a more detailed analysis of the functional properties of projection cells of the EC, as well as different conditions that determine the information transfer by the two separate pathways, from layer II and III of the EC, to the hippocampus, would be timely. In this chapter, we review our recent studies on the properties of the EC neurons projecting to the hippocampus.

MEMBRANE CURRENTS IN RAT MEDIAL EC CELLS

Outward Currents in Stellate and Pyramidal Cells of the Rat EC

Although the morphological properties of different types of EC cells are well established, much less is known about the ionic components underlying the electrical behavior of these cells. Most studies investigating different currents in EC cells, such as Na^+,[43,44] K^+,[45] and Ca^{2+} currents,[46] were carried out on acutely isolated neurons. The superficial layer II stellate cells express a persistent Na^+ current, which is involved in the generation of low threshold membrane potential oscillation in the theta range.[47] EC neurons always exhibit fast activating Na^+ currents, which are characterized by different activation and inactivation behaviors in the different EC layers,[44] whereby the window current of superficial cells is more pronounced than that of deep neurons. Moreover, in addition to the normal tetrodotoxin (TTX)–sensitive currents, Na^+ currents were found in the medial EC that showed a much lower sensitivity to TTX.[43] K^+ currents of the EC cells seem to be under strong metabolic control. During long-time recording (more than 1 h), a rundown of slowly inactivating K^+ currents was observed in stellate neurons that could be prevented by the use of nystatin-perforated patch recordings.[45]

To compare properties of K^+ currents of acutely isolated EC stellate and pyramidal cells, we analyzed their kinetics and pharmacology. Both cell types express a fast transient and a slow inactivating outward K^+ current. In contrast to pyramidal cells, which mainly expressed large A-type currents and only small delayed rectifying currents, stellate cells exhibited prominent delayed rectifying and only small A-type currents.[48] I_A and I_K of pyramidal cells are characterized by activation and inactivation behavior similar to those in stellate cells. In addition, outward currents of both cell types responded in a similar way to all pharmacological drugs tested.[49] I_K values of both cell types were reduced by tetraethylammonium (TEA) in a concentration-dependent manner. Superfusion of 4-AP resulted in a reduction of the amplitudes of I_A and I_K. In addition, extracellularly applied dendrotoxin did not have any effect on EC K^+ currents. Therefore, it can be concluded that, in contrast to Na^+ currents,[43,44] K^+ outward currents of stellate and pyramidal cells in the EC differ only in their current density, but not in their kinetics or pharmacology.

Inward Rectifier Currents in the Rat EC Stellate and Pyramidal Cells

Inward rectifying cation currents (I_H) have been observed in various central neurons.[50] It has been shown that I_H can contribute to the resting membrane potentials[51–53] and to rhythmic membrane potential oscillations.[47,52] As I_H was not measurable in acutely isolated neurons of the EC[45] due to their sensitivity to extracellular proteolysis, we used a slice preparation to study age-dependent changes of I_H in superficial (layer II) stellate and deep layer (layer IV) pyramidal cells using the whole-cell configuration of the patch-clamp technique.[54] The current density of I_H in adult rats was larger in stellate than in pyramidal cells. The current density of inward rectifier currents of the EC neurons changed during postnatal development. I_H of stellate cells exhibited larger amplitudes in adult than in juvenile rats. Interestingly, in contrast to the findings obtained in adult rats, the current density of I_H of pyramidal cells in juvenile animals was significantly larger than that of stellate cells. However, the currents did not differ in their sensitivity to extracellular Cs^+ in both age groups. A similar increase of amplitude or current density of inward rectifying cation currents during maturation has been described for pyramidal cells of the visual cortex.[55]

The presence of prominent inward rectifier current in EC stellate cells of adult animals is well established.[47] Interestingly, blockade of this current with extracellu-

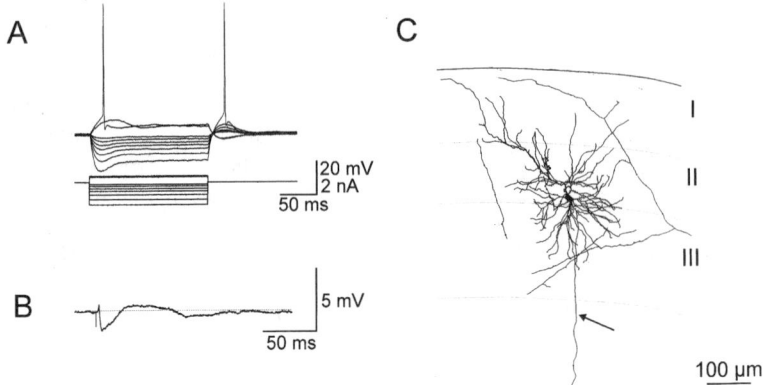

FIGURE 2. Electrophysiology and morphology of a projection stellate cell of EC layer II. (**A**) Typical responses of a cell to hyperpolarizing and depolarizing current injections. (**B**) Layer II cells responded to single synaptic stimulation with a small EPSP followed by a fast and slow IPSP. (**C**) Camera lucida reconstruction of a stellate cell with soma located in layer II of the EC and with an axonal projection to the deep layers (arrow).

lar Cs^+ induced a reduction of frequency and a decrease of rhythmicity of subthreshold membrane potential oscillations.[47] Since robust rhythmic subthreshold oscillations occur in stellate cells,[47] one may argue that the expression of large inward rectifier currents in stellate cells of adult animals is correlated with the development of these oscillations. An increase of the current density of I_H in EC neurons during maturation might be due to either an increase of the number of identical ion channels or an additional expression of a different type of ion channel. 8-Bromo-cAMP increased amplitudes of I_H in stellate cells, while I_H of pyramidal cells remained unchanged (Richter, Heinemann, and Eder; unpublished observation). Therefore, it is suggested that different types of hyperpolarization-activated cation channels are expressed in these two types of EC cells.

INTRINSIC AND SYNAPTIC PROPERTIES OF THE MEDIAL EC LAYER II CELLS

Layer II, in particular of the lateral EC, is among the first region to show neurofibrillary tangles and neuropil threads during the onset of Alzheimer's disease.[56] The loss of layer II cells may in part be responsible for the early cognitive impairments seen in this disorder.[26]

It has been shown that the main projection cells in layer II of the EC are the spine stellate neurons (FIG. 2C).[57–61] Layer II stellate cells in the mEC have characteristic electrophysiological and morphological properties (FIGS. 2A–C).[58,60,61] These cells displayed sag potentials during subthreshold depolarizing or hyperpolarizing current injection as well as rebound depolarization following hyperpolarizing current injection (FIG. 2A).[58,61] These cells responded to synaptic stimulation from deep layers or lateral EC with a rather flat input-output curve, and therefore much larger stimuli are required to elicit action potentials in these cells than layer III projection cells (see below). These cells responded to electrical stimulation with a fast excitatory postsynaptic potential (EPSP) followed by a fast and slow inhibitory postsynaptic potential (IPSP),[60–62] which was interrupted by a depolarizing component (FIG. 2B). The different synaptic components could be pharmacologically identified by their sensitivity to AMPA and NMDA receptor antagonists, as well as to GABA$_A$ and GABA$_B$ receptor antagonists.[60–62] The depolarizing component between the fast and slow inhibitory potential is insensitive to APV and CNQX antagonists for NMDA and AMPA/kainate receptors, respectively (Schmitz, Hetka, Stenkamp, Behr, Gloveli, and Heinemann; unpublished observation). This APV-insensitive NMDA response could reliably be evoked from the lateral and deep EC, but not from the superficial layers and the parasubiculum, while the "classical" APV-sensitive NMDA response could be evoked from all stimulation sites (FIG. 3). Whole cell recordings of both types of NMDA-EPSCs as well as NMDA-induced currents revealed a clear difference in the strength of the voltage-dependent block by [Mg^{2+}]$_o$ ions. In addition, the decay time constant of the less APV-sensitive NMDA-EPSCs was significantly slower than that of the APV-sensitive NMDA-EPSCs. The faster kinetics and stronger Mg^{2+} sensitivity of "classical" APV-sensitive NMDA receptors are suitable for precise temporal coding, while the slower NMDA-EPSCs of less APV-sensitive receptors might be more important for detection of low frequency

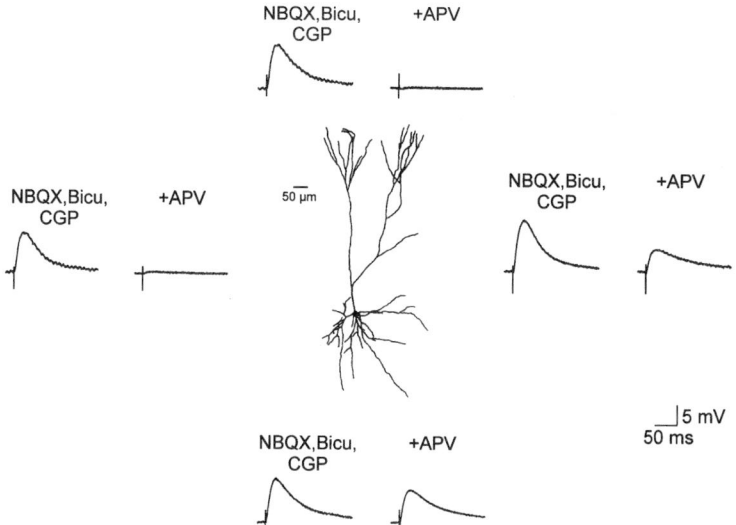

FIGURE 3. Synapse-specificity of two distinct types of NMDA-EPSPs. Stimulation of different synaptic inputs onto layer III EC neurons (camera lucida reconstruction of the biocytin-stained recorded neurons) revealed remarkable differences in the "expression" of the less APV-sensitive NMDA-EPSP. While stimulation of the lateral EC (right-hand) and deep layers of the EC (bottom) evoked a pronounced NMDA-EPSP in the presence of APV, the stimulation sites parasubiculum (left-hand) and superficial layers (top) of the EC did not. Note also slower kinetics of the remaining NMDA-EPSPs.

synchronicity. We suggest that most of the EC neurons express at least two distinct types of functional and molecular NMDA receptors (Schmitz, Hetka, Stenkamp, Behr, Gloveli, and Heinemann; unpublished observation).

INTRINSIC AND SYNAPTIC PROPERTIES OF THE
MEDIAL EC LAYER III CELLS

The glutamatergic projection from layer III cells to area CA1 activates predominantly inhibitory interneurons.[13] This projection may be critically involved in the activation of place cells,[63] which remain responsive after lesioning of the DG.[64] Recent evidence suggests that temporal lobe epilepsy and subforms of schizophrenia share lesions in layer III of the medial EC,[34,65,66] where the number of neurons and the thickness of the gray matter are reduced in comparison to control.[67,68]

Projection cells in layer III have distinctly different properties than layer II stellate neurons. None of the layer III cells presented robust hyperpolarization-activated sag potential or rhythmic membrane potential oscillations. Two types of projection cells within layer III of the mEC have been described.[69] Both type 1 and type 2 cells could be activated antidromically from the deep layers of the EC. In FIGURE 4, we show the morphology of an intracellularly stained, most abundant type 1 projection cell (B) of layer III as well as the intrinsic and synaptic properties (A, C). Type 1

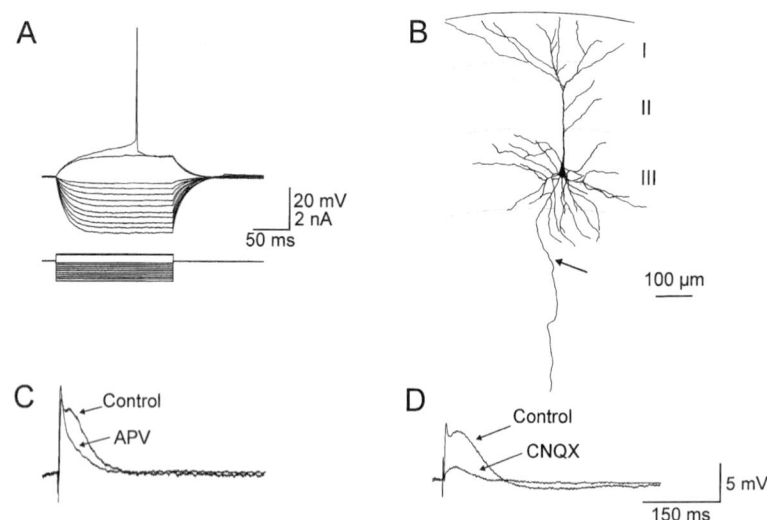

FIGURE 4. Electrophysiological and morphological properties of a typical projection pyramidal neuron of EC layer III. (**A**) Responses of this cell to hyperpolarizing and depolarizing current injection. (**B**) Camera lucida reconstruction of biocytin-stained neuron with soma located in layer II of the EC and with an axonal projection to the deep layers (arrow). (**C**) APV effectively reduced the prominent later part of the EPSPs. (**D**) CNQX reduced both components of the EPSPs and slow IPSP.

neurons responded to both hyperpolarizing and depolarizing intracellular current pulses in an approximately linear fashion until inward rectification occurred with extreme positive and negative current injection (FIG. 4A). The input-output curves were rather steep, with a doubling of the intensity for induction of a threshold EPSP, often bringing these cells above firing threshold.[61] This is in contrast to layer II stellate cells, where the input-output curves were rather flat, and stimulation intensity to evoke EPSP had to be multiplied by a factor of 4–5 in order to generate an action potential. These cells responded to electrical stimulation from the lateral EC with a pronounced EPSP, usually consisting of a distinct fast and slow component, that was then often followed by a small-amplitude slow IPSP (FIGS. 4C, 4D). In contrast to layer II cells, layer III projection cells responded with a long-lasting inhibitory potential to high frequency synaptic stimulation (see below). This slow hyperpolarization lasted up to 20 s.[70] Based on pharmacological evidence, the slow hyperpolarization could be discriminated into three components: (1) an early component sensitive to $GABA_B$ receptor antagonist and with a reversal potential close to -90 mV, representing a slow $GABA_B$-mediated IPSP; (2) a second component, with a reversal potential close to -84 mV, being sensitive to atropine and ($\pm$)-1-amino-cyclopentane-*trans*-1,3-dicarboxylic acid (t-ACPD); and (3) a third component being sensitive to naloxone.

INTRINSIC AND SYNAPTIC PROPERTIES OF DEEP LAYERS (IV–VI) OF THE MEDIAL EC

While the morphological and electrophysiological properties of superficial cells (layer II/III) have been well described, less is known about the properties of deep layer (layer IV–VI) cells. In addition to the "classical" major entorhino-dentate projection, arising from the superficial layers of the EC, the anatomical data demonstrated that a small number of deep layer (IV–VI) neurons of the EC also project to the DG and hippocampus.[14]

The synaptic responses of deep layer cells were composed of a fast AMPA/kainate receptor–mediated EPSP and a fast and slow $GABA_A$ and $GABA_B$ receptor–mediated IPSP, interrupted by a slow EPSP.[71] Our result indicated that not only stellate layer II cells can generate rhythmic membrane potential oscillations,[47] but the neurons of the deep layers are also able to produce them. In our slice preparation, about two-thirds (31 out of 50 neurons) of intracellulary recorded neurons were able to generate voltage-sensitive subthreshold membrane potential oscillations. At a membrane potential of about -50 mV, the mean frequency of the voltage oscillations was 8.1 Hz, while at slightly more positive potential (-44 mV) the frequency was 20 Hz.[71] Pharmacological experiments revealed that the oscillations were not affected by Cs^+, but could be blocked by the fast Na^+-channel blocker TTX. The synaptic stimulation of the subiculum or the DG evoked antidromic responses in these rhythmic cells. The electrophysiological and pharmacological experiments revealed similar mechanisms (voltage and Na^+ dependency) for the deep EC neuron oscillations as reported for the stellate layer II cells.[47,58] Therefore, it seems that these kinds of oscillations are unique to the EC since oscillations in other principal neurons typically rely on the activation of voltage-dependent Ca^{2+} conductances.[72,73]

Since stimulation of the DG leads to antidromic activation in some of the deep layer rhythmic cells, one might argue that at least some of the tested neurons contributed to the newly described pathway from the deep layers to the DG.[15] Our further set of experiments confirms this assumption. A substantial number of pyramidal projection cells to the DG exhibit a low threshold membrane potential oscillation. In addition, deep layer vertical bipolar and few multipolar non-GABAergic cells contribute to this projection (Gloveli, Dugladze, Schmitz, and Heinemann; unpublished observation).

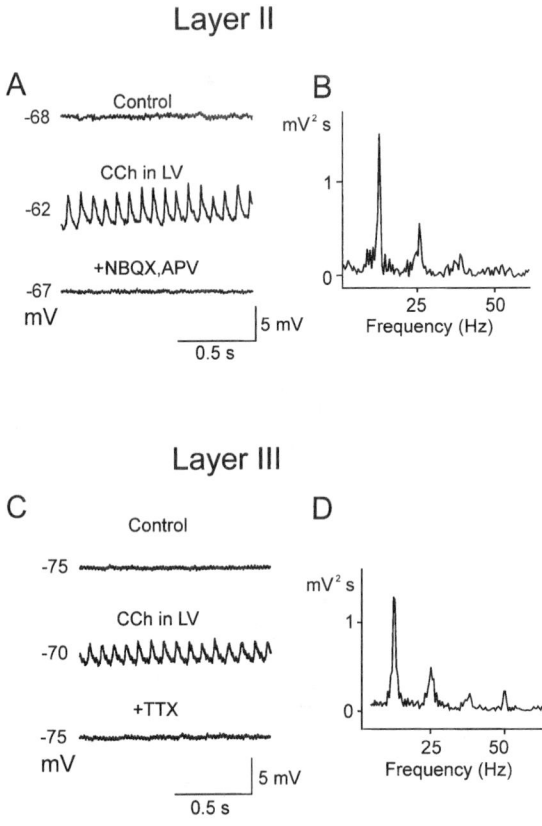

FIGURE 5. Synaptic oscillations in layer II stellate and layer III pyramidal cells. **(A)** Muscarinic receptor activation with CCh application in deep layers leads to prominent rhythmic activity in the layer II stellate cell (CCh in LV), which was abolished by addition of ionotropic glutamate receptor antagonists (10 μM NBQX, 60 μM APV). **(B)** Frequency spectrum of CCh-induced synaptic rhythmic activity in this stellate cell shows three characteristic peaks. Mean frequencies were 11.0 ± 0.5 Hz, 23 ± 1.2 Hz, and 36.7 ± 1.2 Hz. **(C)** CCh application into layer V (CCh in LV) evoked in layer III cells, as in stellate cells, a synaptic oscillation that was blocked in the presence of TTX. **(D)** Frequency spectrum of synaptic oscillation activity in this layer III cell shows three characteristic peaks. Mean frequencies were 10.6 ± 1.2 Hz, 23.8 ± 1.7 Hz, and 40.0 ± 1.0 Hz.

To examine the issue of whether deep layers play a leading role in the generation of epileptiform activity in the EC,[33,74] we used muscarinic receptor activation of the deep layers by pressure-pulse application of carbachol (CCh) in these layers and studied changes on excitability and intracellular Ca^{2+} signaling in layer II stellate and layer III pyramidal cells of the EC. In contrast to pressure-pulse application in layer II or III close to the recorded cells, low concentration of CCh (1 mM) applied into the deep layers consistently evoked a membrane potential fluctuation in the theta and gamma frequency range (FIGS. 5A–D) and in some cells even a prolonged series of epileptiform discharges. These results are in agreement with recent work by Dickson and Alonso,[74] demonstrating CCh-induced epileptiform activity in the EC that was usually driven by deep layers. In both cell classes, the rhythmic membrane potential changes were synaptically mediated by activation of cells in the deep layers of the EC as their frequency was voltage-independent, and they were blocked by the ionotropic glutamate receptor antagonists (NBQX, APV; FIG. 5A).

In contrast to CCh, activation of the serotonergic system evoked suppression of synaptic transmission in the superficial EC. Experiments with serotonin in the EC revealed a dose-dependent suppression of both excitatory[35,75] and polysynaptic IPSP, which contrasts with data from hippocampal pyramidal cells where high concentrations of serotonin are necessary to reduce EPSPs[76] and where lower concentrations can even transiently increase the EPSP amplitude.[76,77] Recent data from our laboratory suggest that the depression of synaptic excitation by 5-HT is caused by a presynaptic reduction of glutamate released from the axonal terminals. The effects of serotonin on layer III cells of the EC, which predominantly activate inhibitory cells in area CA1,[13,78] may well contribute to the disinhibition of area CA1, thereby increasing the excitability in this region.

FREQUENCY-DEPENDENT INFORMATION TRANSFER FROM THE SUPERFICIAL LAYERS OF THE EC TO THE HIPPOCAMPUS

In the hippocampus, storage of information is thought to be promoted during periods where rhythmical activity is generated.[79,80] *In vivo* experiments have shown that layer III of the EC can mediate activation of place cells in the hippocampus, which fire only when the animal is located at a specific location in a complex environment.[81] While place cell activation frequently occurs at a relatively low frequency background EEG,[82] layer II EC cells are rhythmically active during exploratory behavior associated with EEG activity in the theta rhythm range.[38] Therefore, one might speculate that the information transfer from the EC to the hippocampus is regulated in a frequency-dependent manner. To test this hypothesis, we studied how the separate pathways from layers II and III of the medial EC to the hippocampus are activated as a function of stimulation frequency. During low frequency (<10 Hz) stimulation of the lateral EC, layer III neurons are much more likely to fire action potentials than layer II cells (FIGS. 6C, 6F). When high frequency stimulus trains (>10 Hz) were applied, layer III neurons initially fired, but then rapidly ceased to generate action potentials (FIG. 6D). Thus, on high frequency activation, there was only a short firing period of these neurons early during a stimulus train at a time where layer II cells usually did not fire yet action potentials (FIG. 6B). Thus, under low frequency synaptic stimulation, the pathway from layer III to CA1 and to the

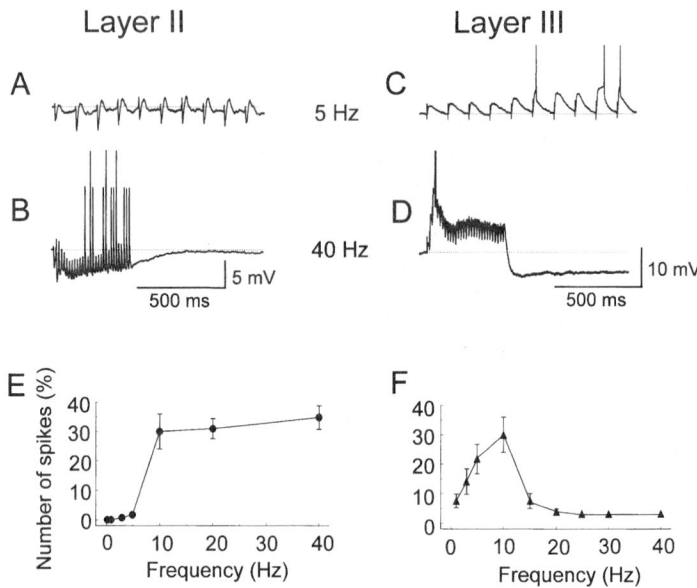

FIGURE 6. Different synaptic responses of layer II and III cells on repetitive stimulation. **(A)** On low frequency (5 Hz or lower) subthreshold stimulation, layer II cells did not produce any action potentials at all during the stimulus train. **(B)** However, when stimulation frequencies were increased (>10 Hz), fast EPSPs often induced action potentials during trains of stimulation, even when cells were hyperpolarized. **(C)** In contrast to layer II cells, EPSPs in layer III cells summated and generated action potentials on low frequency (10 Hz or lower) subthreshold stimulation. **(D)** During high frequency repetitive stimulation (>10 Hz), only one or two action potentials could be elicited. **(E, F)** Average number of action potentials (in percent of applied stimuli) induced by 20 stimuli of lateral EC with indicated frequencies in layer II (E) and layer III (F) cells. Data from 7 and 6 cells, respectively.

subiculum was activated, while the hippocampal trisynaptic loop (via layer II to the DG) remained quiet. In contrast, higher frequency synaptic activation of the EC was more effective in generating action potentials from layer II EC neurons (FIGS. 6B and 6E).

Thus, a frequency switch might operate in the EC regulating output of layer II and III to the hippocampal formation. Although the situation *in vivo* might be different, some of the present results agree well with those from *in vivo* observations. It was consistently shown that layer II cells of the EC *in vivo* display a net hyperpolarization in response to high frequency afferent stimulation[83] similar to the situation in our *in vitro* experiments. It was shown that most DG cells *in vivo* are probably silent or discharged at very low rates[84] and that their intrinsic properties confer a high threshold for synaptic activation (see reference 85). Therefore, high frequency discharges of layer II cells, noted in our study during high frequency stimulation, could be required to pass information via the trisynaptic loop. In contrast, the inhibition of layer III projection cells under the same conditions could relieve the direct inhibitory influence[13,78] on principal cells in area CA1.

ACKNOWLEDGMENTS

This work was supported by the BMBF and the DFG grants INK21/A1-1. We are grateful for technical assistance to A. Düerkop.

REFERENCES

1. WITTER, M.P. *et al.* 1989. Functional organization of the extrinsic and intrinsic circuitry of the parahippocampal region. Prog. Neurobiol. **33:** 161–253.
2. ZOLA-MORGAN, S.M. *et al.* 1989. Lesions of perirhinal and parahippocampal cortex that spare the amygdala and hippocampal formation produce severe memory impairment. J. Neurosci. **9:** 4355–4370.
3. MISHKIN, M. & E.A. MURRAY. 1994. Stimulus recognition. Curr. Opin. Neurobiol. **4:** 200–206.
4. MEUNIER, M. *et al.* 1996. Effects of rhinal cortex lesions combined with hippocampectomy on visual recognition memory in rhesus monkeys. J. Neurophysiol. **75:** 1190–1205.
5. BURWELL, R.D. *et al.* 1995. Perirhinal and postrhinal cortices of the rat: a review of the neuroanatomical literature and comparison with findings from the monkey brain. Hippocampus **5:** 390–408.
6. NABER, P.A. *et al.* 1997. Parallel input to the hippocampal memory system through peri- and postrhinal cortices. NeuroReport **8:** 2617–2621.
7. BURWELL, R.D. & D.G. AMARAL. 1998. Perirhinal and postrhinal cortices of the rat: interconnectivity and connections with the entorhinal cortex. J. Comp. Neurol. **391:** 293–321.
8. STEWARD, O. & S.A. SCOVILLE. 1976. Cells of origin of entorhinal cortical afferents to the hippocampus and fascia dentata of the rat. J. Comp. Neurol. **169:** 347–370.
9. RUTH, R.E. *et al.* 1988. Topographical relationship between the entorhinal cortex and the septotemporal axis of the dentate gyrus in rats: II. Cells projecting from lateral entorhinal subdivisions. J. Comp. Neurol. **270:** 506–516.
10. RUTH, R.E. *et al.* 1982. Topography between the entorhinal cortex and the dentate septotemporal axis in rats: I. Medial and intermediate entorhinal projecting cells. J. Comp. Neurol. **209:** 69–78.
11. STEWARD, O. 1976. Topographic organization of the projections from the entorhinal area to the hippocampal formation of the rat. J. Comp. Neurol. **167:** 285–314.
12. WITTER, M.P. *et al.* 1988. Entorhinal projections to the hippocampal CA1 region in the rat: an underestimated pathway. Neurosci. Lett. **85:** 193–198.
13. EMPSON, R.M. & U. HEINEMANN. 1995. The perforant path projection to hippocampal area CA1 in the rat hippocampal-entorhinal cortex combined slice. J. Physiol. (Lond.) **484:** 707–729.
14. KÖHLER, C. 1985. A projection from the deep layers of the entorhinal area to the hippocampal formation in the rat brain. Neurosci. Lett. **56:** 13–19.
15. DELLER, T. *et al.* 1996. A novel entorhinal projection to the rat dentate gyrus: direct innervation of proximal dendrites and cell bodies of granule cells and GABAergic neurons. J. Neurosci. **16:** 3322–3333.
16. SWANSON, L.W. & W.M. COWAN. 1977. An autoradiographic study of the organization of the efferent connections of the hippocampal formation in the rat. J. Comp. Neurol. **172:** 49–84.
17. KÖHLER, C. 1985. Intrinsic projections of the retrohippocampal region in the rat brain. I. The subicular complex. J. Comp. Neurol. **236:** 504–522.
18. VAN GROEN, T. *et al.* 1986. The organization of the reciprocal connections between the subiculum and the entorhinal cortex in the cat: I. A neuroanatomical tracing study. J. Comp. Neurol. **250:** 485–497.
19. TAMAMAKI, N. & Y. NOJYO. 1995. Preservation of topography in the connections between the subiculum, field CA1, and the entorhinal cortex in rats. J. Comp. Neurol. **353:** 379–390.

20. VAN HAEFTEN, T. *et al.* 1995. Quantitative morphological analysis of subicular terminals in the rat entorhinal cortex. Hippocampus **5:** 452–459.
21. WITTER, M.P. *et al.* 1989. Topographical organization of the entorhinal projection to the dentate gyrus of the monkey. J. Neurosci. **9:** 216–228.
22. EICHENBAUM, H. *et al.* 1994. Two functional components of the hippocampal memory system. Behav. Brain Sci. **17:** 449–518.
23. CHO, Y.H. & R.P. KESNER. 1996. Involvement of entorhinal cortex or parietal cortex in long-term spatial discrimination memory in rats: retrograde amnesia. Behav. Neurosci. **110:** 436–442.
24. GABRIELI, J.D.E. *et al.* 1997. Separate neural bases of two fundamental memory processes in the human medial temporal lobe. Science **276:** 264–266.
25. FLICKER, C. *et al.* 1991. Mild cognitive impairment in the elderly: predictors of dementia. Neurology **41:** 1006–1009.
26. BRAAK, H. & E. BRAAK. 1993. Entorhinal-hippocampal interaction in mnestic disorders. Hippocampus **3**(suppl.)**:** 239–246.
27. CASTRÉN, E. *et al.* 1993. Differential effects of MK-801 on brain-derived neurotrophic factor mRNA levels in different regions of the rat brain. Exp. Neurol. **122:** 244–252.
28. GLOVELI, T. *et al.* 1997. Systemic administration of the phencyclidine compound MK-801 affects stimulus-induced field potentials selectively in layer III of rat medial entorhinal cortex. Neurosci. Lett. **221:** 93–96.
29. LINDÉN, A.M. *et al.* 1997. NMDA receptor 2C subunit is selectively decreased by MK-801 in the entorhinal cortex. Eur. J. Pharmacol. **319:** R1–R2.
30. OLNEY, J.W. *et al.* 1991. NMDA antagonist neurotoxicity: mechanism and prevention. Science **254:** 1515–1518.
31. FARBER, N.B. *et al.* 1993. Antipsychotic drugs block phencyclidine receptor–mediated neurotoxicity. Biol. Psychiatry **34:** 119–121.
32. OLNEY, J.W. & N.B. FARBER. 1995. Glutamate receptor dysfunction and schizophrenia. Arch. Gen. Psychiatry **52:** 998–1007.
33. JONES, R.S.G. & U. HEINEMANN. 1988. Synaptic and intrinsic responses of medial entorhinal cortical cells in normal and magnesium-free medium *in vitro.* J. Neurophysiol. **59:** 1476–1497.
34. DU, F. *et al.* 1995. Preferential neuronal loss in layer III of the medial entorhinal cortex in rat models of temporal lobe epilepsy. J. Neurosci. **15:** 6301–6313.
35. SCHMITZ, D. *et al.* 1997. Serotonin blocks different pattern of low Mg^{2+}-induced epileptiform activity in rat entorhinal cortex, but not hippocampus. Neuroscience **76:** 449–458.
36. INSAUSTI, R. *et al.* 1993. Plasticity in the entorhinal-hippocampal system. Hippocampus **3**(suppl.)**:** 289–292.
37. JONES, R.S.G. 1993. Entorhinal-hippocampal connections: a speculative view of their function. Trends Neurosci. **16:** 58–64.
38. MITCHELL, S.J. & J.B. RANCK, JR. 1980. Generation of theta rhythm in medial entorhinal cortex of freely moving rats. Brain Res. **189:** 49–66.
39. STEWART, M. *et al.* 1992. Firing relations of medial entorhinal neurons to the hippocampal theta rhythm in urethane anesthetized and walking rats. Exp. Brain Res. **90:** 21–28.
40. CHROBAK, J.J. & G. BUZSÁKI. 1994. Selective activation of deep layer (V–VI) retrohippocampal cortical neurons during hippocampal sharp waves in the behaving rat. J. Neurosci. **14:** 6160–6170.
41. YLINEN, A. *et al.* 1995. Sharp wave–associated high-frequency oscillation (200 Hz) in the intact hippocampus: network and intracellular mechanisms. J. Neurosci. **15:** 30–46.
42. CHROBAK, J.J. & G. BUZSÁKI. 1998. Gamma oscillations in the entorhinal cortex of the freely behaving rat. J. Neurosci. **18:** 388–398.
43. WHITE, J.A. *et al.* 1993. A heart-like Na^+ current in the medial entorhinal cortex. Neuron **11:** 1037–1047.
44. FAN, S. *et al.* 1994. Differences in voltage-dependent sodium currents exhibited by superficial and deep layer neurons of guinea pig entorhinal cortex. J. Neurophysiol. **71:** 1986–1991.
45. EDER, C. *et al.* 1991. Outward currents in rat entorhinal cortex stellate cells studied with conventional and perforated patch recordings. Eur. J. Neurosci. **3:** 1271–1280.

46. BRUEHL, C. & W.J. WADMAN. 1999. Calcium currents in acutely isolated stellate and pyramidal neurons of rat entorhinal cortex. Brain Res. **816:** 554–562.
47. ALONSO, A. & R.R. LLINÁS. 1989. Subthreshold Na^+-dependent theta-like rhythmicity in stellate cells of entorhinal cortex layer II. Nature **342:** 175–177.
48. EDER, C. & U. HEINEMANN. 1994. Current density analysis of outward currents in acutely isolated rat entorhinal cortex cells. Neurosci. Lett. **174:** 58–60.
49. EDER, C. & U. HEINEMANN. 1996. Potassium currents in acutely isolated neurons from superficial and deep layers of the rat entorhinal cortex. Pflüg. Arch. Eur. J. Physiol. **432:** 637–643.
50. PAPE, H-C. 1996. Queer current and pacemaker: the hyperpolarization-activated cation current in neurons. Annu. Rev. Physiol. **58:** 299–327.
51. HALLIWELL, J.V. & P.R. ADAMS. 1982. Voltage-clamp analysis of muscarinic excitation in hippocampal neurons. Brain Res. **250:** 71–92.
52. MCCORMICK, D.A. & H-C. PAPE. 1990. Properties of a hyperpolarization-activated cation current and its role in rhythmic oscillation in thalamic relay neurones. J. Physiol. (Lond.) **431:** 291–318.
53. SPAIN, W.J. *et al.* 1987. Anomalous rectification in neurons from cat sensorimotor cortex *in vitro*. J. Neurophysiol. **57:** 1555–1576.
54. RICHTER, H. *et al.* 1997. Developmental changes of inward rectifier currents in neurons of the rat entorhinal cortex. Neurosci. Lett. **228:** 139–141.
55. KASPER, E.M. *et al.* 1994. Pyramidal neurons in layer 5 of the rat visual cortex. II. Development of electrophysiological properties. J. Comp. Neurol. **339:** 475–494.
56. BRAAK, H. & E. BRAAK. 1991. Neuropathological staging of Alzheimer-related changes. Acta Neuropathol. Berl. **82:** 239–259.
57. LINGENHÖHL, K. & D.M. FINCH. 1991. Morphological characterization of rat entorhinal neurons *in vivo*: soma-dendritic structure and axonal domains. Exp. Brain Res. **84:** 57–74.
58. ALONSO, A. & R. KLINK. 1993. Differential electroresponsiveness of stellate and pyramidal-like cells of medial entorhinal cortex layer II. J. Neurophysiol. **70:** 128–143.
59. TAMAMAKI, N. & Y. NOJYO. 1993. Projection of the entorhinal layer II neurons in the rat as revealed by intracellular pressure-injection of neurobiotin. Hippocampus **3:** 471–480.
60. JONES, R.S.G. 1994. Synaptic and intrinsic properties of neurons of origin of the perforant path in layer II of the rat entorhinal cortex *in vitro*. Hippocampus **4:** 335–353.
61. GLOVELI, T. *et al.* 1997. Frequency-dependent information flow from the entorhinal cortex to the hippocampus. J. Neurophysiol. **78:** 3444–3449.
62. JONES, R.S.G. & U. HEINEMANN. 1991. Excitatory Amino Acids and Synaptic Transmission, pp. 265–285. Academic Press. London.
63. QUIRK, G.J. *et al.* 1992. The positional firing properties of medial entorhinal neurons: description and comparison with hippocampal place cells. J. Neurosci. **12:** 1945–1963.
64. MCNAUGHTON, B.L. *et al.* 1989. Hippocampal granule cells are necessary for normal spatial learning, but not for spatially selective pyramidal cell discharge. Exp. Brain Res. **76:** 485–496.
65. DU, F. *et al.* 1993. Preferential neuronal loss in layer III of the entorhinal cortex in patients with temporal lobe epilepsy. Epilepsy Res. **16:** 223–233.
66. JAKOB, H. & H. BECKMANN. 1994. Circumscribed malformation and nerve cell alterations in the entorhinal cortex of schizophrenics: pathogenetic and clinical aspects. J. Neural Transm. **98:** 83–106.
67. BROWN, R. *et al.* 1986. Postmortem evidence of structural brain changes in schizophrenia: differences in brain weight, temporal horn area, and parahippocampal gyrus compared with affective disorder. Arch. Gen. Psychiatry **43:** 36–42.
68. ROBERTS, G.W. 1990. Schizophrenia: the cellular biology of a functional psychosis. Trends Neurosci. **13:** 207–211.
69. GLOVELI, T. *et al.* 1997. Morphological and electrophysiological characterisation of layer III cells of the medial entorhinal cortex of the rat. Neuroscience **77:** 629–648.
70. GLOVELI, T. *et al.* 1997. Prolonged inhibitory potentials in layer III projection cells of the rat medial entorhinal cortex induced by synaptic stimulation *in vitro*. Neuroscience **80:** 119–131.
71. SCHMITZ, D. *et al.* 1998. Subthreshold membrane potential oscillations in neurones of deep layers of the entorhinal cortex. Neuroscience **85:** 999–1004.

72. JAHNSEN, H. & R.R. LLINÁS. 1984. Electrophysiological properties of guinea-pig thalamic neurones: an *in vitro* study. J. Physiol. (Lond.) **349:** 205–226.
73. LLINÁS, R.R. 1988. The intrinsic electrophysiological properties of mammalian neurons: insights into central nervous system function. Science **242:** 1654–1664.
74. DICKSON, C.T. & A. ALONSO. 1997. Muscarinic induction of synchronous population activity in the entorhinal cortex. J. Neurosci. **17:** 6729–6744.
75. SCHMITZ, D. *et al.* 1995. Serotonin reduces synaptic excitation of principal cells in the superficial layers of rat hippocampal-entorhinal cortex combined slices. Neurosci. Lett. **190:** 37–40.
76. SCHMITZ, D. *et al.* 1995. Serotonin and 8-OH-DPAT reduce excitatory transmission in rat hippocampal area CA1 via reduction in presumed presynaptic Ca^{2+} entry. Brain Res. **701:** 249–254.
77. SEGAL, M. 1990. Serotonin attenuates a slow inhibitory postsynaptic potential in rat hippocampal neurons. Neuroscience **36:** 631–641.
78. BUZSÁKI, G. 1984. Feed-forward inhibition in the hippocampal formation. Prog. Neurobiol. **22:** 131–153.
79. HUERTA, P.T. & J.E. LISMAN. 1993. Heightened synaptic plasticity of hippocampal CA1 neurons during a cholinergically induced rhythmic state. Nature **364:** 723–725.
80. MITCHELL, S.J. *et al.* 1982. Medial septal area lesions disrupt theta rhythms and cholinergic staining in medial entorhinal cortex and produce impaired radial arm maze behavioral in rats. J. Neurosci. **2:** 292–302.
81. MULLER, R.U. & J.L. KUBIE. 1989. The firing of hippocampal place cells predicts the future position of freely moving rats. J. Neurosci. **9:** 4101–4110.
82. O'KEEFE, J. & M.L. RECCE. 1993. Phase relationship between hippocampal place units and the EEG theta rhythm. Hippocampus **3:** 317–330.
83. FINCH, D.M. *et al.* 1986. Neurophysiology of limbic system pathways in the rat: projections from the subicular complex and hippocampus to the entorhinal cortex. Brain Res. **397:** 205–213.
84. MCNAUGHTON, B.L. *et al.* 1991. Contribution of granule cells to spatial representation in hippocampal circuits: a puzzle. *In* Kindling and Synaptic Plasticity. F. Morell, Ed.: 110–123. Birkhäuser. Boston.
85. LAMBERT, J.D.C. & R.S.G. JONES. 1990. A reevaluation of excitatory amino acid–mediated synaptic transmission in rat dentate gyrus. J. Neurophysiol. **64:** 119–132.

Oscillatory Activity in Entorhinal Neurons and Circuits

Mechanisms and Function

CLAYTON T. DICKSON,[a] JACOPO MAGISTRETTI,[a,b] MARK SHALINSKY,[a] BASSAM HAMAM,[a] AND ANGEL ALONSO[a,c]

[a]*Department of Neurology and Neurosurgery, Montreal Neurological Institute and McGill University, Montreal, Canada, H3A 2B4*

[b]*Dipartimento di Neurofisiologia Sperimentale, Istituto Nazionale Neurologico "C. Besta," Milan, Italy 20133*

ABSTRACT: Layers II and V of the entorhinal cortex (EC) occupy a privileged anatomical position in the temporal lobe memory system that allows them to gate the main flow of information in and out of the hippocampus, respectively. *In vivo* studies have shown that layer II of the EC is a robust generator of theta as well as gamma activity. Theta may also be present in layer V, but the layer V network is particularly prone to genesis of short-lasting high-frequency oscillations ("ripples"). Interestingly, *in vitro* studies have shown that EC layers II and V, but not layer III, have the potential to act as independent pacemakers of population oscillatory activity. Moreover, it has also been shown that subgroups of principal neurons both within layers II and V, but not layer III, are endowed with autorhythmic properties. These are characterized by subthreshold oscillations where the depolarizing phase is driven by the activation of "persistent" Na^+ channels. We propose that the oscillatory properties of layer II and V neurons and local circuits are responsible for setting up the proper temporal dynamics for the coordination of the multiple sensory inputs that converge onto EC and thus help to generate sensory representations and memory encoding.

OVERVIEW

The importance of the entorhinal cortex (EC) is usually considered in the context of acting as an interface between the hippocampus and the rest of the cortical mantle and, as such, it plays a pivotal role in the functions of the temporal lobe, particularly in the formation of memories.[1,2] The attributed role of the EC as an interface derives from its main extrinsic connections. Via a cascade of cortico-cortical connections, information from polysensory associational areas converges onto the superficial layers of the EC, which then project massively into the hippocampus via the perforant path. In turn, the hippocampus projects back to the deep layers of the EC, which redistribute the information processed by the hippocampus back to the neocortex, in

[c]Address for correspondence: Dr. Angel Alonso, Department of Neurology and Neurosurgery, Montreal Neurological Institute, 3801 University St., Montreal, Quebec, Canada H3A 2B4. Tel.: (514) 398-6901; fax: (514) 398-8106.
e-mail: mdao@musica.mcgill.ca

fact to the very same polysensory associational areas where the loop began.[3–5] On these purely anatomical grounds, the EC has thus been considered an intermediary in the neocortical-hippocampal dialogue.

Neuropsychological studies in humans and monkeys have revealed that although the memory role of the EC is tightly coupled to that of the hippocampus and neighboring regions (such as the perirhinal cortex), the EC also appears to play an independent role.[6,7] In addition, the analysis of the fine morphological and physiological organization of the EC has revealed a high degree of complexity in its local circuit arrangements and synaptic properties, as well as in the intrinsic biophysical properties of its neuronal elements.[8–11]

Since the classical studies of Adey and colleagues,[12,13] it has been known that the electrophysiological behavior of the EC is characterized by the presence of robust rhythmic activity. In particular, the EC shares with the hippocampus the expression of a very robust theta rhythm, which is also co-expressed with trains of gamma waves during exploring behavior in the awake animal as well as during REM sleep.[14–16] Theta and gamma activity in the EC is generated primarily by neurons from layers II and III[14,17] which, via their perforant path projections, rhythmically modulate the excitability of the dentate granule cells and CA1 pyramidal cells, respectively.[18,19] In addition to theta activity, the EC network also expresses, like the hippocampus, "sharp waves" that emerge from a high-frequency oscillatory discharge ("ripple") of the layer V neurons.[20,21] Sharp waves occur predominantly during slow-wave sleep, and EC and hippocampal sharp waves are closely associated in time.

As with other cortical rhythms, considerable controversy exists with respect to the functional significance of entorhinal/hippocampal theta and sharp-wave activity. Multiple lines of evidence have linked the expression of theta oscillations with memory function in rodents[22] as well as in humans.[23] How theta may contribute to memory function is an issue of debate. It is possible that theta oscillations create the appropriate temporal dynamics between presynaptic activity and postsynaptic excitability that favors synaptic plasticity.[24,25] It is also possible that theta oscillations in the EC act by implementing a synchronizing mechanism by which convergent information is temporally coordinated for the ultimate generation of a memory representation (in the form of the population distribution of spike times and patterns).[26–28] With respect to the sharp-waves, perhaps the most currently favored hypothesis is that the high-frequency discharges associated with the sharp wave represent a mechanism by which encoded information in the hippocampal/entorhinal network is transferred back to the neocortex.[29]

From a reductionistic point of view, a way by which we might be able to clarify the functional significance of neuronal oscillations is by dissecting out their basic mechanisms.[30] Over the last 10 years, work carried out by several laboratories using a variety of approaches from *in vitro* to *in vivo* electrophysiological studies and computational modeling analysis has very substantially clarified the mechanisms by which population oscillations emerge in the hippocampus. Knowledge regarding the origin of oscillatory activities in the entorhinal cortex and understanding of the relation of these activities to those of the hippocampus and neocortex lag somewhat behind. Given the key anatomical position of the entorhinal cortex, clarifying these issues seems essential to understand the function(s) of the temporal lobe. By primarily using *in vitro* electrophysiological techniques, much of the work carried out in our laboratory centers on determining the building blocks within the entorhinal neurons and circuits that determine the emergence of population oscillations. Our current state of knowledge is reviewed in this paper. Importantly, both EC layers II and V express a very robust tendency toward intrinsic oscillatory activity, both at the single-cell and circuit levels. In contrast, neurons from layer III do not express intrinsic autorhythmicity, and the local circuits within layer III also do not appear to be able to sustain independent oscillatory activity. Interestingly, the mechanism by which autorhythmicity is generated by layer II and V neurons is similar in that in both cases it depends on the activation of a "persistent" sodium current (and not Ca^{2+} conductances) though it differs in other fundamental aspects. Synchronized activity generated by the deep EC layers also appears to be able to control, and potentially produce plastic changes in, the activity of the superficial layers, but not vice versa. We discuss the potential role of these findings regarding the functional role of the entorhinal cortex in memory function and also their implication for temporal lobe epileptogenesis.

OSCILLATORY PROPERTIES OF LAYER II NEURONS

The most abundant cell type in layer II of the EC is the spiny "stellate cell" of Ramon y Cajal.[31] These neurons give rise to the most prominent component of the perforant path, which terminates on dentate granule cells as well as on CA3 pyramidal cells. Electrophysiological studies *in vivo* have shown that during epochs of theta rhythm most neurons in EC layer II typically fire at a lower frequency than theta although spiking keeps very precise phase relationships with the field theta waves.[17] Importantly, the analysis of the intrinsic electroresponsiveness of the stellate cells has revealed that these neurons in fact possess robust autorhythmic properties. As illustrated in FIGURE 1, while these neurons are typically silent at rest, when the membrane potential is depolarized positive to about −60 mV (either by direct current injection or via modulatory influences), they consistently develop low-amplitude (1–4 mV) rhythmic subthreshold oscillations in the theta range of frequencies (about 8 Hz). These oscillations are persistent in that they are maintained for as long as the membrane potential is set in the subthreshold range. Interestingly, as the membrane potential approaches spike threshold, action potentials invariably occur at the peak of the oscillations though they may skip multiple subthreshold cycles. The fact that the stellate cells display "theta" pacemaker properties suggests that *in vivo* these properties may act in conjunction with the known rhythmic synaptic input from the medial septum to generate the expression of synchronized (or rhythmically orchestrated) population activity.

In order to understand how the subthreshold oscillations may contribute to the processing of synaptic inputs, and interact with some of these inputs to generate synchronized (a timely orchestrated) activity, it is important to understand which the biophysical mechanisms are that generate these oscillations. It was originally shown by Alonso and Llinás[32] that, in contrast to the Ca^{2+}-dependent oscillatory activity expressed by thalamic and other central nervous system (CNS) neurons, the subthreshold oscillations generated by the stellate cells depend on the activation of a TTX-

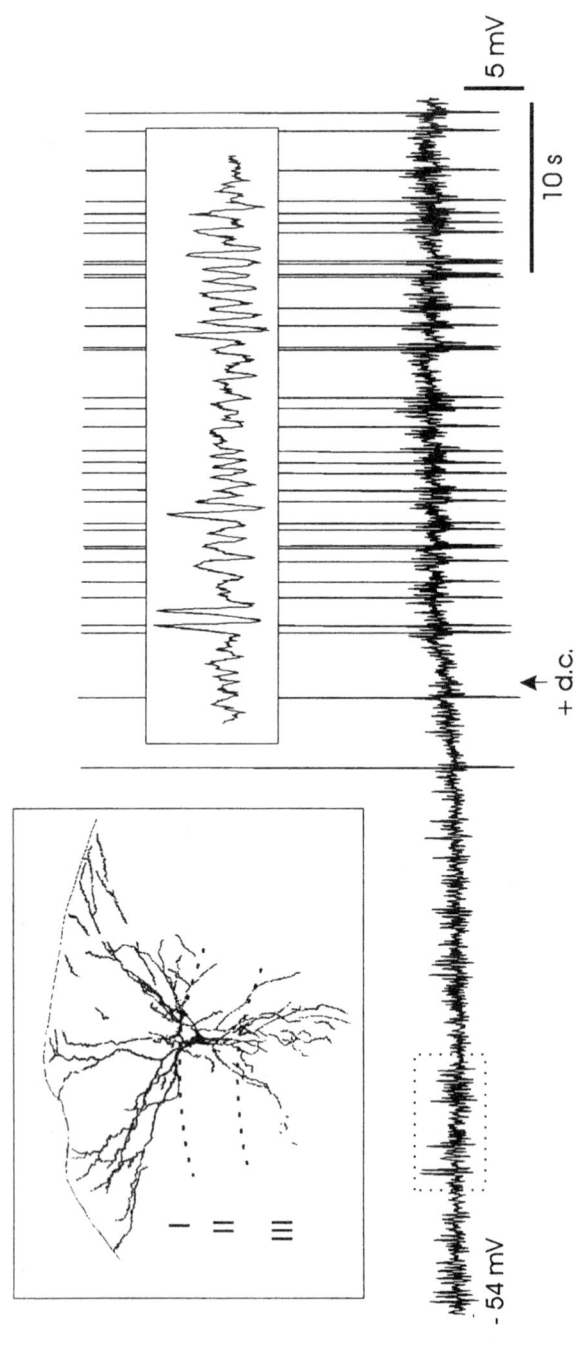

FIGURE 1. Representative subthreshold membrane potential oscillatory behavior of EC layer II stellate cell (*top left inset*), rhythmic subthreshold membrane potential oscillations developed with injection of depolarizing current positive to −55 mV. The boxed region highlighting the rhythmic nature of this oscillatory process is seen expanded in the *upper right inset*. As the cell is further depolarized at the arrow shown, the cell begins to discharge in a characteristic cluster pattern. Note that spikes tend to occur at the peak of subthreshold oscillations.

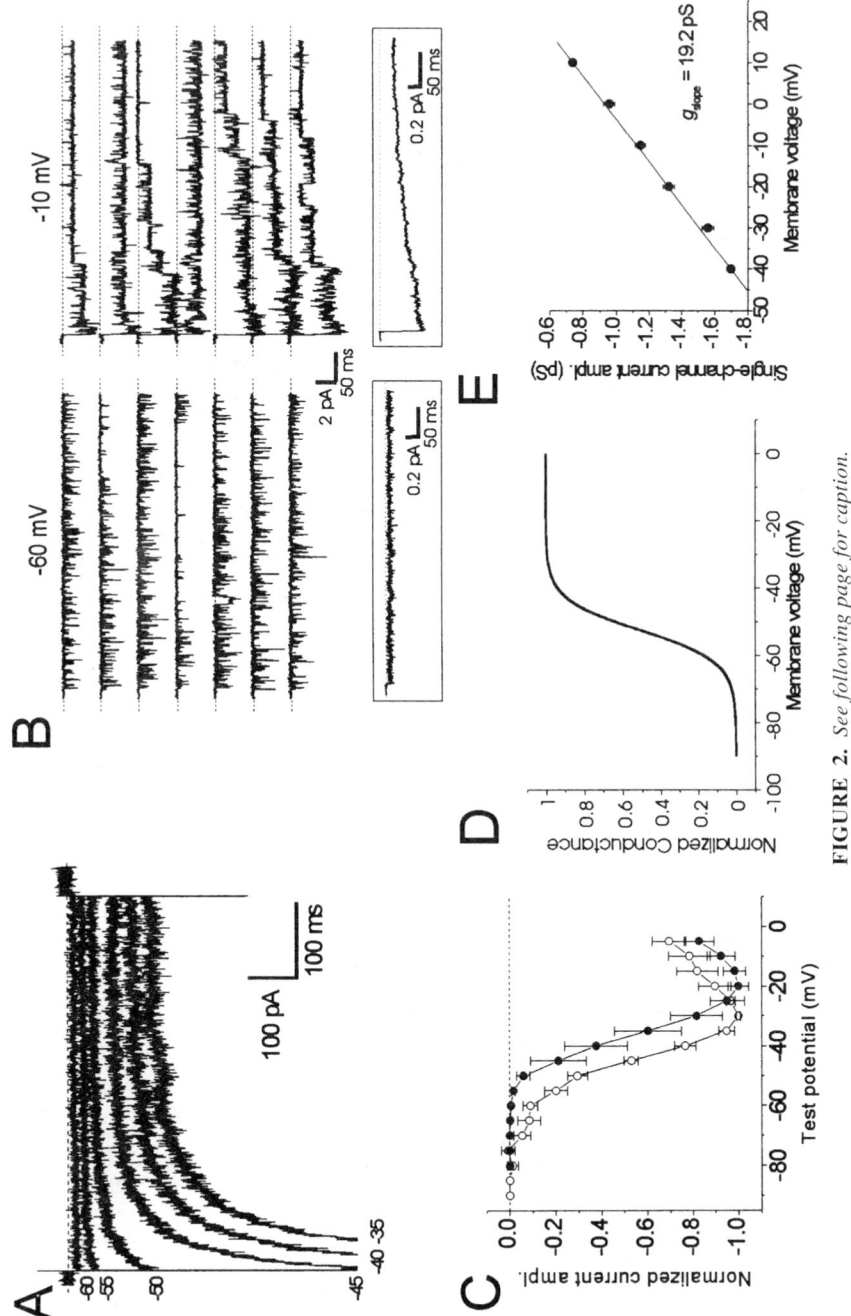

FIGURE 2. *See following page for caption.*

sensitive Na^+ current, and it was proposed that the oscillations emerge from the interaction between this Na^+ current and a hyperpolarization-activated cation current (I_h).

A recent series of whole-cell and single-channel studies of Na^+ currents expressed by the stellate cells has indeed demonstrated that these neurons express a low-threshold persistent Na^+ current (I_{NaP}) that is generated by sustained single-channel activity characterized by a higher conductance than the transient single-channel activity.[33,34] FIGURE 2 summarizes these studies. Panel A depicts the whole-cell Na^+ current evoked by 0.5 s voltage-clamp steps from a holding potential of –80 mV in a dissociated stellate cell. In addition to the large amplitude transient I_{Na} (I_{NaT}), a significant persistent Na^+ current component is apparent. In the stellate cells, I_{NaP} has an activation threshold at about –65 mV, peaks at –30 mV (i.e., 10 mV more negative than I_{NaT}) and a $V_{1/2}$ of –53 mV (panels C and D). Whereas at –20 mV I_{NaP} represents only about 1% of the total Na^+ current, within the oscillatory voltage range (–60 to –50 mV), I_{NaP} accounts for more than 80% of the total Na^+ current. In the cell-attached configuration, persistent Na^+ channel activity that has a low threshold for activation can be observed either in isolation, as shown in panel B, or in combination with transient Na^+ channel activity. The estimated single-channel conductance of persistent Na^+ channels is about 20 pS (panel E), significantly larger than that of transient Na^+ channels (15 pS).[34] Whatever the molecular basis of the persistent Na^+ channels turns out to be (see Ref. 33 for discussion), it seems clear that a rather specialized mechanism governs the excitability of the stellate cells in the subthreshold range controlling the way these neurons approach spike threshold.

I_{NaP} must constitute the inward current that gives rise to the depolarizing phase of the subthreshold oscillations. However, to generate an oscillation, a process is needed whose action, by feedback, slows down the rate of the process itself and, most critically, a delay in the execution of the feedback. By analogy with the repolarizing phase of the action potential, one obvious possibility would be that a slow outward K current, such as the M current, gives rise to the repolarizing phase of the subthreshold oscillatory cycle. However, voltage-clamp analysis gives no indication

---

FIGURE 2. Voltage-clamp recordings characterizing the persistent Na^+ current in acutely dissociated EC layer II stellate cells. (**A**) Representative traces showing both I_{NaT} and I_{NaP} at high gain. Depolarizing voltage steps were delivered at test potentials of –60 to –35 mV in 5 mV steps, from a holding potential of –80 mV. All the traces shown are TTX subtracted (control minus 1 µM TTX). (**B**) Single-channel currents in a patch exhibiting a high level of persistent activity. Na^+ channel currents were evoked by consecutive 500 ms depolarizing pulses to –60 or –10 mV (*left* and *right panels*, respectively). *Insets* below individual traces show ensemble average currents obtained from sets of 20 consecutive sweeps. (**C**) Mean current-voltage relationships for whole-cell currents corresponding to I_{NaT} (*closed circles*; $n = 8$) and I_{NaP} (*open circles*; $n = 5$). I_{NaT} amplitudes were measured at the current peak. I_{NaP} amplitudes were derived by averaging the data points between 400 and 500 ms from the start of each test. Symbols and error bars show means ± SD. (**D**) Activation curve of G_{NaP} as derived from step protocols (I_{NaP} amplitude was measured by averaging the data points between 400 and 500 ms from the pulse onset; $n = 5$). The Boltzmann fit gave a $V_{1/2}$ of –44.4 mV, and a slope factor (k) of –5.2 mV. (**E**) Voltage dependence of persistent single-channel current amplitude. Only openings occurring at least 20 ms after the start of the test pulse were considered. Data points are from eight patches. The *straight line* is a linear least squares fit of the mean data points, with the slope conductance value given in the graph. (Modified from Magistretti *et al.*[34])

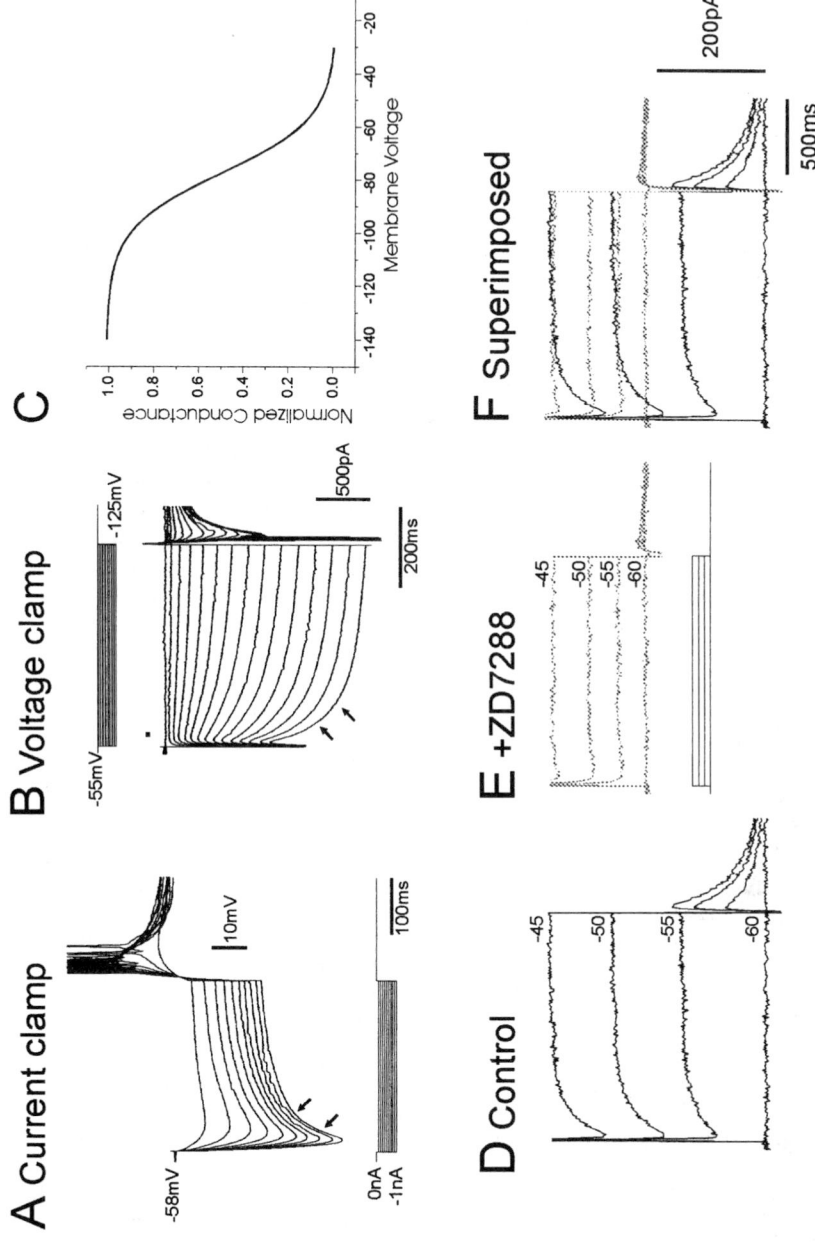

FIGURE 3. *See following page for caption.*

of an M-like current being activated in the oscillatory voltage range and, in addition, muscarinic activation of the stellate cells does not abolish the oscillations.[35] However, the stellate cells do display a very robust time-dependent inward rectification which is generated by a hyperpolarization-activated nonspecific cation current (I_h) (FIG. 3A to C).[36] In the stellate cells, I_h has an activation threshold at about –45 mV and a $V_{1/2}$ at about –75 mV. I_h is thus substantially active in the oscillatory voltage range. How can the inward I_h current cause the repolarizing phase of the oscillation? A time dependence exists not only in the activation process of I_h, but also in its deactivation. As illustrated in FIGURE 3D, membrane depolarization throughout the oscillatory voltage range causes slow outward current relaxations due to the deactivation of I_h. Conceptually, the deactivation of an inward current, as in this case, can be seen as being equivalent to the activation of an outward current. Thus, the net outward current produced by the deactivation of I_h can potentially stop the I_{NaP} driven depolarization and lead to the repolarizing phase of the oscillation. If so, the selective blocker of I_h ZD7288 (FIG. 3D and E) should block the oscillations—which, in fact, is the case.[36]

Given that both I_h and I_{NaP} are necessary for the production of the subthreshold oscillatory properties of EC layer II stellate cells as evidenced above, we wished to further characterize their interaction to test whether their interplay constitutes a sufficient condition for the production of an oscillatory state in the subthreshold range. This was conducted by incorporating the kinetic and voltage-dependent parameters concerning I_h and I_{NaP} in a simplified single-compartment model of the stellate cell, which also included a linear leak conductance. The model, summarized in FIGURE 4, could reproduce with excellent accuracy the characteristics "sags" in membrane potential in response to hyperpolarizing current pulses. In addition, and most importantly, it could also reproduce the generation of subthreshold oscillations upon membrane depolarization. In fact, the model allows us to understand the dynamics of the interactions between I_h and I_{NaP} in the production of membrane potential os-

---

FIGURE 3. Characterization of I_h in EC layer II stellate cells using whole-cell recording methods in the slice preparation. (**A**) In current-clamp conditions, hyperpolarizing current pulses evoke voltage responses with a robust time-dependent depolarizing sag (*arrows*). (**B**) In the same neuron, under voltage-clamp conditions, hyperpolarizing voltage steps evoke a slow inward current (I_h) that grows in amplitude and rate of activation with increasing hyperpolarization. (**C**) Average activation curve of I_h as characterized by normalization of I_h tail currents evoked at a constant potential following steps throughout the range shown. Note that within the oscillatory range of potentials (–60 to –50 mV) a sufficient proportion of I_h is active. (**D**) Voltage-clamp experiment in the presence of 1 μM TTX and 2 mM Co^{2+} showing outward current relaxations (corresponding to I_h deactivation) during depolarizing voltage steps through the oscillatory voltage level (–55, –50, and –45 mV), as well as inward current relaxations (corresponding to I_h activation) upon return to the holding potential (–60 mV). (**E**) Addition of 100 μM ZD7288 eliminated I_h and thus caused a robust outward shift in the holding current and the concomitant disappearance of the outward current relaxations upon depolarization, as well as the inward current relaxations upon return to the holding potential. However, outward rectification is still obvious, especially between the current traces corresponding to –50 and –45 mV. (**F**) Superimposition of traces in B and C. Note that control and ZD7288 current traces to –45 mV overlap perfectly at steady state thus indicating that in the voltage range examined the actions of ZD7288 were selective for I_h. (Modified from Dickson *et al.*[36])

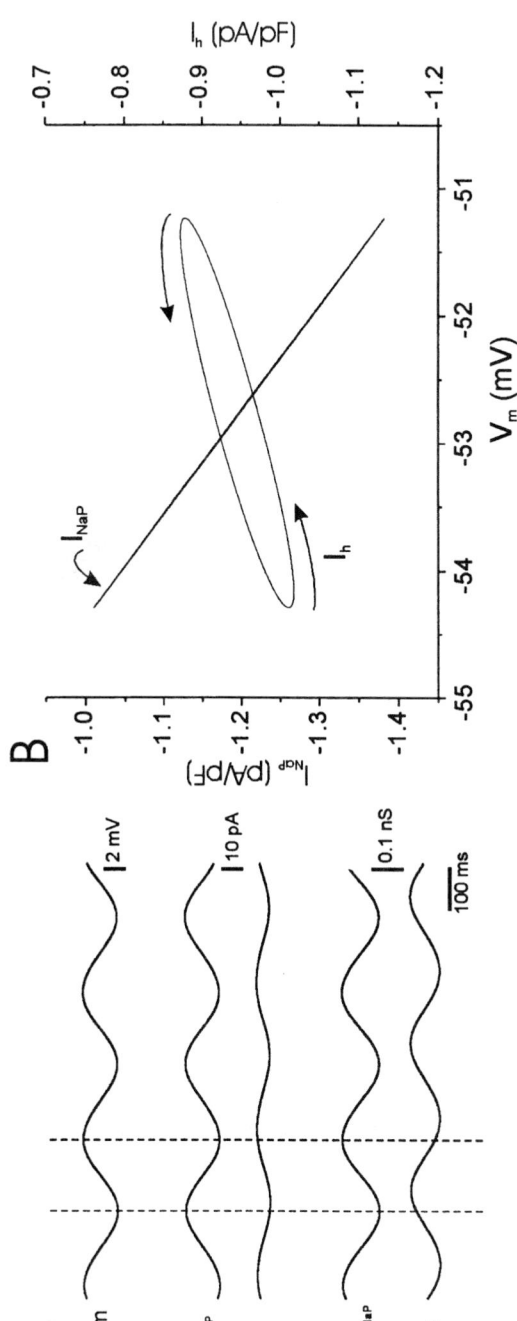

FIGURE 4. The interplay between I_h and I_{NaP} is sufficient to explain the oscillatory behavior of EC layer II cells. (**A**) Simulation of membrane potential oscillations in a single-compartment model evoked by the injection of +0.21 pA/pF and of the behavior of the underlying currents (I_h, I_{NaP}) and conductances (G_h, G_{NaP}). The vertical, dashed lines help in the appraisal of the phase relationships between the membrane potential, the currents, and their conductances. Note the almost perfect phase correspondence between V_m and I_{NaP}. (**B**) Phase plane plot of the simulated membrane potential versus the amplitude of both I_{NaP} and I_h. For the simulation shown in **A**, the amplitude of both I_{NaP} and I_h was plotted with respect to the membrane potential. The plot corresponding to I_{NaP} travels a straight line with negative slope showing no hysteresis. Therefore, during both the upswing and downswing of the oscillation there is a relatively "instantaneous" increase and decrease, respectively, in the amplitude of I_{NaP}. On the other hand, the plot corresponding to I_h demonstrates a large degree of hysteresis. Opposite to I_{NaP} during the upswing and downswing of the oscillation there is a delayed decrease and increase, respectively, in the amplitude of I_h. Due to this delay, the maxima and minima of the amplitude of I_h tend to occur just after the membrane potential has achieved its most hyperpolarized and depolarized values, respectively (i.e., just following the commencement of the upswing and downswing of the oscillation, respectively). (Modified from Dickson *et al.*[36])

cillations. In panel A, note that at the trough of an oscillation, I_{NaP} is at a minimum and that the maximum in I_h coincides with the initiation of the depolarizing phase. As depolarization proceeds, I_{NaP} rapidly increases. In turn, the depolarization boosted by I_{NaP} leads to the deactivation and thus the decrease in I_h, which slows down and eventually stops the depolarization. Note that the minimum in I_h occurs just after the peak. Thus, the deactivation of I_h is now responsible for initiating the repolarizing phase of the oscillation.

Note that in the modeled traces, I_{NaP} essentially changes instantaneously with changes in V_m while changes in I_h follow with a certain delay. When a phase plane plot of the membrane potential versus the amplitude of both I_{NaP} and I_h is constructed (panel B), it becomes apparent that the hysteresis introduced by the kinetic properties of I_h implements a delayed feedback mechanism to the voltage changes led by I_{NaP}. It is this interaction that allows the sustained oscillatory activity to occur.

Each stellate cell generates oscillations, but how can this process contribute to synchronization? A potential mechanism is illustrated in FIGURE 5. Layer II of the entorhinal cortex is very heavily innervated by GABAergic fibers, which are of both local[37,38] as well as extrinsic origin, the latter most likely deriving from the GABAergic projection cells of the medial septum.[39,40] Local stimulation of layer II typically causes an IPSP that is amplified in the subthreshold range by virtue of the gating properties of I_{NaP}. Independently of the phase of the oscillation at which the IPSP occurs, it will invariably cause membrane hyperpolarization accompanied by an "instant" deactivation of I_{NaP} and delayed activation of I_h. The result is a rebound phenomenon boosted now by the activation of I_{NaP}, which triggers the initiation of an intrinsic oscillatory cycle. As a consequence, a reset phenomenon takes place. When a population of stellate cells receives a synchronized inhibitory input, they

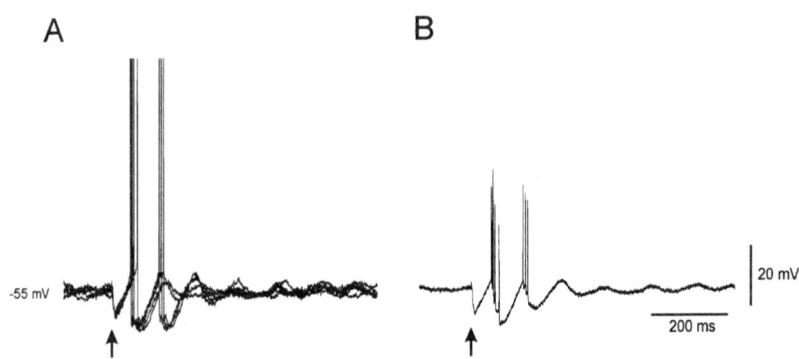

FIGURE 5. Inhibitory reset of subthreshold membrane potential oscillations in EC layer II stellate cells. (**A**) In a cell held at the oscillatory voltage range (in this example, approximately −55 mV), an IPSP evoked by proximal electrical stimulation of layer I results in one to two rebound spikes followed by a train of oscillations. Superimposition of individual traces reveals a good phase correspondence between the oscillations evoked following, but not previous to, the stimulation. (**B**) Averaging over all responses highlights this effect since the membrane potential is flat prior to the stimulus, but oscillates following it.

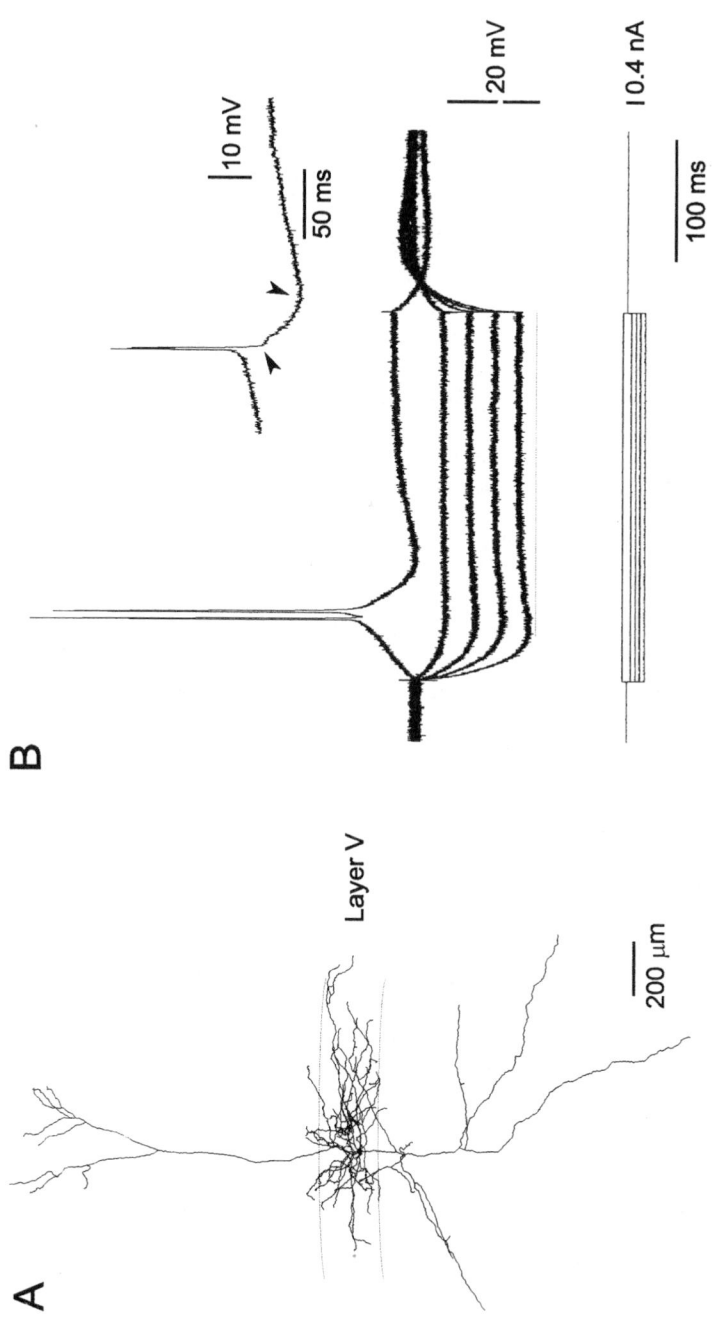

FIGURE 6. Typical electrophysiological profile of EC layer V horizontal cells. (**A**) Neurolucida reconstruction of a horizontal cell showing the vast majority of the basal dendritic tree confined to lamina V. (**B**) In the same neuron, voltage responses to depolarizing and hyperpolarizing current pulses from the resting level. The inset shows a typical bi-phasic hyperpolarizing afterpotential with a small depolarizing afterpotential. (Modified from Hamam *et al.*[45])

will then tend to fire in synchrony in an oscillatory manner. The synchronous inhibitory input could have an extrinsic origin (such as the medial septum) or could be locally generated, as we have recently shown in slices.[41]

OSCILLATORY PROPERTIES OF LAYER V NEURONS

While EC layer II provides the input to the hippocampus via the perforant path, EC layer V is the target of the cortically directed output of the hippocampus which arises primarily from the subiculum.[42,43] Neurons in layer V direct their output, in turn, to the rest of the cortical mantle. However, in addition to their extrinsic connections, layer V neurons also give rise to an important ascending pathway within the EC that appears to terminate on neurons in both layers III and II.[11,41,44] We characterized the morphology and intrinsic electroresponsiveness of layer V neurons expecting to find major differences with respect to layer II. Morphologically, layer V cells are obviously quite different because most of them are pyramidal cells. However, to our surprise we did find a wide spectrum of morphological subtypes that included large pyramidal cells as well as small pyramidal cells and two relatively unique subtypes that we named horizontal cells and polymorphic cells.[45] Like pyramidal cells, horizontal cells have an apical dendrite, but their basal dendritic tree extends almost exclusively in the horizontal plane and within the confines of layer V. Polymorphic cells lacked an apical dendrite and their dendritic tree could extend in all directions, sometimes even reaching the subiculum.

We found that the electrophysiological behavior of layer V neurons is also very heterogeneous, but none of the morphological subtypes could be unequivocally distinguished by their electrophysiological profile. Surprisingly, it appears that EC layer V is devoid of rhythmic bursting cells similar to those that are present in neocortical layer V or in the hippocampal CA3 subfield. The closest approximation to this electrophysiological behavior was found in neurons that fired in spike doublets (FIG. 6), and this activity was dependent on the activation of low-threshold Na^+ conductance. Some layer V neurons displayed time-dependent inward rectification (FIG. 6) but to a much lesser degree than the layer II stellate cells. The presence of I_h in these cells was not associated with the expression of subthreshold oscillations. However, to our surprise, we did find a large percentage (about 30%) of layer V neurons that did display a robust rhythmic subthreshold oscillatory activity similar to that expressed by the stellate cells. A typical example is illustrated in FIGURE 7. Note, in panel A, the subthreshold oscillations gradually develop as the cell is depolarized toward spike threshold, becoming very robust and of relatively large amplitude (3–5 mV) at about −55 mV. The frequency of these oscillations was constant for every cell, but varied from cell to cell and ranged from about 5 to 15 Hz.

Importantly, and as noted above, the expression of subthreshold oscillations by the layer V neurons was not associated at all with the presence of I_h. On the contrary, cells that lacked any trace of I_h tended to express more robust oscillatory activity. Preliminary work that we have carried out indicates that the layer V oscillations depend on the activation of I_{NaP} and an outward K^+ current. Thus, different ionic mechanisms appear to generate a similar pattern of rhythmicity in different neuronal populations.

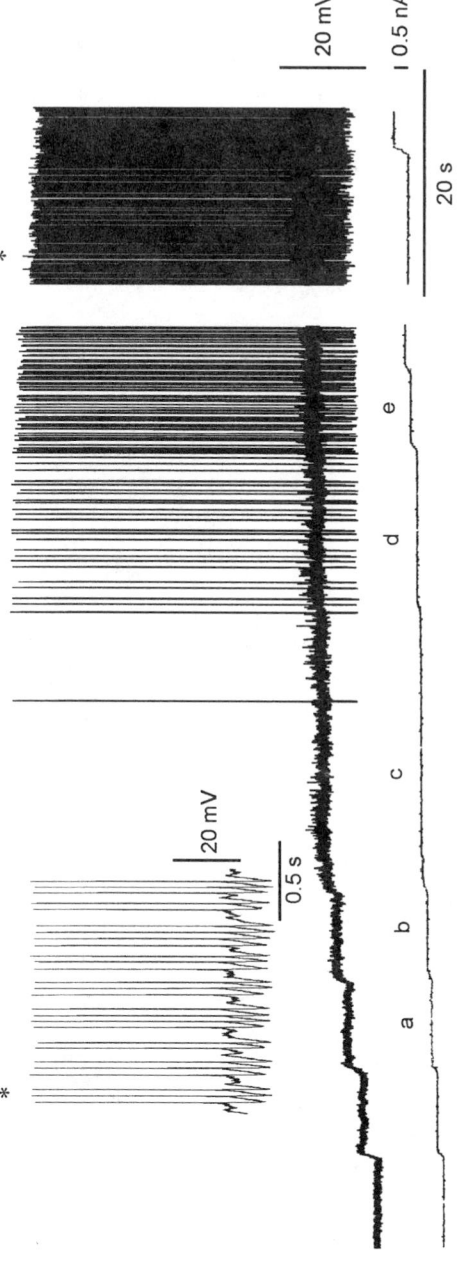

FIGURE 7. *See following pge for caption.*

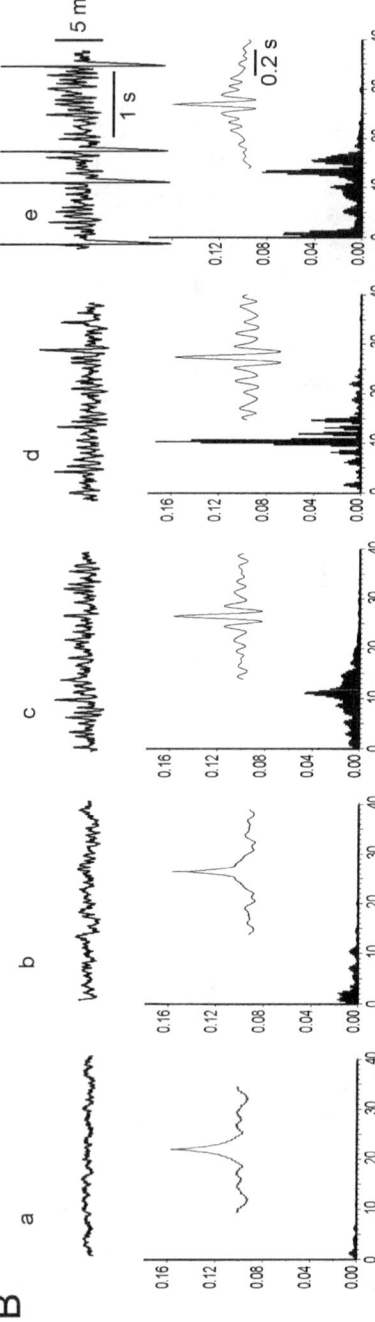

FIGURE 7. Representative subthreshold membrane potential oscillatory behavior of EC layer V horizontal cells. (**A**) Long-lasting trace demonstrating the changes in membrane potential as the cell is progressively depolarized by D.C. current injection from its resting level (about –64 mV). The increase in the voltage trace noise is a reflection of the emergence of subthreshold oscillations (as detailed in panel **B**). Note that at the most depolarized level the cell does not display tonic repetitive discharge, but rather intermittent spiking consisting of spike clusters interspersed by subthreshold oscillations (*inset to the right, asterisk*). (**B**) Expanded traces from **A** taken at the times indicated (a to e) demonstrating the appearance of robust subthreshold oscillations with membrane depolarization. The lower graphs are the power spectrum of the membrane potential and the corresponding autocorrelation function for each period. Note that the membrane potential is most rhythmic when the membrane potential is just below firing threshold (c and d). (Modified from Hamam *et al.*[45])

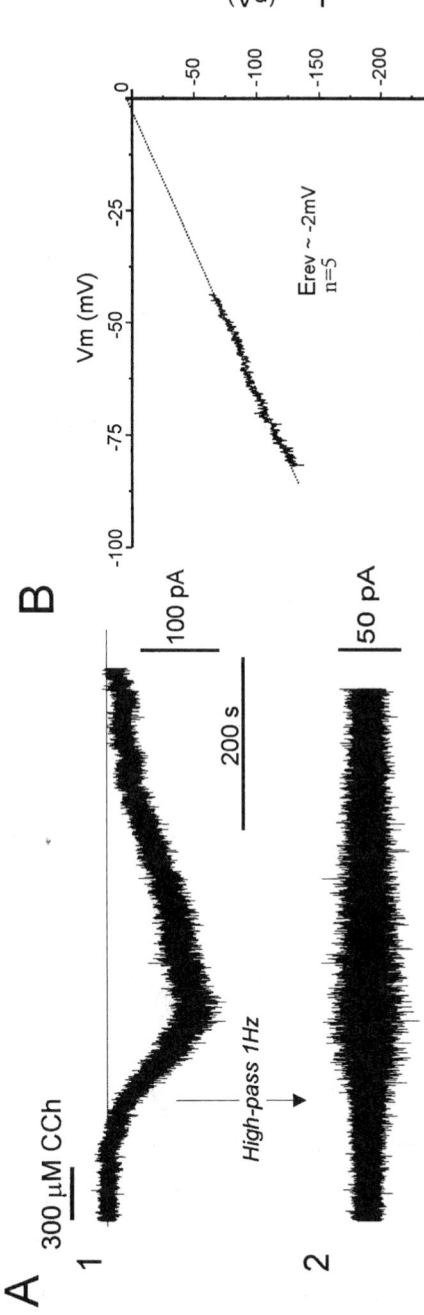

FIGURE 8. Muscarinic activation induces an inward current in EC layer II neurons. (**A**) (1) In the presence of 1 μM TTX and 2 mM Cs⁺, pressure pulse application of carbachol (CCh) evokes an inward current at a holding potential of −60 mV (approximately resting membrane potential). When the current trace is high-pass filtered, (2) the resulting trace shows a substantial increase in high-frequency noise following the application of CCh, suggesting an increase in channel openings. (**B**) Extrapolating the linear portion of the average IV curve of this current as calculated by subtraction of ramp protocols before and after CCh application reveals a reversal potential of approximately 0 mV, suggesting that the inward current has a mixed ionic nature.

CHOLINERGIC MODULATION OF OSCILLATORY DYNAMICS

The EC receives a very robust cholinergic innervation from the basal forebrain which distributes primarily on layers II and V. Since the cholinergic system is implicated in cortical activation and promotes the emergence of limbic theta rhythm, we explored the effects that muscarinic receptor activation would have on the subthreshold oscillations of both layer II and layer V cells, as well as on the induction of synchronized population activity.

At the single-cell level, we found, not surprisingly, that M1 receptor activation depolarizes both layer II and layer V cells. However, two issues were of importance. First, the mechanism for depolarization is not simply through a block of a K^+ conductance but also depends upon the activation of a nonspecific cation current that is modulated by a rise in the intracellular Ca^{2+} concentration.[46] Second, the expression of subthreshold oscillations becomes facilitated by the cholinergic activation, and is particularly prominent in layer V.

The mechanism of cholinergic action has been explored in great detail both under current-clamp and voltage-clamp conditions in layer II neurons. FIGURE 8 illustrates the point that during block of Na^+ channels with TTX, leak K^+ conductance block with Ba^{2+}, and, in the presence of glutaminergic and GABAergic synaptic transmission blockers, muscarinic receptor activation with carbachol (CCh) induces an inward current (panel A1) associated with a large increase in total transmembrane current noise (panel A2), thus indicating that the muscarinic-induced inward current is due to the opening of cation channels. By applying ramp protocols (not shown), we estimated the reversal potential of the muscarinic-induced inward current to be at about 0 mV (panel B).

The fact that in entorhinal neurons the muscarinic-induced cationic current is enhanced by a rise in intracellular Ca^{2+} [46] facilitates the emergence of a bi-stable behavior. Depolarization to a suprathreshold level elicits spiking, which in turn results in Ca^{2+} influx. This influx, illustrated in FIGURE 9, enhances the current and sustains a plateau depolarization. The figure shows the same layer V cell as that from FIGURE 7 during continuous superfusion with 30 μM CCh. There are a number of noteworthy observations to make. First, the application of CCh depolarized the membrane potential to the range at which subthreshold oscillations are expressed. Second, the application of CCh did not abolish the oscillations, suggesting that an M-type K^+ current is not involved in their generation. Finally, when a minor direct current injection is applied to initiate firing, this firing persists following removal of the injected current; and it can only be stopped following application of a long-duration hyperpolarizing current.

In addition to facilitating oscillatory dynamics at the single-cell level, muscarinic receptor activation also induces the emergence of synchronized population activity in the slice preparation. The spatiotemporal dynamics of this activity is complex and has been described in detail by Dickson and Alonso.[41] FIGURES 10 and 11 summarize some of the aspects that are perhaps more relevant in the context of this paper. The first point, shown in FIGURE 10, is that within the EC both layers V and layer II have the independent capacity to generate synchronous population activity with muscarinic receptor activation. Layer III, however, lacks the appropriate cellular and/or network properties to do so. Note in panel D that a microinjection of CCh centered in

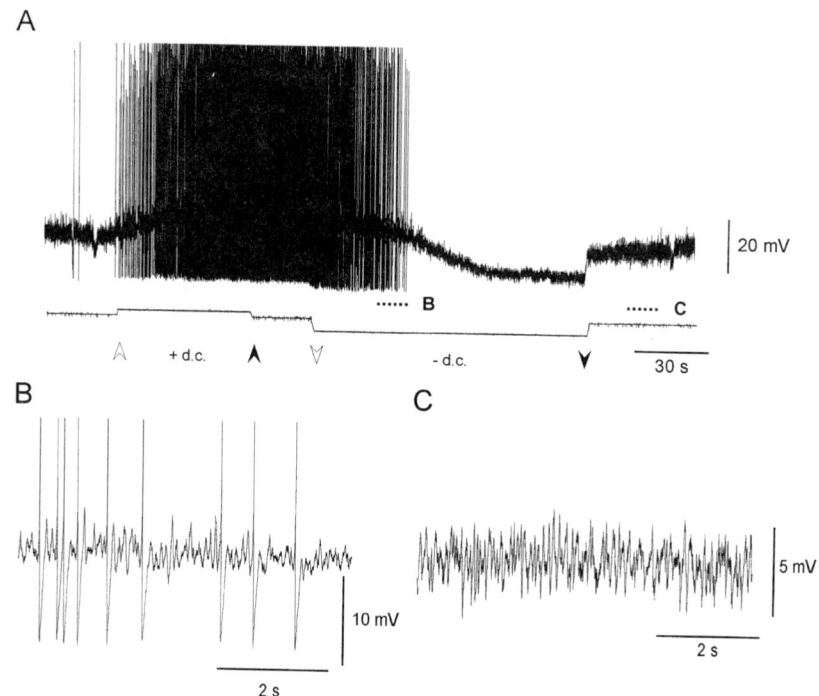

FIGURE 9. Muscarinic activation induces bi-stable membrane behavior in EC layer V neurons. (**A**) Current-clamp intracellular recording in a layer V neuron during a continuous (20 min) perfusion with 30 μM CCh. The initial effect of CCh was to depolarize the cell to the level at which intrinsic oscillations were expressed (shown at higher magnification in **B** and **C**). Further depolarization of the cell by injection of depolarizing current (*open arrowhead*) brings the cell to spike firing threshold and induces an afterdepolarization which was sustained following removal of depolarizing current (*closed arrowhead*). Restoration of the original membrane potential was achieved following a substantial and long-lasting injection of hyperpolarizing current (shown between the *open* and *closed asterisks*).

layer V generates bursts of activity that are then propagated toward layer II. Panel B shows how a microinjection centered in layer II can also generate population activity in layer II, but that in that case the activity does not propagate ventrally. On the other hand, a microinjection centered on layer III does not induce any population activity. Interestingly, as shown in previous figures, both neurons within layers II and V do express robust autorhythmic properties whereas neurons from layer III do not.[10,47,48]

A second important point illustrated in FIGURE 11 is that the activity triggered in layer V can frequently consist of population bursts that always propagate synaptically and excite neurons in layers III and II. Interestingly, as it can be noticed in the field potential trace (panel B, white trace) as well as in the CSD profile, these bursts of layer V activity typically consist of a high-frequency oscillation at about 200 Hz. This activity is reminiscent of the high-frequency "ripples" that are generated by EC layer V *in vivo*.

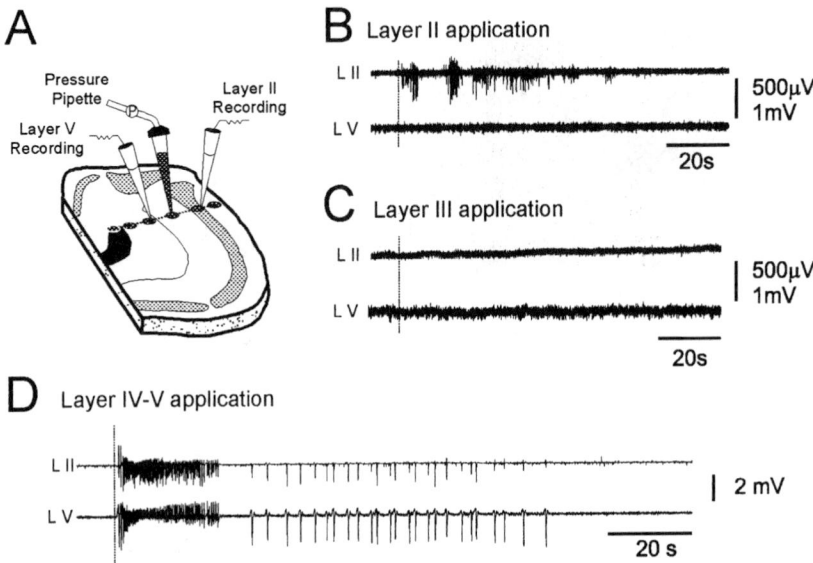

FIGURE 10. Field effects of laminar-localized pressure pulse applications of CCh (10 mM) in the entorhinal slice. (**A**) Diagrammatic representation of the recording and application arrangement. Two stationary recording electrodes were located in layers II and V. A pressure pipette was placed consecutively in layers I, II, III, V, and VI and in the angular bundle, and a 10 ms pulse was administered at each point. (**B**) Layer II application (denoted by the *vertical line*). After only a short delay, small-amplitude epileptiform activity was recorded in layer II. Note the absence of activity in layer V. (**C**) Layer III application. No activity was elicited. (**D**) Layer V application. A long-lasting series of large-amplitude epileptiform events of both long and short duration were elicited in layer V and propagated to layer II. These events are remarkably similar to those engendered by bath perfusion of CCh. (Modified from Dickson & Alonso.[41])

CONCLUSIONS

In parallel with the robust tendency of the entorhinal network to display oscillatory activity, specific subpopulations of entorhinal neurons also display very robust autorhythmic "pacemaker" properties. Importantly, one of the main populations is constituted by the stellate cells from layer II, which give rise to the main component of the perforant path projection that terminates on principal neurons in both the dentate gyrus and area CA3. Equally significant, the second main population of oscillatory neurons is constituted by projection neurons from EC layer V. These cells give rise to long-range projections that return entorhinal-hippocampal information to the neocortex and also give off collaterals that innervate more superficial EC cell layers (III and II). The oscillatory tendency of EC layers II and V neurons is matched by a similarly robust tendency of the local networks in layers II and V that have the potential to, independently, generate population oscillatory activity. It thus appears that

A

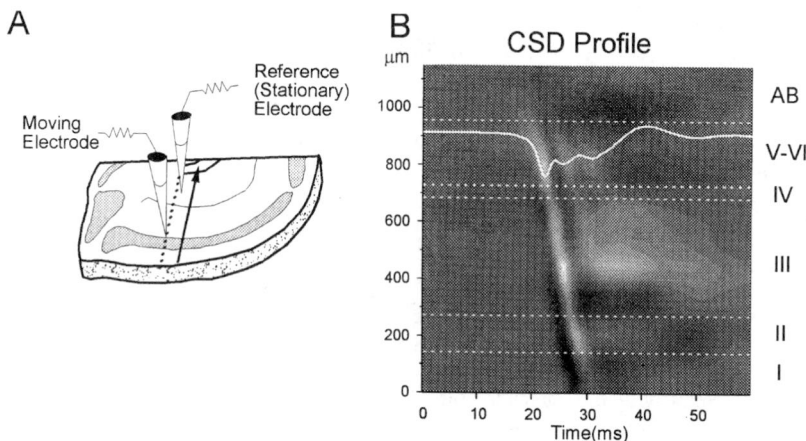

B

FIGURE 11. Current source density (CSD) analysis of the initiation of synchronized activity induced by CCh in the EC slice. (**A**) Representation of the experimental scheme. A stationary (reference) electrode was located in layers V–VI while another electrode (moving) was advanced from the pial surface (layer I) to the deep layers (angular bundle, AB) in 50-μm increments. (**B**) Grayscale surface contour plot of the CSD (*right panel*) profile (*light shades* indicate sinks, whereas *dark shades* indicate sources). The field potential negativity (as shown by the superimposition of the extracellular potential trace, in white) is typically first observed in layers V–VI from where it propagates to layers III and II. Associated with the field negativity in each region are spatially distinct current sinks lasting for approximately 2 ms, seen first in layers V–VI and subsequently in layer III, and last in layer II. Following the initial sink there is a rhythmic reappearance of sinks in layers V–VI (approximate frequency 200 Hz), whereas a more tonic sink of elongated duration (12 ms) appears in layer III, far outlasting those observed in either layers V–VI or layer II. (Modified from Dickson & Alonso.[41])

oscillatory behavior in the main input/output layers of the hippocampal/entorhinal system may constitute, at least, an important gating mechanism.

Nevertheless, *in vivo* studies have shown that the dominant rhythmic behaviors of entorhinal layers II and V seem to be distinct not only in terms of frequency but also in terms of behavioral correlates. The main rhythmic activity associated with layer II is theta accompanied by gamma during exploratory behavior in waking and during REM sleep.[14,15,49] On the other hand, the most salient rhythmic behavior of layer V is short-lasting, high-frequency bursts (ripples) that occur mainly during slow-wave sleep and immobility in the awake animal.[20,21,29] The ways by which the intrinsic rhythmicity of neurons contributes to these population rhythms remains to be determined. Future analysis of the local synaptic interactions within layers II and V may be essential to understand this process.

The sustained oscillatory activity in layer II stellate cells depends on the dynamic interactions between I_h and a low-threshold persistent Na$^+$ current, I_{NaP}. Although I_h is well known to play an important pacemaker role in heart,[50] as well as in some neuronal populations such as thalamic[51] or inferior olivary neurons,[52] this pacemaker role typically depends on the depolarizing influence of the activation of I_h and its interaction with low-threshold Ca^{2+} conductances. To our knowledge, the stellate cells are the first case in which both the depolarizing and hyperpolarizing influences of the activation and deactivation, respectively, of an h current have been shown to generate persistent oscillatory activity by interacting with a sustained Na^+ current. Because of the voltage-dependent gating properties of I_h and I_{NaP} expressed by the stellate cells, subthreshold oscillations occur around 5 mV below firing threshold. Integrative events in this subthreshold range would have a most important impact in shaping firing pattern.

Because of the rebound phenomena that the voltage-dependent properties of I_h and I_{NaP} implement, distributed synchronous synaptic input on a population of stellate cells will tend to "reset" the intrinsic oscillatory activity in each, thus potentially establishing a population timing device. The stellate cells funnel convergent information from polysensory associational areas into the hippocampus. If the hippocampal machinery does in fact construct a sort of a "memory code" from such convergent polysensory input, one might expect that an oscillatory network, such as that of EC layer II, can provide the means to "bind" together in time what can be considered as multidimensional information associated with an "explicit" memory event.

A different issue is that of the oscillatory activity in layer V neurons. Several aspects were surprising with respect to the intrinsic oscillatory activity of these neurons. First, the subthreshold oscillatory activity of the layer V cells is remarkably similar to that of the stellate cells in terms of its morphology and frequency range (2–7 mV in amplitude and 5–15 Hz in frequency). However, in spite of the fact that, similarly to layer II cells, subthreshold oscillations in layer V cells depend on the activation of I_{NaP}, I_h is not involved in the oscillatory process in layer V cells. Thus, it would appear that different mechanisms can generate the same pattern of activity in different neuronal populations. Second, while the dominant oscillatory tendency of the network of layer V neurons appears to be the production of high-frequency ripples, the intrinsic oscillations of the layer V cells occur at a much lower frequency. This would suggest that they are not involved in ripple generation. It might be that this low-frequency oscillatory activity has more to do with theta generation in spite of the fact that theta, as recorded by extracellular field and single-unit methods,[14,16,17,53,54] dominates in layers II and III. Indeed, *in vivo* recordings have shown that some layer V units do in fact fire at theta frequencies.[17] In addition, EC layer V is a main target for medial septal input to the EC, and is richly innervated by medial-septum cholinergic cell fibers.[55] Theta activity promoted by the cholinergic system could thus guarantee the coordinated flow of information in and out of the hippocampus. Alternatively, or in addition to the above, the intrinsic subthreshold oscillations of layer V cells may act as the initial synchronizing trigger for the emergence of a high-frequency population event largely dependent on recurrent excitatory synaptic interactions.[56] The emergence of theta or ripples could depend on the level of cholinergic activation and the interaction of this system with other modulatory influences, such as those emanating from the brainstem serotoninergic nuclei.[57] While high levels of cortical activation, which are associated with the highest level of cortical acetylcholine release,[58,59] might promote a theta state, lower levels of cortical activation may facilitate the emergence of ripples.

Another issue of discussion is the relationship between the oscillatory properties of entorhinal neurons and circuits that we observe *in vitro* in the slice preparation and the role of the entorhinal cortex in temporal lobe epileptogenesis. Our analysis of synchronous population activity in the slice preparation has supported previous studies suggesting that the local circuits within EC layer V are capable of generating epileptiform discharges.[11] However, in addition, we have also shown that EC layer II is also capable of independently generating epileptiform activity.[41] This might be related to the fact that populations of neurons both within layers II and V possess intrinsic oscillatory mechanisms, but also that the local circuitry within each layer must also be capable of engaging each population into an oscillatory state. In fact, anatomical studies based on the intracellular labeling of neurons in the EC have revealed that layer V and particularly layer II cells form extensive nets of recurrent axon collaterals.[9] Because of the key anatomical position that both EC layers II and V occupy as input and output channels, respectively, of the hippocampus, the fact that these two layers have the intrinsic ability of generating hypersynchronous activity makes the EC a potential site of critical importance for the generation and/or maintenance of temporal lobe epileptogenesis. In fact, recent studies both in animal models as well as in humans do point to this critical role of the entorhinal cortex in epilepsy.[60–64]

A final aspect we would like to consider is that of the role of the cholinergic system in the activation of entorhinal circuits. While acetylcholine is well known to activate cortical neurons via modulation (block) of K^+ conductances, we have found that in entorhinal neurons, in addition to this moderate and long-lasting K^+-conductance block, the dominant action of acetylcholine is the activation of a nonspecific cation conductance (I_{CAN}), which is enhanced by a rise in intracellular Ca^{2+} concentration.[46,65] In this way, neurons are depolarized to the oscillatory voltage range without major changes in their input resistance. In addition, the dependence and potentiation of I_{CAN} by an increase in intracellular Ca^{2+} enable the generation of plateau-potentials that sustain oscillatory dynamics. In this way, the properties of I_{CAN} can be considered to introduce a Hebbian paradigm whereby pairing of muscarinic receptor stimulation with suprathreshold neuronal activity (and thus Ca^{2+} influx) is necessary to evoke a large change in the intrinsic properties of the postsynaptic cell. This introduces a new aspect for the production of plasticity in the entorhinal neurons that can participate in their memory functions.

ACKNOWLEDGMENTS

This work was supported by the Medical Research Council of Canada and the Human Frontier Science Program Organization.

REFERENCES

1. SQUIRE, L.R. 1998. Memory systems. C. R. Acad. Sci. III. **321**(2–3): 153–156.
2. SCOVILLE, W.B. & B. MILNER. 1957. Loss of recent memory after bilateral hippocampal lesions. J. Neurol. Neurosurg. Psychiatry **20**: 11–21.
3. SUZUKI, W. & D.G. AMARAL. 1994. Topographic organization of the reciprocal connections between the monkey entorhinal cortex and the perirhinal and parahippocampal cortices. J. Neurosci. **14**: 1856–1857.
4. VAN HOESEN, G.W. 1982. The parahippocampal gyrus. New observations regarding its cortical connections in the monkey. Trends Neurosci. **5**: 345–350.
5. SWANSON, L.W. & C. KOHLER. 1986. Anatomical evidence for direct projections from the entorhinal area to the entire cortical mantle in the rat. J. Neurosci. **6**: 3010–3023.

6. MEUNIER, M., J. BACHEVALIER, et al. 1993. Effects on visual recognition of combined and separate ablations of the entorhinal and perirhinal cortex in rhesus monkeys. J. Neurosci. **13**(12): 5418–5432.
7. SUZUKI, W.A., E.K. MILLER, et al. 1997. Object and place memory in the macaque entorhinal cortex. J. Neurophysiol. **78**(2): 1062–1081.
8. ALONSO, A. & R. KLINK. 1993. Differential electroresponsiveness of stellate and pyramidal-like cells of medial entorhinal cortex layer II. J. Neurophysiol. **70**: 128–143.
9. KLINK, R. & A. ALONSO. 1997. Morphological characteristics of layer II projection neurons in the rat medial entorhinal cortex. Hippocampus **7**: 571–583.
10. VAN DER LINDEN, S. & F.H. LOPES DA SILVA. 1998. Comparison of the electrophysiology and morphology of layers III and II neurons of the rat medial entorhinal cortex *in vitro*. Eur. J. Neurosci. **10**(4): 1479–1489.
11. JONES, R.S.G. & V. HEINEMANN. 1988. Synaptic and intrinsic responses of medial entorhinal cortical cells in normal and magnesium-free medium "*in vitro*." J. Neurophysiol. **59**: 1476–1496.
12. ADEY, W.R., S. SUNDERLAND, et al. 1957. The entorhinal area: electrophysiological studies of its interrelations with rhinencephalic structures and the brainstem. Electroenceph. Clin. Neurophysiol. **9**: 309–324.
13. ADEY, W.R., C.W. DUNLOP, et al. 1960. Hippocampal slow waves: distribution and phase relationships in the course of approach learning. Arch. Neurol. **3**: 74–90.
14. ALONSO, A. & E. GARCÍA-AUSTT. 1987. Neuronal sources of theta rhythm in the entorhinal cortex. I. Laminar distribution of theta field potentials. Exp. Brain Res. **67**: 493–501.
15. CHROBAK, J.J. & G. BUZSAKI. 1998. Gamma oscillations in the entorhinal cortex of the freely behaving rat. J. Neurosci. **18**(1): 388–398.
16. DICKSON, C.T., I.J. KIRK, et al. 1995. Classification of theta-related cells in the entorhinal cortex: cell discharges are controlled by the ascending brainstem synchronizing pathway in parallel with hippocampal theta-related cells. Hippocampus **5**: 306–319.
17. ALONSO, A. & E. GARCÍA-AUSTT. 1987. Neuronal sources of theta rhythm in the entorhinal cortex of the rat. II. Phase relations between unit discharges and theta field potentials. Exp. Brain Res. **67**: 502–509.
18. KOCSIS, B., A. BRAGIN, et al. 1999. Interdependence of multiple theta generators in the hippocampus: a partial coherence analysis. J. Neurosci. **19**(14): 6200–6212.
19. BUZSÁKI, G., L.-W. LEUNG, et al. 1983. Cellular bases of hippocampal EEG in the behaving rat. Brain Res. Rev. **6**: 139–171.
20. CHROBAK, J.J. & G. BUZSAKI. 1996. High-frequency oscillations in the output networks of the hippocampal-entorhinal axis of the freely behaving rat. J. Neurosci. **16**(9): 3056–3066.
21. CHROBAK, J.J. & G. BUZSAKI. 1994. Selective activation of deep layer (V–VI) retrohippocampal cortical neurons during hippocampal sharp waves in the behaving rat. J. Neurosci. **14**: 6160–6170.
22. WINSON, J. 1978. Loss of hippocampal theta rhythm results in spatial memory deficit in the rat. Science **201**: 160–163.
23. KAHANA, M.J., R. SEKULER, et al. 1999. Human theta oscillations exhibit task dependence during virtual maze navigation. Nature **399**(6738): 781–784.
24. HUERTA, P.T. & J.E. LISMAN. 1993. Heightened synaptic plasticity of hippocampal CA1 neurones during a cholinergically induced rhythmic state. Nature **19**: 723–725.
25. LARSON, J. & G. LYNCH. 1986. Induction of synaptic potentiation in hippocampus by patterned stimulation involves two events. Science **232**: 985–988.
26. BUZSÁKI, G. 1989. A two-stage model of memory trace formation: a role for "noisy" brain states. Neuroscience **31**: 551–570.
27. ABELES, M. 1982. Role of the cortical neuron: integrator or coincidence detector? Isr. J. Med. Sci. **18**(1): 83–92.
28. HOPFIELD, J.J. 1995. Pattern recognition computation using action potential timing for stimulus representation. Nature **376**(6): 33–36.
29. BUZSÁKI, G. 1996. The hippocampo-neocortical dialogue. Cereb. Cortex. **6**(2): 81–92.
30. LLINAS, R.R. 1988. The intrinsic electrophysiological properties of mammalian neurons: insights into central nervous system function. Science **242**: 1654–1664.

31. RAMON Y CAJAL, S. 1902. Sobre un ganglio especial de la corteza esfeno-occipital. Trab. del Lab. de Invest. Biol. Univ. Madrid. Spain **1:** 189–201.
32. ALONSO, A. & R.R. LLINAS. 1989. Subthreshold Na^+-dependent theta-like rhythmicity in stellate cells of entorhinal cortex layer II. Nature **342:** 175–177.
33. MAGISTRETTI, J. & A. ALONSO. 1999. Biophysical properties and slow voltage-dependent inactivation of a sustained sodium current in entorhinal cortex layer-II principal neurons. A whole-cell and single-channel study. J. Gen. Physiol. **114**(4)**:** 491–509.
34. MAGISTRETTI, J., D.S. RAGSDALE, *et al.* 1999. High conductance sustained single-channel activity responsible for the low-threshold persistent Na^+ current in entorhinal cortex neurons. J. Neurosci. **19**(17)**:** 7334–7341.
35. KLINK, R. & A. ALONSO. 1997. Muscarinic modulation of the oscillatory and repetitive firing properties of entorhinal cortex layer II neurons. J. Neurophysiol. **77:** 1813–1828.
36. DICKSON, C.T., J. MAGISTRETTI, *et al.* 2000. Properties and role of Ih in the pacing of subthreshold oscillations in entorhinal cortex layer II neurons. J. Neurophysiol. In press.
37. WOUTERLOOD, P.G., W. HÄRTIG, *et al.* 1995. Parvalbumin-immunoreactive neurons in the entorhinal cortex of the rat: localization, morphology, connectivity and ultra-structure. J. Neurocytol. **24:** 135–153.
38. KOHLER, C., J.Y. WU, *et al.* 1985. Neurons and terminals in the retrohippocampal region in the rat's brain identified by anti-gamma-aminobutyric acid and anti-glutamic acid decarboxylase immunocytochemistry. Anat. Embryol. (Berl). **173**(1)**:** 35–44.
39. KOHLER, C., V. CHAN-PALAY, *et al.* 1984. Septal neurons containing glutamic acid decarboxylase immunoreactivity project to the hippocampal region. Anat. Embryol. **169:** 41–44.
40. ALONSO, A. & C. KÖHLER. 1984. A study of the reciprocal connections between the septum and the entorhinal area using anterograde and retrograde axonal transport methods in the rat brain. J. Comp. Neurol. **225:** 327–343.
41. DICKSON, C.T. & A. ALONSO. 1997. Muscarinic induction of synchronous population activity in the entorhinal cortex. J. Neurosci. **17:** 6729–6744.
42. AMARAL, D.G. & M.P. WITTER. 1989. The three-dimensional organization of the hippocampal formation: a review of anatomical data. **31**(3)**:** 571–591.
43. LOPES DA SILVA, F.H., M.P. WITTER, *et al.* 1990. Anatomic organization and physiology of the limbic cortex. Physiol. Rev. **76**(2)**:** 453–511.
44. SCHARFMAN, H.E., J.H. GOODMAN, *et al.* 1998. Chronic changes in synaptic responses of entorhinal and hippocampal neurons after amino-oxyacetic acid (AOAA)-induced entorhinal cortical neuron loss. J. Neurophysiol. **80**(6)**:** 3031–3046.
45. HAMAM, B.N., T.E. KENNEDY, *et al.* 1999. Morphological and electrophysiological characteristics of layer V neurons of the rat entorhinal cortex. J. Comp. Neurol. In press.
46. KLINK, R. & A. ALONSO. 1997. Ionic mechanisms of muscarinic depolarization in entorhinal cortex layer II neurons. J. Neurophysiol. **77:** 1829–1843.
47. DICKSON, C.T., A.R. MENA, *et al.* 1997. Electroresponsiveness of medial entorhinal cortex layer III neurons *in vitro*. Neuroscience **81:** 937–950.
48. GLOVELI, T., D. SCHMITZ, *et al.* 1997. Morphological and electrophysiological characterization of layer III cells of the medial entorhinal cortex of the rat. Neuroscience **77:** 629–648.
49. CHROBAK, J.J. & G. BUZSAKI. 1997. Gamma oscillations in the input network of the entorhinal-hippocampal axis of the freely-behaving rat. J. Neurosci. **18**(1)**:** 388–398.
50. DIFRANCESCO, D. 1993. Pacemaker mechanisms in cardiac tissue. Annu. Rev. Physiol. **55:** 455–472.
51. MCCORMICK, D.A. & H.-C. PAPE. 1990. Properties of a hyperpolarization-activated cation current and its role in rhythmic oscillation in thalamic relay neurones. J. Physiol. (Lond.) **431:** 291–318.
52. BAL, T. & D. MCCORMICK. 1997. Synchronized oscillations in the inferior olive are controlled by the hyperpolarization-activated cation current I(h). J. Neurophysiol. **77**(6)**:** 3145–3156.

53. MITCHELL, S.J. & J.B.J. RANCK. 1980. Generation of theta rhythm in medial entorhinal cortex of freely moving rats. Brain Res. **189:** 49–66.
54. DICKSON, C.T., C. TREPEL, et al. 1994. Extrinsic modulation of theta field activity in the entorhinal cortex of the anesthetized rat. Hippocampus **4:** 37–52.
55. AMARAL, D.G. & J. KURZ. 1985. An analysis of the origins of the cholinergic and non-cholinergic septal projections to the hippocampal formation of the rat. J. Comp. Neurol. **240:** 37–59.
56. TRAUB, R.D., R. MILES, et al. 1989. Model of the origin of rhythmic population oscillations in the hippocampal slice. Science **243:** 1319–1325.
57. VANDERWOLF, C.H. 1988. Cerebral activity and behavior: control by central cholinergic and serotoninergic systems. Int. Rev. Neurobiol. **30:** 225–340.
58. KANAI, T. & J.C. SZERB. 1965. Mesencephalic reticular activating system and cortical acetylcholine output. Nature **205:** 80–82.
59. KUROSAWA, M., A. SATO, et al. 1989. Stimulation of the nucleus basalis of Meynert increases acetylcholine release in the cerebral cortex in rats. Neuroscience Lett. **98:** 45–50.
60. RUTECKI, P.A., R.G. GROSSMAN, et al. 1989. Electrophysiological connections between the hippocampus and entorhinal cortex in patients with complex partial seizures. J. Neurosurg. **70:** 667–675.
61. DASHEIFF, R.M. & J.O. MCNARMARA. 1982. Electrolytic entorhinal lesions cause seizures. Brain Res. **231:** 444–450.
62. WALTHER, H., J.D.C. LAMBERT, et al. 1986. Epileptiform activity in combined slices of the hippocampus, subiculum and entorhinal cortex during perfusion with low magnesium medium. Neurosci. Lett. **69:** 165–161.
63. BRAGIN, A., J. CSICSVARI, et al. 1997. Epileptic afterdischarge in the hippocampal-entorhinal system: Current source density and unit studies. Neuroscience **76:** 1187–1203.
64. SCHARFMAN, H.E. 1996. Hyperexcitability of entorhinal cortex and hippocampus after application of aminooxyacetic acid (AOAA) to layer III of the rat entorhinal cortex in vitro. J. Neurophysiol. **76:** 2986–3001.
65. SHALINSKY, M.H., C.T. DICKSON, et al. 1988. Voltage-clamp analysis of muscarinic-induced depolarizing currents in entorhinal cortex layer II neurons. Soc. Neurosci. Abstr. **24:** 1339.

Differential Information Processing by Hippocampal and Subicular Neurons

ROBERT E. HAMPSON,[a] THOMAS HEDBERG,[b] AND SAM A. DEADWYLER[a,c]

[a]Department of Physiology and Pharmacology, Neuroscience Program, Wake Forest University School of Medicine, Winston-Salem, North Carolina 27157, USA

[b]Department of Neurology/Neuroscience, Albert Einstein College of Medicine, Bronx, New York 10461, USA

ABSTRACT: It has been known for some years that hippocampal neurons are critically involved in processing of information necessary for encoding memories. What is less understood is the role of the subiculum in this process. We describe here differential response characteristics of subicular and hippocampal neurons in rats during execution of a delayed-nonmatch-to-sample short-term memory task. Subicular neurons, unlike hippocampal neurons, fire primarily in the delay interval of the task and appear to provide a temporal linkage between events encoded in hippocampus during the sample and nonmatch phases. Indeed, a large proportion of subicular neurons fire robustly for the entire duration of the delay only. Further analyses using electrical activation methods indicate that subicular neurons that receive short latency inputs from the anterior thalamus and do not project to cingulate cortex are the most responsive to stimuli with behavioral significance.

INTRODUCTION

The retrohippocampal areas are composed of several structures, many of which are described in this volume. These structures include the perirhinal and postrhinal cortices, the entorhinal cortex, and perhaps regions adjacent to these including the parasubicular region. However, one area not classically included in this dichotomization is the subiculum, the allocortical structure immediately adjacent to the hippocampus and the one to which a majority of hippocampal output is directed.[1–4] Current theories of hippocampal information processing suggest that patterned activity must arrive in the hippocampus from the parahippocampal structures via major inputs to the dentate gyrus and CA1 regions (i.e., perforant path) and exit through projections to the subiculum and deep layers of the entorhinal cortex.[2,3,5–7] It is therefore important to understand the nature of information encoding and retrieval in the subicular region with respect to how these processes are modified from those recently characterized in the hippocampus.

[c]Corresponding author: Sam A. Deadwyler, Ph.D., Department of Physiology and Pharmacology, Wake Forest University School of Medicine, Medical Center Boulevard, Winston-Salem, NC 27157-1800. Tel.: (336) 716-8540; fax: (336) 716-8501.
e-mail: sdeadwyl@wfubmc.edu

HIPPOCAMPAL PROCESSING

The encoding of task-relevant information in the hippocampus has been studied primarily in short-term memory paradigms, such as delayed-match and nonmatch-to-sample tasks as well as other variants in which stimuli are associated and retained across delay intervals.[8–13] In these cases, it has been demonstrated that hippocampal neurons process information about the task by encoding critical features across the different neurons in the ensemble. Thus, while all of the information in the task may

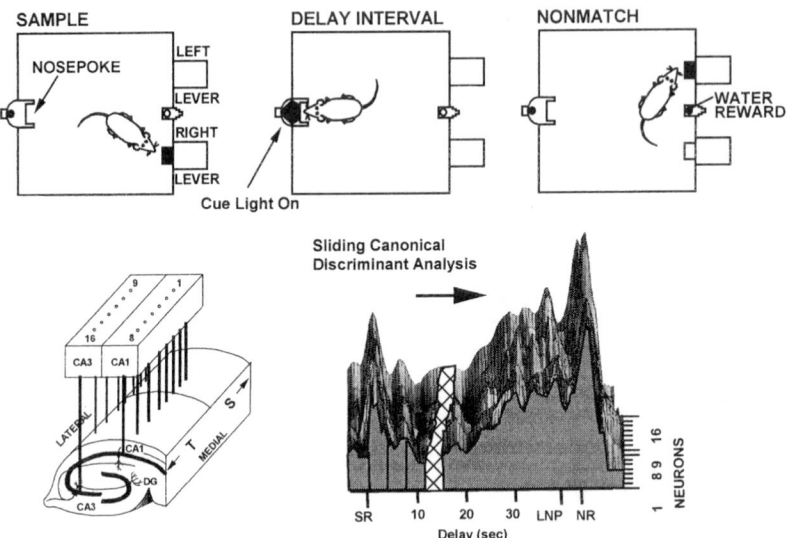

FIGURE 1. Delayed-nonmatch-to-sample (DNMS) task. **(Top)** Three principal phases of the DNMS task. During sample phase, a single lever is extended and a response retracts the lever and initiates the delay phase, in which a cue light is illuminated for 1–40 s, designating the duration of the delay interval. The animal must nosepoke at least once in the delay interval to terminate the preprogrammed delay period, which turns off the cue light and initiates the nonmatch phase. In this phase, both levers are extended and a response on the lever opposite the "sample lever" (i.e., a nonmatch response) produces a water reward. An incorrect (i.e., match) response results in no reward, and the chamber light is turned off for 5 s. Delay intervals are presented randomly from 1 to 40 s with 1.0-s resolution and the intertrial interval (ITI) is 10 s. **(Bottom left)** Diagram of hippocampal recording array.[13] Two rows of 40-μm-diameter stainless steel wires are positioned to traverse the CA1 and CA3 subfields of hippocampus. Electrode tips are positioned 200 μm apart within a row and 800 μm apart in CA1 and CA3 recording sites within a row. **(Bottom right)** Ensemble histogram of 16 individual hippocampal neurons recorded from the electrode array during DNMS performance. The histogram reflects the average firing of the 16 neurons over 100 DNMS trials shown in three dimensions (3D) to illustrate individual neuron activity within the ensemble. Note peak firing at sample (SR) and nonmatch (NR) phases and progressive increase in firing across the delay phase (LNP). Canonical discriminant analysis was performed across the entire trial by computing canonical discriminant functions at SR, LNP, and NR, and then "sliding" (i.e., reevaluating) the functions in 3-s increments (shaded band) along the histograms to compute associated discriminant scores across the entire DNMS trial. LNP: Last nosepoke in the delay interval.

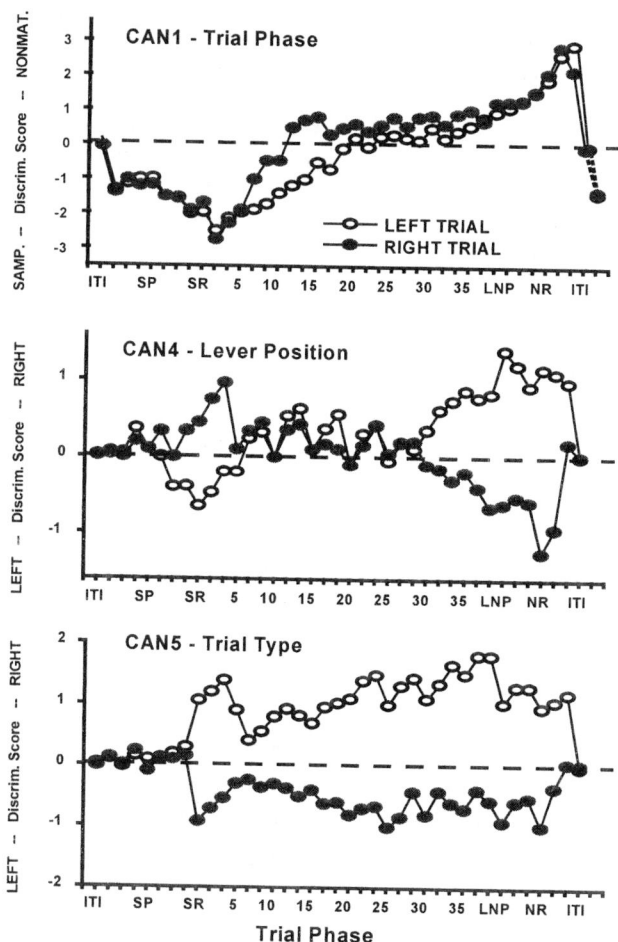

FIGURE 2. Three discriminant functions derived from "sliding" CDA across DNMS trials. **(Top)** First discriminant function (CAN1) accounted for 46% of the variance and produced scores that discriminated between sample and nonmatch phases (negative vs. positive scores, respectively), but were not different for left (filled circles) vs. right (unfilled circles) DNMS trials. **(Center)** Fourth discriminant function (CAN4) accounted for 12% of the variance and discriminated left from right position during sample and nonmatch responses. It is critical that the crossover as shown from positive to negative score, or vice versa, reflects the behavioral contingency in which the appropriate nonmatch response is associated as determined by the position of the sample response. Note that sample or nonmatch phase is not discriminated independent of position by this CAN4 component. **(Bottom)** Fifth discriminant function (CAN5) accounted for 9% of the variance and produced differential scores according to trial type, but did not discriminate trial phase or lever position. Trial identity was based on the sample lever response. Note lack of crossover during the trial as with CAN4. Terms—ITI: intertrial interval; SP: sample presentation; SR: sample response; LNP: last nosepoke in the delay; NR: nonmatch response.

not be encoded by a single neuron, certain specific events are encoded either individually or in conjunction with others such that, across the entire population of cells, all of the elements necessary to successfully perform the task are reflected in the activity of the ensemble.[11,13–16] This is shown in FIGURE 1 with respect to DNMS performance. In this task, individual neurons encode the two relevant dimensions of the task—position (of lever) and phase (match or nonmatch)—as well as combinations or conjunctions of those dimensions (i.e., left-sample, right-nonmatch, etc). At the ensemble or population level, analyses across all neurons using multivariate statis-

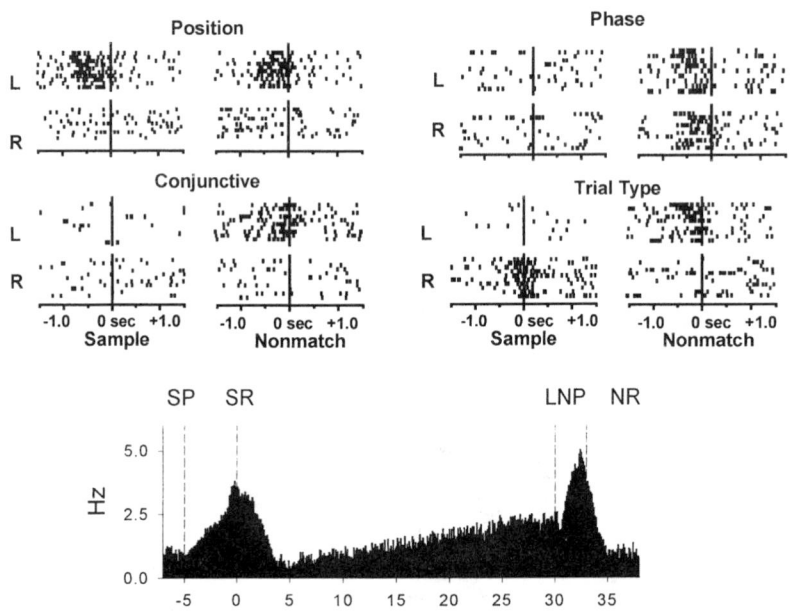

FIGURE 3. Examples of functional hippocampal cell types. **(Top)** Single-trial rastergrams of individual hippocampal neurons identified with respect to firing characteristics on DNMS trials. Each row of dots represents the occurrence of action potentials for a single trial displayed 1.5 s before and after the indicated lever press response (0 s). Ten trials are shown for each cell type. *Position cell* increased firing only when the response was in a specific position (left) in either phase of the task and did not fire when responses occurred on the opposite (right) lever. *Phase cell* increased firing to responses during a specific phase (nonmatch), irrespective of position of the lever response. *Conjunctive cell* increased firing in response to a specific combination or "conjunction" of position and phase events (i.e., left nonmatch) and did not alter firing to other combinations. *Trial-type cell* fired for a given DNMS trial type (i.e., right sample, left nonmatch) in a manner that resembled two "coupled" conjunctive cells. Note the correspondence of functional cell types to the canonical discriminant functions shown in FIGURE 2. **(Bottom)** Mean overall trial-based histogram averaged over all neurons in the ensemble. Sample and nonmatch peaks in the ensemble histogram illustrate the combined activity of all functional cell types across the DNMS trial. Note distinct depression in firing in the delay interval at 5–15 s and ramplike increase in firing until terminated by the LNP. Terms—SP: sample presentation; LNP: last nosepoke in the delay; NR: nonmatch response.

tics extract sources of variance that are associated with these individual cell types, and such sources of variance indicate the nature of the encoding process (FIGS. 2 and 3). Thus, it appears that the hippocampus sorts and categorizes information required to perform the task in much the same fashion as demonstrated in standard neural networks.[17–19]

The above scheme adequately describes the encoding process; however, with respect to the memory aspect of retention and retrieval of task information, it is important to understand the manner in which the encoding process gets utilized within the delay to "allow" accurate recognition or recall of trial-specific items. FIGURE 3 shows that, from an ensemble perspective, delay firing is suppressed to background levels for 5–10 s after initial encoding during the sample phase of the task, after which activity across the ensemble increases in a linear manner until the delay is terminated and firing specific to the correct decision occurs in association with the nonmatch response. The decrease in sample activity and the "ramplike" acceleration of firing in the delay reflect the encoding, retention, and (perhaps most importantly) *utilization* of information in terms of the nonmatch decision rule. In terms of population dynamics, there must thus be a transition from activity present at the time of the sample response to activity in the set of neurons that encode the appropriate information required for the nonmatch phase. We presume that this entails activation of a different set of position, phase, and conjunctive neurons in the ensemble specific for the nonmatch response.[20] How this transition occurs is not understood, so it is important to examine in more detail the activity of neurons that encode sample and nonmatch information during the delay phase of the task. FIGURE 3 shows ensemble codes in the form of different sources of variance as extracted by multivariate analyses[13] that display differential patterns during the delay. Ensemble activity specific to encoding "trial type" increases after 10 s into the delay and is sustained until the occurrence of the nonmatch response. Activity in the ensemble specific for "lever position" and "phase" is not sustained but becomes differentiated after 30–35 s into the delay.

The three-dimensional trial-based histograms shown in FIGURE 4 were constructed from the firing of individual hippocampal neurons, all of which were a given functional cell type (FIG. 3). The histograms on the left show the firing tendencies of position (right/left) encoding cells across the DNMS trial. Firing of these elements in the ensemble during the delay reflects selection of the lever position that is *going to be* correct on that trial as dictated by the nonmatch-to-sample decision rule. Firing of inappropriate position cells is not increased on this type of trial. Trial-type cells show a similar delay and nonmatch firing pattern, except *they also fire in the sample phase*, which means that the encoding is specific only for the type of trial (i.e., LS-RN or RS-LN, FIG. 4, trial type), not the correct nonmatch "decision", since these cells fire in both phases of the task. In hippocampus, these are the only two cell types that fire during the delay. In both cases, however, firing is near background levels for the initial 5–15 s of the delay interval (FIG. 1); hence, ensemble firing is not discretionary with respect to trial-specific information at this point in the delay interval. The hippocampus with respect to cell firing correlates is essentially information "silent" during this interval, suggesting that some other brain region must be "holding" or representing the information in a manner that would allow the hippocampal ensemble to become "reactivated" with the appropriate *nonmatch* pattern in the latter stages of the delay interval.

Position Cells   Trial-type Cells

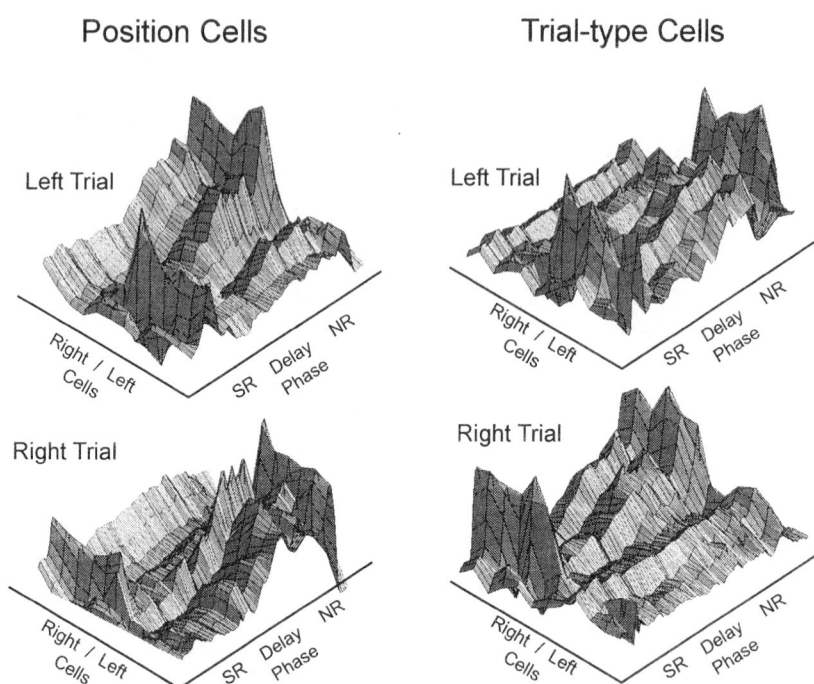

FIGURE 4. Three-dimensional (3D) histograms of delay interval firing patterns of functional hippocampal cell types. Distinct firing patterns during the delay phase were demonstrated by *position cells* and *trial-type cells*. Left: 3D trial-based histograms of 12 neurons each, constructed to illustrate the respective functional cell type firing patterns for left and right sample trials. Histograms of 6 left and 6 right position cells shown for left and right DNMS trials. Right position cell responses are shown in the "back" of the 3D histogram, with left position responses in front. Compare upper and lower trial types. Note that position cells appropriate to the NR increase firing during the delay, while position cells that fired to the sample rapidly decrease firing in the delay. Trial type: 3D histograms showing 6 left and 6 right trial-type cells on the left (upper) and right (lower) DNMS trials as with position cells. Note decrease at 5–15 s and lack of firing on inappropriate trials.

SUBICULAR NEURONS EXHIBIT DELAY-DEPENDENT ACTIVITY

FIGURE 5 shows the approach utilized to make multineuron recordings simultaneously in the subiculum and CA1 subfield of the hippocampus. The same electrode array was utilized, but reversed (FIG. 1), so that one row was placed in the subiculum instead of CA3. At the right are shown trial-based histograms of the types of firing patterns recorded from different neurons in the subiculum during the same DNMS task. The top histogram is the combined (averaged) for hippocampal cells shown in FIGURE 3. Below are histograms from the various subicular cell types. About 40% of cells fell into the type 1 and 1a categories (FIG. 5, top), in which bursts of firing occurred at primarily two different latencies (just prior to the sample response) (type

1) and 3–5 s after its completion (type 1a). The next most prominent (35%) cell firing pattern was that labeled type 2 (4th trace in FIG. 5), which exhibited a pronounced threefold increase in firing for the entire duration of the delay that abruptly ended prior to the execution of the nonmatch response. Two other cell types were noted, type 3 and 4 (3rd and 5th traces, respectively, in FIG. 5) which made up the smallest percentage (10% and 5%, respectively) of subicular neurons, with different but complementary firing patterns to the other types. Thus, it is immediately obvious that the different temporal firing characteristics of subicular cells are capable of "bridging" the 5–15 s period of "nondifferentiation" in hippocampal ensemble firing during the delay interval (see above). Therefore, in marked contrast to hippocampal cells, the

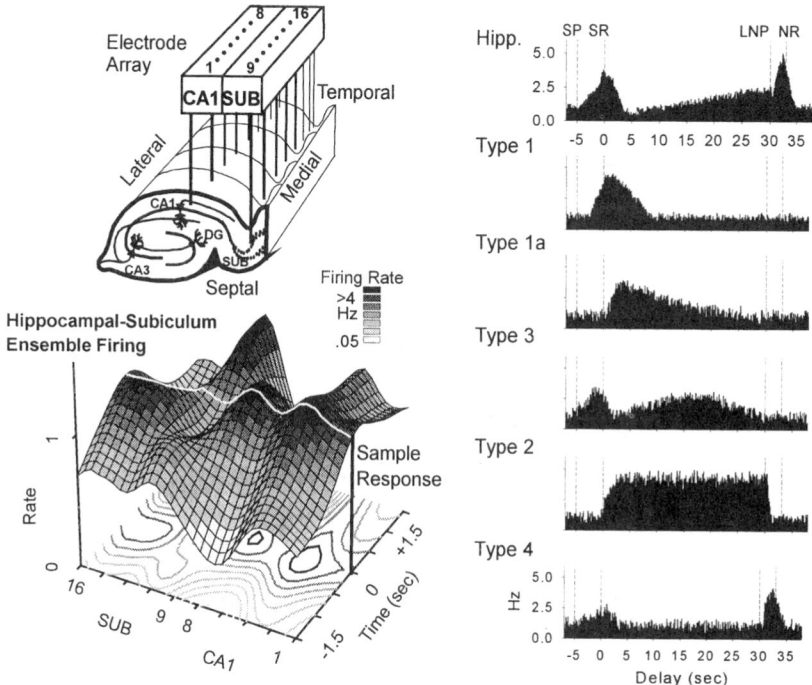

FIGURE 5. Simultaneous recordings from dorsal hippocampus and subiculum. (**Top left**) Modification of array electrode (FIG. 1) for recording in CA1 and subiculum. Electrodes have same relation to each other as in FIGURE 1. (**Bottom left**) 3D surface showing mean ensemble firing in CA1 and subiculum constructed at ±1.5 s around the sample response (0 s) for a single animal. Vertical deflections and shadings represent firing rate (see scale). CA1 neurons are 1–8; dorsal subiculum neurons are 9–16. (**Right**) Functional cell types from identified subicular neurons ($n = 67$) recorded during DNMS performance. Mean hippocampal ensemble trial-based histogram (Hipp.) is shown at top (FIG. 3). Each trial-based histogram below shows firing for a single neuron as an example of each type, averaged over 100 DNMS trials. Cell types were categorized by similarity in firing pattern and number of cells encountered with that pattern. Type 1 cells were then further split into separate categories according to peak latency and rate of decay in firing (see text for details).

majority of subicular cell firing occurred during the delay period and not during the sample or nonmatch phases of the task, denoting a clear separation of function.

SUBICULAR CELLS DO NOT ENCODE TASK-RELEVANT EVENTS

The predominance of delay-specific firing raised the question of whether the information specific for a given trial was retained within subicular cell firing during the delay. This was found not to be the case. In general, discharge patterns were obtained regardless of trial type (LS-RN, RS-LN) over the five different types of subicular neurons. The only clear evidence of differential encoding of trial-specific information was detected in type 1 and type 2 cells, which exhibited shifts in the latency of onset to firing in the sample and early delay period (FIG. 6). Thus, shifts in latency corresponded to similar patterns in individual hippocampal neurons that fire during the sample phase of the task.[20] The significance of these latency shifts between trial types is not understood. However, such temporal codes in subicular neurons would only be of value if they persisted or were translated in some form to the generation of the response in the nonmatch phase of the task,[20] which has not as yet been determined. Therefore, given the percentage (25%) of subicular cell firings that show trial-specific differentiated latencies, it appears as though some cells are influenced by encoding of within-trial events.

SUBICULAR CELLS SUSTAIN HIPPOCAMPAL ENSEMBLE ACTIVITY ACROSS THE DNMS DELAY

Given the fact that subicular cells do not appear to encode task-relevant information in the same manner as hippocampal cells and that the majority of subicular cell

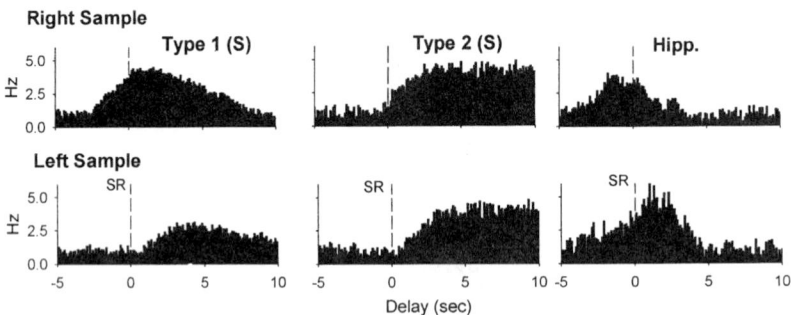

FIGURE 6. Position encoding by subicular neurons. Only type 1 and 2 subicular (S) neurons showed differences when sorted by trial type. **Left:** Perievent histograms for a single type 1 cell constructed from right (top) and left (bottom) DNMS trials. Note latency and amplitude differences. **Center:** Perievent histograms for a single type 2 (FIG. 5) subicular cell that showed a similar latency difference between trial types. **Right:** Hippocampal *ensemble* that differentially encoded left vs. right sample responses by similar peak latency shifts (see Hampson *et al.*, 1998).

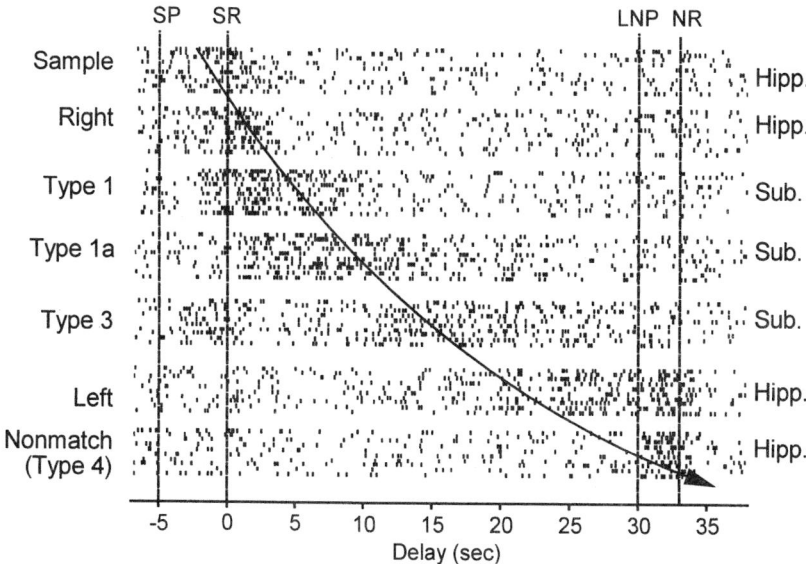

FIGURE 7. Single trial rastergrams showing temporal sequence of firing of different functional cell types recorded from dorsal hippocampus and subiculum. Ten trials for each indicated cell type are illustrated as rastergrams as in FIGURE 3. Cell types are organized by latency of firing peaks, with hippocampal sample *phase* and right *position cells* initiating the trial, and left *position* and nonmatch *phase cells* terminating the trial. Various subicular cell types (type 1, 1a, and 3) fire at successive intervals during the delay when hippocampal cells are quiescent.

firing is in the delay interval, it appears that the function of cells in this region is to generate various temporally patterned firing sequences that sustain activity during the delay until hippocampal ensemble firing is reinitiated and accelerates toward nonmatch firing peaks (FIG. 5, top). FIGURE 7 shows an example of how this sequential firing across regions could occur with respect to the various cell types in hippocampus and subiculum. The different cell types are illustrated as continuous trial-based rastergrams for each cell type, arranged to indicate peak firing times over 10 DNMS trials with 30-s delays. The density of "dots" represents frequency of firing and shows the progression of activity from hippocampal cells to subicular cells and back to a different set of hippocampal cells over the course of the trial. Given this scheme, it is apparent that there is no interval of time within the trial that cells within either the hippocampus or subiculum are not active. Thus, sequential activation of different "temporally tuned" cell types in the subiculum could be a key factor in re-activation of the appropriate cell types within hippocampal ensembles. However, the mechanism by which subicular cell firing "captures" the appropriate hippocampal nonmatch cells during the delay (FIGS. 5 and 7), a key element in this scheme, remains unresolved.

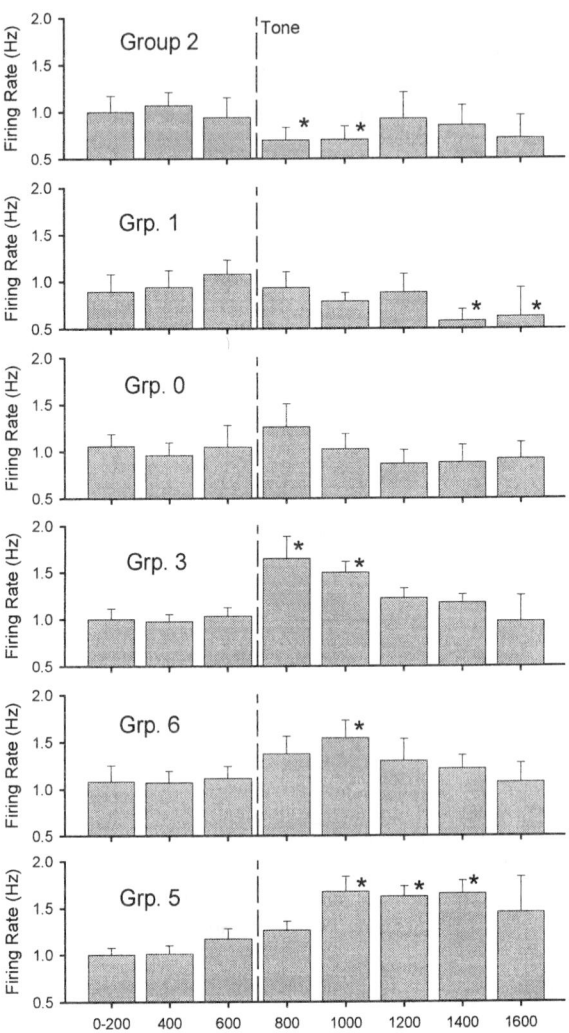

FIGURE 8. Tone-response characteristics of a different set of subiculum cells recorded in animals performing a differential tone-discrimination task. Cells ($n = 62$) were sorted into six groups according to tone-response characteristics. Bar graphs show mean firing rate (Hz) within 200-ms increments; error bars represent SEM across cells. The dashed line indicates tone presentation at 600 ms into the trial. Asterisks indicate significant z-scores for altered firing to pretone rates ($z > 3.19$, $p < 0.001$). Group (0) showed no significant change to the tone stimulus. Groups 3, 6, and 5 showed increased firing at various time intervals following the tone. Asterisks indicate significant rate increases over pretone firing. Group 2, $n = 5$; group 1, $n = 16$; group 0, $n = 6$; group 3, $n = 17$; group 6, $n = 6$; group 5, $n = 12$.

INPUTS AND PROJECTIONS OF BEHAVIORALLY RESPONSIVE
SUBICULAR NEURONS

An important issue related to activation of subicular neurons in conditioning tasks such as DNMS is how such activity is generated with respect to connectivity with other brain regions. This was examined in a study in which individual subicular cells were recorded in animals responding on a simple single or dual tone discrimination task (Hedberg *et al.*, in preparation). The task was the same as reported in earlier studies from this laboratory requiring rats to withhold responding into a nosepoke device until the onset of an audible tone stimulus.[21] Cells were identified, however, not only on the basis of whether they showed an increase in firing to the conditioned tone stimulus (CS), but also if that same cell elicited a short or long latency discharge to electrical stimulation delivered to either (1) the anterior dorsal (AD)/anterior ventral (AV) nuclei of the thalamus or (2) area 29c of the cingulate cortex. Electrical stimulation parameters were adjusted in an attempt to activate either anti- or orthodromically (i.e., monosynaptically) subicular neurons recorded in the tone discrimination task. A small number of cells tested revealed that the short latency activation via stimulation of area 29c satisfied criteria for antidromic activation; that is, spikes could be collided and cells followed at high frequencies with short invariant latencies.[3,22,23] Cells were therefore classified into categories of electrical stimulus driving (i.e., activation) at either short (possibly antidromic) or long (orthodromic) latency.

Sixty-two cells were recorded and identified as to type of electrical activation and pattern of discharge during performance of the tone discrimination task. FIGURE 8 shows the arrangement of all cells into one of six categories based on firing tendency to the tone stimulus. It is clear that the discharge patterns of the various cells ranged from inhibition (groups 1 and 2, $F_{2496} = 4.72$, $p < 0.001$), through lack of significant change (group 0), to highly significant increases in groups 3, 5, and 6 ($F_{2496} = 3.99$, $p < 0.001$) at different times during the 800 ms following the onset of the tone stimulus. This distribution of temporally specific firing tendencies resembles that shown in FIGURES 5 and 7 for delay firing of subicular neurons in the DNMS task. This difference in firing latency did not result from differences in behavioral response latencies since cells with different latencies were recorded in the same animals. The high degree of variability in peak firing latencies in subicular neurons suggests that these cells, as in the DNMS task, were encoding inherent (unidentified) temporal aspects of the tone discrimination task.

The above firing characteristics in the tone discrimination task were then compared with observations on area and type of electrical activation. A double dissociation was obtained with respect to the likelihood of activation by the tone stimulus and region of electrical stimulation (29c or AD/AV). This is shown in FIGURE 9. Cells activated at a long latency via AD/AV and not activated via area 29c showed robust responding to the tone stimulus as well as a characteristic "tapering off" of firing at the end of the 800-ms analysis period (FIG. 9: upper right and lower left). In contrast, cells that were least responsive to the tone stimulus were effectively driven at short latencies from area 29c and not via AD/AV (FIG. 9: upper left and lower right). Closer inspection revealed that the pretone firing in the cells that were more responsive to the tone stimulus and activated by AD/AV stimulation was significant-

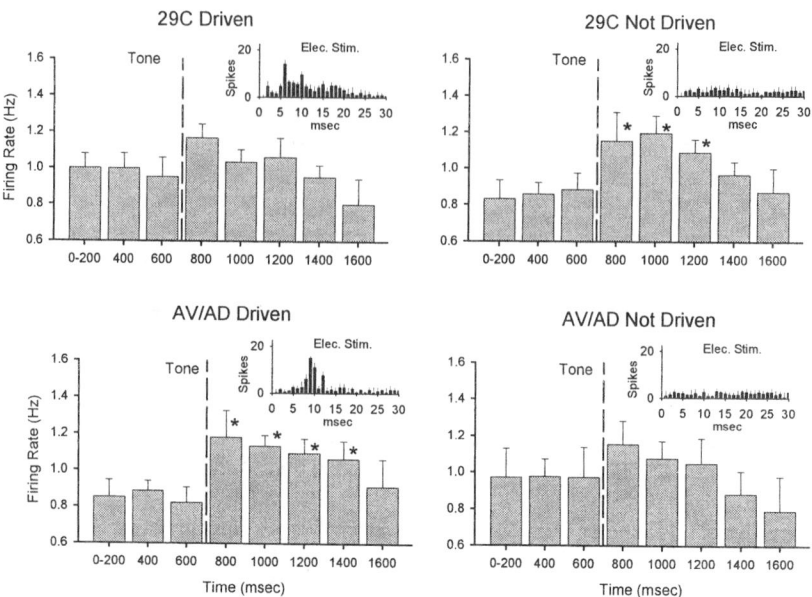

FIGURE 9. Differentiation of tone response for subicular cells antidromically activated by neocortex (area 29c) or thalamus (AD/AV). Large bar graphs indicate mean firing rate in response to tone presentation as in FIGURE 8. Cells were sorted this time according to electrical stimulation ("driving") characteristics and not tone response. Insets represent histograms of mean spikes/pulse to electrical stimulation at time = 0 s of area 29c or AD/AV. **Top left:** Subicular cells driven at short latency (5–8.0 ms) via area 29c stimulation were not significantly activated by the tone stimulus. **Top right:** Subicular cells that were not driven by 29c stimulation showed a decreased pretone firing relative to driven cells and also exhibited a significant increase ($z > 3.19$, $p < 0.001$) in posttone firing. **Bottom left:** Cells driven at longer latency (~10.0 ms) from AD/AV showed a significant increase in firing to the tone, similar to cells not driven by area 29c (upper right). **Bottom right:** In contrast, cells not driven by AD/AV showed no significant change in posttone firing. Area 29c driven, $n = 13$ cells; area 29c not driven, $n = 47$; AD/AV driven, $n = 19$; AD/AV not driven, $n = 27$.

ly lower ($F_{3496} = 3.51$, $p < 0.02$) than that of cells that were less responsive to the tone and activated at short latency via area 29c.

TABLE 1 shows the breakdown of cells with respect to tone response electrical driving from one of the two areas. It is clear that a significant difference existed between cells that were driven and not driven from areas 29c and AV/AD thalamus, which provided one basis for the double dissociation. TABLE 1 also shows that an equal portion of subicular cells in the AD/AV thalamus group were driven at long and short latencies, and these cells tended to be responsive to the tone. Curiously, a similar percentage of cells not driven by stimulation of AV/AD responded significantly in the tone discrimination task (TABLE 1). Six subicular neurons were activated by stimulation of both areas (short latency 29c and long latency AD/AV) and all showed significant increases in firing to the tone stimulus. Thus, cells that received

TABLE 1. Proportion of tone-responsive cells driven by thalamic or cortical stimulation

Percent of Cells	AV/AD			29C		
	Short Latency	Long Latency	Not Driven	Short Latency	Long Latency	Not Driven
Tone response	21%[a]	24%	24%	10%	3%	55%
No tone response	10%	11%	19%	11%	2%	21%

[a]Six cells showed both long- and short-latency activation. Total = 62 cells; 6 cells were activated from 29C and AV/AD.

inputs from AD/AV and apparently *did not* project to area 29c (i.e., were not activated antidromically) were the most responsive to the tone, while cells with putative projections to area 29c were not activated via stimulation of AV/AD and also were not responsive to the tone stimulus.

SUMMARY

The above description of hippocampal and subicular cell firing tendencies during short-term memory and conditioning tasks indicates that there is a marked distinction between the functional characteristics of the cells in both of these regions.[4,24] The "timing circuit" controlled by either the sustained (type 2) or sequential (types 1 and 3) activation of subicular cells that allows reactivation of the appropriate subset of ensemble neurons in hippocampus at the end of the delay in the nonmatch phase of the DNMS task suggests a circuit that somehow runs in synchrony with the task-specific processing going on in hippocampus. Finally, the findings with respect to subicular neurons and their connections to other brain regions, although preliminary, indicate that information specific to associatively conditioned stimuli is encoded via inputs from the thalamus primarily onto cells that do not project to cingulate cortex area 29c.[2,7,25–28]

ACKNOWLEDGMENTS

We wish to acknowledge the assistance of Joanne Konstantopoulos, Doug Byrd, Erica Jordan, John Simeral, and Tom Smulders. The research was supported by NIDA Grant Nos. DA03502 and DA00119 to S.A. Deadwyler and NIDA Grant No. DA08549 to R.E. Hampson.

REFERENCES

1. COMMINS, S., J. GIGG, M. ANDERSON & S.M. O'MARA. 1998. The projection from hippocampal area CA1 to the subiculum sustains long-term potentiation. Neuroreport **9:** 847–850.
2. WITTER, M.P. & H.J. GROENEWEGEN. 1990. The subiculum: cytoarchitectonically a simple structure, but hodologically complex. Prog. Brain Res. **83:** 47–58.

3. STEWART, M. 1997. Antidromic and orthodromic responses by subicular neurons in rat brain slices. Brain Res. **769:** 71–85.
4. YOUNG, B.J., T. OTTO, G.D. FOX & H. EICHENBAUM. 1997. Memory representation within the parahippocampal region. J. Neurosci. **17:** 5183–5195.
5. AMARAL, D.G., C. DOLORFO & P. ALVAREZ-ROYO. 1991. Organization of CA1 projections to the subiculum: a PHA-L analysis in the rat. Hippocampus **1:** 415–435.
6. NABER, P.A. & M.P. WITTER. 1998. Subicular efferents are organized mostly as parallel projections: a double-labeling, retrograde-tracing study in the rat. J. Comp. Neurol. **393:** 284–297.
7. VAN GROEN, T., F.J. VAN HAREN, M.P. WITTER & H.J. GROENEWEGEN. 1986. The organization of the reciprocal connections between the subiculum and the entorhinal cortex in the cat: I. A neuroanatomical tracing study. J. Comp. Neurol. **250:** 485–497.
8. EICHENBAUM, H., T. PARIKH & N.J. COHEN. 1985. Delayed non-match to sample with trial-unique odor stimuli in intact and fornix-damaged rats: a new test for recognition memory and model of temporal-lobe amnesia. Soc. Neurosci. Abstr. **15:** 1047.
9. GAFFAN, D., C. SHIELDS & S. HARRISON. 1984. Delayed matching by fornix-transected monkeys: the sample, the push, and the bait. Q. J. Exp. Psychol. **36B:** 305–317.
10. IWASAKI, T., S. FURUKAWA & K. KAWASAKI. 1990. Effects of hippocampal, amygdaloid, and caudate lesions on spatial delayed responses in rats. In Visual Memory and the Temporal Lobe, pp. 163–167. Elsevier. New York.
11. OTTO, T. & H. EICHENBAUM. 1992. Neuronal activity in the hippocampus during delayed non-match to sample performance in rats: evidence for hippocampal processing in recognition memory. Hippocampus **2:** 323–334.
12. WATANABE, T. & H. NIKI. 1985. Hippocampal unit activity and delayed response in the monkey. Brain Res. **325:** 241–254.
13. DEADWYLER, S.A., T. BUNN & R.E. HAMPSON. 1996. Hippocampal ensemble activity during spatial delayed-nonmatch-to-sample performance in rats. J. Neurosci. **16:** 354–372.
14. DEADWYLER, S.A. & R.E. HAMPSON. 1997. The significance of neural ensemble codes during behavior and cognition. In Annual Review of Neuroscience. Vol. 20, pp. 217–244. Annual Reviews, Inc. Palo Alto, CA.
15. HAMPSON, R.E. & S.A. DEADWYLER. 1999. Pitfalls and problems in the analysis of neuronal ensemble recordings during performance of a behavioral task. In Methods for Simultaneous Neuronal Ensemble Recordings, pp. 229–248. Academic Press. New York.
16. EICHENBAUM, H. 1993. Thinking about cell assemblies. Science **261:** 993–994.
17. ANDERSON, J.A. & G.E. HINTON. 1981. Models of information processing in the brain. In Parallel Models of Associative Memory, pp. 9–47. Erlbaum. Hillsdale, NJ.
18. HOPFIELD, J.J. 1995. Pattern recognition computation using action potential timing for stimulus representation. Nature **376:** 33–36.
19. KOHONEN, T. & R. HARI. 1999. Where the abstract feature maps of the brain might come from. Trends Neurosci. **22:** 135–139.
20. HAMPSON, R.E., J.D. SIMERAL & S.A. DEADWYLER. 1999. Distribution of spatial and nonspatial information in dorsal hippocampus. Nature **402:** 610–614.
21. FOSTER, T.C., R.E. HAMPSON, M.O. WEST & S.A. DEADWYLER. 1988. Control of sensory activation of granule cells in the fascia dentata by extrinsic afferents: septal and entorhinal inputs. J. Neurosci. **8:** 3869–3878.
22. WHITE, T.D., A.M. TAN & D.M. FINCH. 1990. Functional reciprocal connections of the rat entorhinal cortex and subicular complex with the medial frontal cortex: an in vivo intracellular study. Brain Res. **533:** 95–106.
23. CHRISTIAN, E.P. & S.A. DEADWYLER. 1986. Behavioral functions and hippocampal cell types: evidence for two nonoverlapping populations in the rat. J. Neurophysiol. **55:** 331–348.
24. EICHENBAUM, H., T. OTTO & N.J. COHEN. 1994. Two functional components of the hippocampal memory system. Behav. Brain Sci. **17:** 449–518.
25. BEHR, J., T. GLOVELI & U. HEINEMANN. 1998. The perforant path projection from the medial entorhinal cortex layer III to the subiculum in the rat combined hippocampal-entorhinal cortex slice. Eur. J. Neurosci. **10:** 1011–1018.

26. INO, T., T. KANEKO & N. MIZUNO. 1998. Direct projections from the entorhinal cortical layers to the dentate gyrus, hippocampus, and subicular complex in the cat. Neurosci. Res. **32:** 241–265.
27. SHI, C.J. & M.D. CASSELL. 1999. Perirhinal cortex projections to the amygdaloid complex and hippocampal formation in the rat. J. Comp. Neurol. **406:** 299–328.
28. KANG, E. & M. GABRIEL. 1998. Hippocampal modulation of cingulo-thalamic neuronal activity and discriminative avoidance learning in rabbits. Hippocampus **8:** 491–510.

The Parahippocampal Region and Object Identification

E.A. MURRAY,[a] T.J. BUSSEY, R.R. HAMPTON, AND L.M. SAKSIDA

Laboratory of Neuropsychology, National Institute of Mental Health, Bethesda, Maryland 20892, USA

ABSTRACT: The hippocampus has long been thought to be critical for memory, including memory for objects. However, recent neuropsychological studies in nonhuman primates have indicated that other regions within the medial temporal lobe, specifically, structures in the parahippocampal region, are primarily responsible for object recognition and object identification. This article reviews the behavioral effects of removal of structures within the parahippocampal region in monkeys, and cites relevant work in rodents as well. It is argued that the perirhinal cortex, in particular, contributes to object identification in at least two ways: (i) by serving as the final stage in the ventral visual cortical pathway that represents stimulus features, and (ii) by operating as part of a network for associating together sensory inputs within and across sensory modalities.

INTRODUCTION

This article reviews the contributions of the parahippocampal region to learning and memory in nonhuman primates, with special emphasis on its role in *object identification*: the knowledge that a particular object or class of objects is one and the same across the different instances in which it is experienced. In macaque monkeys, the parahippocampal region consists of three main cortical fields, located on the ventromedial aspect of the temporal lobe: entorhinal cortex, perirhinal cortex, and parahippocampal cortex (see FIG. 1). Currently, much more information is available regarding the contributions of the perirhinal cortex to learning and memory than for either the entorhinal cortex or parahippocampal cortex. Accordingly, although future studies might consider whether the functions of the cortical fields comprising the parahippocampal region can be understood within a unified framework, the present article focuses on the functions of just one portion of this region, namely, the perirhinal cortex.

We cover two main topics. First, we discuss the specific behavioral impairments that follow ablations of perirhinal cortex in macaque monkeys. Parallel findings in rats are also noted. Second, taking into account the results from these ablation studies, we discuss a tentative framework for understanding many of the behavioral effects of perirhinal cortex removal. Finally, we briefly summarize the contributions

[a]Address for correspondence: Elisabeth A. Murray, Ph.D., Laboratory of Neuropsychology, National Institute of Mental Health, Building 49, Room 1B80, 49 Convent Drive, Bethesda, MD 20892-4415. Tel.: (301) 496-5625, ext. 227; fax: (301) 402-0046.

e-mail: eam@ln.nimh.nih.gov

of the perirhinal cortex to visual perception and memory, and the way in which these promote object identification.

WHAT BEHAVIORAL IMPAIRMENTS FOLLOW DAMAGE TO THE PARAHIPPOCAMPAL REGION?

One of the earliest reported deficits found after damage to the parahippocampal region was an impairment in visual object recognition memory, as measured by the delayed nonmatching-to-sample (DNMS) or delayed matching-to-sample (DMS) tasks. In DNMS, each trial has two parts: a sample presentation followed by a choice test. During the sample presentation, the monkey sees a single object, which covers the central well of a three-well test tray. The monkey then displaces the object to obtain a small piece of food hidden in the well underneath. A few seconds later the monkey sees the same, now-familiar object plus a novel one, with one object covering the left well of the test tray and the other covering the right well. The monkey can obtain a second piece of food by displacing the novel object, but not by pushing aside the familiar one. Thus, on the choice test, the monkey solves the problem by applying a "nonmatching" rule, that is, by choosing the object that does not match the sample. If the monkey consistently chooses the novel object on the choice test, one can infer that the monkey *recognizes* the sample. In DMS, the monkey is trained on the "matching" rule rather than the nonmatching rule. These tasks can also be administered using a computerized apparatus that presents two-dimensional pictures on a touch-sensitive video screen rather than using actual objects on a test tray.

Monkeys with combined removals of the entorhinal cortex and perirhinal cortex are severely impaired on visual DNMS[1] and DMS.[2] Monkeys with such lesions perform at high levels of accuracy when delay intervals between the sample presentation and choice are short (~10 s), but perform at near chance levels when given a choice test only 60 seconds or so after presentation of the sample. By contrast, unoperated control monkeys perform over 90% correct responses at these and longer delay intervals.[1] Although alternative accounts have been proposed,[3] this pattern of results is traditionally interpreted as demonstrating rapid forgetting in the operated group. The precise nature of the deficit aside, these experiments show that, within the medial temporal lobe, the perirhinal cortex and the entorhinal cortex are important for visual recognition memory.

The perirhinal cortex, in particular, appears to play a central role in visual recognition. Within the parahippocampal region, ablation or reversible cooling of this cortical field yields the most devastating effects on visual recognition memory.[1,4,5] Removals restricted to the entorhinal cortex yield only mild, transient deficits on visual recognition.[1,6] Preliminary data indicate that removals restricted to the parahippocampal cortex yield no deficits.[7] Finally, even though ablations of entorhinal cortex alone produce little or no disruption of visual recognition, circumstantial evidence suggests that the entorhinal cortex, as well as area TE (a cortical field just lateral to the perirhinal cortex), can contribute to visual recognition: Monkeys with combined damage either to the entorhinal cortex plus perirhinal cortex, or to area TE plus the perirhinal cortex, have greater recognition impairments than do monkeys with damage to the perirhinal cortex alone.[8] Importantly, these group differences in the magnitude of the recognition impairment cannot be accounted for by differences

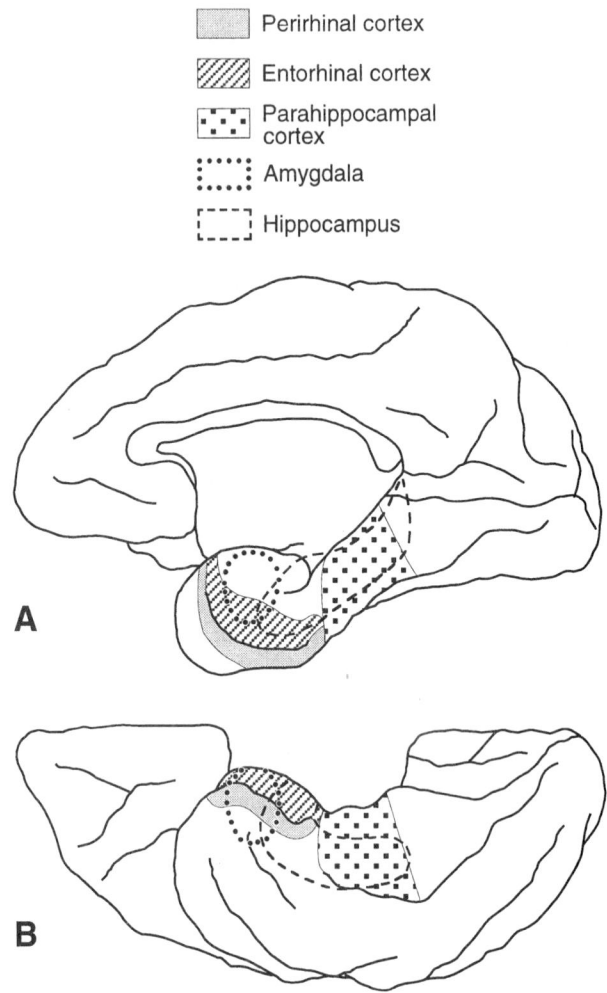

FIGURE 1. Diagrams of the medial (**A**) and ventral (**B**) views of the right hemisphere of a macaque brain showing the location and extent of various structures in the medial temporal lobe. The amygdala and the hippocampus are buried deep within the temporal lobe, whereas the perirhinal, entorhinal, and parahippocampal cortical fields are located on the surface of the brain.

across groups in the size of the perirhinal cortex removal itself, indicating that the cortex outside the perirhinal field is indeed making a contribution.

Impairments in recognition memory after combined damage to the perirhinal and entorhinal cortex have now been reported under several different conditions. For example, impairments are found in studies using either DNMS or DMS tasks in monkeys, using either a manual[1] or an automated[2] test apparatus, and using either visual[9] or olfactory[10] versions of DNMS in rats. In addition, monkeys with removals of perirhinal plus parahippocampal cortex are impaired on a tactual version of DNMS.[11] Selective perirhinal cortex damage can also affect tactual DNMS.[5] Thus, the recognition impairment after perirhinal cortex damage is robust, and affects more than one sensory modality.

Currently, there is controversy about the way in which various medial temporal lobe structures (including the entorhinal cortex, perirhinal cortex, parahippocampal cortex, amygdala and hippocampus) contribute to visual recognition memory. Although there is widespread agreement that the perirhinal and entorhinal cortex play a central role in recognition memory, and also that the amygdala is not important for this type of memory, no such consensus of opinion exists about the potential contribution of the hippocampus. Many studies have reported that damage to the hippocampus or fornix produces little or no impairment on visual recognition. For example, such damage produces either a mild impairment or no impairment on visual DNMS in monkeys,[12–14] as well as on olfactory[10] or visual recognition memory tasks[9,15–17] in rats. Recently, however, two additional studies have examined the effects of excitotoxic lesions of the hippocampus in monkeys, and both found impairments on DNMS.[18,19] Two points are worth making in this regard. First, the impairment that follows hippocampal lesions, when it is found, is much milder than that which follows perirhinal and entorhinal cortex damage. Second, for the hippocampus, there is no evidence for a positive correlation between magnitude of the recognition impairment and volume of the lesion, as one would predict if a given structure were mediating a given function. Indeed, one study has reported a significant inverse correlation,[13] and the two others likewise yielded negative correlations, although they do not attain statistical significance. By contrast, a positive correlation exists between the amount of damage to the entorhinal and perirhinal cortex, considered together, and magnitude of the recognition memory impairment.[1] Although a detailed discussion of this set of findings is beyond the scope of this article, we note that the data are consistent with the idea that partial hippocampal lesions might yield an indirect, adverse effect on other brain structures,[20,21] perhaps including the entorhinal and perirhinal cortex. In sum, damage to the hippocampus produces an impairment in visual recognition memory in some studies but not in others, and the manner in which the deficit arises remains uncertain.

Recognition memory, however, is not the only function disrupted by damage to the parahippocampal region. Monkeys with lesions of the entorhinal and perirhinal cortex have been found to be impaired in the learning or retention of stimulus-stimulus associations, including visual-visual associations or "paired associates,"[22] tactile-visual associations,[23] and flavor-visual associations.[24] In addition, rats with lesions of the entorhinal and perirhinal cortex are poor at an olfactory version of paired-associate learning.[25] As was the case for visual recognition memory, it appears that, within the parahippocampal region, the perirhinal cortex is especially critical for this kind of association learning.[26] Whether the perirhinal cortex is essential for all types of stimulus-stimulus associations in nonhuman primates, or only for those involving visual stimuli, remains uncertain. Future studies should address this question experimentally.

As was the case for recognition, stimulus-stimulus associations can proceed in the absence of the hippocampus. For example, learning of visual–visual associations[22] and retention of tactual-visual associations[27] in monkeys is unaffected by hippocampal removals. Although there are no studies assessing the effects of removal of the parahippocampal cortex alone, both studies cited above used aspiration removals of the hippocampus that included the underlying parahippocampal cortex. Thus, it is unlikely that selective removals of the parahippocampal cortex would disrupt this kind of stimulus-stimulus associative learning.

A third class of task on which there are impairments after removals within the parahippocampal region is pair-wise discrimination learning. Lesions of the perirhinal cortex alone, or of the entorhinal and perirhinal cortex together, have yielded mixed results; in some cases no impairment has been found,[2,28–30] and, in others, impairments have been reported.[5,30–32] Buckley and Gaffan[30] conducted a study to test the possibility that the deficits in concurrent visual discrimination learning following perirhinal cortex removals were related to the number of items to be discriminated (i.e., stimulus set size). Although the results as reported appear somewhat equivocal, a reanalysis restricted to the data from novel discriminations reveals stronger evidence for a relationship between set size and the magnitude of the deficit. These results thus lend some support to the hypothesis that the number of items to be discriminated is a factor underlying the impairments in concurrent discrimination learning. Another type of impairment in discrimination learning observed after perirhinal cortex removal is a severe deficit in configural discrimination learning,[26] even when small stimulus sets are used. Finally, either removals of the perirhinal plus entorhinal cortex, or removals of the perirhinal cortex alone, have been reported to disrupt retention of preoperatively learned discrimination problems in both monkeys[28,29,32] and rats.[33–35]

WHAT ARE THE CONTRIBUTIONS OF THE PARAHIPPOCAMPAL REGION TO PERCEPTION AND MEMORY?

As we have seen, perirhinal cortex lesions produce a variety of effects on visual learning and memory tasks, and yield some disruption in cross-modal associative tasks as well. Recently, Saksida and Bussey[36] have suggested that many of the effects of perirhinal cortex lesions described above may be understood by a consideration of the organization of visual representations in inferior temporal cortex, including the perirhinal cortex. Specifically, it has been proposed[36,37] that as one proceeds rostrally within the ventral visual processing stream, or "what" pathway, neurons code stimulus representations of increasing complexity. On this view, neurons in perirhinal cortex (and perhaps entorhinal cortex) represent complex conjunctions of features of visual stimuli, whereas neurons in earlier regions in the visual processing pathway represent simpler features from which the conjunctions are formed. This view is supported by anatomical and electrophysiological studies, which suggest a hierarchical organization of visual information processing in the inferior temporal cortex.[38,39] In this sense, perirhinal cortex might be considered to be the final station in the ventral visual processing stream.

If this supposition concerning the hierarchical organization of visual representations is correct, then perirhinal cortex should be particularly important for discriminations requiring the use of the complex visual representations stored there. For example, such representations would be required when the discrimination could not be solved on the basis of simple features of the discriminanda, a situation that arises in "configural" learning tasks. If one considers a configural task such as the biconditional discrimination, AB+, CD+, BC−, AD− (where AB can be thought of as an object, A and B as features of that object, and + and − as indicating whether a given object is rewarded or not), it can easily be seen that such a discrimination cannot be solved on the basis of simple features alone: sometimes A is rewarded; sometimes it is not. However, by associating representations of the *conjunctions* of features such as AB with reward or nonreward, the task can be solved. Consistent with this analysis, Buckley and Gaffan[26] found that perirhinal cortex lesions severely disrupted configural learning in monkeys. This analysis can also account for impairments in concurrent discrimination learning with large stimulus sets. This is because as the number of objects to be discriminated increases, the probability increases that a given feature might be rewarded in one case (i.e., one object) but not in another. A prediction that follows is that deficits in configural discriminations—in which the amount of feature ambiguity is at a maximum—should be obtainable using a smaller set size than that required to obtain impairments in concurrent discrimination learning. Although this has not been tested directly in a single experiment, comparison across studies supports this prediction.[26,30]

Other predictions follow from the proposal that visual representations in inferior temporal cortex are organized hierarchically. For example, in cases where the discriminanda have many visual features in common, even discrimination of a single pair of objects could be disrupted in monkeys with perirhinal cortex removals relative to controls. Preliminary results support this idea. Bussey *et al.*[40] first taught monkeys to discriminate complex greyscale picture stimuli. By use of a computer algorithm, the pictures were then "morphed" (blended) together in a manner that increased the number of features the discriminanda had in common. Although perirhinal cortex lesions did not disrupt the acquisition of the original discrimination, performance in these animals was impaired, relative to controls, when the number of common features was increased. By contrast, performance of the same operated monkeys did not differ from that of controls after the same types of picture stimuli were made more difficult to discriminate, not by increasing the number of common features, but by manipulating their size.

The studies reviewed above indicate an important role for the perirhinal cortex in object identification. The case for a role for perirhinal cortex in object identification has been made even stronger by the results of experiments by Buckley and Gaffan, who showed that perirhinal cortex lesions can disrupt object discrimination when objects are presented in new views, or presented within a complex scene.[41] Similar findings have been reported in rodents. For example, E.A. Gaffan *et al.*[42] found that rats with perirhinal cortex lesions had a specific difficulty in discriminating objects embedded in scenes. In their task, rats were required to discriminate a "constant negative," nonrewarded scene from positive, rewarded scenes. In brief, when spatial cues were available, the operated rats could discriminate the scenes, but when only stimulus quality cues were available, the rats were impaired, suggesting a specific difficulty with object identification. There are, however, some limitations on the conditions under which the perirhinal cortex is essential for object identification. Recently, Hampton and Murray[32] tested the effects of perirhinal cortex removals on various aspects of object identification, including, among other things, discrimination of rotated objects, shrunken or enlarged objects, and degraded objects presented on a monitor screen. Whereas the manipulations of the images were effective in substantially increasing the difficulty of the discriminations, monkeys with perirhinal cortex removals performed at the same level of accuracy as the unoperated controls. In contrast to these negative findings, the same operated monkeys were impaired in the learning of both concurrent and single pair visual object discriminations, so the lack of impairment on the earlier tests cannot be accounted for by ineffective lesions. These results constrain the ways in which the perirhinal cortex can be said to contribute to object identification, by showing that the perirhinal cortex is not necessary for the identification and selection of familiar objects under certain challenging conditions.

SUMMARY

    For the present, it appears that the perirhinal cortex contributes to object identification in at least two different ways. First, it is thought to process information in much the same way as other parts of inferior temporal cortex, and may serve as the final stage in the ventral visual processing pathway devoted to visual perception and memory. Its special contribution is held to be in the representation of complex conjunctions of stimulus features. To the extent that the perirhinal cortex serves to represent stimuli, it can be said to contribute to object identification. Second, the perirhinal cortex operates as part of a network for associating together sensory inputs within and across sensory modalities. In addition, the perirhinal cortex, together with other cortical fields, also serves as a site of long-term storage of such knowledge. Thus, the perirhinal cortex in monkeys, together with other brain regions, appears to comprise a network analogous to a semantic network in humans, specialized for representing objects and object-related information.

ACKNOWLEDGMENT

    This work is supported by the Intramural Research Program of the National Institute of Mental Health.

REFERENCES

1. MEUNIER, M., J. BACHEVALIER, M. MISHKIN & E.A. MURRAY. 1993. Effects on visual recognition of combined and separate ablations of the entorhinal and perirhinal cortex in rhesus monkeys. J. Neurosci. **13:** 5418–5432.
2. EACOTT, M.J., D. GAFFAN & E.A. MURRAY. 1994. Preserved recognition memory for small sets, and impaired stimulus identification for large sets, following rhinal cortex ablations in monkeys. Eur. J. Neurosci. **6:** 1466–1478.
3. RINGO, J.L. 1991. Memory decays at the same rate in macaques with and without brain lesions when expressed in d' or arcsine terms. Behav. Brain Res. **42:** 123–134.
4. HOREL, J.A., D.E. PYTKO-JOINER, M.L. VOYTKO & K. SALSBURY. 1987. The performance of visual tasks while segments of the inferotemporal cortex are suppressed by cold. Behav. Brain Res. **23:** 29–42.
5. BUFFALO, E.A., S.J. RAMUS, R.E. CLARK, E. TENG, L.R. SQUIRE & S.M. ZOLA. 1999. Dissociation between the effects of damage to perirhinal cortex and area TE. Learn. Memory **6:** 572–599.

6. LEONARD, B.W., D.G. AMARAL, L.R. SQUIRE & S. ZOLA-MORGAN. 1995. Transient memory impairment in monkeys with bilateral lesions of the entorhinal cortex. J. Neurosci. **15:** 5637–5659.
7. RAMUS, S.J., S. ZOLA-MORGAN & L.R. SQUIRE. 1994. Effects of lesions of perirhinal cortex or parahippocampal cortex on memory in monkeys. Soc. Neurosci. Abstr. **20:** 1074.
8. MURRAY, E.A. 2000. Memory for objects in nonhuman primates. *In* The New Cognitive Neurosciences. M.S. Gazzaniga, Ed.: 753–763. MIT Press. Cambridge, MA.
9. MUMBY, D.G. & J.P.J. PINEL. 1994. Rhinal cortex lesions and object recognition in rats. Behav. Neurosci. **108:** 11–18.
10. OTTO, T. & H. EICHENBAUM. 1992. Complementary roles of the orbital prefrontal cortex and the perirhinal-entorhinal cortices in an odor-guided delayed-nonmatching-to-sample task. Behav. Neurosci. **106:** 762–775.
11. SUZUKI, W.A., S. ZOLA-MORGAN, L.R. SQUIRE & D.G. AMARAL. 1993. Lesions of the perirhinal and parahippocampal cortices in the monkey produce long-lasting memory impairment in the visual and tactual modalities. J. Neurosci. **13:** 2430–2451.
12. BACHEVALIER, J., R.C. SAUNDERS & M. MISHKIN. 1985. Visual recognition in monkeys: effects of transection of fornix. Exp. Brain Res. **57:** 547–553.
13. MURRAY, E.A. & M. MISHKIN. 1998. Object recognition and location memory in monkeys with excitotoxic lesions of the amygdala and hippocampus. J. Neurosci. **18:** 6568–6582.
14. GAFFAN, D. 1994. Dissociated effects of perirhinal cortex ablation, fornix transection and amygdalectomy: evidence for multiple memory systems in the primate temporal lobe. Exp. Brain Res. **99:** 411–422.
15. ROTHBLAT, L.A. & L.F. KROMER. 1991. Object recognition memory in the rat: the role of the hippocampus. Behav. Brain Res. **42:** 25–32.
16. STEELE, K. & J.N.P. RAWLINS. 1993. The effects of hippocampectomy on performance by rats of a running recognition task using long lists of non-spatial items. Behav. Brain Res. **54:** 1–10.
17. BUSSEY, T.J., J. DUCK, J.L. MUIR & J.P. AGGLETON. 2000. Distinct patterns of behavioural impairments resulting from fornix transection or neurotoxic lesions of the perirhinal and postrhinal cortices in the rat. Behav. Brain Res. In press.
18. BEASON-HELD, L.L., D.L. ROSENE, R.J. KILLIANY & M.B. MOSS. 1999. Hippocampal formation lesions produce memory impairment in the rhesus monkey. Hippocampus **9:** 562–574.
19. ZOLA, S.M., L.R. SQUIRE, E. TENG, L. STEFANACCI, E.A. BUFFALO & R.E. CLARK. 2000. Impaired recognition memory in monkeys after damage limited to the hippocampal region. J. Neurosci. **20:** 451–463.
20. BACHEVALIER, J. & M. MISHKIN. 1989. Mnemonic and neuropathological effects of occluding the posterior cerebral artery in *Macaca mulatta*. Neuropsychologia **27:** 83–105.
21. MISHKIN, M. & E.A. MURRAY. 1994. Stimulus recognition. Curr. Opin. Neurobiol. **4:** 200–206.
22. MURRAY, E.A., D. GAFFAN & M. MISHKIN. 1993. Neural substrates of visual stimulus-stimulus association in rhesus monkeys. J. Neurosci. **13:** 4549–4561.
23. GOULET, S. & E.A. MURRAY. 1995. Effects of lesions of either the amygdala or anterior rhinal cortex on crossmodal DNMS in rhesus macaques. Soc. Neurosci. Abstr. **21:** 1446.
24. PARKER, A. & D. GAFFAN. 1998. Lesions of the primate rhinal cortex cause deficits in flavour-visual associative memory. Behav. Brain Res. **93:** 99–105.
25. BUNSEY, M. & H. EICHENBAUM. 1993. Critical role of the parahippocampal region for paired-associate learning in rats. Behav. Neurosci. **107:** 740–747.
26. BUCKLEY, M.J. & D. GAFFAN. 1998. Perirhinal cortex ablation impairs configural learning and paired–associate learning equally. Neuropsychologia **36:** 535–546.
27. MURRAY, E.A. & M. MISHKIN. 1985. Amygdalectomy impairs crossmodal association in monkeys. Science **228:** 604–606.
28. GAFFAN, D. & E.A. MURRAY. 1992. Monkeys (*Macaca fascicularis*) with rhinal cortex ablations succeed in object discrimination learning despite 24-hr intertrial intervals and fail at matching to sample despite double sample presentations. Behav. Neurosci. **106:** 30–38.

29. THORNTON, J.A., L.A. ROTHBLAT & E.A. MURRAY. 1997. Rhinal cortex removal produces amnesia for preoperatively learned discrimination problems but fails to disrupt postoperative acquisition and retention in rhesus monkeys. J. Neurosci. **17:** 8536–8549.

30. BUCKLEY, M.J. & D. GAFFAN. 1997. Impairment of visual object-discrimination learning after perirhinal cortex ablation. Behav. Neurosci. **111:** 467–475.

31. BAXTER, M.G., W.S. HADFIELD & E.A. MURRAY. 1999. Rhinal cortex lesions produce mild deficits in visual discrimination learning for an auditory secondary reinforcer in rhesus monkeys. Behav. Neurosci. **113:** 243–252.

32. HAMPTON, R.R. & E.A. MURRAY. 1999. Stimulus representations in rhesus monkeys with perirhinal cortex lesions. Soc. Neurosci. Abstr. **25:** 789–789.

33. WIIG, K.A., L.N. COOPER & M.F. BEAR. 1996. Temporally graded retrograde amnesia following separate and combined lesions of the perirhinal cortex and fornix in the rat. Learn. Memory **3:** 313–325.

34. KORNECOOK, T.J., A. ANZARUT & J.P.J. PINEL. 1999. Rhinal cortex, but not medial thalamic, lesions cause retrograde amnesia for objects in rats. Neuroreport **10:** 2853–2858.

35. MACHIN, P.E. & M.J. EACOTT. 1999. Perirhinal cortex and visual discrimination learning in the rat. Psychobiology **27:** 470–479.

36. SAKSIDA, L.M. & T.J. BUSSEY. 1998. Toward a neural network model of visual object identification in primate inferotemporal cortex. Soc. Neurosci. Abstr. **24:** 1906.

37. MURRAY, E.A. & T.J. BUSSEY. 1999. Perceptual-mnemonic functions of the perirhinal cortex. Trends Cognit. Sci. **3:** 142–151.

38. TANAKA, K. 1996. Inferotemporal cortex and object vision. Annu. Rev. Neurosci. **19:** 109–139.

39. LOGOTHETIS, N.K. 1998. Object vision and visual awareness. Curr. Opin. Neurobiol. **8:** 536–544.

40. BUSSEY, T.J., L.M. SAKSIDA & E.A. MURRAY. 1999. Overgeneralization in monkeys with perirhinal cortex lesions. Soc. Neurosci. Abstr. **25:** 789.

41. BUCKLEY, M.J. & D. GAFFAN. 1998. Perirhinal cortex ablation impairs visual object identification. J. Neurosci. **18:** 2268–2275.

42. GAFFAN, E.A., M.J. EACOTT & E.L. SIMPSON. 2000. Perirhinal cortex ablation in rats selectively impairs object identification in a simultaneous visual comparison task. Behav. Neurosci. **114:** 18–31.

The Neurophysiology of Memory

WENDY A. SUZUKI[a,c] AND HOWARD EICHENBAUM[b]

[a]Center for Neural Science, New York University, 4 Washington Place, Room 809, New York, New York 10003, USA

[b]Laboratory of Cognitive Neurobiology, Department of Psychology, Boston University, 64 Cummington Street, Boston, Massachusetts 02215, USA

ABSTRACT: How do the structures of the medial temporal lobe contribute to memory? To address this question, we examine the neurophysiological correlates of both recognition and associative memory in the medial temporal lobe of humans, monkeys, and rats. These cross-species comparisons show that the patterns of mnemonic activity observed throughout the medial temporal lobe are largely conserved across species. Moreover, these findings show that neurons in each of the medial temporal lobe areas can perform both similar as well as distinctive mnemonic functions. In some cases, similar patterns of mnemonic activity are observed across all structures of the medial temporal lobe. In the majority of cases, however, the hippocampal formation and surrounding cortex signal mnemonic information in distinct, but complementary ways.

INTRODUCTION

The landmark study of the amnesic patient H.M. first showed that bilateral damage to the medial temporal lobe severely impairs the ability to form and retain new long-term declarative memories (i.e., memories for facts and events).[1] Since that description, the development of animal models of medial temporal lobe amnesia in both monkeys and rats, together with detailed neuroanatomical studies of this region, have helped identify the individual areas important for normal declarative memory.[2,3] These structures include the hippocampal formation (defined here as the dentate gyrus, areas CA3, CA1, and the subiculum) and the entorhinal, perirhinal, and parahippocampal cortices. While these studies have contributed substantially to our understanding of the brain basis of memory, neuropsychological studies on brain-damaged patients or experimental animals can provide only indirect insights into the specific patterns of neural activity that allow us to form and retain new long-term declarative memories. Instead, characterizations of behavior-related neural activity offer the most direct insight into the neural processes that underlie memory. How do medial temporal lobe neurons signal the acquisition, retention, or recall of a particular stimulus, fact, or event? Do neurons throughout the medial temporal lobe signal memory in a similar way or are different regions of the medial temporal lobe specialized for different aspects of memory? Findings from neurophysiological studies in monkeys, rats, and humans have begun to provide answers to these questions.

[c]Address for correspondence: Wendy A. Suzuki, Ph.D., Center for Neural Science, New York University, 4 Washington Place, Room 809, New York, NY 10003. Phone: (212) 998-3734; fax: (212) 995-4011.

e-mail: wendy@cns.nyu.edu

Although the neurophysiological correlates of memory in rats and monkeys have been studied for over 20 years, early comparisons in the two species provided few points of contact. Comparisons in the two species were limited by an emphasis on studies of spatial learning in rats and by a focus on visual recognition memory in monkeys. More recently, however, a broader range of tasks, especially those designed for rats, has allowed more direct comparisons of the patterns of neural responses both across species and across different medial temporal lobe areas.

These comparative neurophysiological findings make two main points. First, the mnemonic signals observed throughout the medial temporal lobe are largely conserved across species. Second, neurons throughout the medial temporal lobe can perform both similar as well as distinctive mnemonic functions that usually operate cooperatively in signaling declarative memory. In most cases, the hippocampal formation and surrounding cortex signal mnemonic information in different but complementary ways. New evidence indicates that in some situations the same recognition memory signals are apparent throughout the medial temporal lobe.

In this chapter, we review the neurophysiological findings that address these two main points. We focus on findings from neurophysiological studies of recognition and associative memory in both monkeys and rats. We also discuss relevant findings from studies on neuronal activity and functional imaging in humans. These mnemonic signals can be further illuminated by considering the patterns of parallel and serial connections between the structures of the medial temporal lobe. Thus, we begin with a brief overview of the neuroanatomical organization of this region.

ANATOMY OF THE MEDIAL TEMPORAL LOBE

A large body of tract tracing studies in monkeys and rats have provided detailed information about the neuroanatomical organization of the medial temporal lobe.[4–11] Although some notable differences exist in the details of the cortical and subcortical connections of these structures across species, the general principles of organization of medial temporal lobe connections are highly conserved.

FIGURE 1 illustrates two major organizing principles of the medial temporal lobe. First, the connections of the medial temporal lobe are organized in a hierarchy of increasing amounts of sensory convergence. At the lowest "rung" of the hierarchy are the perirhinal (areas 35 and 36) and parahippocampal (areas TH and TF) cortices. The parahippocampal cortex in monkeys and humans is considered homologous to the postrhinal cortex in rats.[12] The perirhinal and parahippocampal/postrhinal cortices are distinguished by receiving not only inputs from other higher order association areas (including regions of the prefrontal cortex and other polymodal areas within the temporal and parietal lobes), but also unimodal sensory input from visual, somatosensory, olfactory, and auditory association areas. Although the perirhinal and parahippocampal/postrhinal cortices in monkeys and rats receive a similar convergence of unimodal sensory inputs, the two species differ in the relative proportions of the various sensory modalities they receive. For example, the perirhinal cortex in monkeys receives the strongest projections from visual area TE, reflecting the prominent role of visual information processing in this species. By contrast, the perirhinal cortex of rats receives a more even distribution of information from visual,

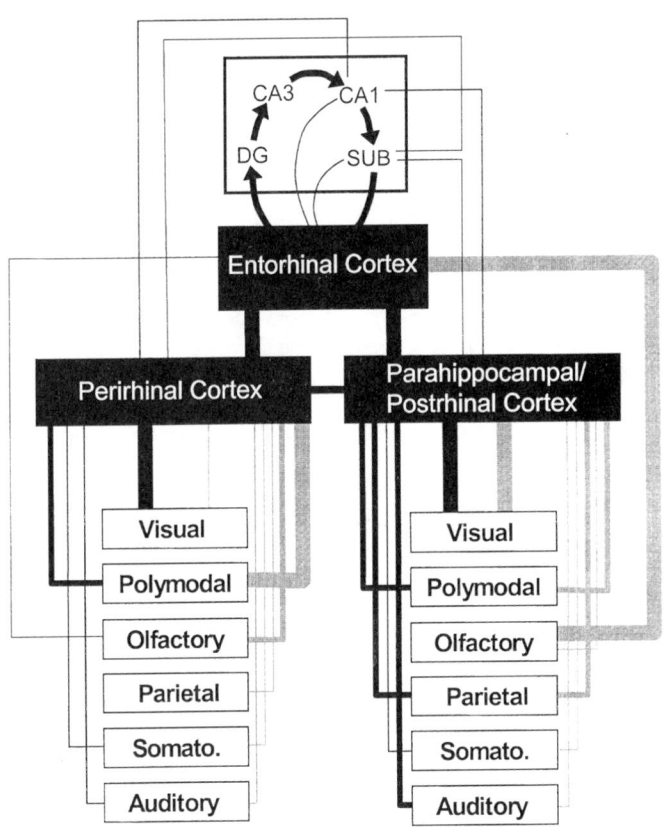

FIGURE 1. Summary of the sensory connections and interconnections of the structures of the medial temporal lobe. The lower half of the figure illustrates the pattern and relative strength of projections from various unimodal and polymodal sensory areas to the perirhinal cortex, parahippocampal/postrhinal cortex, and entorhinal cortex. Projections in the monkey are shown in *black* and the projections in rats are shown in *gray*. The thickness of the lines corresponds to the relative strength of the projections, where the thickest line represents approximately 30% of all cortical inputs or higher, the medium thick line represents between approximately 10 and 29% of projections, and the thinnest line represents less than 10% of inputs. All projections between the perirhinal, parahippocampal/postrhinal, entorhinal, and hippocampus are similar in monkey and in rats and are shown in *black* (except for one instance described in the text). All projections are reciprocal except those between subfields of the hippocampus, which are denoted with an *arrowhead*. Quantitative estimates for monkey data were taken from Suzuki *et al.*[18] and those from the rat were taken from Burwell *et al.*[12]

somatosensory, as well as auditory and olfactory areas, reflecting the more prominent role of these other sensory modalities in this species. This difference across species can be appreciated by comparing the patterns of cortical inputs to the perirhinal cortex in monkeys (black lines) to those in rats (gray lines) in the lower portion of FIGURE 1. Projections from other unimodal and polymodal sensory areas to the parahippocampal cortex in monkeys and the postrhinal cortex in rats are roughly similar.

The perirhinal and parahippocampal/postrhinal cortices then provide the major input to the next "rung" of the hierarchy, the entorhinal cortex. A second notable difference between monkeys and rats is the organization of the direct olfactory inputs to the entorhinal cortex. In monkeys, for example, the entorhinal cortex receives only a small direct projection from olfactory areas.[13] The entorhinal cortex in rats is distinguished by receiving more extensive olfactory inputs.[11,14] Consistent with these differences in the pattern and strength of visual and olfactory inputs to the medial temporal lobe, behavioral studies of memory in monkeys have most often used visual stimuli, whereas studies in rats have commonly used olfactory stimuli.

The entorhinal cortex then provides the major cortical input to the hippocampal formation via a series of well-described serial and parallel projections.[15] In addition to the prominent projections from the entorhinal cortex to various components of the hippocampal formation, there is also a direct, though weaker, projection from both the perirhinal and parahippocampal cortices to the CA1/subicular border region in monkeys.[16] In rats, while evidence indicates that the perirhinal cortex provides a similar direct projection to both area CA1 and the subiculum,[12] postrhinal projections terminate only in the subiculum (Naber and Witter, personal communication).

A second prominent feature of the connections of the medial temporal lobe is that all projections (except those between the different subregions of the hippocampal formation) are strongly reciprocal. For example, the perirhinal and parahippocampal cortices not only have strong and reciprocal connections with the entorhinal cortex, but also have weaker interconnections with the CA1/subicular border region. Thus, the medial temporal lobe is made up of a complex series of both serial and parallel projections in which any level of the hierarchy has either direct or indirect access to all other levels of the system.

What do these neuroanatomical data tell us about the functional organization of these structures? These data make at least two predictions. On the one hand, the fact that each of these structures differs markedly in the amount and content of convergent cortical input suggests that each area may be able to process or combine information to encode, store, or retrieve memory in different ways. This view suggests that each area may be characterized by distinct patterns of mnemonic activity. On the other hand, the strong parallel projections from the perirhinal and parahippocampal/postrhinal cortices to both the entorhinal cortex and area CA1 suggest that neurons in all of these regions have access to similar kinds of sensory/mnemonic information. This raises the possibility that in certain situations, each of these structures may encode or store memory in similar ways. The available neurophysiological data support both functional predictions. For example, evidence is strong that the hippocampal formation combines information in memory in ways not observed in the adjacent cortex. In other situations, similar patterns of mnemonic activity have been observed across many medial temporal lobe structures. These patterns of mnemonic activity will be described in greater detail below.

NEURAL SIGNALS OF RECOGNITION MEMORY

Perhaps the largest body of work on the neurophysiology of memory has been done using variants of the delayed match to sample task. This classic task of recognition memory typically consists of three phases. First, a to-be-remembered sample stimulus is presented. The sample stimulus is then followed by a delay period and finally by a "test" or recognition phase in which one or more items are presented. Animals are rewarded for responding to either the stimulus that matches the sample (delayed match to sample) or the stimulus that does not match the sample (delayed nonmatch to sample). Another commonly used version of this task is the "continuous" delayed nonmatch to sample task.[17] In this task, stimuli are presented to the animal sequentially, separated by delay intervals. Animals are rewarded for responding if the stimulus is different from the preceding stimulus. In this version of the task, each stimulus is both the sample for the following item and the test stimulus for the preceding item. Other variations of the task include the use of either highly familiar or novel stimuli, the use of varying numbers of "test" stimuli presented between the sample stimulus and the final match, or variations in the length of the delay intervals used.

How do medial temporal lobe neurons signal recognition memory? To approach this question, it is useful to ask what the animal must do to solve a typical recognition memory task. To perform such a task, the animal must first successfully discriminate between the stimuli being used. Second, the animal must maintain a representation of the to-be-remembered sample stimulus throughout the trial including during the delay interval(s). Third, the animal must determine whether the current "test" stimulus matches the stimulus held in memory. Neurons throughout the medial temporal lobe exhibit firing properties consistent with each of these three key task requirements. The most extensively characterized medial temporal lobe regions have been the perirhinal and the entorhinal cortices. We begin with a description of the recognition memory signals observed in these cortical areas. The patterns of neural activity underlying each of the three recognition task requirements just outlined will be discussed in turn. We will then compare the patterns of activity observed in the perirhinal and entorhinal cortices to the patterns seen in the hippocampal formation. Much less is known about the patterns of mnemonic activity in the parahippocampal/postrhinal cortex, and therefore this region will not be discussed.

Recognition Memory in Perirhinal and Entorhinal Cortices

An important requirement to solve any recognition memory task is the ability to discriminate between the different sensory stimuli being shown. A defining characteristic of neurons throughout the entorhinal and perirhinal cortices of rats and monkeys is that they respond with a high firing rate to certain sensory stimuli and not to others (i.e., sensory-selective response). For example, in monkeys, 47% of the visually responsive neurons in the entorhinal cortex[18] and 94% of the visually responsive neurons in the perirhinal cortex[19] respond selectively to particular visual stimuli. In rats, 35% of the sampled lateral entorhinal neurons and 11% of the sampled perirhinal neurons exhibit odor-specific firing properties.[20] Visually responsive neurons have been reported in the rat perirhinal and entorhinal cortices,[21] although the selectivity of these responses has not been extensively characterized.

A second requirement of a typical recognition memory task is the ability to maintain the representation of the to-be-remembered sample stimulus throughout the duration of the trial including the delay interval. Consistent with this task requirement, some neurons in the perirhinal and entorhinal cortices either sustain or reactivate their stimulus-selective response for the to-be-remembered sample stimulus during the delay interval. For example, in rats, some neurons in the perirhinal and entorhinal cortices respond robustly during the delay interval of a delayed nonmatching to sample task if the to-be- remembered stimulus is one particular odor (i.e., odor A), but not if it is any other odor from a set of alternative stimuli.[20] Other cells in these same areas appear to reactivate their selective response only at the very end of the delay period immediately before the choice phase of the task.[20] In monkeys, some perirhinal or entorhinal neurons exhibit stimulus-selective activity during the delay period that begins immediately following the sample stimulus of a delayed match to sample task.[18,22] In the entorhinal cortex, this selective activity was maintained in the delay intervals following multiple intervening test stimuli.[18] By contrast, selective delay activity in the perirhinal cortex was disrupted by the presentation of even a single intervening stimulus.[22] The effect of intervening stimuli on the selective delay activity in the perirhinal or entorhinal cortices of rats has not been examined.

A third requirement of a typical delayed match to sample task is the ability to determine if the current stimulus matches or does not match the stimulus held in memory. In other words, is a neuron's response to a particular stimulus influenced by whether that stimulus is held in memory or not? To address this question, comparisons have been made between the response of a neuron to its preferred stimulus when it was presented as a match and the response to the same stimulus when it was presented as a nonmatch in other trials.[18–20] Importantly, the physical characteristics of the stimulus were identical in both the "match" and the "nonmatch" conditions. The only difference between the two stimulus presentations was that in the match condition (and not in the nonmatch condition), the animals carried a memory of having seen the stimulus at the beginning of the trial. This analysis showed that neurons in the entorhinal and perirhinal cortices signaled the occurrence of a matching stimulus with either a suppressed (decreased) or an enhanced (increased) response. These so-called match-suppression or match-enhancement signals convey information about the previous occurrence of a particular stimulus on a given trial. The match-suppression response cannot be explained by sensory fatigue or habituation, because the suppression disappears when the same stimulus is shown as a sample on the following trial.[19] The match-suppression or match-enhancement effects occurred very early in the sensory response and well before the animal's behavioral response, suggesting that these suppressed or enhanced sensory signals could be used by the animals to perform the task.

Studies conducted in the entorhinal and perirhinal cortex in both monkeys and rats typically find varying proportions of neurons with selectively suppressed or enhanced responses.[18,19,23–26] In general, more neurons tend to respond to a repeated stimulus with a suppressed response. One intriguing question concerns which factors determine whether a neuron signals a remembered stimulus with an enhanced or a suppressed response. One study found that a seemingly minor change in the task demands resulted in a significant shift in the ratio of enhanced versus suppressed responses observed in the perirhinal cortex.[25] This study compared the pattern of neural activity in two different versions of a delayed match to sample task. In the "standard" version of the task, a sample stimulus was followed by a variable number of unique "nonmatching" test items, and the animals were required to respond to the repetition of the sample stimulus (i.e., the match). If **A**, **B**, and **C** refer to different visual stimuli, a typical trial in the standard version of the task would be **A**...**B**...**C**...**A**. The animals were always rewarded for responding to the second **A**, and none of the intervening "test" stimuli (i.e., **B** and **C**) were ever repeated. In the second version of the task, the sample stimulus was also followed by a variable number of nonmatching test items, but in this case the nonmatching test items could also repeat. This was termed the "ABBA" version of the task, where BB refers to the repeated nonmatch. In this version of the task, the animals had to learn to ignore the repeated nonmatch and respond only when the sample was repeated. Match suppression and match enhancement were observed as animals performed both versions of the task. However, the proportion of neurons exhibiting match enhancement was substantially higher during performance of the ABBA version of the task compared to the standard version. Moreover, an important difference was noted in the pattern of responses of the match-suppression and match-enhancement neurons on the ABBA version of the task. That is, neurons exhibiting match suppression showed suppressed responses to any repeated stimulus including the repeated nonmatch. By contrast, the match-enhancement neurons were enhanced only when the behaviorally relevant stimulus was repeated. Thus, match enhancement may represent an "active" form of working or recognition memory that is associated with signaling the behaviorally relevant stimulus.[25]

If match enhancement signals active or working memory, then what does match suppression represent? One possibility is that match suppression also represents a form of active memory in that it resets between trials of the standard version of the DMS task.[19] This recognition memory signal may be used in situations different from those that engage the match-enhancement signal. An alternative possibility, however, is that match suppression does not reflect a form of active memory, but instead reflects a passive or implicit form of memory. Priming is one possible candidate. Priming is defined as an improvement in the ability to detect or identify stimuli as the result of previous experience with the stimuli. The improvement in performance is observed independent of whether subjects are consciously aware of the learning experience (i.e., it is a form of implicit memory). Consistent with the idea that match suppression may be associated with a priming-like memory signal, functional imaging studies have shown that priming is associated with decreased brain activation.[27,28] Although many forms of priming are intact following medial temporal lobe lesions, a recent study showed that one form of implicit memory was impaired in patients with medial temporal lobe amnesia.[29] This finding raises the possibility that the medial temporal lobe can participate in certain forms of priming or implicit memory. If match suppression was a form of implicit or unconscious memory, one would expect the mnemonic signal to occur with any repeated stimulus irrespective of whether the animal consciously recognized the stimulus as familiar or repeated (i.e., whether the animal got the trial correct or not). On the other hand, if match suppression represents a more active or "conscious" form of memory, the prediction would be that match suppression should be robust on correct trials and diminished on error trials. Unfortunately, this prediction has not been extensively tested, because animals typically perform these recognition tasks at very high levels of accuracy. Therefore, few if any error trials have been available for analysis. Additional studies are needed to examine the relationship between match suppression, match enhancement, and conscious or unconscious forms of memory.

While the studies just described used familiar sets of stimuli to test recognition memory, robust patterns of match suppression are also observed when novel visual stimuli are used. In general, neurons in the entorhinal and perirhinal cortex respond with their highest firing rate to particular novel (or rarely seen) stimuli, and these stimulus-selective responses continue to diminish gradually as the novel stimulus becomes more familiar with repeated exposure. For some neurons, the firing rate is suppressed when the novel stimulus is repeated, even after a delay interval of 24 hours.[24,26] This pattern of activity (referred to as the familiarity effect) is seen as animals passively view repeated stimuli[24] or when animals perform a simple novel/familiar discrimination task.[26] This kind of robust stimulus-selective response suppression could be used to perform one widely used recognition memory task in which novel or rarely seen objects are used for each trial (i.e., the trial unique version of the delayed nonmatching to sample task). Performance of the trial-unique version of the delayed nonmatching to sample task is impaired in monkeys following lesions that include the perirhinal and entorhinal cortices.[30–32]

Recognition Memory in the Hippocampal Formation

Early neurophysiological studies of recognition memory in the hippocampal formation of rats and monkeys reported no evidence of the stimulus-selective recognition signals just described for perirhinal and entorhinal neurons. Recordings in the monkey hippocampal formation tended to include neurons throughout the dentate gyrus, CA3, CA1, and the subiculum,[23,26,33–35] whereas recordings in rats tended to be limited to area CA1.[17,36,37] Although the neurons of the hippocampal formation do not convey robust stimulus-selective recognition signals, they do indeed signal mnemonic information during the performance of various recognition memory tasks. The nature of these mnemonic signals, however, is distinctly different from the patterns of activity typically observed in the adjacent cortex. Two different kinds of memory signals have been described in the hippocampal formation. First, some neurons in this region respond differentially to stimuli when they are shown as matches compared to when the same stimuli are shown as nonmatches (15 of 120 or 12.5% of the responsive neurons).[17] Unlike neurons in the entorhinal or perirhinal cortex that signal this match-nonmatch difference for *particular* stimuli (i.e., stimulus-selective match-nonmatch responses), neurons in the hippocampal formation signaled this match-nonmatch difference for *all* stimuli.[17] This pattern of activity has been referred to as an "abstracted" recognition signal in the sense that these hippocampal neurons do not convey specific information about particular stimuli but, instead, appear to signal the outcome of the match-nonmatch comparison (i.e., the answer) for all stimuli. Importantly, control experiments showed that these abstracted match-nonmatch signals could be clearly dissociated from activity related to the behavioral (i.e., motor) response the animals made.[17] Like the selective match-suppression and match-enhancement cells observed in the cortex, these abstracted match-nonmatch signals observed in the hippocampus could be used by the animal to signal stimulus recognition. Although direct comparisons are difficult because of differences in analyses, similar patterns of activity have also been described in other studies of recognition memory in monkeys.[35,36]

A second pattern of mnemonic activity was observed in hippocampal (areas CA3 and CA1) neurons as rats performed an olfactory recognition task (continuous delayed nonmatching to sample) in which odors were presented in cups of odorized sand at many different locations on an open platform.[37] Animals learned to dig in a cup of odorized sand to retrieve a food reward if the odor did not match the previous sample stimulus. If the odor matched the previous sample, no reward was present and the rats learned to turn away from the cup. The location of the odor presentation changed on each trial but did not predict whether the trial was a nonmatch or a match. All recordings in this study were limited to areas CA1 and CA3 of the hippocampus. Consistent with the study described above, some neurons signaled the match-nonmatch status of an odor irrespective of the odor identity ("abstracted" match-nonmatch signal; 13 of 91 or 14% of the responsive neurons). A second subset of neurons in this task signaled the abstracted match-nonmatch signals in conjunction either with the position in which it occurred (18 of 91 or 20% of the responsive neurons) or with both position as well as odor identity (4 of 91 or 4%). The pattern of activity exhibited by the second subset of neurons has been referred to as "conjunctive coding" and can be considered a form of associative memory (see below). Similar patterns of conjunctive coding in hippocampal neurons were also reported by Hampson et al.[38] in a spatial delayed match to sample task and by Wiebe and Staubli[39] in an olfactory delayed nonmatching to sample task. Conjunctive coding neurons in the hippocampal formation that carry abstract information about the match-nonmatch status of a stimulus could also be used by the animal to perform a recognition memory task. Conjunctive coding is consistent with a recently outlined theoretical framework in which hippocampal activity is characterized as reflecting a sequence of episodic representations including the many complex conjunctions or associations unique to a particular episode.[40]

Although the majority of neurons in the hippocampal formation signal recognition memory either with the abstracted match-nonmatch signal or in conjunction with other aspects of the task, two recent studies[37,39] report a small number of stimulus-selective match-suppression or match-enhancement neurons in the rat hippocampal formation. Although these neurons were a minority, these findings suggest that in certain situations, hippocampal neurons can also signal "cortex-like" recognition memory signals. This kind of selective recognition memory signal has also been observed in the human hippocampus (see below). In no case has selective delay activity been reported in the hippocampal formation.

Contrasting Recognition Memory Signals in Cortex and Hippocampal Formation

The neurophysiological data described herein show that the entorhinal and perirhinal cortex, on the one hand, and the hippocampal formation, on the other, both signal recognition memory in different but complementary ways. The patterns of mnemonic activity observed in the entorhinal and perirhinal cortices can be summarized by two general principles. First, some cortical neurons signal recognition memory by either suppressing or enhancing their sensory-selective responses. Thus, if a neuron responds selectively to odor A, it might signal the repetition of odor A (i.e., a "match") with an enhanced response. Second, neurons in these cortical medial temporal lobe areas signal memory by sustaining or reactivating their activity in the delay period associated with a remembered stimulus. Thus, an entorhinal neuron might respond with an increased firing rate in the delay interval when odor A was presented as the sample, but not if any other odor was presented as the sample.

In contrast to the stimulus-selective recognition signals observed in cortex, neurons of the hippocampal formation convey abstracted recognition memory signals. For example, hippocampal neurons might signal any matching stimulus with a significantly enhanced or suppressed response. In other cases, hippocampal neurons signal stimulus recognition in conjunction with other aspects or elements of the task (i.e., conjunctive coding). It has been suggested that conjunctive coding may represent elements of unique episodes held in memory (e.g., an odor sampled in a particular place).[40] By this account, the "abstract" representations may provide access to all the episodic memories that include that abstraction. Thus, cells whose activity reflects, for example, a nonmatch, may provide a link to recent episodic memories of nonmatch trials. The more abstracted or conjunctive nature of the signal in the hippocampal formation compared to the cortex can be understood in terms of the connectivity of these areas. Whereas the cortex has prominent access to unimodal sensory information, the hippocampus is characterized by receiving input from other polymodal association areas. The hippocampus is in a privileged position to either combine the stimulus-selective mnemonic information in cortex into more complex conjunctions or to abstract, from the stimulus-selective information, a more general "output" signal. In certain task situations, a small number of neurons in the hippocampal formation signal the stimulus-selective match suppression or match enhancement similar to that observed in the entorhinal or perirhinal cortex. These "cortex-like" recognition signals may be conveyed via the direct projections from both the perirhinal and the entorhinal cortices to area CA1. Taken together, these findings suggest that all these medial temporal lobe areas work cooperatively to signal many forms of recognition memory.

Recognition Memory Signals in the Human Medial Temporal Lobe

While the majority of the information concerning neuronal activity in the medial temporal lobe during memory tasks comes from experimental studies in animals, there are also relevant data from the human literature. For example, a single unit physiology study in human neurological patients reported prominent recognition signals in the hippocampus (subregions of the hippocampus not specified), entorhinal cortex, and amygdala. In this study, individual neurons in all three areas were recorded during the encoding and retrieval phases of a yes-no recognition task in which faces and objects were used as stimuli.[41] Unlike most experimental studies in animals in which stimuli are only remembered for a maximum of several seconds, the retrieval phase in this task occurred between 1 and 10 hours after the encoding phase. Importantly, this is a delay interval known to challenge amnesic patients with selective hippocampal damage.[42] Despite the relatively small number of neurons examined (74 neurons in 3 regions), the overall pattern of activity was strikingly similar to the findings described for the perirhinal and entorhinal neurons in rats and monkeys. That is, neurons in the human hippocampus and entorhinal cortex responded selectively during the encoding phase of the task. Moreover, neural responses during the recognition phase were influenced not only by stimulus identity but also by whether the stimulus had been seen before. The responses of 35% (10 of 29) of cells recorded in the human hippocampus and 40% (8 of 20) of cells recorded in the entorhinal cortex in the retrieval phase were influenced by whether a stimulus was new or old. The majority of these cells exhibited enhanced activity in response to previously seen stimuli. These findings support the idea that neurons in the human hippocampus and entorhinal cortex signal long-term stimulus recognition for objects or faces. These findings are also consistent with findings from human neuropsychological studies[42] showing that discrete lesions limited to the hippocampus can impair performance on a wide variety of recognition tasks.

Another relevant set of findings derives from human functional imaging literature. A growing body of studies has shown that the hippocampal formation signals the relative novelty or familiarity of stimuli during the encoding phase of various tasks. Several studies compared responses during the encoding phase of recognition memory tasks of items that had been seen before (OLD conditions) to novel items (NEW). Irrespective of whether the to-be-remembered stimuli were pictures,[43,44] auditory sentences,[45] common words,[46,47] or nonpictorial visual stimuli,[47] significant activations were observed in the hippocampal formation and parahippocampal gyrus when the OLD condition was subtracted from the NEW. These findings are reminiscent of the patterns of activity of entorhinal and perirhinal neurons that respond best to particular novel stimuli and give increasingly suppressed responses to the same stimulus as it becomes familiar. Based on these findings, Tulving and colleagues[43] have argued that the medial temporal lobe is part of a novelty detection network. These patterns of activity could participate in many different forms of recognition memory, including the kind of recognition memory required to perform delayed nonmatching to sample with novel stimuli.[48] In this task, animals must discriminate a novel stimulus from one that has been seen once before. Indeed, lesions limited to the hippocampus produce a significant recognition memory impairment on this task that is most striking at the longest delay intervals.[48–50] In another study, however, no recognition impairment was observed following selective lesions of both the hippocampus and the amygdala.[51] Taken together, findings from the human functional imaging literature support the idea that the hippocampus signals information useful for certain forms of recognition memory.

NEURAL SIGNALS OF ASSOCIATIVE MEMORY

A second form of memory that has been examined at a neurophysiological level is associative memory. We define associative memory in a broad sense to include any memory about the relationship between two or more items. Unlike recognition memory, very little exists in the way of direct comparisons between firing patterns of neurons in the perirhinal and entorhinal cortex versus those in the hippocampal formation in tasks of associative memory. In a study explicitly designed to evaluate associative responses, Sakai and Miyashita[52] examined responses of anterior inferotemporal and perirhinal neurons to 24 fractal stimulus patterns. These stimuli were arbitrarily paired so that on each trial one stimulus of a pair was presented as a sample cue, and after a delay period was followed by a choice between the assigned paired cue and one of the other stimuli. After acquisition of this paired associate task over a series of training sessions, two different associative correlates were observed in the firing of these neurons. "Pair-coding" neurons fired maximally associated with presentations of either of the two cues that were paired associates, more so than for any of several other cues involved in different paired associates. "Pair-recall" neurons increased their firing rate during the delay period following presentation of the associate of the optimal cue, leading up to a robust response to that cue. Thus, within these cortical areas, stimulus-stimulus associations may be represented by the acquired capacity of a stimulus to generate the neural representation of another stimulus with which it has been associated.

In addition, in the study by Fried et al.[41] described above, single entorhinal and hippocampal neurons were recorded as human subjects viewed different faces in the encoding phase of the task. They found that some cells responded during the presentation of faces in both areas and that many of these neurons were activated differentially associated with the conjunction of particular facial expressions and gender and between facial expression and the identity of the face. These conjunctive (i.e., associative) responses were observed in both the entorhinal cortex and the hippocampus.

Other studies on humans using brain imaging methods have also shed light on neural activity in the hippocampus and neighboring parahippocampal cortex during associative learning. Henke et al.[53] measured activation of the medial temporal lobe using PET in subjects learning about pictures of people and houses. Subjects were trained in two conditions. In one condition they learned separately about a person and about a house, while making independent judgments about the gender of a person (single item learning condition) or whether the view of a house was inside or outside. In the other condition they were encouraged to learn an association between a person and a house while making a judgment about whether a particular person was likely to live in a particular house (associative learning condition). Participation in the associative learning condition led to better subsequent recognition of previously presented person-house pairings, suggesting this kind of processing indeed resulted in learning associations between particular persons and houses. In addition, both the parahippocampal gyrus and the hippocampus showed increased PET activation in the associative learning condition as compared to the single item learning condition, showing selective activation of both areas during this type of associative learning.

On the other hand, Gabrieli et al.[54] dissociated parahippocampal from hippocampal activation using fMRI. They found that the parahippocampal gyrus, but not the hippocampus, was selectively activated during the encoding of novel pictures. Conversely, the hippocampus (specifically the subiculum), but not the parahippocampal gyrus, was selectively activated during retrieval of a previously seen picture cued by the name of the pictured item or during retrieval of previously seen names of items cued by a picture of the item. Thus, under these conditions, activation of the parahippocampal cortex was differentially associated with encoding novel materials, whereas activation of the hippocampus was differentially associated with retrieval based on name-and-picture associations.

Findings from single unit recording studies in rodents also shed light on the issue of associative learning.[40] A common finding in this large literature is that hippocampal principal neurons fire when an animal is in a particular location in its environment. The firing patterns of many of these so-called place cells are dependent on the spatial configuration of multiple environmental cues and therefore are an example of conjunctive (i.e., associative) encoding. In addition, as described above, recent work has shown that the firing patterns of hippocampal principal neurons also incorporate a broad variety of nonspatial stimuli and behavioral events into their representations[37] and encode conjunctions of spatial and nonspatial information.[55] Thus, conjunctive/associative coding is particularly prominent in rodent hippocampal neurons.

Quirk et al.[56] directly compared the spatial firing properties of entorhinal neurons with those of principal cells of the hippocampus in rats foraging for food in each of two different environments. One environment was a circular open field surrounded by a plain cylinder with a contrasting vertical stripe that provided a salient orienting cue. The other environment was a square open field of the same area surrounded by a rectangular set of walls, one of which had the same contrasting color and therefore provided a similar orienting cue. Place cells were observed in both the entorhinal cortex and the hippocampus. In addition, many of the entorhinal place cells had similar spatial firing patterns in the two environments, so that translation of the "place field" from the circular to the square produced a close correspondence in the activity pattern of the cells in the two environments. By contrast, hippocampal neurons nearly always showed different and independent patterns of spatial activity in the two environments. These findings were interpreted as evidence that entorhinal cells were more strongly controlled by particular salient sensory cues (e.g., the orienting stripe), whereas hippocampal neurons were more strongly controlled by differences in the spatial geometry of the environments.

To summarize, consistent with the studies of recognition memory, evidence exists both for similarities in the types of associative memory coding apparent in the perirhinal and entorhinal cortex and the hippocampal formation under some testing conditions and for differences under other conditions. A compelling direct comparison that reveals the critical aspects of these different testing conditions has yet to be made. Yet the evidence showing differences between these areas suggests that parahippocampal cortical neurons may participate in associative memory by developing representations of complex perceptual stimuli that can be activated by their associates (i.e., pair-coding neurons of Sakai and Miyashita[52]), whereas neurons of the hippocampal formation participate in associative memory by representing conjunctions of independent perceptual stimuli as well as behavioral events (i.e., conjunctive coding neurons of Wood et al.[37]).

SUMMARY AND CONCLUSIONS

How do the structures of the medial temporal lobe signal the formation, retention, and recall of declarative memories? Far from a simple division of labor within the medial temporal lobe, the available neurophysiological evidence suggests that all medial temporal lobe areas can signal information relevant for all forms of declarative memory, from recognition to association. There are key differences, however, in the level or character of those signals, suggesting evidence for certain functional dissociations. These findings are also consistent with a large body of results from experimental lesion studies. For example, numerous studies have shown that damage including the entorhinal and perirhinal cortices produces impairment on tasks of recognition memory detectable even at short delay intervals (on the order of several seconds). This memory impairment is exacerbated as the delay intervals increase.[32,57,58] Importantly, the severe memory impairment following damage to the entorhinal or perirhinal cortex does not appear to be a perceptual deficit, because animals with large medial temporal lobe lesions including these structures can perform normally on recognition tasks when there is no delay interval between the sample and choice phases (zero-second delay interval).[59] Consistent with these findings from lesion studies, robust match-suppression and match-enhancement signals are observed with short delay intervals (on the order of several seconds), and these recognition signals persist for intervals as long as 24 hours.[26] Thus, these stimulus-selective recognition signals appear to be used at both short as well as longer delay intervals. In contrast to lesion studies involving the cortical medial temporal lobe areas, damage limited to the hippocampus produces the most striking recognition impairments when delay intervals are long (many minutes to hours).[48-50] At longer delay intervals, when interference can play a detrimental role, information about the context or episode in which the stimulus was seen could be particularly helpful to successful performance. By this view, the conjunctive signals conveyed by the hippocampus may be particularly useful when contextual or episodic information is needed to solve recognition tasks with long delay intervals. These findings support the view that the prominent selective recognition signals observed in the cortex as well as the robust conjunctive signals observed in the hippocampus contribute to successful recognition performance. Depending on the particular mnemonic demands of the task (long- vs. short-term memory or high vs. low interference), one or the other mnemonic signal may be preferentially used. Whereas less is known about the neural correlates of associative memory, differential patterns of associative coding have been described in the cortex on the one hand (pair-coding and pair-recall neurons) and in the hippocampus on the other (conjunctive signals). Additional comparative studies are needed to determine the full scope of neural signals underlying associative memory across the medial temporal lobe.

REFERENCES

1. SCOVILLE, W.B. & B. MILNER. 1957. Loss of recent memory after bilateral hippocampal lesions. J. Neurol. Neurosurg. Psychiatry **20:** 11–21.
2. EICHENBAUM, H. 1992. The hippocampal system and declarative memory in animals. J. Cognit. Neurosci. **4:** 217–231.50.
3. SQUIRE, L.R. & S.M. ZOLA. 1996. Structure and function of declarative and nondeclarative memory systems. Proc. Natl. Acad. Sci. USA **93:** 13515–13522.
4. VAN HOESEN, G.W. et al. 1972. Cortical afferents to the entorhinal cortex of the rhesus monkey. Science **175:** 1471–1473.
5. VAN HOESEN, G.W. et al. 1975. Some connections of the entorhinal (area 28) and perirhinal (area 35) cortices of the rhesus monkey. II. Frontal lobe afferents. Brain Res. **95:** 25–38.
6. VAN HOESEN, G.W. & D.N. PANDYA. 1975. Some connections of the entorhinal (area 28) and perirhinal (area 35) cortices of the rhesus monkey. I. Temporal lobe afferents. Brain Res. **95:** 1–24.
7. VAN HOESEN, G.W. & D.N. PANDYA. 1975. Some connections of the entorhinal (area 28) and perirhinal (area 35) cortices of the rhesus monkey. III. Efferent connections. Brain Res. **95:** 48–67.
8. DEACON, T.W. et al. 1983. Afferent connections of the perirhinal cortex in the rat. J. Comp. Neurol. **220:** 168–190.

9. MARTIN-ELKINS, C.L. & J.A. HOREL. 1992. Cortical afferents to behaviorally defined regions of the inferior temporal and parahippocampal gyri as demonstrated by WGA-HRP. J. Comp. Neurol. **321:** 177–192.
10. SUZUKI, W.A. & D.G. AMARAL. 1994. Perirhinal and parahippocampal cortices of the macaque monkey: cortical afferents. J. Comp. Neurol. **350:** 497–533.
11. BURWELL, R.D. & D.G. AMARAL. 1998. Cortical afferents of the perirhinal, postrhinal and entorhinal cortices. J. Comp. Neurol. **398:** 179–205.
12. BURWELL, R.D. et al. 1995. The perirhinal and postrhinal cortices of the rat: a review of the neuroanatomical literature and comparison with findings from the monkey brain. Hippocampus **5:** 390–408.
13. INSAUSTI, R. et al. 1987. The entorhinal cortex of the monkey: II. Cortical afferents. J. Comp. Neurol. **264:** 356–395.
14. BECKSTEAD, R.M. 1978. Afferent connections of the entorhinal area in the rat as demonstrated by retrograde cell-labeling with horseradish peroxidase. Brain Res. **152:** 249–264.
15. AMARAL, D.G. & M.P. WITTER. 1995. Hippocampal Formation. In The Rat Nervous System. G. Paxinos, Ed. Academic Press Inc. New York.
16. SUZUKI, W. & D.G. AMARAL. 1990. Cortical inputs to the CA1 field of the monkey hippocampus originate from the perirhinal and parahippocampal cortex but not from area TE. Neurosci. Lett. **115:** 43–48.
17. OTTO, T. & H. EICHENBAUM. 1992. Neuronal activity in the hippocampus during delayed nonmatch to sample performance in rats: evidence for hippocampal processing in recognition memory. Hippocampus **2:** 323–334.
18. SUZUKI, W.A. et al. 1997. Object and place memory in the macaque entorhinal cortex. J. Neurophysiol. **78:** 1062–1081.
19. MILLER, E.K. et al. 1993. Activity of neurons in anterior inferior temporal cortex during a short-term memory task. J. Neurosci. **13:** 1460–1478.
20. YOUNG, B.J. et al. 1997. Memory representation within the parahippocampal region. J. Neurosci. **17:** 5183–5195.
21. ZHU, X.O. et al. 1995. Neuronal signaling of information important to visual recognition memory in rat rhinal and neighboring cortices. Eur. J. Neurosci. **7:** 753–765.
22. MILLER, E.K. et al. 1996. Neural mechanisms of visual working memory in prefrontal cortex of the macaque. J. Neurosci. **16:** 5154–5167.
23. RICHES, I.P. et al. 1991. The effects of visual stimulation and memory on neurons of the hippocampal formation and the neighboring parahippocampal gyrus and inferior temporal cortex of the primate. J. Neurosci. **11:** 1763–1779.
24. FAHY, F.L. et al. 1993. Neuronal activity related to visual recognition memory: long-term memory and the encoding of recency and familiarity information in the primate anterior and medial inferior temporal and rhinal cortex. Exp. Brain Res. **96:** 457–472.
25. MILLER, E.K. & R. DESIMONE. 1994. Parallel neuronal mechanisms for short-term memory. Science **263:** 520–522.
26. XIANG, J.Z. & M.W. BROWN. 1998. Differential neuronal encoding of novelty, familiarity and recency in regions of the anterior temporal lobe. Neuropharmacology **37:** 657–676.
27. UNGERLEIDER, L.G. 1995. Functional brain imaging studies of cortical mechanisms for memory. Science **270:** 769–775.
28. SCHACTER, D.L. & R.L. BUCKNER. 1998. On the relations among priming, conscious recollection, and intentional retrieval: evidence from neuroimaging research. Neurobiol. Learn. Mem. **70:** 284–303.
29. CHUN, M.M. & E.A. PHELPS. 1999. Memory deficits for implicit contextual information in amnesic subjects with hippocampal damage. Nature Neurosci. **2:** 844–847.
30. GAFFAN, D. & E.A. MURRAY. 1992. Monkeys (*Macaca fascicularis*) with rhinal cortex ablations succeed in object discrimination learning despite 24-hr intertrial intervals and fail at matching to sample despite double sample presentations. Behav. Neurosci. **106:** 30–38.
31. MEUNIER, M. et al. 1993. Effects on visual recognition of combined and separate ablations of the entorhinal and perirhinal cortex in rhesus monkeys. J. Neurosci. **13:** 5418–5432.

32. MEUNIER, M. *et al.* 1996. Effects of rhinal cortex lesions combined with hippocampectomy on visual recognition memory in rhesus monkeys. J. Neurophys. **75:** 1190–1205.
33. BROWN, M.W. *et al.* 1987. Neuronal evidence that inferomedial temporal cortex is more important than hippocampus in certain processes underlying recognition memory. Brain Res. **409:** 158–162.
34. COLOMBO, M. & C.G. GROSS. 1994. Responses of inferior temporal cortex and hippocampal neurons during delayed matching to sample in monkeys (*Macaca fascicularis*). Behav. Neurosci. **108:** 443–455.
35. WILSON, F.A. *et al.* 1990. Hippocampus and medial temporal cortex: neuronal activity related to behavioural responses during the performance of memory tasks by primates. Behav. Brain Res. **40:** 7–28.
36. SAKURAI, Y. 1990. Hippocampal cells have behavioral correlates during the performance of an auditory working memory task in the rat. Behav. Neurosci. **104:** 253–263.
37. WOOD, E.R. *et al.* 1999. The global record of memory in hippocampal neuronal activity. Nature **397:** 613–616.
38. HAMPSON, R.E. *et al.* 1993. Hippocampal cell firing correlates of delayed-matching-to-sample performance in the rat. Behav. Neurosci. **107:** 715–739.
39. WIEBE, S. & U. STAUBLI. 1999. Dynamic filtering of recognition memory codes in the hippocampus. J. Neurosci. **19:** 10562–10574.
40. EICHENBAUM, H. *et al.* 1999. The hippocampus, memory, and place cells: is it spatial memory or a memory space? Neuron **23:** 209–226.
41. FRIED, I. *et al.* 1997. Single neuron activity in human hippocampus and amygdala during recognition of faces and objects. Neuron **18:** 753–765.
42. REED, J.M. & L.R. SQUIRE. 1997. Impaired recognition memory in patients with lesions limited to the hippocampal formation. Behav. Neurosci. **111:** 667–675.
43. TULVING, E. *et al.* 1996. Novelty and familiarity activations in PET studies of memory encoding and retrieval. Cereb. Cortex **6:** 71–79.
44. STERN, C.E. *et al.* 1996. The hippocampal formation participates in novel picture encoding: evidence from functional magnetic resonance imaging. Proc. Natl. Acad. Sci. USA **93:** 8660–8665.
45. TULVING, E. *et al.* 1994. Neuroanatomical correlates of retrieval in episodic memory: auditory sentence recognition. Proc. Natl. Acad. Sci. USA **91:** 2012–2015.
46. KAPUR, S. *et al.* 1995. Functional role of the prefrontal cortex in memory retrieval: a PET sutdy. NeuroReport **6:** 1880–1884.
47. MARTIN, A. *et al.* 1997. Modulation of human medial temporal lobe activity by form, meaning and experience. Hippocampus **7:** 587–593.
48. ZOLA, S.M. *et al.* 2000. Impaired recognition memory in monkeys after damage limited to the hippocampal region. J. Neurosci. **20:** 451–463.
49. BEASON-HELD, L. *et al.* 1999. Hippocampal formation lesions produce memory impairment in the rhesus monkey. Hippocampus **9:** 562–574.
50. HAMPSON, R.E. *et al.* 1999. Effects of ibotenate hippocampal and extrahippocampal destruction on delayed-match and -nonmatch-to-sample behavior in rats. J. Neurosci. **19:** 1492–1507.
51. MURRAY, E.A. & M. MISHKIN. 1998. Object recognition and location memory in monkeys with excitotoxic lesions of the amygdala and hippocampus. J. Neurosci. **18:** 6568.
52. SAKAI, K. & Y. MIYASHITA. 1991. Neural organization for the long-term memory of paired associates. Nature **354:** 152–155.
53. HENKE, K. *et al.* 1997. Human hippocampus establishes associations in memory. Hippocampus **7:** 249–256.
54. GABRIELI, J.D.E. *et al.* 1997. Separate neural basis of two fundamental memory processes in the human medial temporal lobe. Science **276:** 264–266
55. DEADWYLER, S.A. *et al.* 1996. Hippocampal ensemble activity during spatial delayed-nonmatch-to-sample performance in rats. J. Neurosci. **16:** 354–372.
56. QUIRK, G.J. *et al.* 1992. The positional firing properties of medial entorhinal neurons: description and comparison with hippocampal place cells. J. Neurosci. **12:** 1945–1963.
57. ZOLA-MORGAN, S. *et al.* 1989. Lesions of perirhinal and parahippocampal cortex that spare the amygdala and hippocampal formation produce severe memory impairment. J. Neurosci. **9:** 4355–4370.

58. SUZUKI, W.A. *et al.* 1993. Lesions of the perirhinal and parahippocampal cortices in the monkey produce long-lasting memory impairment in the visual and tactual modalities. J. Neurosci. **13:** 2430–2451.
59. OVERMAN, W.H. *et al.* 1990. Picture recognition vs. picture discrimination learning in monkeys with medial temporal removals. Exp. Brain Res. **79:** 18–24.

Involvement of Non-Neuronal Cells in Entorhinal-Hippocampal Reorganization Following Lesions

INGO BECHMANN AND ROBERT NITSCH[a]

Institute of Anatomy, Department of Cell and Neurobiology, Humboldt-University Hospital Charité, Berlin, Germany

ABSTRACT: Entorhinal lesion leads to anterograde degeneration of perforant path fibers in their main hippocampal termination zones. Subsequently, remaining fibers sprout and form new synapses on the denervated dendrites. This degeneration and reorganization is accompanied by sequential changes in glial morphology and function. Within a few hours following the lesion, amoeboid microglia migrate into the zone of denervation. Some hours later, signs of activation can be seen on astrocytes in the zone of denervation, where both cell types proliferate and remain in an activated state for more than two weeks. These activated glial cells might be involved in lesion-induced plasticity in at least two ways: (1) by releasing cytokines and growth factors which regulate layer-specific sprouting and (2) by phagocytosis of axonal debris, because myelin sheaths act as obstacles for sprouting fibers in the central nervous system. Whereas direct evidence for the former is still missing, the latter was investigated using phagocytosis-dependent labeling techniques. Both microglial cells and astrocytes incorporate axonal debris. Phagocytosing microglial cells develop the immune phenotype of antigen-presenting cells, whereas astrocytes strongly express FasL (CD95L), which induces apoptosis of activated lymphocytes. Thus, the interaction of glial cells with immune cells might be another, previously underestimated, aspect of reorganization following entorhinal lesion.

INTRODUCTION

Stereotaxic entorhinal cortex lesion (ECL) disconnects the hippocampal formation from its main afferent input, that is, the perforant path. Following ECL, intrinsic, associational, and commissural fibers sprout in the denervated outer molecular layers of the fascia dentata, a process that shows a high degree of layer specificity.[1–8] This process of reactive synaptogenesis had been considered to reflect the capability of functional reorganization following brain injury.[9–12] In spite of almost 30 years of research on plasticity following ECL, the molecular mechanisms regulating sprouting and reactive synaptogenesis are still not understood. Along with the numerous changes described in the denervated dentate gyrus after ECL, an early notion was a

[a]Address for correspondence: Robert Nitsch, M.D., Institute of Anatomy, Department of Cell and Neurobiology, Humboldt-University Hospital Charité, 10098 Berlin, Germany. Tel.: 0049-30-2802-3547; fax: 0049-30-2802-1460.
e-mail: robert.nitsch@charite.de

sequential activation of both astrocytes and microglial cells.[13–20] Interestingly, the onset of changes in glial morphology precedes the onset of sprouting, suggesting an active role for glial cells in inducing synaptic plasticity.[14] Although clear-cut evidence of such a role for glial cells is still missing, various studies contributed to a more detailed picture of the complex functional glial changes following ECL. From the data reviewed in this article, it now seems possible to design promising experiments to determine the function of glial cells in reorganization following hippocampal deafferentation. This kind of understanding might be helpful to counter putative harmful effects of glial responses without abrogating their helpful contributions to remodeling following brain lesions.

MORPHOLOGICAL CHANGES OF MICROGLIAL CELLS AND ASTROCYTES IN THE COURSE OF ANTEROGRADE DEGENERATION

Several studies have reported changes in glial cell morphology and distribution following ECL. A rapid transformation of ramified microglia to an amoeboid form in the zone of denervation can be observed as early as 1 day post lesion (dpl). The density of microglial cells increases in the zone of anterograde degeneration and decreases in adjacent hippocampal subfields, suggesting migration of microglia in the denervated area. These migratory cells show increased immunoreactivity for several microglial markers including 5′-nucleotidase,[20] OX-42 and GSI-B4,[18] VLA-4, ICAM-1 and LFA-1,[21] as well as MHC-I and LCA.[22] During the second and third week following ECL, microglial cells return to their resting state. In contrast, astrocytes exhibit a delayed, but long-lasting, hypertrophy and increased immunoreactivity for acidic glial fibrillary acidic protein (GFAP), first visible at about 2 dpl and lasting until at least 20 dpl.[14–16,23,24] The early notion of reactive glial cells was regarded as a sign of *activation*, but only recent findings enabled some of the functional implications of these morphological changes to be defined.

IDENTIFICATION OF PHAGOCYTIC GLIAL CELLS IN THE ZONE OF ANTEROGRADE DEGENERATION

The first step toward tissue repair in the course of anterograde degeneration is phagocytosis of axonal debris. This is of functional relevance because removal of degenerated material provides space for sprouting axons, and phagocytosis is the first step of interaction with the specific immune system. Moreover, myelin is known to act as a potential inhibitor of neurite growth and subsequent repair.[25] It was therefore necessary to determine the capacity and time schedule of debris removal, and to identify the cellular populations involved in phagocytosis. For that purpose, we established a phagocytosis-dependent labeling technique. The main idea behind this approach is that pretracing of neuronal structures and subsequent lesion-induced degeneration will lead to labeling of those cells that take up degenerated labeled debris. Subsequent immunocytochemistry then determines the type of phagocytic cell. Similar experimental designs have been applied to investigate the glial reaction in models of retrograde degeneration using carbocyanine dyes and Fluoro-Gold.[26–32] In

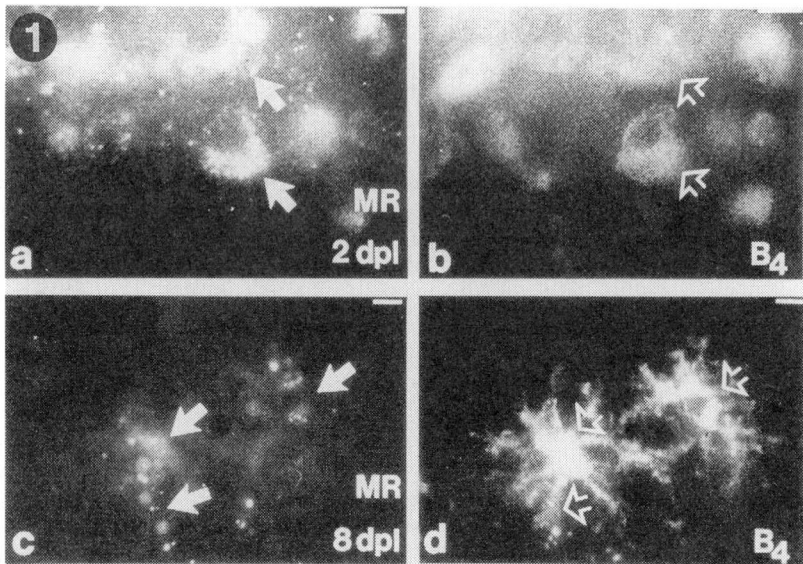

FIGURE 1. Identification of phagocytic microglial cells. (**a,b**) Arrows point to two cell-like structures loaded with rhodamine-fluorescent granules at 2 dpl. These cell-like structures can clearly be identified as Isolectin B4-positive cells exhibiting the typical morphology of activated microglial cells (*open arrows*, **b**). Scale bars = 10 µm. (**c,d**) Several MR-labeled granules (*arrows*, **c**) can be co-localized with ramified B4-positive microglial cells (*open arrows,* **d**) at 8 dpl. These cells exhibit the typical morphology of resting microglia. Scale bars = 5 µm. (From Bechmann & Nitsch.[18] Reprinted with permission from *Glia*.)

order to identify phagocytic glial cells following ECL, the perforant path was prelabeled with the biotin- and rhodamine-conjugated 10,000 D dextran amine Mini Ruby (MR).[33–36] Using double-fluorescence light and confocal as well as electron microscopy, this approach identified both microglial cells and astrocytes as scavengers of axonal debris.[18,19]

Phagocytic microglia exhibiting the typical morphology of amoeboid cells were first found at 1 dpl. Formerly phagocytic cells returned to a resting state and decreased in number until 15 dpl (FIG. 1). The first astrocytes that had incorporated degenerating fibers were found on day 3 post lesion (FIG. 2). After long survival times, virtually all GFAP-positive cells in the zone of anterograde degeneration exhibited phagocytosed granules. Conversely, phagocytic and non-phagocytic microglial cells were found close together, and no morphologic differences were seen between the two cell types.[18] This raises the possibility that different microglial subtypes exist or develop during brain diseases.

Besides the identification of phagocytosing cells, these experiments allowed us to follow the uptake of degenerated material. The phagocytosis of labeled debris could be followed by observing its translocation from extracellular to intracellular sites. After about two weeks following the lesion, the debris was almost completely located within phagocytosing cells (FIG. 3). This shows the capacity of glial cells to

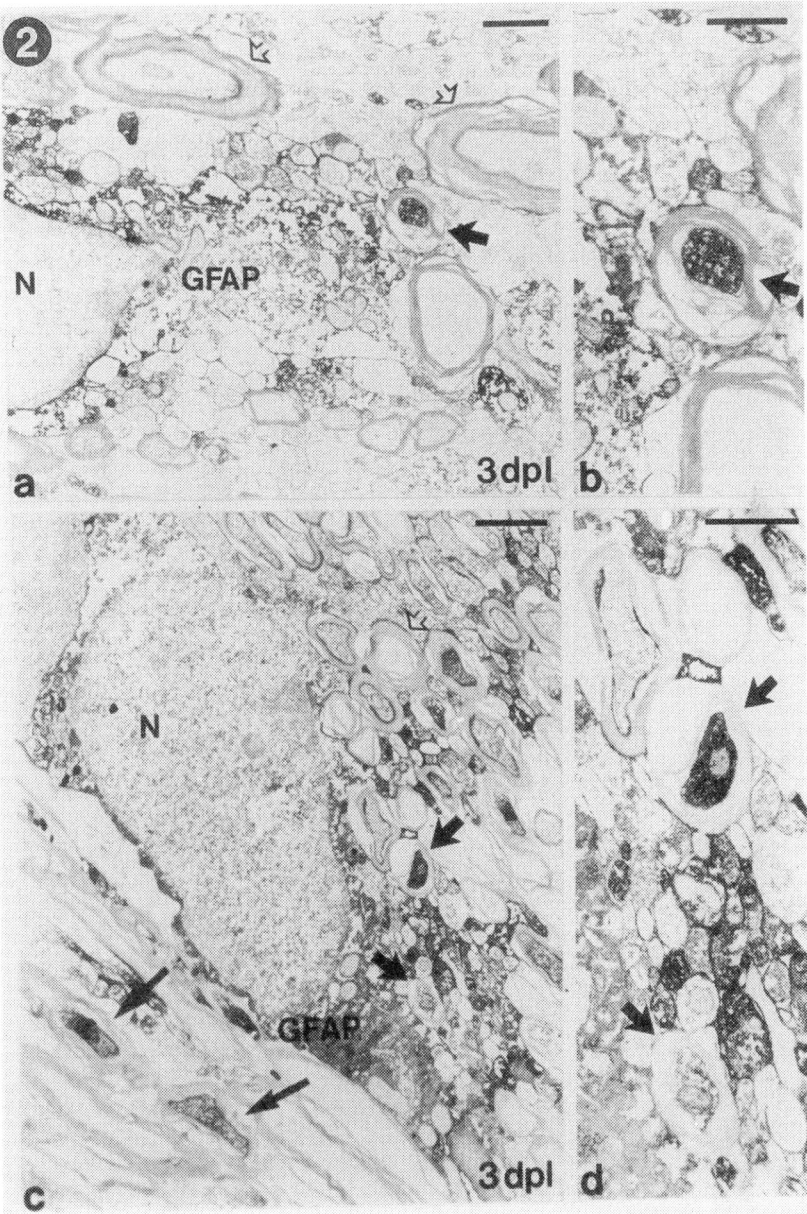

FIGURE 2. Identification of phagocytic astrocytes. (**a,b**) Electron micrographs show a GFAP-positive astrocyte at 3 dpl engulfing a traced myelinated fiber (*solid arrows,* **a** and **b**). *Open arrows* point to untraced myelinated axons. Note that GFAP immunoreactivity cannot be distinguished unequivocally from the intra-axonal DAB-converted Mini Ruby. Scale bars = 1 μm. (**c,d**) GFAP-positive astrocyte at 3 dpl has incorporated two traced axons (*thick arrows,*

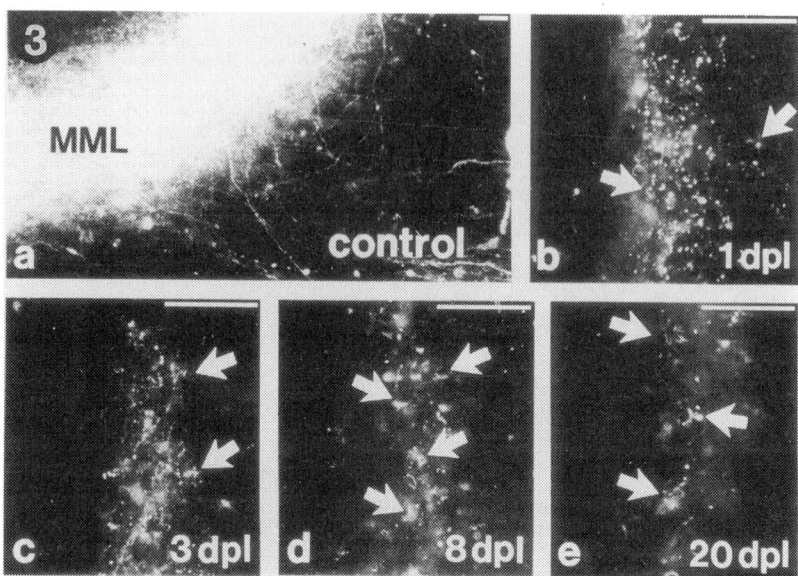

FIGURE 3. Uptake of debris. Translocation from extracellular to intracellular sites. (**a**) MR-traced fibers perforate the hippocampal fissure and form a dense plexus in their termination zone, i.e., the middle molecular layer (MML) of an unlesioned control animal. Scale bar = 10 μm. (**c,d,e**) In the course of degeneration, axons, as observed in **c**, convert to small fluorescent granules and appear as cell-like structures (*arrows*). As early as 1 dpl, the first cell-like structures can be seen (**b**). The MR-labeled debris is increasingly confined to cellular structures from 3 dpl (**c**) to 8 dpl (**d**). After 20 dpl, the fluorescent signal is for the most part located intracellularly (**e**). Scale bars = 50 μm. (From Bechmann & Nitsch.[18] Reprinted with permission from *Glia*.)

remove myelin sheath following ECL. This is of importance because degenerated axons are an obstacle to outgrowing fibers by inhibitory properties of myelin,[25] and an inhibited capacity of phagocytes to remove debris in the central nervous system (CNS) was linked to its limited ability to regenerate compared to peripheral nerves.[37–39] Experiments using stripe assays to determine the effects of myelin on outgrowing fibers in fact revealed that myelin-associated factors have a strong inhibitory effect on the outgrowth length of entorhinal axons.[40] Currently, drugs to selectively inhibit glial phagocytosis are not available. It will be of great interest to learn whether inhibited phagocytosis following ECL hinders sprouting and reactive synaptogenesis. The presence of peripheral macrophages might also enhance sprouting following ECL, as shown for optic fibers following nerve crush.[38]

---

c and **d**) and engulfs several others. O*pen arrow* points to an untraced axon, and thin arrows show traced, nonincorporated fibers. N, nucleus; GFAP, glial fibrillary acidic protein. Scale bar = 0.5 μm. (From Bechmann & Nitsch.[18] Reprinted with permission from *Glia*.)

FITC RHODAMINE

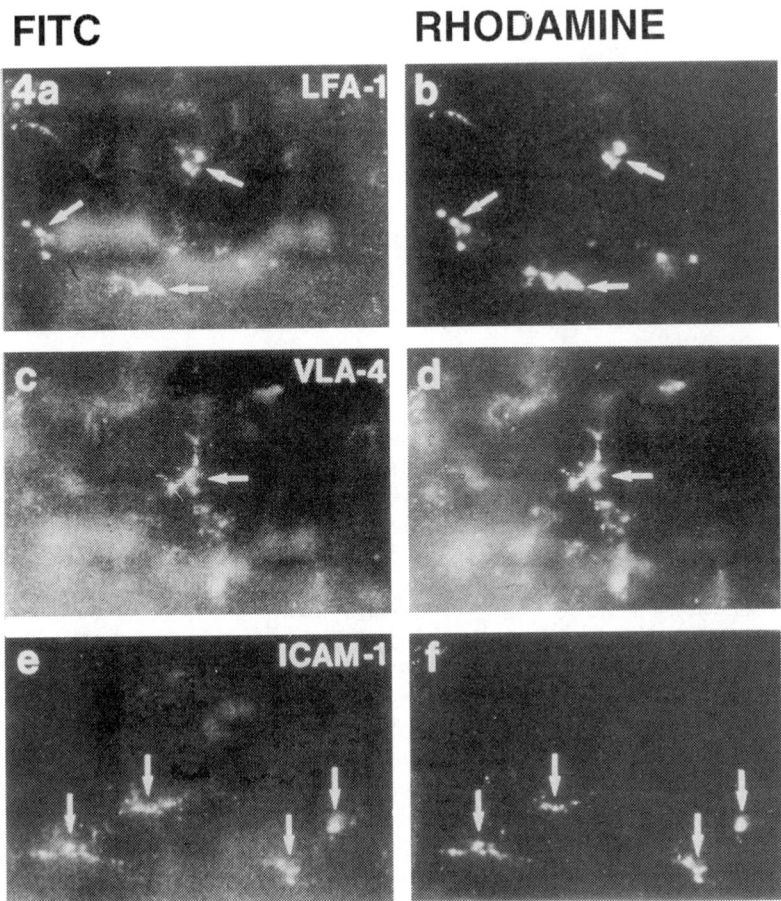

FIGURE 4. Expression of LFA-1a, VLA-4, and ICAM-1 on phagocytic microglial cells in the deafferented outer molecular layer (OML). (**a,c,e**) FITC-filter fluorescence photographs show activated microglial cells (*arrows*) following staining for LFA-1a (**a**), VLA-4 (**c**), or ICAM-1 (**e**). (**b,d,f**) Rhodamine-filter fluorescence photographs show corresponding regions to FITC-filter fluorescence photographs (a 4 b, c 4 d, and e 4 f), displaying double-labeled microglial cells (*arrows*) with incorporated, rhodamine-conjugated tracer that was previously contained in perforant path axons. (From Hailer *et al.*[21] Reprinted with permission from *Hippocampus*.)

CHANGES IN THE IMMUNE PHENOTYPE OF PHAGOCYTOSING GLIAL CELLS FOLLOWING ECL

Phagocytosis performed by astrocytes following ECL was an astonishing finding, because in models of retrograde degeneration using phagocytosis-dependent labeling, only microglial cells and perivascular cells were identified as neuronophages.[26–32] Since both cell types can stimulate naive T cells *in vitro*, the question of whether astrocytic and/or microglial phagocytosis is accompanied by the expression of molecules involved in antigen presentation became an important issue. Combinations of phagocytosis-dependent labeling and immunocytochemistry for the integrin adhesion molecules leukocyte function antigen-1 LFA-1, very late antigen-4 VLA-4 and the ligand of LFA-1, the intercellular adhesion molecule ICAM-1, demonstrated that microglial cells exclusively express these proteins[21] (FIG. 4).

Since myelin-associated proteins can induce immune responses, it will be of particular interest to see why the degeneration of myelinated fibers after ECL is not followed by autoimmune attacks. One possibility is that following ECL antigen-presenting cells in the brain lack co-stimulatory signals, leading to lymphocytic anergy, thus preventing immune responses. However, LFA-1 is a co-stimulatory molecule. Moreover, we recently detected the expression of B 7.1 (CD 80) on phagocytic microglia following ECL. Binding of B 7.1 to its receptor CD28 induces proliferation of naive T cells. Therefore, it appears that microglial cells are capable of presenting antigens and stimulating T cells following ECL. It will therefore be of interest to examine whether a direct contact of microglial cells with T lymphocytes occurs. Only one study has so far addressed this issue.[16] The authors reported that HRP injected in veins, and DiI-HDL labeled monocytes injected intraperitoneally, did not cross brain vessels in the zone of anterograde degeneration until 72 hours post lesion. From these findings, it was concluded that the blood-brain barrier is not disrupted following ECL. This conclusion is contradictory in several ways. First, it was shown that activated T cells permanently cross brain vessels[41,42] even though the blood-brain barrier remains impermeable for HRP.[43] Such an invasion does not necessarily take place within the first 72 hours following a lesion, but can occur weeks later, at least during retrograde degeneration.[43] Moreover, antigen presentation can occur at the glia limitans and thus without a previous infiltration of T cells.[44] For this reason, the issue of antigen presentation following ECL remains an open question. This became even more interesting because a possible role of (autoimmune) T cells in tissue healing and axonal growth was reported following optic nerve and spinal cord trauma.[45,46] A possible model to study the effects of autoimmune T cells in sprouting following ECL is discussed below.

PROLIFERATION OF ASTROCYTES AND MICROGLIAL CELLS FOLLOWING ECL

Another important question regarding glial roles following ECL was whether anterograde degeneration in this setting comprises signals that stimulate glial cells to proliferate. Thymidine injections before and shortly after ECL revealed a massive appearance of labeled cells in the ipsilateral and the contralateral hippocampus.[14] Using combined BrdU-labeling and immunocytochemistry for glial markers, both microglial cells and astrocytes were found to proliferate.[47] An increase in microglial counts was first observed at 3 dpl and ceased at 10 dpl. Astroglial cell numbers increased slightly later and were still elevated at 30 dpl. The total number of microglial cells in the hippocampus returned to control level at dpl 30. At dpl 100, astroglial counts also returned to pre-lesion levels in all dentate layers. The picture of microglial cells being quickly activated rather than delayed, combined with long-lasting astrocytic reactivity, is based on several phenomena including proliferation, phago-cytosis, and expression of various activation markers. However, both cell types show signs of activation well before the onset of sprouting, which starts at 4 dpl. This could indicate that (1) microglial signals are important for astrocytic activation, and (2) glial activation is a prerequisite for reactive synaptogenesis. A possible link be-tween microglia-induced activation of astrocytes and sprouting has been suggested by Gage and Fagan.[48,49] In their view, phagocytosing microglial cells could secrete IL-1,[50] which in turn stimulates astrocytes to release nerve growth factor (NGF).[51,52] As discussed below, various factors that provided instructive, permissive, and inhib-itory axonal guidance signals were found on glial cells following ECL. Whether the expression of such factors on astrocytes is indeed triggered by microglial cells re-mains to be determined. It is noteworthy that Gall and colleagues[14] described prolif-erative cells at the hilar border of the granule cell layer following ECL, an area which is not directly affected by the entorhinal lesion. This was 20 years before progenitor cells were found in this area.[53] As to how far these thymidine-labeled cells in the hi-lus derive from progenitors and further differentiate into glial cells or even neurons remains to be seen.

EXPRESSION OF FASL (CD95L) AND FAS FOLLOWING ECL (CD95)

Interestingly, the total number of glial cells returns to control levels after longer survival times. Following proliferation, one would expect increased numbers in the zone of denervation and, if migration does occur, also in the adjacent hippocampal subfields; this, however, is not the case.[47] The total number of microglia declines to pre-lesion levels at 30 dpl, the total number of astrocytes at 100 dpl. If migration is not responsible for this effect, the programmed cell death of activated glial cells could be an alternative explanation. We therefore studied glial apoptosis and the ex-pression and putative function of Fas (CD95) and FasL (CD95L) following ECL. Fas is a cell surface receptor that mediates apoptosis after cross-linking with its ligand FasL.[54–56] In the immune system, the growth of lymphocytes is regulated via Fas-mediated apoptosis, and deficiencies in this system lead to severe lymphoprolifera-tive diseases. Activated lymphocytes upregulate the expression of both proteins, leading to cell death both by suicide and fratricide. Whether glial populations are controlled in the same way is unknown. However, the expression of Fas and FasL on glial cells has been described,[57–63] rendering them putative targets of Fas-induced lysis. Indeed, we found a strong increase of both Fas and FasL on reactive, prolifer-ative astrocytes in the first 10 days following the lesion, yet this was not accompa-nied by astrocytic cell death until at least 14 dpl. However, few apoptotic bodies were found in the zone of anterograde degeneration. From the size and morphology of these cells, it is tempting to speculate that they belong to the hematopoetic lin-eage.[64] From these data, one can conclude that astrocytes do not die in the first two weeks following the lesion, supporting the concepts of them providing a growth-supportive environment.

Because astrocytic FasL does not act upon astrocytes themselves, other cells might be targets of FasL-mediated lysis. One possible candidate is lymphocytes be-cause intrinsic FasL expression was shown to act upon infiltrating T cells.[57,65] Our current data, using FasL-deficient and nondeficient astrocytes in co-culture with activated T cells, show that the capacity of astrocytes to kill T cells is FasL-dependent. Thus, astrocytes might form an immunological brain barrier for infiltrating immune cells, thereby contributing to the maintenance of the immune privilege in the intact and the injured central nervous system.[57]

EXPRESSION OF MOLECULES RELEVANT FOR FIBER GROWTH INHIBITION AND SUPPORT

One astonishing feature of plasticity following ECL is the laminar specificity of growing fibers. Originally, it was believed that the source of sprouting fibers was the inner molecular layer. Using *Phaseolus vulgaris* leucoagglutinin to visualize single sprouting axons, it recently became possible to demonstrate that this is not the case. In fact, it was shown that remaining fibers of the outer molecular layer expand and form new synapses on denervated dendrites.[66–68] The border between inner and outer molecular layers seems to be a barrier for growing fibers. Whereas establishing new synapses might be regulated by differential expression of (adhesion) molecules along intact and denervated parts of dendrites,[69] growth-promoting and guidance molecules were found on astrocytes following ECL. Ciliary neurotrophic factor (CNTF) and its receptor, CTNF-α, were found on astrocytes in the outer molecular layer following ECL. CNTF has been shown to ameliorate axotomy-induced degeneration of CNS neurons. Since its receptor is expressed on granule cells, the astrocytic CNTF may act upon these neurons in a neurotrophic manner following lesions.[70,71] Another interesting protein that might regulate the layer specificity is tenascin-C. Growth cone-deflecting, as well as neurite outgrowth-promoting, isoforms of tenascin-C were upregulated after ECL. Thus, a tenascin-C-rich substrate is present in the outer molecular layer during the time of sprouting, and a sharp boundary is formed against the inner molecular layer. Neurite outgrowth may be promoted within the denervated zone, whereas axons trying to grow into the denervated outer molecular layer, for example, from the inner molecular layer, would be deflected by a tenascin-C-rich barrier.[72] These data suggest that astrocytes might well secrete factors that regulate axonal reorganization.

ENTORHINAL-HIPPOCAMPAL ORGANOTYPIC SLICE CULTURES AS A MODEL TO STUDY HIPPOCAMPAL REORGANIZATION FOLLOWING LESIONS

Although the expression of various factors related to axonal sprouting was reported following ECL, their functional relevance still awaits conclusive determination because of technical restrictions. Blocking experiments using antisense strategies or blocking antibodies are hindered by the *in vivo* situation. It was therefore necessary to establish an *in vitro* system that maintains the complexity of the entorhinal-hippocampal system, while allowing the easy application of drugs, for example, inhibitors of receptors and their ligands or cytokines. In an attempt to provide such an *in vitro* model, organotypic entorhinal-hippocampal complex slice cultures were es-

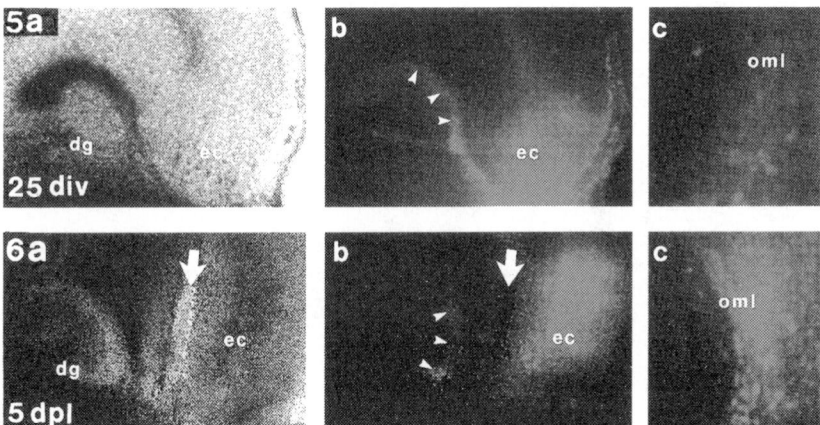

FIGURES 5 and 6. Tracing of the perforant path *in vitro.* **Top row (FIG. 5):** At 5 days after a Mini Ruby application and 25 days *in vitro* (div), the perforant path is apparent by fluorescence and light microscopy. **Bottom row (FIG. 6):** Slice culture 5 days after perforant path transsection after 8 days *in vitro* and 8 days after Mini Ruby application on the entorhinal cortex. Phase contrast microscopy (**a**) and epifluorescence microscopy (**b**) of the same slice culture with entorhinal cortex (ec), Hippocampus with dentate gyrus (dg), and the visible transsection cut (*arrow*). At 5 days post lesion (dpl), a change in the distribution of Mini Ruby in the outer molecular layers (oml) (*arrowheads*) of the dentate gyrus can be observed. (**c**) The formerly fluorescent band in the outer molecular layer at higher magnification developed into a more cellular arrangement of the fluorescent tracer reflecting the uptake of debris. (From Kluge *et al.*[75] Reprinted with permission of *Hippocampus.*)

tablished.[73] These complex slice cultures contain the cells of origin located in the EC, the maintained perforant path, and its target structures—for example, neurons in the dentate gyrus—but depend upon a proper preparatory approach. The projection of the perforant path perpendicular to the longitudinal axis of the hippocampus[74] leads to problems in maintaining the perforant path in slice preparations. Therefore, we developed an *in situ* tracing technique that allows observation of perforant path fibers in living slices.[75] In this way, slices containing this pathway can be selected, and its maintenance following various stimuli can be monitored at any time point during tissue cultivation (FIG. 5). After an initial glial activation as a result of slice preparation, the inner zone of the tissue provides an environment inducing deactivation of glial cells at the beginning of the second week *in vitro.*[76,77] Thus, about this time, slice cultures can be used as a model of intact brain tissue. We have shown that knife lesions in the entorhinal cortex of slices lead to the same glial responses observed *in vivo*, that is, activation, proliferation, migration, and phagocytosis.[75] Using these slice cultures, it is now possible to study the influence of molecules such as cytokines, receptors and their ligands. Present data suggest that the role of glial cells in hippocampal reorganization, such as changes in dendritic arborization, can be addressed. Factors deactivating the glial response allow to answer the important question of whether the post lesional activation is a detrimental or helpful event (Eyüpoglu *et al.*, in preparation).

CONCLUDING REMARKS

In the last three decades of studying degeneration and reorganization following entorhinal cortex lesion, important lessons have been learned. It is now clear that reactive synaptogenesis is not solely a neuronal issue. Glial cells contribute by removing debris, thereby providing space for outgrowing fibers. More specifically, they participate by secreting growth-promoting molecules. New technical approaches are now available to test the relevant factors in this setting. In contrast to the peripheral nervous system, the capability of the CNS to regenerate is limited to small distances. Understanding the factors that regulate these events might help to develop new strategies to overcome this limitation and finally enable better treatment of brain trauma.

ACKNOWLEDGMENTS

The authors wish to thank Dr. N. P. Hailer and A. Kluge who contributed substantially to this work. We also thank S. J. Letham and A. Kovac for carefully reviewing the manuscript. Our studies reviewed in this paper were supported by DFG: SFB 507/C1 and DFG project BE 2272/1-1.

REFERENCES

1. LYNCH, G., D.A. MATTHEWS, S. MOSKO, T. PARKS & W. COTMAN. 1972. Induced acetylcholine-rich layer in rat dentate gyrus following entorhinal lesion. Brain Res. **42:** 311–318.
2. LYNCH, G., S.A. DEADWYLER & G. COTMAN. 1973. Postlesion axonal growth produces permanent functional connections. Science **180:** 1364–1368.
3. MATTHEWS, D.A., C.W. COTMAN & G. LYNCH. 1976. An electron microscopical study of lesion-induced synaptogenesis in the dentate gyrus of the adult rat. I. Magnitude and time course of degeneration. Brain Res. **115:** 1–21.
4. MATTHEWS, D.A., C.W. COTMAN & G. LYNCH. 1976. An electron microscopical study of lesion induced synaptogenesis in the dentate gyrus of the adult rat. II. Reappearance of morphologically normal synaptic contacts. Brain Res. **115:** 23–41.
5. STEWARD, O. & J.A. MESSENHEIMER. 1978. Histochemical evidence for a postlesion reorganization of cholinergic afferents in the hippocampal formation of the mature cat. J. Comp. Neurol. **178:** 697–709.
6. FROTSCHER, M. 1991. Target cell specificity of synaptic connections in the hippocampus. Hippocampus **1:** 123–130.
7. DELLER, T., M. FROTSCHER & R. NITSCH. 1995. Morphological evidence for the sprouting of inhibitory commissural fibers in response to the lesion of excitatory entorhinal input to the rat dentate gyrus. J. Neurosci. **15:** 6868–6878.
8. DELLER, T., M. FROTSCHER & R. NITSCH. 1996. Sprouting of crossed entorhinodentate fibers after unilateral entorhinal lesion: anterograde tracing of fiber reorganization with *Phaseolus vulgaris*-leucoagglutinin (PHAL). J. Comp. Neurol. **365:** 42–55.
9. MYHRER, T. 1975. Maze performance in rats with hippocampal perforant path lesion: some aspects of functional recovery. Physiol. Behav. **15:** 433–437.
10. LOESCHE, J. & O. STEWARD. 1977. Behavioral correlates of the denervation and reinnervation of the hippocampal formation of the rat: recovery of alteration performance following unilateral entorhinal lesion. Brain Res. Bull. **2:** 31–39.
11. STEWARD, O., J. LOESCHE & W.C. HORTON. 1977. Behavioral correlates of denervation and reinnervation of the hippocampal formation of the rat: open field activity and cue utilization following bilateral entorhinal cortex lesions. Brain Res. Bull. **2:** 41–48.

12. COTMAN, C.W. & M. NIETO-SAMPEDRO. 1985. Progress in facilitating the recovery of function after central nervous system trauma. Ann. N.Y. Acad. Sci. **457:** 83–104.
13. ADAMS, I. & D.G. JONES. 1982. Synaptic remodeling and astrocytic hypertrophy in rat cerebral cortex from early to late adulthood. Neurobiol. Aging **3:** 179–186.
14. GALL, C., G. ROSE & G. LYNCH. 1979. Proliferative and migratory activity of glial cells in the partially deafferentated hippocampus. J. Comp. Neurol. **183:** 539–550.
15. GEHRMANN, J., S.W. SCHOEN & G.W. KREUTZBERG. 1991. Lesion of the rat entorhinal cortex leads to a rapid microglial reaction in the dentate gyrus. Acta Neuropathol. **82:** 442–455.
16. FAGAN, A.M. & F.H. GAGE. 1994. Mechanism of sprouting in the adult nervous system: cellular responses in areas of terminal degeneration and reinnervation of the hippocampus. Neuroscience **58:** 705–725.
17. JENSEN, M.B., B. GONZALEZ, B. CASTELLANO & J. ZIMMER. 1994. Microglial and astroglial reactions to anterograde axonal degeneration: a histochemical and immunocytochemical study of the adult rat fascia dentata after entorhinal perforant path lesion. Exp. Brain Res. **98:** 245–260.
18. BECHMANN, I. & R. NITSCH. 1997. Astrocytes and microglial cells incorporate degenerating fibers following entorhinal lesion: a light, confocal, and electron microscopical study using a phagocytosis-dependent labeling technique. Glia **20(2):** 145–154.
19. BECHMANN, I. & R. NITSCH. 1997. Identification of phagocytic glial cells after lesion-induced anterograde degeneration using double-fluorescence labeling: combination of axonal tracing and lectin or immunostaining. Histochem. Cell Biol. **107(5):** 391–397.
20. SCHOEN, S.W. & G.W. KREUTZBERG. 1994. Synaptic 5′-nucleotidase activity reflects lesion-induced sprouting within the adult rat dentate gyrus. Exp. Neurol. **127(1):** 106–118.
21. HAILER, N.P., I. BECHMANN, S. HEIZMANN & R. NITSCH. 1997. Adhesion molecule expression on phagocytic microglial cells following anterograde degeneration of perforant path axons. Hippocampus **7:** 341–349.
22. JENSEN, M.B., B. FINSEN & J. ZIMMER. 1997. Morphological and immunophenotypic microglial changes in the denervated fascia dentata of adult rats: correlation with blood-brain barrier damage and astroglial reactions. Exp. Neurol. **143:** 103–116.
23. JENSEN, M.B., B. GONZALEZ, B. CASTELLANO & J. ZIMMER. 1994. Microglial and astroglial reactions to anterograde axonal degeneration: a histochemical and immunocytochemical study of the adult rat fascia dentata after entorhinal perforant path lesion. Exp. Brain Res. **98:** 245–260.
24. STEWARD, O., M.S. KELLEY & E.R. TORRE. 1993. The process of reinnervation in the denate gyrus of adult rats: temporal relationsship between changes in the level of glial fibrillary acidic protein (GFAP) and GFAP mRNA in reactive astrocytes. Exp. Neurol. **124:** 167–183.
25. SCHNELL, L. & M.E. SCHWAB. 1990. Axonal regeneration in the rat spinal cord produced by an antibody against myelin-associated neurite growth inhibitors. Nature **343:** 269–272.
26. RINAMAN, L., C.E. MILLIGAN & P. LEVITT. 1991. Persistence of fluoro-gold following degeneration of labeled motoneurons is due to phagocytosis by microglia and macrophages. Neuroscience **44(3):** 765–776.
27. THANOS, S. 1991. Specific transcellular carbocyanine-labeling of rat retinal microglia during injury-induced neuronal degeneration. Neurosci. Lett. **127:** 108–112.
28. THANOS, S. 1992. Sick photoreceptors attract activated microglia from the ganglion cell layer: a model to study the inflammatory cascades in rats with inherited retinal dystrophy. Brain Res. **588:** 21–28.
29. THANOS, S., J. MEY & M. WILD. 1993. Treatment of adult retina with microglia-suppressing factor retards axotomy induced neuronal degradation and enhances axonal regeneration *in vivo* and *in vitro*. J. Neurosci. **13:** 455–466.
30. THANOS, S., J. KASCA, J. SEEGER & J. MEY. 1994. Old dyes for new scopes: phagocytosis-dependent long-term fluorescence labeling of microglial cells *in vivo*. TINS **17:** 1994.
31. STREIT, W.J. & M.B. GRAEBER. 1993. Heterogeneity of microglial and perivascular cell populations: insights gained from the facila nucleus paradigm. Glia **7:** 68–74.

32. ANGELOV, D.N., W.F. NEISS, M. STREPPEL, M. WALTHER, O. GUNTINAS-LICHIUS & E. STENNERT. 1996. ED2-positive perivascular cells act as neuronophages during delayed neuronal loss in the facial nucleus of the rat. Glia **16:** 129–139.
33. FRITZSCH, B. 1993. Fast axonal diffusion of 3000 molecular weight dextran amines. J. Neurosci. Methods **50:** 95–103.
34. FRITZSCH, B. & C. WILM. 1990. Dextran amines in neuronal tracing. TINS **13:** 14 (letter).
35. BOULTON, C.L., D. VON HAEBLER & U. HEINEMANN. 1992. Tracing of axonal connections by rhodamine-dextranamine in the rat hippocampal-entorhinal cortex slice preparation. Hippocampus **2:** 99–106.
36. OHM, T.G. & S. DIEKMANN. 1994. The use of lucifer yellow and mini ruby for intracellular staining in fixed brain tissue. Methodological considerations evaluated in rat and human autopsy brains. J. Neurosci. Methods **55:** 105–110.
37. CADELLI, D.S., C.E. BANDTLOW & M.E. SCHWAB. 1992. Oligodendrocyte- and myelin-associated inhibitors of neurite outgrowth: their involvement in the lack of CNS regeneration. Exp. Neurol. **115:** 189–92.
38. LAZAROV-SPIEGLER, O., A.S. SOLOMON, S. BENN ZEEV-BRANN, M. BELKIN, S. RUMELT & M. SCHWARTZ. 1996. Transplantation of activated macrophages overcomes central nervous system regrowth failure. FASEB J. **10:** 1296–1302.
39. ZEEV-BRANN, A.B., O. LAZAROV-SPIEGLER, T. BRENNER & M. SCHWARTZ. 1998. Differential effects of central and peripheral nerves on macrophages and microglia. Glia **23:** 181–190.
40. SAVASKAN, N.E., M. PLASCHKE, O. NINNEMANN, A.A. SPILLMANN, M.E. SCHWAB, R. NITSCH & T. SKUTELLA. 1999. Myelin does not influence the choice behaviour of entorhinal axons but strongly inhibits their outgrowth length *in vitro*. Eur. J. Neurosci. **11**(1)**:** 316–326.
41. HICKEY, W.F., B.L. HSU & H. KIMURA. 1991. T-lymphocyte entry into the central nervous system. J. Neurosci. Res. **28:** 254–260.
42. WEKERLE, H. 1993. Lymphocyte traffic to the brain. *In* The Blood-Brain Barrier. W.M. Pardridg, Ed.: 67–85. Raven Press. New York.
43. RAIVICH, G., L.L. JONES, C.U. KLOSS, A. WERNER, H. NEUMANN & G.W. KREUTZBERG. 1998. Immune surveillance in the injured nervous system: T-lymphocytes invade the axotomized mouse facial motor nucleus and aggregate around sites of neuronal degeneration. J. Neurosci. **18**(15)**:** 5804–5816.
44. LASSMANN, H., F. ZIMPRICH, K. VASS & W.F. HICKEY. 1991. Microglial cells are components of the perivascular glia limitans. J. Neurosci. Res. **28:** 236–243.
45. RAPALINO, O., O. LAZAROV-SPIEGLER, E. AGRANOV, G.J. VELAN, E. YOLES, M. FRAIDAKIS, A. SOLOMON, R. GEPSTEIN, A. KATZ, M. BELKIN, M. HADANI & M. SCHWARTZ. 1998. Implantation of stimulated homologous macrophages results in partial recovery of paraplegic rats. Nature Med. **4**(7)**:** 814–821.
46. MOALEM, G., R. LEIBOWITZ-AMIT, E. YOLES, F. MOR, I.R. COHEN & M. SCHWARTZ. 1999. Autoimmune T cells protect neurons from secondary degeneration after central nervous system axotomy. Nature Med. **5**(1)**:** 49–55.
47. HAILER, N.P., A. GRAMP & R. NITSCH. 1999. Proliferation of microglia and astrocytes in the dentate gyrus following entorhinal lesion: a quantitative bromodeoxyuridine-labeling study. Eur. J. Neurosci. In press.
48. GAGE, F.H., P. OLEJNICZAK & D.M. ARMSTRONG. 1988. Astrocytes are important for sprouting in the septohippocampal circuit. Exp. Neurol. **102:** 2–13.
49. FAGAN, A.M. & F.H. GAGE. 1990. Cholinergic sprouting in the hippocampus: a proposed role for IL-1. Exp. Neurol. **110**(1)**:** 105–120.
50. GIULIAN, D. & L.B. LACHMANN. 1985. Interleukin-1 stimulation of astroglial proliferation after brain injury. Science **228:** 497–498.
51. LINDSAY, R.M. 1979. Adult rat brain astrocytes support survival of both NGF-dependent and NGF-insensitive neurons. Nature **282:** 80–82.
52. WUJEK, J.R. & R.A. AKESON. 1987. Extracellular matrix derived from astrocytes stimulates neuritic outgrowth from PC12 cells *in vitro*. Brain Res. **431:** 87–97.
53. GAGE, F.H., G. KEMPERMANN, T.D. PALMER, D.A. PETERSON & J. RAY. 1998. Multipotent progenitor cells in the adult dentate gyrus. J. Neurobiol. **36**(2)**:** 249–266.

54. MIYAWAKI, T., T. VEHARA, R. NIBU, T. TSUJI, A. YACHIE, S. YONEHARA & N. TAGUCHI. 1992. Differential expression of apoptosis-related Fas antigen on lymphocyte subpopulations in human peripheral blood. J. Immunol. **149:** 3753–3758.

55. OWEN-SCHAUB, L.B., S. YONEHARA, W.L. CRUMP III & E.A. GRIMM. 1992. DNA fragmentation and cell death is selectively triggered in activated human lymphocytes by Fas antigen engagement. Cell. Immunol. **140**(1): 197–205.

56. DHEIN, J., H. WALCZAK, C. BAUMLER, K.M. DEBATIN & P.H. KRAMMER. 1995. Autocrine T-cell suicide mediated by APO-1/(Fas/CD95). Nature **373**(6513): 438–441.

57. BECHMANN, I., G. MOR, J. NELSON, M. ELIZA, R. NITSCH & F. NAFTOLIN. 1999. FasL (CD95L, APO1L) is expressed in the normal rat and human brain: evidence for the existence of an immunological brain barrier. Glia **27:** 62–74.

58. D'SOUZA, S., B. BONETTI, V. BALASINGMAN, N. CASHMAN, P. BARKER, A. TROUTT, C. RAINE & J. ANTEL. 1996. Multiple sclerosis: Fas signaling in oligodendrocyte cell death. J. Exp. Med. **184:** 2361–2370.

59. SPANAUS, K.S., R. SCHLAPBACH & A. FONTANA. 1998. TNF–alpha and IFN-gamma render microglia sensitive to Fas ligand-induced apoptosis by induction of Fas expression and down-regulation of Bcl-2 and Bcl-xL. Eur. J. Immunol. **28**(12): 4398–4408.

60. NISHIMURA, T., H. AKIYAMA, S. YONEHARA, H. KONDO, K. IKEDA, M. KATO, E. ISEKI & K. KOSAKA. 1995. Fas antigen expression in brains of patients with Alzheimer-type dementia. Brain Res **695**(2): 137–145.

61. BECHER, B., S.D. D'SOUZA, A.B. TROUTT & J.P. ANTEL. 1998. Fas expression on human fetal astrocytes without susceptibility to Fas-mediated cytotoxicity. Neuroscience **4**(2): 627–634.

62. CHOI, C., J.Y. PARK, J. LEE, J.H. LIM, E.C. SHIN, Y.S. AHN, C.H. KIM, S.J. KIM, J.D. KIM, I.S. CHOI & I.H. CHOI. 1999. Fas ligand and Fas are expressed constitutively in human astrocytes and the expression increases with IL-1, IL-6, TNF-alpha, or IFN-gamma. J. Immunol. **162**(4): 1889–1895.

63. SAAS, P., J. BOUCRAUT, A.L. QUIQUEREZ, V. SCHNURIGER, G. PERRIN, S. DESPLAT JEGO, D. BERNARD, P.R. WALKER & P.Y. DIETRICH. 1999. CD95 (Fas/Apo-1) as a receptor governing astrocyte apoptotic or inflammatory responses: a key role in brain inflammation? J. Immunol. **162**(4): 2326–2333.

64. BECHMANN, I., B. LOSSAU, B. STEINER, G. MOR, U. GIMSA & R. NITSCH. 1999. Reactive astrocytes upregulate Fas (CD95) and FasL (CD95L) expression, but do not undergo apoptosis in the course of anterograde degeneration. Submitted.

65. SABELKO-DOWNES, K.A., A.H. CROSS & J.H. RUSSELL. 1999. Dual role for Fas ligand in the initiation of and recovery from experimental allergic encephalomyelitis. J. Exp. Med. **189**(8): 1195–1205.

66. DELLER, T., M. FROTSCHER & R. NITSCH. 1995. Morphological evidence for the sprouting of inhibitory commissural fibers in response to the lesion of the excitatory entorhinal input to the rat dentate gyrus. J. Neurosci. **15**(10): 6868–6878.

67. FROTSCHER, M., B. HEIMRICH & T. DELLER. 1997. Sprouting in the hippocampus is layer-specific. Trends Neurosci. **20**(5): 218–222.

68. DELLER, T. 1998. The anatomical organization of the rat fascia dentata: new aspects of laminar organization as revealed by anterograde tracing with *Phaseolus vulgaris-*leucoagglutinin (PHAL). Anat. Embryol. **197:** 89–103.

69. MILLER, P.D., S.D. STYREN, C.F. LAGENAUR & S.T. DEKOSKY. 1994. Embryonic neural cell adhesion molecule (N-CAM) is elevated in the denervated rat dentate gyrus. J. Neurosci. **14**(7): 4217–4225.

70. GUTHRIE, K.M., A.G. WOODS, T. NGUYEN & C.M. GALL. 1997. Astroglial ciliary neurotrophic factor mRNA expression is increased in fields of axonal sprouting in deafferented hippocampus. J. Comp. Neurol. **386**(1): 137–148.

71. LEE, M.Y., T. DELLER, M. KIRSCH, M. FROTSCHER & H.D. HOFMANN. 1997. Differential regulation of ciliary neurotrophic factor (CNTF) and CNTF receptor alpha expression in astrocytes and neurons of the fascia dentata after entorhinal cortex lesion. J. Neurosci. **17**(3): 1137–1146.

72. DELLER, T., C.A. HAAS, T. NAUMANN, A. JOESTER, A. FAISSNER & M. FROTSCHER. 1997. Up-regulation of astrocyte-derived tenascin-C correlates with neurite outgrowth in

the rat dentate gyrus after unilateral entorhinal cortex lesion. Neuroscience **81**(3): 829–846.

73. DIEKMANN, S., R. NITSCH & T.G. OHM. 1994. The organotypic entorhinal-hippocampal complex slice culture of adolescent rats. A model to study transcellular changes in a circuit particularly vulnerable in neurodegenerative disorders. J. Neural Transm. Suppl. **44:** 61–71.

74. AMARAL, D.G. & M.P. WITTER. 1989. The three-dimensional organization of the hippocampal formation: a review of anatomical data. Neuroscience **31**(3): 571–591.

75. KLUGE, A., N.P. HAILER, T.L. HORVATH, I. BECHMANN & R. NITSCH. 1998. Tracing of the entorhinal-hippocampal pathway *in vitro*. Hippocampus **8:** 57–68.

76. HAILER, N.P., J. JARHULD & R. NITSCH. 1996. Resting microglial cells *in vitro*: analysis of morphology and adhesion molecule expression in organotypic hippocampal slice cultures. Glia **18:** 319–331.

77. HAILER, N.P., F.L. HEPPNER, D. HAAS & R. NITSCH. 1997. Fluorescent dye prelabeled microglial cells migrate into organotypic hippocampal slice cultures and ramify. Eur. J. Neurosci. **9:** 863–866.

Reorganization of the Rat Fascia Dentata after a Unilateral Entorhinal Cortex Lesion

Role of the Extracellular Matrix

THOMAS DELLER,[a] CAROLA A. HAAS, AND MICHAEL FROTSCHER

Institute of Anatomy, University of Freiburg, D-79001 Freiburg, Germany

ABSTRACT: Entorhinal cortex lesion (ECL) partially denervates the fascia dentata of the hippocampus. This is said to induce the sprouting of intact fibers from neighboring layers that invade the zone of the degenerating axons. However, recent studies using anterograde tracing failed to demonstrate sprouting across laminar boundaries. Sprouting does occur, but it mainly involves unlesioned fiber systems terminating within the layer of fiber degeneration. It is now of interest to identify the cues that could underlie this layer-specific sprouting response. Since extracellular matrix (ECM) molecules delineate boundaries of axonal growth during development, it was tested whether these molecules play a similar role during the sprouting process following ECL. After ECL, reactive astrocytes rapidly synthesize and secrete growth-inhibiting ECM molecules, such as tenascin-C and the chondroitin sulfate proteoglycan neurocan, into the ECM of the outer molecular layer. These molecules form a sharp border against the nondenervated inner molecular layer. This pattern of ECM molecule expression may contribute to the layer-specific sprouting response of surviving afferents after ECL: axons trying to grow into the denervated outer molecular layer, for example, from the inner molecular layer, would be deflected by a growth-inhibiting ECM barrier.

INTRODUCTION

Following an injury of the central nervous system, complex cellular changes take place in the denervated brain areas. Reactive gliosis, transneuronal degeneration of denervated neurons, as well as lesion-induced sprouting of surviving axons occur and result in a fundamental reorganization of the deafferented brain regions (see references 1–3 for review). Although these processes are observed in many regions of the brain after a lesion, they were most intensively investigated in the rat fascia dentata after a unilateral entorhinal cortex lesion (ECL). The fascia dentata is particularly suitable for this purpose because its major afferents, that is, the entorhinal and the commissural/associational (C/A) fiber systems, terminate in a lamina-specific fashion in the outer and inner molecular layers of the fascia dentata, respectively. Following ECL, the entorhinal afferents to the outer molecular layer are lost and this zone is heavily denervated, whereas the C/A afferents to the inner molecular layer remain intact.[4,5] As a consequence of this layer-specific denervation, lesion-induced

[a]Address for correspondence: Thomas Deller, Anatomisches Institut I, Postfach 111, 79001 Freiburg, Germany. Tel.: +49-761-203-5077; fax: +49-761-203-5054.
e-mail: dellerth@uni-freiburg.de

changes primarily occur within the denervated zone and cellular events that take place at the laminar boundary between the denervated outer and the nondenervated inner molecular layer can readily be analyzed.

A particularly interesting aspect of the reorganization of the fascia dentata after ECL is the reinnervation of the denervated outer molecular layer by surviving afferents (see reference 6 for review). This reinnervation process is quite extensive and occurs within the first weeks postlesion.[5,7] It is said to involve surviving fibers within the outer molecular layer, such as cholinergic septohippocampal and crossed entorhino-dentate fibers, which sprout within their normal termination zone. In addition, a robust expansion of the C/A fiber plexus in the inner molecular layer was observed postlesion,[8] and electron microscopic and histochemical data suggested that these fibers participate in the reinnervation of the denervated outer molecular layer. Since it was not known at that time that some commissural fibers normally terminate within the outer molecular layer,[9] and sprouting could not yet be demonstrated at the level of single identified axons using sensitive anterograde tracing methods, these data were taken as evidence for a translaminar sprouting response of C/A fibers. Thus, it was assumed that sprouting C/A fibers are able to cross the border between the inner and outer molecular layer, the main laminar boundary of the fascia dentata that is so precisely respected by these fibers in normal rats. Many details of this sprouting process have recently been reviewed[10] and, therefore, we will focus on the specific question as to what extent C/A fibers are capable of leaving their home layer and invading the neighboring entorhinal termination zone. We will propose that molecules located in the extracellular matrix (ECM) of the denervated fascia dentata provide some of the cues that guide the sprouting process.

ANTEROGRADE TRACING OF SPROUTING COMMISSURAL FIBERS AFTER ECL

The concept of translaminar sprouting C/A fibers dominated the ECL model system for many years, although other explanations were also provided. For example, Storm-Mathisen (1974)[11] and Steward (1991)[1] pointed out that the expansion of the C/A fiber plexus in the inner molecular layer can also be explained by the growth of proximal granule cell dendrites associated with a shift of the laminar boundaries outwards toward the hippocampal fissure. Thus, an intralaminar expansion of C/A fibers within their normal home territory would be an alternative explanation for the widening of the inner molecular layer postlesion. In the same line, a series of *in vitro* experiments cast doubts on the concept of translaminar sprouting after ECL. In these experiments, it was shown that entorhinal and C/A fibers are guided into their appropriate layers by highly layer-specific molecular cues.[12] Clearly, such a molecular concept of axon guidance within the fascia dentata is difficult to bring into agreement with the concept of a translaminar sprouting response that postulates that C/A fibers can sprout into a territory not normally available to them. Therefore, it appeared to be timely to directly analyze the sprouting C/A fibers.

In more recent years, highly sensitive anterograde tracers such as *Phaseolus vulgaris*–leucoagglutinin (PHAL)[13] were developed that made the identification of projections at the level of single axons possible, a resolution capability not achieved by any of the classical techniques. With this technique, new insights were gained into normal hippocampal connectivity and topography (see references 14 and 15 for review), and it became possible to directly visualize and analyze individual sprouting axons.[16,17] Therefore, we used anterograde tracing with PHAL to analyze the sprouting commissural[16] and crossed entorhinal[18] fibers. We chose these projection systems as paradigms for putative translaminar (commissural) and intralaminar (crossed entorhinal) sprouting fiber systems and compared the morphology, arborization pattern, and bouton density of individual sprouting axons of these projections with those of the same axon type in unlesioned animals.

Using this technique, we could demonstrate that commissural fibers after ECL remain within their expanded home territory and do not normally invade the outer molecular layer (FIG. 1).[19] Postlesion, these fibers form a sharp and quite distinct border between the inner and outer molecular layer that is difficult to explain with a diffuse axonal invasion of the denervated zone. If such a translaminar fiber invasion had occurred, we would have seen a severe disruption of the outer border of the commissural fiber plexus, as is in fact the case in mice after ECL.[20,20A] Thus, our PHAL tracing revealed that the commissural fibers to the inner molecular layer expand their termination field outwards, but that this altered zonal organization of the fascia dentata is unlikely to be due to translaminar sprouting.

However, what about the commissural synapses and fibers that were observed beyond the expanded inner molecular layer? In normal rats that were used as controls for the lesioned animals, we found a previously unknown commissural projection to the outer molecular layer. These fibers could be followed from the hilus into the outer molecular layer of the fascia dentata where they arborized.[9,21] This projection is fairly weak in normal rats, which might explain why it was missed with less sensitive tracing techniques. After ECL, these fibers sprout within their normal home territory, the outer molecular layer (FIG. 2),[16] and the intralaminar sprouting of these fibers readily explains the presence of commissural fibers and synapses within the denervated zone. Taken together, these tracing data indicate that sprouting of C/A fibers in the denervated fascia dentata after ECL is not translaminar, but rather that it is layer-specific.[10,19]

ARE THE SPROUTING FIBERS GUIDED BY THE SAME SET OF CUES AS FIBERS DURING DEVELOPMENT?

Clearly, the next logical step is to identify the molecular cues that underlie this layer-specific sprouting response. This question appeared to be closely linked to the question of which signals underlie the formation of hippocampal layers during development, and we expected that a better understanding of these developmental processes could help us to understand some of the molecular cues that guide sprouting fibers after denervation. Recently, some of the molecules involved in the formation of hippocampal layers have been identified,[22–24] and some of these data have been reviewed (see reference 25 for review). In these studies, Cajal-Retzius cells located in the outer molecular layer of the fascia dentata were implicated as pioneer neurons for the ingrowing entorhinal fibers during development.[22,26] These cells synthesize the ECM molecule, reelin, which can affect the branching pattern of ingrowing entorhinal fibers.[22] Thus, it was attractive to test whether reelin may in fact play a role in the reinnervation of the denervated fascia dentata, for example, for the sprouting

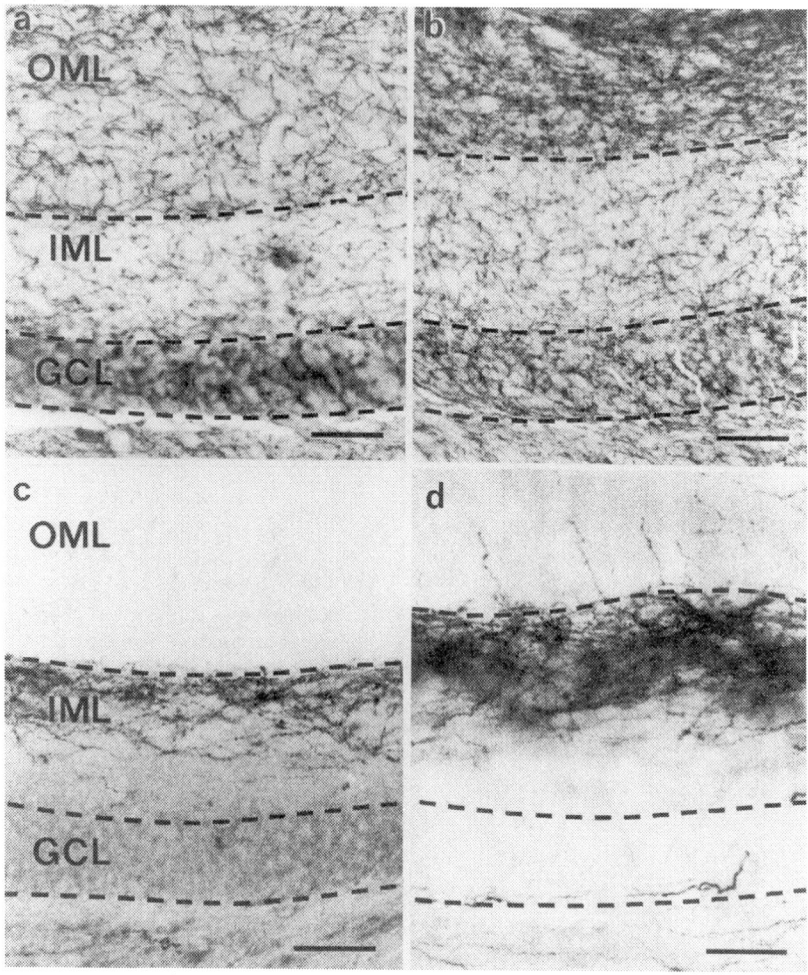

FIGURE 1. Expansion of the commissural fibers plexus in the inner molecular layer of the dentate gyrus after ECL. (a) Acetylcholinesterase (AChE)–stained section of the dentate gyrus in a control animal. The width of the inner molecular layer is approximately 70 μm. GCL, granule cell layer; IML, inner molecular layer; OML, outer molecular layer. (b) AChE-stained section of the dentate gyrus four weeks after entorhinal cortex lesion. Note that a densely AChE-stained fiber plexus is present in the outer molecular layer, which is characteristic for a complete lesion. The weakly AChE-stained inner molecular layer has expanded by 30–40 μm. (c) Section of the dentate gyrus immunostained for PHAL in a control animal. The commissural projection to the inner molecular layer terminates within 70 μm from the granule cell layer. (d) Section of the dentate gyrus of an animal four weeks after entorhinal cortex lesion. The termination field of commissural fibers to the inner molecular layer has expanded by 30–40 μm. Scale bars: 50 μm. Reprinted from reference 19 with permission from Elsevier Science.

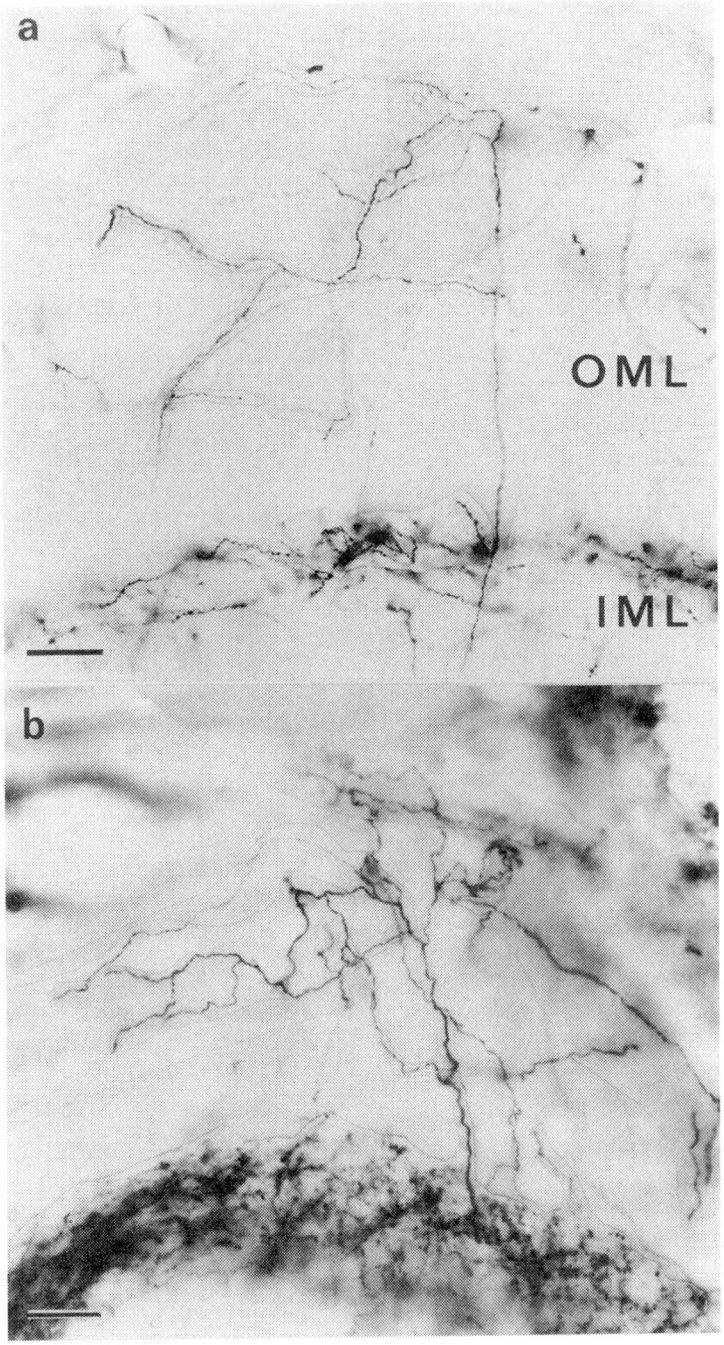

FIGURE 2. *See following page for caption.*

of the crossed entorhinal fiber system. To our surprise, reelin expression was not altered in the fascia dentata after ECL,[27] which makes it unlikely that reelin is a relevant signal for the sprouting fibers. In addition, the majority of reelin-expressing Cajal-Retzius cells as well as other pioneer neurons implicated in the formation of hippocampal layers disappear shortly after birth[23,28] and are fairly scarce in adult animals. Taken together, these data indicate that the set of molecular and cellular cues that guide sprouting fibers after ECL in adult animals may differ from those guiding the same fiber systems during development.

ASTROCYTES MAY FORM A BOUNDARY FOR SPROUTING AXONS AFTER ECL

Which other cellular and molecular candidates could be relevant for the layer-specific sprouting of C/A fibers after ECL? It has been pointed out very early by Rose and coworkers (1976)[29] that astrocytes might play a crucial role for the expansion of C/A fibers in the inner molecular layer. Astrocytes undergo hypertrophy within one day postlesion, migrate to the denervated zone, and form a row of astrocyte cell bodies right at the border between the inner molecular layer and the denervated outer molecular layer (FIGS. 3a, 3b). This astrocytic reaction occurs before the onset of the sprouting response, and the row of astrocytes shifts outwards approximately as much as the C/A fibers expand their termination field. For this reason, it was proposed that the cellular arrangement of the astroglial cells might determine the extent of the C/A sprouting response.[29] More recent data support this concept, and astrocytes have been implicated in the formation of growth boundaries during development (see reference 30 for review) and in the regulation of lesion-induced axonal growth processes.[31–33]

However, it is quite surprising that the row of astrocytes shifts outwards postlesion. Since astrocytes participate in the phagocytosis of degenerating terminals after ECL,[1,4,34] it would be reasonable to expect them to migrate right up to the *original* laminar boundary where they should encounter numerous degenerating terminals. Furthermore, the distance that the row of astrocytes shifts outwards is the same as that reported for dendritic growth after a lesion (i.e., 30–40 μm). Taken together, these data suggest an outward expansion of the entire neuropil, which is not yet fully understood. The growth of granule cell dendrites, the outward migration of astrocytes, as well as the expansion of the C/A fibers to the inner molecular layer may all be involved in this outward shift.

FIGURE 2. Commissural fibers to the outer molecular layer sprout after ECL. (a) Commissural fiber to the outer molecular layer in a control animal. These fibers do not give off branches to the inner plexus, and the number of collaterals in the outer molecular layer is low. IML, inner molecular layer; OML, outer molecular layer. (b) Commissural fiber to the outer molecular layer four weeks after ECL. The number of axonal collaterals has considerably increased in the OML. Note that this axon does not branch in the inner molecular layer similar to the axon shown in part a. Scale bars: 30 μm. Reprinted from reference 16 with permission.

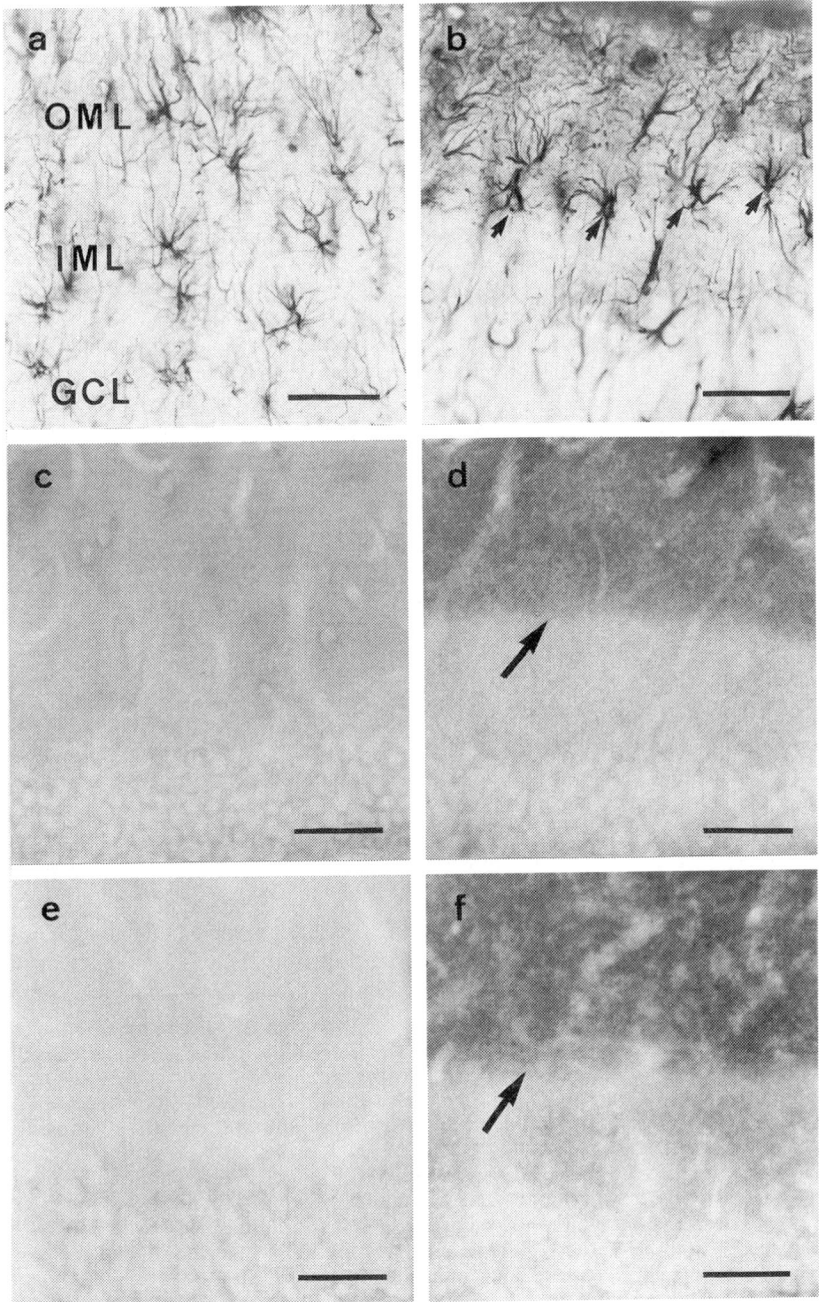

FIGURE 3. *See following page for caption.*

REACTIVE ASTROCYTES CHANGE THE COMPOSITION OF THE ECM

It is unlikely that the row of astrocytes at the inner molecular layer/outer molecular layer border represents some kind of mechanical barrier through which the C/A fibers cannot grow after ECL. Rather, molecules secreted by these cells or molecules located on their surface could play such a role. One of the most interesting groups of molecules in this respect are ECM molecules synthesized by reactive astrocytes. This heterogeneous and versatile group of molecules can regulate cell migration, axonal growth, and axonal pathfinding during development and after brain injury (see references 35–41 for review). Some of these molecules, such as the ECM molecule tenascin-C and the chondroitin sulfate proteoglycan (CSPG) neurocan, delineate boundaries of axonal growth during development and have been implicated in neuronal pattern formation.[35,42] Since the reorganization of the fascia dentata after ECL results in a new "neuronal pattern", that is, an altered zonal organization in which laminar boundaries are sharply defined, we hypothesized that these ECM molecules could also play a role in the reorganization process following ECL. Therefore, we investigated the postlesional expression of tenascin-C (TN-C)[34] and neurocan (NC),[43] and compared the distribution of these molecules to that of the sprouting C/A fibers after ECL.

The ECM molecule TN-C is abundant in the developing and in the adult central nervous system. Several different splice variants of TN-C are known and some of these splice variants show neurite outgrowth promoting effects, whereas others show considerable growth cone repulsive properties *in vitro*. For this reason, we used monoclonal antibodies generated against the different functional domains of TN-C and studied changes in TN-C immunoreactivity in the denervated fascia dentata after ECL.[34] In these experiments, we found that neurite outgrowth promoting splice variants as well as growth cone repulsive splice variants of TN-C are upregulated in the denervated zone by two days postlesion, that is, several days before the expansion of the C/A fiber plexus occurs. Interestingly, the upregulation of TN-C occurred in the outer molecular layer with a sharp boundary towards the inner molecular layer (FIGS. 3c, 3d). As could be demonstrated using *in situ* hybridization in combination with glial fibrillary acidic protein (GFAP)–immunohistochemistry, TN-C was synthesized and released into the ECM by reactive astrocytes.[34]

FIGURE 3. Extracellular matrix molecules are upregulated in the denervated outer molecular layer. (a, b) Immunoreactivity for GFAP in a control animal (a) and in an animal 10 days postlesion (b). In the control (a), astrocytes are fairly evenly distributed throughout the molecular layer. After ECL (b), GFAP immunoreactivity is increased in the outer molecular layer (OML), and astrocytes form a row of cells (short arrows) at the border between the inner molecular layer (IML) and the OML. GCL, granule cell layer. (c, d) Immunoreactivity for a growth-promoting splice variant of tenascin-C (mAb J1/tn2) in a control animal (c) and in an animal 10 days postlesion (d). In the control (c), tenascin-C immunoreactivity is weak. After ECL (d), a distinct tenascin-C immunoreactive band is visible in the OML with a sharp border against the IML (arrow). (e, f) Immunoreactivity for the chondroitin sulfate proteoglycan neurocan in a control animal (e) and in an animal 10 days postlesion (f). In the control (e), neurocan immunoreactivity is not above background level. After ECL (f), a distinct neurocan immunoreactive band is visible in the OML with a sharp border against the IML (arrow). Scale bars: (a–f) 50 μm.

The CSPG neurocan is a very tightly developmentally regulated molecule[44] that inhibits axonal growth *in vitro* (see reference 39 for review). It appears to play an important role during development,[45] but is strongly downregulated shortly after birth. Using antisera specific for the core protein of the molecule, an upregulation of NC throughout the denervated outer molecular layer could be demonstrated as early as two days postlesion. Again, a sharp boundary was maintained between the NC-rich denervated outer molecular layer and the NC-poor inner molecular layer of the fascia dentata (FIGS. 3e, 3f). Using *in situ* hybridization for NC in combination with GFAP-immunohistochemistry, a strong astroglial neurocan expression could be demonstrated throughout the denervated zone (FIG. 4).[43]

These data demonstrate that the ECM of the outer molecular layer is profoundly altered following ECL. These changes are long-lasting since the two molecules referred to here could still be detected in the outer molecular layer of the fascia dentata by half a year postlesion. This indicates that at least some of these molecules have an extremely long half-life once they have been deposited into the ECM of the denervated zone, similar to the long half-life of ECM molecules reported at a lesion site after brain injury.[41,46] Thus, the denervated zone does not revert to its prelesion state even after reorganization of the fascia dentata following ECL is complete.

MOLECULES OF THE ECM DELINEATE BOUNDARIES OF AXONAL GROWTH AFTER ECL

What is the functional role of these molecules within the denervated zone? The role of growth-promoting splice variants of TN-C within the outer molecular layer is likely to contribute to a growth-promoting environment in which sprouting can occur. In contrast, it is more difficult to understand the presence of growth-inhibiting molecules within the denervated outer molecular layer, that is, within the layer where sprouting occurs *in spite* of the presence of these molecules. At least as far as NC is concerned, this situation is fairly similar to the expression pattern of NC during development, when NC is strongly expressed in regions of axonal growth (see reference 35 for review). For this reason, it was suggested that the biological effects of NC or other ECM molecules on growing axons depend on their relative concentration as well as on the order of assembly of the various ECM and cell adhesion molecules present within a given brain region.[38,47] When expressed in regions containing low levels of adhesion molecules, growth-inhibiting ECM molecules may act as a barrier to axonal growth. However, when expressed in regions containing high levels of adhesion molecules, these molecules may still allow axonal extension to occur. After ECL, a whole battery of growth-promoting ECM molecules and cell adhesion molecules are upregulated in the denervated zone (see reference 3 for review) and, thus, the denervated outer molecular layer of the fascia dentata contains many growth-promoting molecules that may balance the growth-inhibiting effects of NC or of inhibitory splice variants of TN-C on the sprouting axons.

The interpretation outlined above does not explain the function of these inhibitory molecules within the ECM. Rather, it explains why axonal growth can occur in these regions *in spite* of the presence of these molecules. A recent study that focused on the role of CSPGs during axonal regeneration[48] has provided an attractive hypothe-

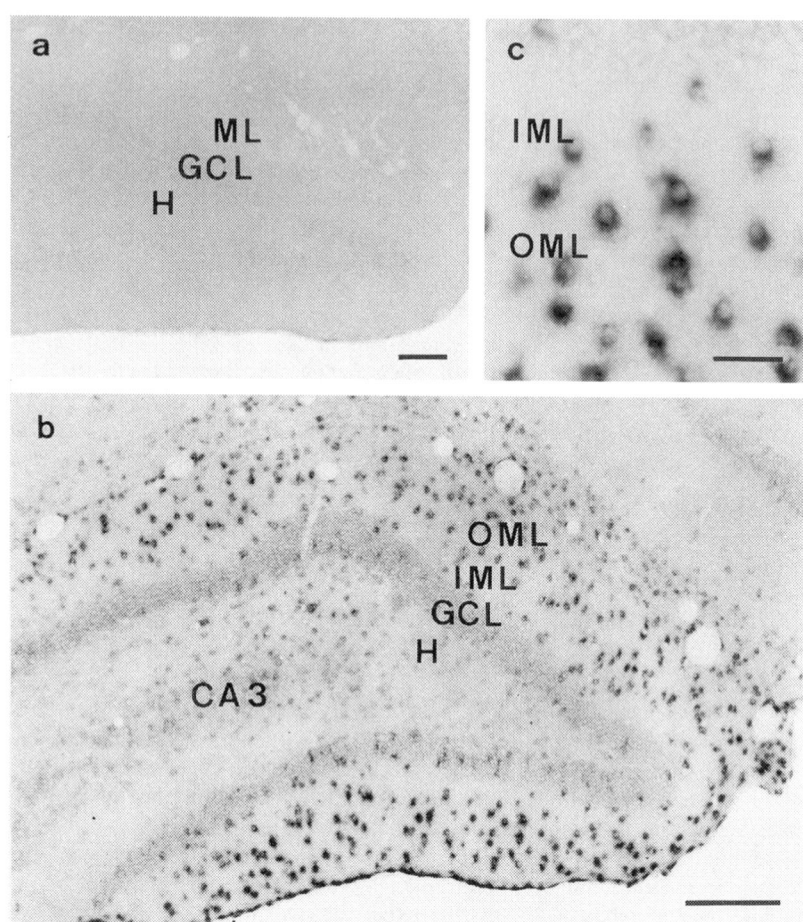

FIGURE 4. Neurocan mRNA expression in the fascia dentata after ECL. (a) Control animal. No labeling for neurocan mRNA can be observed. ML, molecular layer; GCL, granule cell layer; H, hilus. (b) Neurocan mRNA expression in the fascia dentata four days postlesion. Many cellular profiles are observed in the outer molecular layer of the fascia dentata and in stratum lacunosum-moleculare of CA1 and CA3. Portion of the infrapyramidal blade shown at higher magnification in part c. OML, outer molecular layer; IML, inner molecular layer. (c) Higher magnification of a portion of the outer molecular layer. Heavily labeled cells are restricted to the OML. Scale bars: (a) 150 μm; (b) 200 μm; (c) 40 μm.

sis for the role of inhibitory CSPGs during the sprouting process after ECL. Davies *et al.* (1999)[48] demonstrated that regenerating axons that grow inward from the edge of a lesion site grow up a gradient of increasingly CSPG-rich ECM. These axons become more branched as they enter more deeply into the CSPG-rich environment, before coming to a complete stop at the center of the lesion. These data indicate that increasing concentrations of CSPGs can promote the formation of local branches before stopping the elongating axons.[48] In this line, the upregulation of NC in the denervated outer molecular layer could contribute to the branching of sprouting axons and, therefore, to the formation of new axonal collaterals within the denervated zone.

After considering the functional role of ECM molecules within the denervated outer molecular layer, it is now logical to discuss their possible role for the layer-specific sprouting response of the C/A fibers after ECL. As has been mentioned above, earlier studies suggested that ECM molecules expressed in regions of axonal growth may act to define boundaries for growing fibers during development (see references 30 and 35 for review), and we hypothesized that these molecules[45,49] could act in a similar fashion after ECL. Indeed, the distribution of TN-C and NC after ECL correlates nicely with the laminar termination pattern of the sprouting fiber populations. This pattern suggests that afferents trying to invade the denervated zone, for example, C/A fibers in the inner molecular layer, suddenly hit an inhibitory boundary that could prevent further ingrowth into the outer molecular layer. At this point, it should be emphasized that this situation is very different from that observed at a CSPG-rich lesion site, where regenerating axons can grow up a gradient of CSPG-containing ECM before they stop their advance.[48] Following ECL, no gradient of ECM molecules exists that would make a limited ingrowth of axons possible. Rather, a steep increase in inhibitory molecule concentration occurs right at the border between the inner and outer molecular layer of the fascia dentata. As has been convincingly demonstrated, such inhibitory boundaries are quite effective in their ability to prevent the ingrowth of axons (see reference 30 for review).

It should be pointed out that the studies reviewed above do not yet prove that TN-C and NC are causally involved in the formation of an altered zonal organization of the fascia dentata. Although the concept that lesion-induced ECM molecules define boundaries within the denervated outer molecular layer is certainly attractive, it will be necessary to demonstrate that some of these molecules are in fact essential for this process *in vivo*. This is not a trivial problem because many standard experimental approaches cannot be used. For example, it is doubtful that knockout mice lacking TN-C or NC can help to determine the role of these molecules for the layer-specific sprouting process because sprouting in mice differs considerably from that observed in rats.[20] Further, the fact that at least two different inhibitory molecules are upregulated in the denervated outer molecular layer, that is, inhibitory splice variants of TN-C as well as NC, complicates experiments with knockout mice and makes it necessary to use double or even triple knockout animals. For quite similar reasons, strategies involving the injection of antibodies directed against ECM do not appear to be promising. Thus, new experimental strategies aimed, for example, at the ECM molecule synthesizing astrocytes themselves, will have to be developed to tackle this problem.

CONCLUSIONS

In the studies reported here, we analyzed sprouting fiber systems in the rat fascia dentata after ECL using direct anterograde tracing with PHAL. These studies revealed that the sprouting process mainly involves unlesioned fiber systems terminating within the layer of fiber degeneration, for example, crossed entorhino-dentate fibers and a subset of commissural fibers that normally terminate within the outer molecular layer. The main C/A fiber projection to the inner molecular layer, which was believed to invade the outer molecular layer, remains within its home lamina. In order to identify some of the cues that prevent the ingrowth of C/A fibers into the denervated outer molecular layer, we analyzed several ECM molecules implicated in the formation of laminar boundaries and of neuronal pattern during development. Inhibitory splice variants of TN-C as well as NC were upregulated throughout the outer molecular layer after ECL and formed a sharp boundary toward the inner molecular layer. This expression pattern suggests that these molecules could prevent the ingrowth of C/A fibers into the outer molecular layer. These fibers do sprout after ECL but remain within their home territory.

ACKNOWLEDGMENTS

    Some of the studies reviewed here were part of a collaboration with Andreas Faissner (Strasbourg, France), Robert Nitsch (Berlin, Germany), and Uwe Rauch (Lund, Sweden). We thank Regina Hertweck and Marianne Winter for help with the illustrations. This work was supported by the Deutsche Forschungsgemeinschaft (SFB 505).

REFERENCES

1. STEWARD, O. 1991. Synapse replacement on cortical neurons following denervation. Cereb. Cortex **9:** 81–132.
2. STEWARD, O. 1994. Reorganization of neuronal circuitry following central nervous system trauma: naturally occurring processes and opportunities for therapeutic intervention. *In* The Neurobiology of Central Nervous System Trauma, pp. 266–287. Oxford University Press. London/New York.
3. DELLER, T. & M. FROTSCHER. 1997. Lesion-induced plasticity of central neurons: sprouting of single fibers in the rat hippocampus after unilateral entorhinal lesion. Prog. Neurobiol. **53:** 687–727.
4. MATTHEWS, D.A., C.W. COTMAN & G. LYNCH. 1976. An electron microscopic study of lesion-induced synaptogenesis in the dentate gyrus of the adult rat. I. Magnitude and time course of degeneration. Brain Res. **115:** 1–21.
5. STEWARD, O. & S.L. VINSANT. 1983. The process of reinnervation in the dentate gyrus of the adult rat: a quantitative electron microscopic analysis of terminal proliferation and reactive synaptogenesis. J. Comp. Neurol. **214:** 370–386.
6. COTMAN, C.W. & J.V. NADLER. 1978. Reactive synaptogenesis in the hippocampus. *In* Neuronal Plasticity, pp. 227–271. Raven Press. New York.
7. MATTHEWS, D.A., C.W. COTMAN & G. LYNCH. 1976. An electron microscopic study of lesion-induced synaptogenesis in the dentate gyrus of the adult rat. II. Reappearance of morphologically normal synaptic contacts. Brain Res. **115:** 23–41.
8. LYNCH, G., B. STANFIELD & C.W. COTMAN. 1973. Developmental differences in post-lesion axonal growth in the hippocampus. Brain Res. **59:** 155–168.
9. DELLER, T., R. NITSCH & M. FROTSCHER. 1995. *Phaseolus vulgaris* leucoagglutinin (PHAL) tracing of commissural fibers to the rat dentate gyrus: evidence for a previously unknown commissural projection to the outer molecular layer. J. Comp. Neurol. **352:** 55–68.
10. FROTSCHER, M., B. HEIMRICH & T. DELLER. 1997. Sprouting in the hippocampus is layer-specific. Trends Neurosci. **20:** 218–223.
11. STORM-MATHISEN, J. 1974. Choline acetyltransferase and acetylcholinesterase in fascia dentata following lesion of the entorhinal afferents. Brain Res. **80:** 181–197.
12. FROTSCHER, M. & B. HEIMRICH. 1993. Formation of layer-specific fiber projections to the hippocampus *in vitro*. Proc. Natl. Acad. Sci. U.S.A. **90:** 10400–10403.

13. GERFEN, C.R. & P.E. SAWCHENKO. 1984. An anterograde neuroanatomical tracing method that shows the detailed morphology of neurons, their axons, and terminals: immunohistochemical localization of an axonally transported plant lectin, *Phaseolus vulgaris* leucoagglutinin (PHAL). Brain Res. **290**: 219–238.

14. AMARAL, D.G. & M.P. WITTER. 1995. The hippocampal formation. *In* The Rat Nervous System. Second edition, pp. 443–494. Academic Press. San Diego.

15. DELLER, T. 1998. The anatomical organization of the rat fascia dentata—new aspects of laminar organization as revealed by anterograde tracing with *Phaseolus vulgaris*–leucoagglutinin. Anat. Embryol. **197**: 89–103.

16. DELLER, T., M. FROTSCHER & R. NITSCH. 1995. Morphological evidence for the sprouting of inhibitory commissural fibers in response to the lesion of the excitatory entorhinal input to the rat dentate gyrus. J. Neurosci. **15**: 6868–6878.

17. ROSSI, F., L. WIKLUND, J.J.L. VAN DER WANT & P. STRATA. 1991. Reinnervation of cerebellar Purkinje cells by climbing fibres surviving a subtotal lesion of the inferior olive in the adult rat. I. Development of new collateral branches and terminal plexuses. J. Comp. Neurol. **308**: 513–535.

18. DELLER, T., M. FROTSCHER & R. NITSCH. 1996. Sprouting of crossed entorhinodentate fibers after a unilateral entorhinal lesion: anterograde tracing of fiber reorganization with *Phaseolus vulgaris*–leucoagglutinin (PHAL). J. Comp. Neurol. **365**: 42–55.

19. DELLER, T., R. NITSCH & M. FROTSCHER. 1996. Layer-specific sprouting of commissural fibers to the rat fascia dentata after unilateral entorhinal cortex lesion: a *Phaseolus vulgaris* leucoagglutinin tracing study. Neuroscience **71**: 651–660.

20. WOODS, A.G. & T. DELLER. 2000. Reactive axonal sprouting in mouse hippocampus following entorhinal cortex lesion [abstract]. Ann. Anat. **182**: 91.

20A. SHI, B. & B.B. STANFIELD. 1996. Differential sprouting responses in axonal fiber systems in the dentate gyrus following lesions of the perforant path in *Wlds* mutant mice. Brain Res. **740**: 89–101.

21. DELLER, T., R. NITSCH & M. FROTSCHER. 1996. Heterogeneity of the commissural projection to the rat dentate gyrus: a *Phaseolus vulgaris* leucoagglutinin tracing study. Neuroscience **75**: 111–121.

22. DEL RIO, J.A., B. HEIMRICH, V. BORRELL, E. FÖRSTER, A. DRAKEW, S. ALCANTARA, K. NAKAJIMA, T. MIYATA, M. OGAWA, K. MIKOSHIBA, P. DERER, M. FROTSCHER & E. SORIANO. 1997. A role for Cajal-Retzius cells and reelin in the development of hippocampal connections. Nature **385**: 70–74.

23. SUPÈR, H., A. MARTINEZ, J.A. DEL RIO & E. SORIANO. 1998. Involvement of distinct pioneer neurons in the formation of layer-specific connections in the hippocampus. J. Neurosci. **18**: 4616–4626.

24. DELLER, T., A. DRAKEW & M. FROTSCHER. 1999. Different primary target cells are important for fiber lamination in the fascia dentata: a lesson from reeler mutant mice. Exp. Neurol. **156**: 239–253.

25. FROTSCHER, M. 1998. Cajal-Retzius cells, reelin, and the formation of layers. Curr. Opin. Neurobiol. **8**: 570–575.

26. CERANIK, K., J. DENG, B. HEIMRICH, J. LÜBKE, S. ZHENG, E. FÖRSTER & M. FROTSCHER. 1999. Hippocampal Cajal-Retzius cells project to the entorhinal cortex: retrograde tracing and intracellular labeling studies. Eur. J. Neurosci. **11**: 4278–4290.

27. HAAS, C.A., T. DELLER, Z. KRSNIK, A. TIELSCH, A. WOODS & M. FROTSCHER. 2000. Entorhinal cortex lesion does not alter reelin mRNA expression in the dentate gyrus of young and adult rats. Neuroscience **97**: 25–31.

28. DEL RIO, J.A., B. HEIMRICH, H. SUPÈR, V. BORRELL, M. FROTSCHER & E. SORIANO. 1996. Differential survival of Cajal-Retzius cells in organotypic cultures of hippocampus and neocortex. J. Neurosci. **16**: 6896–6907.

29. ROSE, G., G. LYNCH & C.W. COTMAN. 1976. Hypertrophy and redistribution of astrocytes in the deafferented dentate gyrus. Brain Res. Bull. **1**: 87–92.

30. FAISSNER, A. & D. STEINDLER. 1995. Boundaries and inhibitory molecules in developing neural tissues. Glia **13**: 233–254.

31. KAWAJA, M.D. & F.H. GAGE. 1991. Reactive astrocytes are substrates for the growth of adult CNS axons in the presence of elevated levels of nerve growth factor. Neuron **7**: 1019–1030.

32. STEWARD, O. 1992. Signals that induce sprouting in the central nervous system: sprouting is delayed in a strain of mouse exhibiting delayed axonal degeneration. Exp. Neurol. **118:** 340–351.

33. STEWARD, O. 1994. Cholinergic sprouting is blocked by repeated induction of electroconvulsive seizures, a manipulation that induces a persistent reactive state in astrocytes. Exp. Neurol. **129:** 103–111.

34. DELLER, T., C.A. HAAS, T. NAUMANN, A. JOESTER, A. FAISSNER & M. FROTSCHER. 1997. Upregulation of astrocyte-derived tenascin-C correlates with neurite outgrowth in the rat dentate gyrus after unilateral entorhinal cortex lesion. Neuroscience **81:** 829–846.

35. PEARLMAN, A.L. & A.M. SHEPPARD. 1996. Extracellular matrix in early cortical development. Prog. Brain Res. **108:** 117–134.

36. HÖKE, A. & J. SILVER. 1996. Proteoglycans and other repulsive molecules in glial boundaries during development and regeneration of the nervous system. Prog. Brain Res. **108:** 149–163.

37. YAMADA, H., B. FREDETTE, K. SHITARA, K. HAGIHARA, R. MIURA, B. RANSCHT, W.B. STALLCUP & Y. YAMAGUCHI. 1997. The brain chondroitin sulfate proteoglycan brevican associates with astrocytes ensheathing cerebellar glomeruli and inhibits neurite outgrowth from granule neurons. J. Neurosci. **17:** 7784–7795.

38. MARGOLIS, R.U. & R.K. MARGOLIS. 1997. Chondroitin sulfate proteoglycans as mediators of axon growth and pathfinding. Cell Tissue Res. **290:** 343–348.

39. RAUCH, U. 1997. Modeling an extracellular environment for axonal pathfinding and fasciculation in the central nervous system. Cell Tissue Res. **290:** 349–356.

40. FAISSNER, A. 1997. The tenascin gene family in axon growth and guidance. Cell Tissue Res. **290:** 331–341.

41. STICHEL, C.C. & H.W. MÜLLER. 1998. The CNS lesion scar: new vistas on an old regeneration barrier. Cell Tissue Res. **294:** 1–9.

42. FAISSNER, A., B. GÖTZ, A. JOESTER, F. WIGGER, A. SCHOLZE & K. SCHÜTTE. 1996. Tenascin-C glycoproteins in neural pattern formation and plasticity. Sem. Neurosci. **8:** 347–356.

43. HAAS, C.A., U. RAUCH, N. THON, T. MERTEN & T. DELLER. 1999. Entorhinal cortex lesion in adult rats induces the expression of the neuronal chondroitin sulfate proteoglycan neurocan in reactive astrocytes. J. Neurosci. **19:** 9953–9963.

44. MILEV, P., P. MAUREL, A. CHIBA, M. MEVISSEN, S. POPP, Y. YAMAGUCHI, R.K. MARGOLIS & R.U. MARGOLIS. 1998. Differential regulation of expression of hyaluronanbinding proteoglycans in developing brain: aggrecan, versican, neurocan, and brevican. Biochem. Biophys. Res. Commun. **247:** 207–212.

45. MILLER, B., A.M. SHEPPARD, A.R. BICKNESE & A.L. PEARLMAN. 1995. Chondroitin sulfate proteoglycans in the developing cerebral cortex: the distribution of neurocan distinguishes forming afferent and efferent axonal pathways. J. Comp. Neurol. **355:** 615–628.

46. LIPS, K., C.C. STICHEL & H.W. MÜLLER. 1995. Restricted appearance of tenascin and chondroitin sulphate proteoglycans after transection and sprouting of adult rat postcommissural fornix. J. Neurocytol. **24:** 449–464.

47. GRUMET, M., D.R. FRIEDLANDER & T. SAKURAI. 1996. Functions of brain chondroitin sulfate proteoglycans during development: interactions with adhesion molecules. Perspect. Dev. Neurobiol. **3:** 319–330.

48. DAVIES, S.J.A., D.A. GOUCHER, C. DOLLER & J. SILVER. 1999. Robust regeneration of adult sensory axons in degenerating white matter of the adult rat spinal cord. J. Neurosci. **19:** 5810–5822.

49. KATOH-SEMBA, R., M. MATSUDA, K. KATO & A. OOHIRA. 1995. Chondroitin sulphate proteoglycans in the rat brain: candidates for axon barriers of sensory neurons and the possible modification by laminin of their actions. Eur. J. Neurosci. **7:** 613–621.

Pathological Changes in the Parahippocampal Region in Select Non-Alzheimer's Dementias

HEIKO BRAAK,[a,d] KELLY DEL TREDICI,[a] JÜRGEN BOHL,[b]
HANSJÜRGEN BRATZKE,[c] AND EVA BRAAK[a]

[a]*Department of Anatomy, J.W. Goethe University, D-60590 Frankfurt, Germany*

[b]*Department of Neuropathology, J.Gutenberg University, D-55101 Mainz, Germany*

[c]*Department of Forensic Medicine, J.W. Goethe University,
D-60590 Frankfurt, Germany*

ABSTRACT: The transentorhinal and entorhinal regions of the human brain extend over the ambient gyrus and anterior portions of the parahippocampal gyrus. They are important components of the limbic loop which receives its major afferents from the neocortical sensory association areas and generates powerful efferent projections both directly and via intermediary relay stations to the prefrontal cortex. The bilateral structural preservation of limbic loop components is a prerequisite for the maintenance of intact memory functions. In progressive neurodegenerative diseases, such as Alzheimer's disease, argyrophilic grain disease, Pick's disease, idiopathic Parkinson syndrome, and Huntington's disease, the transentorhinal and entorhinal regions are particularly susceptible to severe pathological changes. The transentorhinal region typically registers the initial alterations and becomes the most severely involved. From this transitional region of the mesocortex, the alterations usually invade with decreasing severity both the entorhinal region and temporal proneocortex. Each type of lesion that develops in the above-mentioned neurodegenerative disorders hampers or even interrupts data-transport from the sensory neocortex to the prefrontal neocortex, thereby contributing to the insidious development of progressive changes in personality, cognitive decline, and, ultimately, dementia.

THE NEOCORTEX, ALLOCORTEX, AND LIMBIC LOOP

The human cerebral cortex consists of an extensive neocortex and a small allocortex. Higher-order centers of the limbic system, such as the hippocampal formation as well as the presubicular and entorhinal regions, belong to the allocortex. Closely related is the subcortical amygdala. Transitional zones exist between the mature neocortex and allocortical regions. A belt of periallocortical areas accompanies the allocortex proper, whereas proneocortical fields are allied with the mature neocortex (periallocortex and proneocortex = mesocortex; FIG. 1).[2,7,8,46,58]

[d]Address for correspondence: Prof. Dr. med. Heiko Braak, Department of Anatomy, Theodor Stern Kai 7, D-60590 Frankfurt, Germany. Tel.: +49 69 6301 6900; fax: +49 69 6301 6425.
e-mail: Braak@em.uni-frankfurt.de

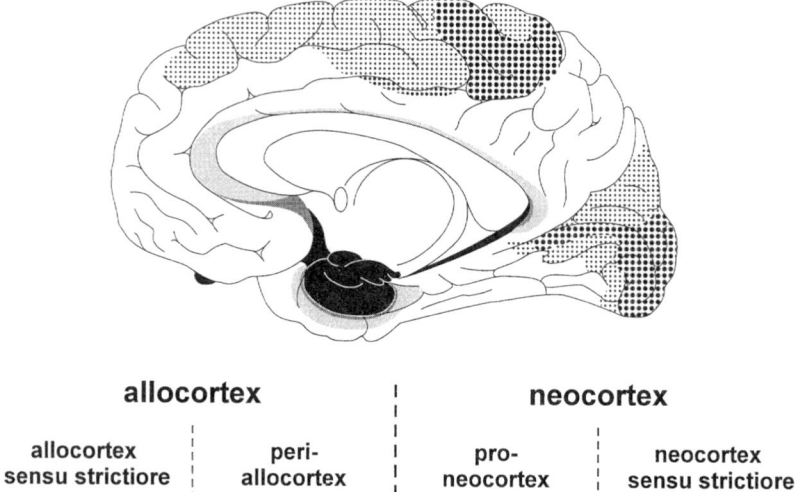

allocortex		neocortex	
allocortex sensu strictiore	peri- allocortex	pro- neocortex	neocortex sensu strictiore

FIGURE 1. The human cerebral cortex consists of two basic types of gray matter—neocortex and allocortex. The allocortex is small and located chiefly in the anteromedial portions of the temporal lobe. A belt of periallocortical areas (*dark gray*) accompanies the allocortex proper (*black*), whereas proneocortical fields (*light gray*) are allied with the mature neocortex (*white*). Periallocortex and proneocortex constitute the mesocortex. The neocortex is particularly extensive. The frontal, parietal, occipital, and temporal neocortices each comprise a primary field (marked by *large dots*), a belt of secondary fields (marked by *small dots*), and related higher-order processing areas (*white*).

Somatosensory, auditory, and visual exteroceptive information normally proceed through primary sensory fields of the neocortex to a variety of related association areas and then are conveyed to the prefrontal neocortex. The data is transferred from this highest deliberative instance in the human brain through the premotor areas to the primary motor field. The major routes for this data-flow are the striatal and the cerebellar loops.[1,13,43] Their task is to integrate into the regulation of cortical output the basal ganglia, many nuclei of the lower brain stem, and the cerebellum (FIG. 2).

The limbic system participates in data-transfer and is involved at a key point where exteroceptive information is transferred from the sensory association areas to the prefrontal cortex. One contingent of information leaves the mainstream to converge upon the transentorhinal periallocortex, entorhinal allocortex, and amygdala (FIG. 2). The neocortex thus is the chief source of input to the human limbic system. It should be noted that those components of the limbic loop that process neocortical data are a late development both phylogenetically and ontogenetically. In the course of evolution from macrosmatic mammals to microsmatic higher primates and humans, there is not only a remarkable expansion of the neocortex but also a thoroughgoing internal reorganization of centers of the limbic loop. The hallmark of this change is a massive expansion of components receiving input from and generating output to the neocortex. This increase occurs at the expense of components process-

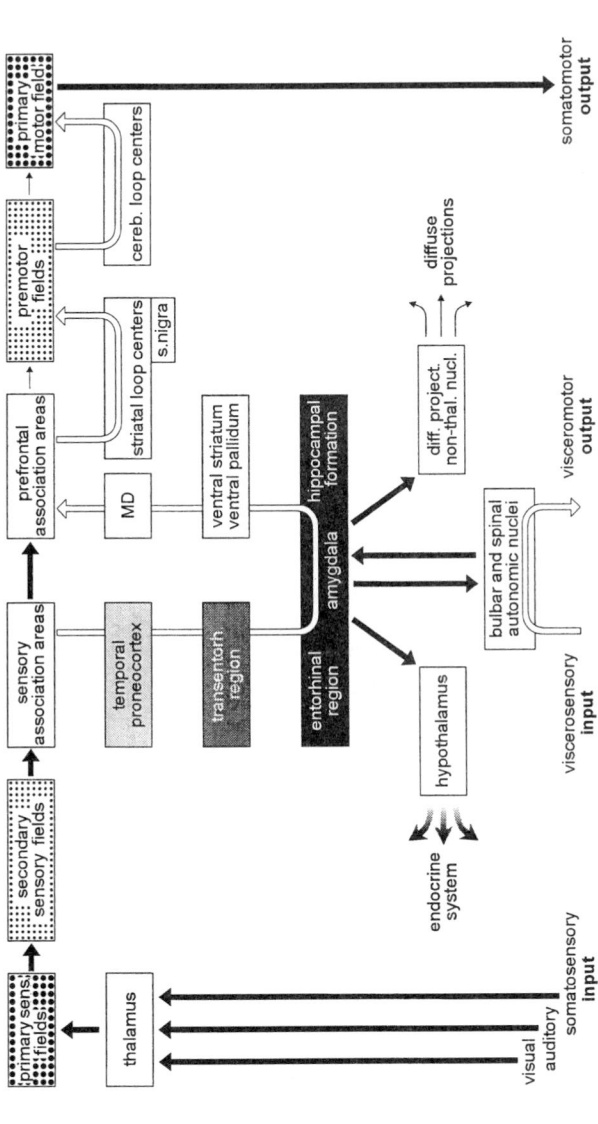

FIGURE 2. Somatosensory, visual, and auditory information proceeds through the respective neocortical primary and secondary areas to a variety of related association fields. From there, data is transported via long corticocortical pathways to the prefrontal cortex. Tracts generated from this highest organizational level of the brain guide the information back—chiefly via the striatal and cerebellar loops—to the primary motor field. Part of this stream of data running from the sensory association areas to the prefrontal cortex branches off to eventually converge—via the temporal proneocortex and periallocortical transentorhinal region—upon the entorhinal region and the amygdala (the afferent trunk of the limbic loop). Projections from the entorhinal region, amygdala, and hippocampal formation (the efferent trunk of the limbic loop) exert important influence upon the prefrontal cortex. cereb. loop centers, cerebellar loop centers; diff. project. non-thal. nuclei, diffusely projecting nonthalamic nuclei; MD, mediodorsal thalamic nuclei; primary sens. fields, primary sensory fields; s. nigra, substantia nigra; transentorhin. region, transentorhinal region.

ing olfactory data. The highest directive entities of the limbic loop consist of the entorhinal region, amygdala, and hippocampal formation. Projections from all three contribute to the efferent trunk of the limbic loop which exerts an important influence upon the prefrontal cortex.[19,30]

In addition, the components of the limbic loop receive interoceptive stimuli from many nuclei processing viscerosensory data. On the output side, they influence the endocrine system via the hypothalamo-hypophyseal axis and direct both brain stem and spinal cord nuclei regulating visceromotor functions (FIG. 2). Integration of exteroceptive and interoceptive data, together with the regulation of endocrine, visceromotor, and somatomotor functions, is important for the initiation of affect-related patterns of movements.[21] The centers of the limbic loop also are crucial for the maintenance of emotional stability, learning abilities, and memory.[33,59]

THE TRANSENTORHINAL AND ENTORHINAL REGIONS

The transentorhinal and entorhinal regions extend over the ambient gyrus and anterior portions of the parahippocampal gyrus. The lateral entorhinal border roughly coincides with the rhinal sulcus anteriorly and the collateral sulcus posteriorly. Wartlike elevations often are found on the free surface of the entorhinal region.

The lamination pattern in the transentorhinal and entorhinal regions is remarkably complex. No cellular layer of the entorhinal cortex corresponds to any layer of the neocortex.[7,11] To avoid confusion, Rose's terminology[46] is used throughout in this text (FIG. 3). The entorhinal cortex is composed of two main strata (stratum principale externum and internum, pre and pri, respectively) which are separated from each other by a lamina dissecans. Nissl-stained paraffin sections usually permit recognition of only two external and two internal cellular layers. Counterstaining for lipofuscin deposits, however, depicts the unequivocal existence of three layers in both the external and internal main strata. Large multipolar projection cells of the external layer pre-α agglomerate to form cellular islands.[2,35,47] The external cellular layers pre-α, pre-β, and pre-γ give rise to the perforant path, an important limbic tract, which pierces the subiculum, crosses the obliterated hippocampal fissure, and terminates in the external two-thirds of the dentate molecular layer, as well as in the subiculum and the first sector of the Ammon's horn.[57]

The periallocortical transentorhinal region mediates between the entorhinal cortex (Brodmann's areas 34 and 28) and the temporal proneocortex (Brodmann's area 35), and is largely hidden in the depths of the rhinal sulcus. It is characterized by the gradual descent of layer pre-α through the outer main stratum (FIG. 3). The beginning of the descent and the abrupt cessation of the layer define the clear-cut boundaries of the region.

The transentorhinal region is most extensive in the human brain and decreases markedly in size going down the primate scale.[11] Together with some of the other components of the parahippocampal region, it is probably the major port of entry for the stream of neocortical data in transit to the entorhinal cortex (for further details see chapter by Burwell, this volume). Information from limbic circuits may reach the entorhinal cortex either directly or by way of the presubiculum, whereas projections from olfactory areas are sparse and rudimentary.

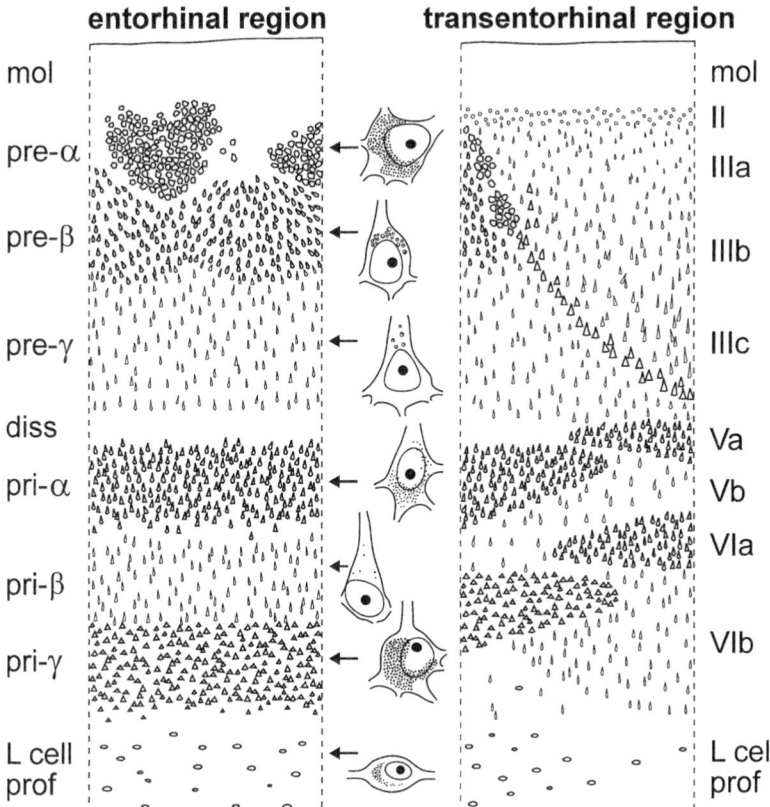

FIGURE 3. Schematic drawings of projection neurons forming the cellular layers of the allocortical entorhinal region (*left lane*) and periallocortical transentorhinal region (*right lane*) as seen in pigment Nissl-stained sections; note the gradual descent of layer pre-α. The lipofuscin pigment pattern of the different types of projection neurons (*central lane*) facilitates recognition of the individual layers. The lipofuscin pigment granules are compact or contain small light droplets (*small circles*). diss, lamina dissecans; mol, molecular layer; pre-α, pre-β, pre-γ, layers of the external main stratum; pri-α, pri-β, pri-γ, layers of the internal main stratum. L cell prof, lamina cellularis profunda, layer of nerve cells located in the white matter beneath layer pri-γ; II, III, V, VI, layers of the neocortex.

THE TRANSENTORHINAL AND ENTORHINAL REGIONS IN NEURODEGENERATIVE DISEASES

Many degenerative disorders of the human brain are associated with severe destruction of the transentorhinal and entorhinal regions. None of these disorders results in random deterioration of the brain. Rather, specific neuronal types as well as select cortical areas and subcortical nuclei become involved and deteriorate according to a predictable sequence. The lesional pattern develops more or less symmetrically in both hemispheres, accrues slowly over time, and remains consistent across

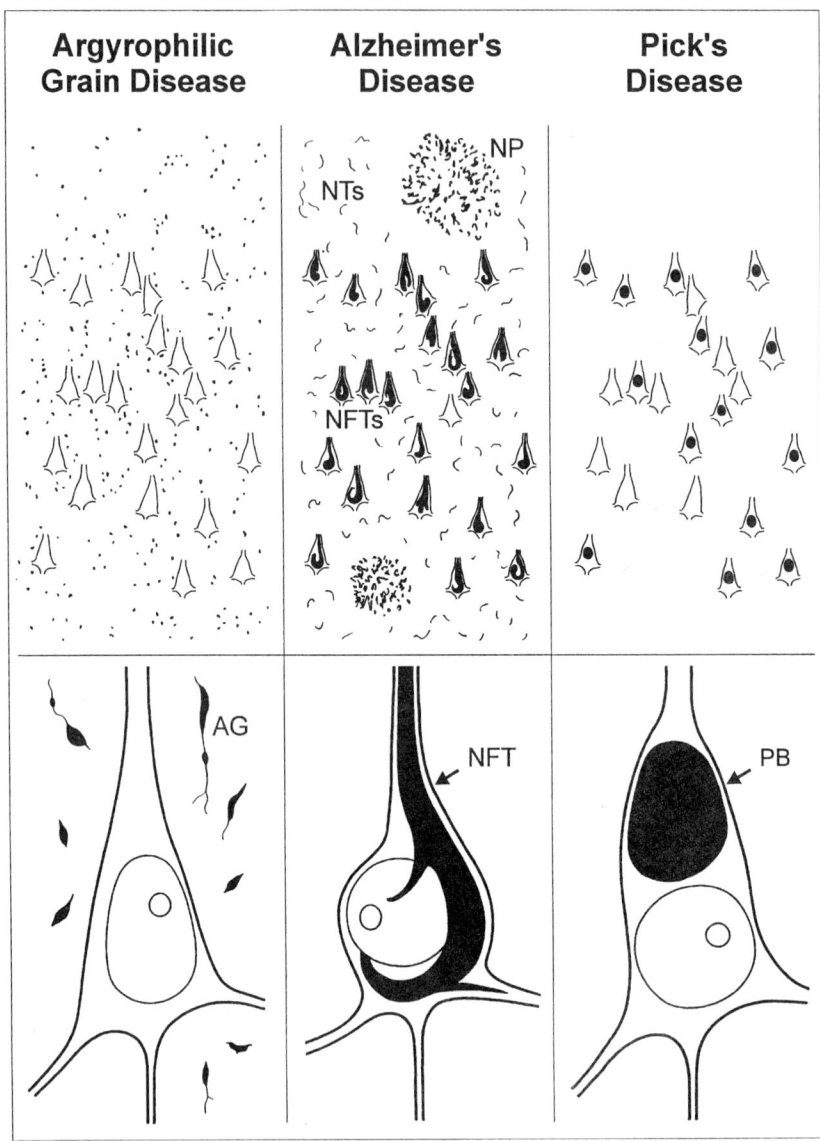

FIGURE 4. Key characteristics of three tauopathies: argyrophilic grain disease, Alzheimer's disease, and Pick's disease. The pathological material developing in all three disorders consists of both nonargyrophilic abnormal tau protein and argyrophilic fibrillary intraneuronal inclusions. The latter constitute the distinguishing features of the three disorders and permit their easy differentiation from each other as well as from other neurodegenerative diseases at post mortem examination. AG, argyrophilic grain; NFT, neurofibrillary tangle; NP, neuritic plaque; NTs, neuropil threads; PB, Pick body.

cases. Remarkably, the centers of the limbic loop, with their pivotal role in the transfer of information between the neocortical sensory association areas, higher-order components of the limbic system, and the prefrontal cortex, are susceptible to particularly grave pathological changes.[10–12,14,16,17,20,34,39,53,54]

Characteristic alterations of the tau-protein, a component of the cellular cytoskeleton, occur in patients with Alzheimer's disease, argyrophilic grain disease, and Pick's disease. In all three disorders susceptible nerve cells produce an initially soluble and non-argyrophilic pathological material which consists mostly of an abnormal and hyperphosphorylated tau protein. In a second facultative step, the pathological material converts into virtually insoluble non-biodegradable deposits which then adopt a pronounced argyrophilia. All of the degenerative illnesses sharing this sequence in the modification of the tau protein are referred to as "tauopathies."[4,6,16,17,22,26,28,36,44,51] The argyrophilic components of the pathological material are represented in Alzheimer's disease by neurofibrillary tangles and neuropil threads, in argyrophilic grain disease by the oat-shaped grains, and in Pick's disease by Pick bodies and Pick neurites (FIG. 4).

EARLY STAGES OF ALZHEIMER'S DISEASE

The transentorhinal region is the first cortical area to register the Alzheimer's disease-related cytoskeletal changes. The first cytoskeletal alterations develop in a few projection neurons residing in the transentorhinal layer pre-α. Further advance of the disease leads to severe affliction of layer pre-α in both the transentorhinal and the entorhinal pre–α layers.[29,32] Subsequently, one of the deep entorhinal layers becomes involved (pri-α). The lesions then encroach upon the amygdala and the first sector of the Ammon's horn (FIG. 5). In general, the early pathological changes develop in the absence of clinical symptoms, thereby marking the preclinical phase of the disease. Once the disease has commenced, however, it progresses relentlessly and clinical symptoms generally begin to appear with the affection of the neocortical association areas.[15]

The brain tissue of elderly nondemented individuals often shows the presence of mild pathological changes corresponding to one of the early stages of the Alzheimer's disease-related cytoskeletal alterations.[15]

ARGYROPHILIC GRAIN DISEASE

Argyrophilic grain disease is a tauopathy which becomes increasingly prevalent with advancing age. It entails multiple neuronal systems and chiefly damages allocortical areas, periallocortex, and proneocortex, but does not extend widely into the neocortex. The disorder merits attention because it occurs frequently and has a marked potential to cause severe brain dysfunction.[9,16,49–51]

Immunoreactions for abnormally phosphorylated tau protein permit identification of the disease-specific changes. Only a fraction of the emerging abnormal fibrillary material becomes argyrophilic. Many projection neurons in the affected regions develop a marked immunoreactivity for abnormal tau protein, but remain in non-argyrophilic status. The hallmark of the disease, the small spindle- or comma-shaped

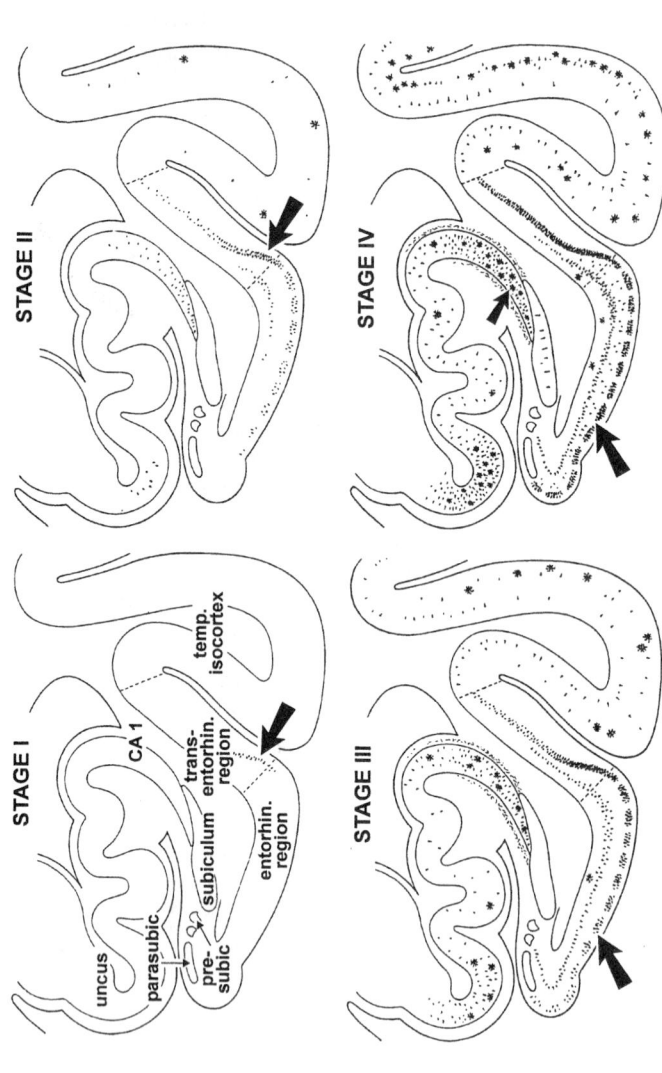

FIGURE 5. Summary diagram of neurofibrillary changes gradually evolving in the hippocampal formation, entorhinal and transentorhinal regions, and the adjoining temporal proneocortex in early stages of Alzheimer's disease seen at the level of the uncus in the hippocampal formation. Note the changes in the lesional distribution pattern that occur with progress of the disease from stage I to stage IV. Stages I and II usually correspond to the preclinical phase of the disorder and stages III and IV to incipient Alzheimer's disease. The *arrows* indicate key features. CA1, first sector of the Ammon's horn; entorhin., entorhinal; parasubic, parasubiculum; presubic, presubiculum; temp., temporal; transentorhin., transentorhinal. (From Braak & Braak.[10] Reprinted with permission from *Acta Neuropathologia*.)

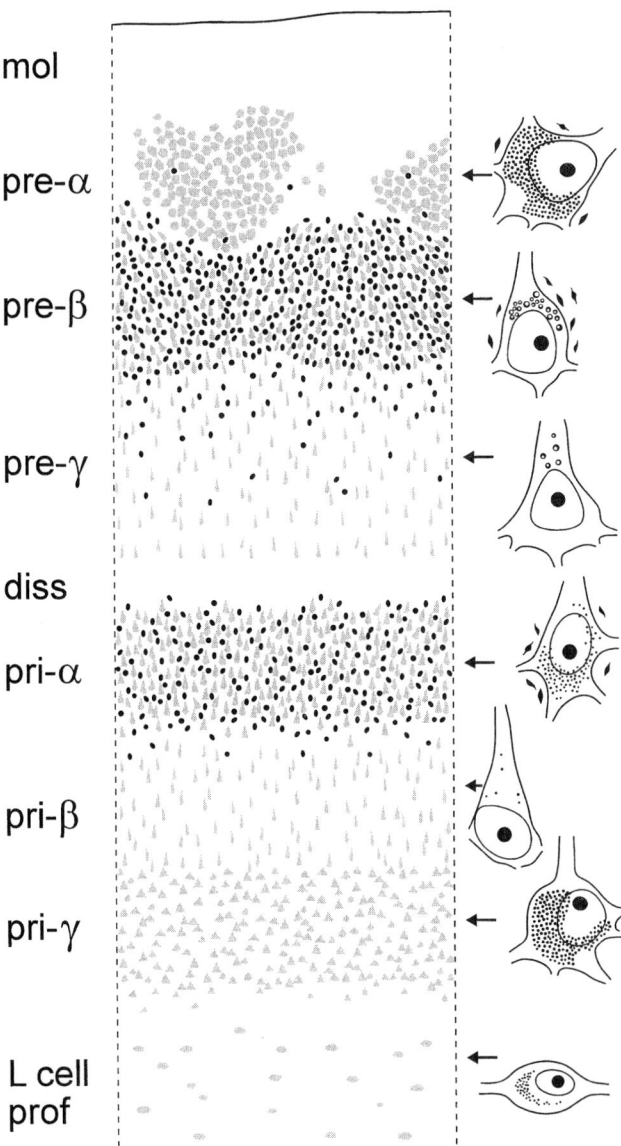

FIGURE 6. Argyrophilic grain disease. Characteristic distribution pattern of argyrophilic grains throughout the various cellular layers of the entorhinal region. Note the particularly severe involvement of layer pre-β. A less dense scattering of grains occurs in layer pri-α. In general, the density of lesions reaches a peak close to the transentorhinal-entorhinal border.

grains, however, convert into argyrophilic structures which usually are loosely scattered throughout the neuropil of select cortical layers and areas, and a few subcortical nuclei. Owing to the characteristic grains, the disorder easily can be differentiated from other tauopathies.[16]

The argyrophilic grains possess a uniform distribution pattern. The highest density of grains usually is encountered in layer pre-ß close to the transentorhinal-entorhinal border (FIG. 6). A somewhat less dense scattering of grains also occurs in the deep entorhinal cellular layers. From the transentorhinal region, the pathological changes invade the temporal proneocortex, and both regions show a high density of grains in layer IIIab. The lesions eventually encroach upon anterobasal portions of the insula, but no further. The first sector of the Ammon's horn, the amygdala, and, in particular, the hypothalamic lateral tuberal nucleus reveal a high density of grains. An interesting feature shared by argyrophilic grain disease, Pick's disease, and other tauopathies is the frequent occurrence of ballooned achromatic pyramidal cells in the neocortical layers IIIc and V.[24,51]

Brains of elderly individuals often show pathological changes which result from the presence of more than one disorder. Frequently, cases of argyrophilic grain disease display concomitant neurofibrillary tangles and neuropil threads in a density and distribution pattern corresponding to one of the early stages of Alzheimer's disease.[16]

PICK'S DISEASE

Pick's disease is a tauopathy which causes macroscopically detectable local atrophies of the frontal and temporal lobes while skirting the central gyri and posterior portions of the superior temporal gyrus.[23,42,45,52,55] Assessment of intraneuronal inclusions in the form of Pick bodies and Pick neurites is essential for the neuropathological diagnosis. The more or less spherical Pick bodies consist largely of hyperphosphorylated tau protein.[17,44,45]

Susceptible nerve cells initially develop pathological material in the form of small granules immunoreactive for abnormal tau protein that generally fill the soma and the cellular processes. Next, part of the material condenses to form argyrophilic inclusion bodies. Again, only a small fraction of the abnormal tau protein becomes argyrophilic in the course of the disease.[45]

The transentorhinal and entorhinal regions bear the brunt of the cortical pathology (FIG. 7). The projection neurons in layers of the external stratum, pre-α, pre-β, and pre-γ, and thereafter those of the internal stratum, pri-α, pri-β, and pri-γ, become affected. The undermost cellular layer (lamina cellularis profunda), which is located in the white matter beneath layer pri-γ, also is affected in Pick's disease. Involved projection cells of the entorhinal region eventually die and disappear from the cortical tissue. The neuronal loss commences in layer pre-α, and the subjacent layers gradually become denuded of projection neurons from top to bottom (FIG. 7). Simultaneously, the cortical tissue shrinks, and increasing numbers of astrocytes partially fill the space left behind by the lost nerve cells.

Very severe affection of the first sector of the Ammon's horn, the granule cell layer of the fascia dentata, amygdala, temporal and frontal proneocortical, and adjacent neocortical areas supplements the transentorhinal and entorhinal involvement.

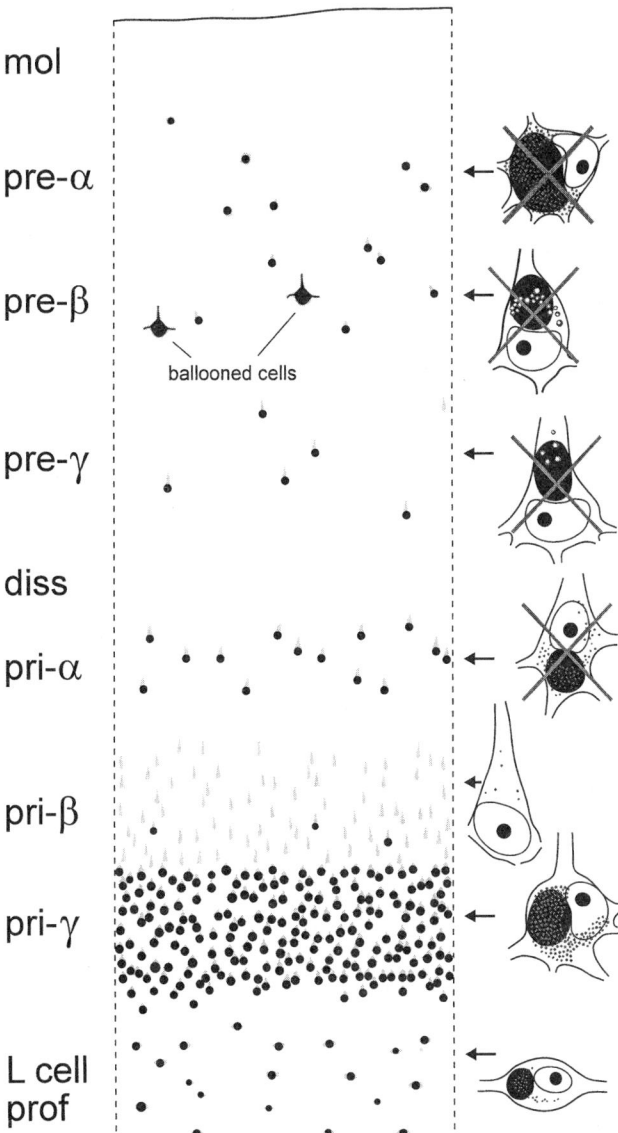

mol

pre-α

pre-β

ballooned cells

pre-γ

diss

pri-α

pri-β

pri-γ

L cell
prof

FIGURE 7. Neuronal loss and pattern of projection neurons containing Pick bodies in Pick's disease. The projection neurons of the entorhinal region are particularly badly stricken by the pathological process. Cytoskeletal alterations begin to evolve in the superficial cellular layer pre-α. Thereafter, they develop gradually in the subjacent layers until the undermost cellular layer located deep in the white matter exhibits the pathological changes as well. The diagram shows a relatively late phase of the illness with a high density of pyramidal cells in layer pri-γ and the undermost cellular layer containing Pick bodies. The formerly involved nerve cells of the outer main stratum and of layer pri-α already have almost totally disappeared from the cortical tissue.

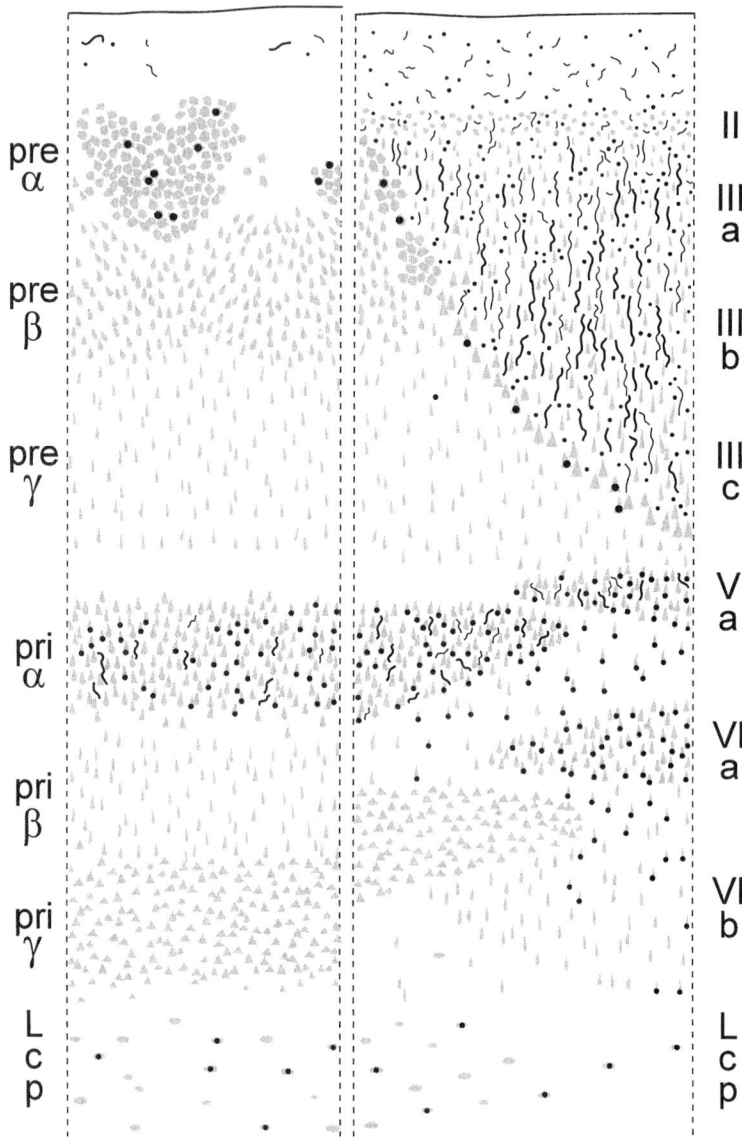

FIGURE 8. Parkinson's disease chiefly affects the frontal, insular, and temporal meso-cortex. This schematic diagram shows Parkinson-specific alterations in the periallocortical transentorhinal region. Note the characteristic and very dense network of Lewy neurites in layers III a–c. The internal layers V and VI harbor mainly Lewy body-bearing projection neurons. The adjoining portions of the temporal proneocortex generally exhibit a degree of damage similar to that seen in the transentorhinal region. The density of Lewy neurites decreases with growing distance from the transentorhinal, proneocortical border.

PARKINSON'S DISEASE

The pathological process underlying Parkinson's disease affects only a few types of nerve cells and manifests itself in thoroughgoing alterations of the cytoskeleton. The disorder entails multiple neuronal systems and leads to particularly severe destructions in periallocortical and proneocortical areas as well as in many subcortical nuclei belonging to both the limbic and the motor systems.[18,20,21,37]

As a result of the cytoskeletal alterations, Lewy bodies appear in the somata of nerve cells and Lewy neurites in their cellular processes. These inclusion bodies consist primarily of abnormally phosphorylated neurofilaments. Additional components include ubiquitin and α-synuclein, a protein which normally occurs in presynaptic structures.[3,5,27,41,48,52] The nerve cells affected by this kind of pathology survive for a long time in spite of damage. Nevertheless, they perish prematurely and lose much of their functional integrity long before actual cell death occurs.

The transentorhinal region together with the adjoining temporal proneocortex and other cingulate, subgenual, and insular proneocortical areas are devastatingly afflicted. The mesocortical lesions typically evolving in the course of Parkinson's disease are depicted in FIG. 8. A remarkably dense network of Lewy neurites extends throughout layer IIIab, whereas the layers V and VI harbor abundant projection neurons bearing Lewy bodies. The entorhinal region proper is far less severely involved and shows a moderate number of Lewy neurites and Lewy bodies in the deep layer pri-α.

The stratum oriens of the second sector of the Ammon's horn exhibits a thick web of long Lewy neurites.[25] Abundant Parkinson's disease-specific alterations generally are seen in the mesocortex, amygdala, limbic nuclei of the thalamus, and lower brain stem nuclei, including the substantia nigra and many nuclei integrated into the limbic system.[18,20,21] This lesional pattern explains the endocrine and autonomic dysregulation gradually developing in the course of Parkinson's disease. The specific involvement on the part of the limbic loop paves the way for a decline of intellectual faculties together with deficits of the affect-related voluntary motor system.

Similar to the situation seen in many cases of argyrophilic grain disease, there is a remarkable tendency for Parkinson-specific alterations to occur in tandem with neurofibrillary changes of the Alzheimer type.[38] In most cases the Alzheimer's disease-related lesions remain nearly confined to the transentorhinal and entorhinal regions. Despite their mild degree of severity, these additional lesions are likely to aggravate the situation, particularly in the transentorhinal cortex. The combined types of lesions almost certainly interfere with the normal exchange of vital data between sensory neocortex, higher-order centers of the limbic system, and the prefrontal neocortex.

HUNTINGTON'S DISEASE

Huntington's disease is featured mainly by a conspicuous atrophy of the striatum. The severe neuronal loss in this subcortical gray matter most probably accounts for the motor dysfunctions accompanying this disorder. Less obvious destruction consistently develops in other parts of the brain as well, which in all likelihood contributes to the patient's personality changes and cognitive decline.[31,40,56]

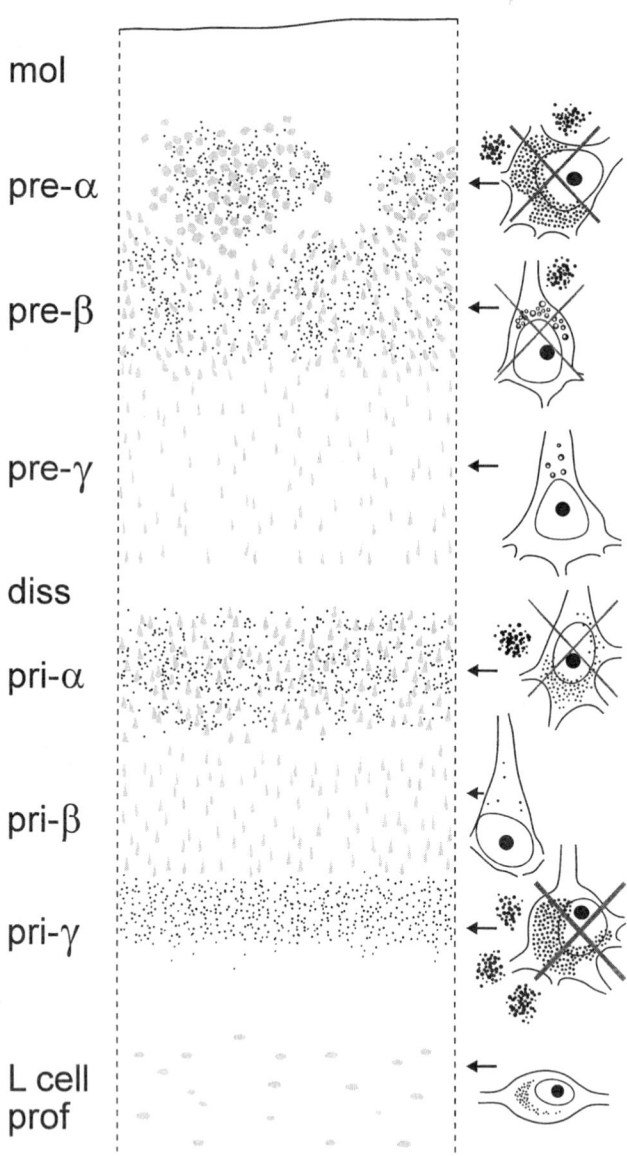

mol

pre-α

pre-β

pre-γ

diss

pri-α

pri-β

pri-γ

L cell
prof

FIGURE 9. Huntington's disease leads to severe and selective layer-specific devastation confined to the transentorhinal and entorhinal regions. Most conspicuous is the nearly total loss of nerve cells in the deep entorhinal layer pri-γ. A slightly less severe loss of cells occurs in the external layer pre-α and comparatively mild neuronal loss in layer pre-β. Recognition of this pathology requires clear differentiation of the three deep layers pri-α, pri-β, and pri-γ. Unequivocal distinction of these is facilitated by using Nissl-stained sections counterstained for lipofuscin pigment. Extraneuronal dots of lipofuscin pigment indicate the former position of the lost nerve cells.

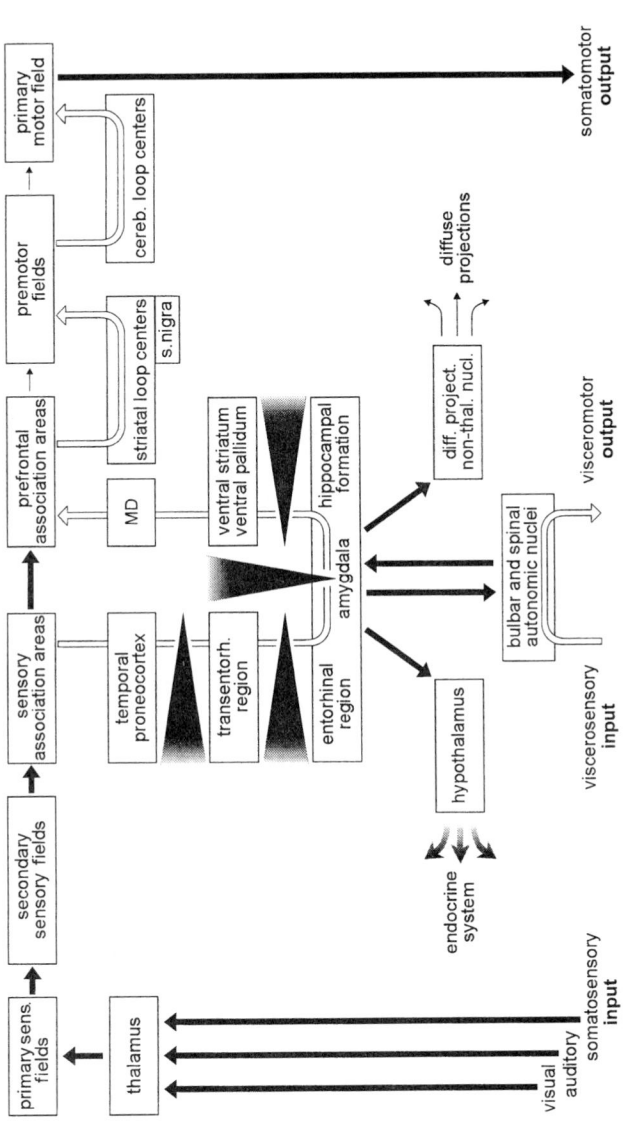

FIGURE 10. Components of the limbic loop play a significant role in the maintenance of memory functions. Precisely these higher-order centers of the limbic system are susceptible to grave pathological changes in many neurodegenerative diseases. Transfer of data from neocortical sensory association areas via the temporal proneocortex, transentorhinal periallocortex, entorhinal region, hippocampal formation, and amygdala to the prefrontal cortex is severely impaired in the course of these disorders. For abbreviations see FIGURE 2.

It is a widely accepted fact that the cerebral cortex somehow is involved in Huntington's disease. The details, however, surrounding the nature of the cortical affection are still an issue for debate. An unambiguously severe and selective layer-specific devastation, however, evolves in Huntington's disease which is limited to the transentorhinal and entorhinal regions. Cases with Huntington's disease present with drastic destruction of layer pri-γ which either is completely denuded of nerve cells or marked by pronounced neuronal loss. A somewhat less, yet still severe, change can be seen in the external layers pre-α and pre-β. Extraneuronal dots of lipofuscin pigment indicate the former position of the lost nerve cells.[12] Such a degree of neuronal loss almost certainly hampers the stream of data being funneled through the limbic loop.

Studies in the subprimate mammalian brain show the existence of projections from the lowermost entorhinal cellular layer to the striatum. Given the fact that such projections exist in the human brain, it may well be that the almost total loss of nerve cells in layer pri-γ reflects the devastation of the striatum in Huntington's disease.[12]

CONCLUDING REMARKS

The summary diagram emphasizes the importance of the transentorhinal and entorhinal regions as cortical predilection sites for select degenerative diseases of the human brain (FIG. 10). The most important among these is certainly Alzheimer's disease; still, the specific changes evolving in the course of argyrophilic grain disease, Pick's disease, idiopathic Parkinson syndrome, and Huntington's disease merit attention as well.

The transentorhinal region generally registers the initial changes and is the most severely involved. From this transitional mesocortical region, the lesions usually invade with decreasing severity the entorhinal region and temporal proneocortex. All of the lesional types described here result in severe dysfunctions entailing data-transport from the sensory neocortex via the limbic loop to the prefrontal neocortex, thereby contributing to the insidious development of personality changes and cognitive decline.

ACKNOWLEDGMENTS

This work was supported by the Deutsche Forschungsgemeinschaft and the Bundesministerium für Bildung, Wissenschaft, Forschung und Technologie, the Alzheimer Research Center Frankfurt (AFZF), and Degussa, Hanau. The skillful assistance in graphics by Ms. Szasz is gratefully acknowledged.

REFERENCES

1. ALHEID, G.F., M.D. CRUTCHER, et al. 1990. Basal ganglia. In The Human Nervous System. G. Paxinos, Ed.: 483–582. Academic Press. San Diego, CA.
2. AMARAL, D.G. & R. INSAUSTI. 1990. Hippocampal formation. In The Human Nervous System. G. Paxinos, Ed.: 711–755. Academic Press. San Diego, CA.

3. BANCHER, C. & H. LASSMANN, *et al.* 1989. An antigenic profile of Lewy bodies: immunocytochemical indication for protein phosphorylation and ubiquitination. J. Neuropathol. Exp. Neurol. **48:** 81–93.
4. BANCHER, C. & C. BRUNNER, *et al.* 1989. Accumulation of abnormally phosphorylated τ precedes the formation of neurofibrillary tangles in Alzheimer's disease. Brain Res. **477:** 90–99.
5. BERGERON, C. & M.S. POLLANEN. 1996. Pathogenesis of the Lewy body. *In* Dementia with Lewy Bodies. R. Perry, I. Mc Keith, *et al.*, Eds.: 302–308. Cambridge University Press. New York.
6. BRAAK, E., H. BRAAK, *et al.* 1994. A sequence of cytoskeleton changes related to the formation of neurofibrillary tangles and neuropil threads. Acta Neuropathol. **87:** 554–567.
7. BRAAK, H. 1980. Architectonics of the Human Telencephalic Cortex. Springer. Berlin.
8. BRAAK, H. & E. BRAAK. 1985. On areas of transition between entorhinal allocortex and temporal isocortex in the human brain. Normal morphology and lamina-specific pathology in Alzheimer's disease. Acta Neuropathol. **68:** 325–332.
9. BRAAK, H. & E. BRAAK. 1989. Cortical and subcortical argyrophilic grains characterize a disease associated with adult onset dementia. Neuropathol. Appl. Neurobiol. **15:** 13–26.
10. BRAAK, H. & E. BRAAK. 1991. Neuropathological stageing of Alzheimer-related changes. Acta Neuropathol. **82:** 239–259.
11. BRAAK, H. & E. BRAAK. 1992. The human entorhinal cortex: Normal morphology and lamina-specific pathology in various diseases. Neurosci. Res. **15:** 6–31.
12. BRAAK, H. & E. BRAAK. 1992. Allocortical involvement in Huntington's disease. Neuropathol. Appl. Neurobiol. **18:** 539–547.
13. BRAAK, H. & E. BRAAK. 1993. Anatomy of the human basal ganglia. *In* Inhibitors of Monoamine Oxidase. B.I. Szelenyi, Ed.: 3–23. Birkhäuser. Basel.
14. BRAAK, H. & E. BRAAK. 1994. Pathology of Alzheimer's disease. *In* Neurodegenerative Diseases. D.B. Calne, Ed.: 585–613. Saunders. Philadelphia, PA.
15. BRAAK, H. & E. BRAAK. 1997. Frequency of stages of Alzheimer-related lesions in different age categories. Neurobiol. Aging **18:** 351–357.
16. BRAAK, H. & E. BRAAK. 1998. Argyrophilic grain disease: frequency of occurrence in different age categories and neuropathological diagnostic criteria. J. Neural Transm. **105:** 801–819.
17. BRAAK, H. & E. BRAAK. 1998. Involvement of precerebellar nuclei in Pick's disease. Exp. Neurol. **153:** 351–365.
18. BRAAK, H., E. BRAAK, *et al.* 1994. Amygdala pathology in Parkinson's disease. Acta Neuropathol. **88:** 493–500.
19. BRAAK, H., E. BRAAK, *et al.* 1996. Functional anatomy of the human hippocampal formation and related structures. J. Child Neurol. **11:** 265–275.
20. BRAAK, H., R.A.I. DE VOS, *et al.* 1998. Neuropathological hallmarks of Alzheimer's and Parkinson's diseases. Prog. Brain Res. **117:** 267–285.
21. BRAAK, H., U. RÜB, *et al.* 2000. Parkinson's disease: affection of brain stem nuclei controlling premotor and motor neurons of the somatomotor system. Acta Neuropathol. **99:** 489–495.
22. DICKSON, D.W. 1997. Neurodegenerative diseases with cytoskeletal pathology: a biochemical classification. Ann. Neurol. **42:** 541–544.
23. DICKSON, D.W. 1998. Pick's disease: a modern approach. Brain Pathol. **8:** 339–354.
24. DICKSON, D.W., S.H. YEN, *et al.* 1986. Ballooned neurons in select neurodegenerative diseases contain phosphorylated neurofilament epitopes. Acta Neuropathol. **71:** 216–223.
25. DICKSON, D.W., M.L. SCHMIDT, *et al.* 1994. Immunoreactivity profile of hippocampal CA2/3 neurites in diffuse Lewy body disease. Acta Neuropathol. **87:** 269–276.
26. FEANY, M.B. & D.W. DICKSON. 1996. Neurodegenerative disorders with extensive tau pathology: a comparative study and review. Ann. Neurol. **40:** 139–148.
27. GOEDERT, M. 1997. The awakening of α-synuclein. Nature **388:** 232–233.
28. GOEDERT, M., J.Q. TROJANOWSKI, *et al.* 1997. The neurofibrillary pathology of Alzheimer's disease. *In* The Molecular and Genetic Basis of Neurological Disease, 2nd edit. R.N. Rosenberg, Ed.: 613–627. Butterworth-Heinemann. Boston, MA.

29. GOMEZ-ISLA, T., J.L. PRICE, et al. 1996. Profound loss of layer II entorhinal neurons occurs in very mild Alzheimer's disease. J. Neurosci. **16**: 4491–4500.
30. HEIMER, L., J. DE OLMOS, et al. 1991. "Perestroika" in the basal forebrain: opening the border between neurology and psychiatry. Prog. Brain Res. **87**: 109–165.
31. HEINSEN, H., M. STRIK, et al. 1994. Cortical and striatal neurone number in Huntington's disease. Acta Neuropathol. **88**: 320–333.
32. HYMAN, B.T., G.W. VAN HOESEN, et al. 1984. Alzheimer's disease: cell-specific pathology isolates the hippocampal formation. Science **225**: 1168–1170.
33. HYMAN, B.T., G.W. VAN HOESEN, et al. 1990. Memory-related neural systems in Alzheimer's disease: an anatomic study. Neurology **40**: 1721–1730.
34. HYMAN, B.T. & T. GOMEZ-ISLA. 1994. Alzheimer's disease is a laminar, regional, and neural system specific disease, not a global brain disease. Neurobiol. Aging **15**: 353–354.
35. INSAUSTI, R., T. TUNON, et al. 1995. The human entorhinal cortex: a cytoarchitectonic analysis. J. Comp. Neurol. **335**: 171–198.
36. IQBAL, K., A.C. ALONSO, et al. 1994. Mechanism of neurofibrillary degeneration in Alzheimer's disease. Mol. Neurobiol. **9**: 119–123.
37. JELLINGER, K. 1991. Pathology of Parkinson's disease. Changes other than the nigrostriatal pathway. Mol. Chem. Neuropathol. **14**: 153–197.
38. JELLINGER, K., H. BRAAK, et al. 1991. Alzheimer lesions in the entorhinal region and isocortex in Parkinson's and Alzheimer's diseases. Ann. New York Acad. Sci. **640**: 203–209.
39. KEMPER, T.L. 1978. Senile dementia: a focal disease in the temporal lobe. In Senile Dementia: a Biomedical Approach. E. Nandy, Ed.: 105–113. Elsevier. Amsterdam.
40. KOWALL, N.W. & R.J. FERRANTE. 1998. Huntington's disease. In Neuropathology of Dementing Disorders. W.R. Markesbery, Ed.: 219–256. Arnold. London.
41. LOWE, J. 1994. Lewy bodies. In Neurodegenerative Diseases. D.B. Calne, Ed.: 51–69. Saunders. Philadelphia, PA.
42. MARKESBERY, W.R. 1998. Pick's disease. In Neuropathology of Dementing Disorders. W.R. Markesbery, Ed.: 142–157. Arnold. London.
43. PARENT, A. & L.N. HAZRATI. 1995. Functional anatomy of the basal ganglia. I. The cortico-basal ganglia-thalamo-cortical loop. Brain Res. Rev. **20**: 91–127.
44. PROBST, A., B. ANDERTON, et al. 1983. Pick's disease: an immunocytochemical study of neuronal changes. Monoclonal antibodies show that Pick bodies share antigenic determinants with neurofibrillary tangles and neurofilaments. Acta Neuropathol. **60**: 175–182.
45. PROBST, A., M. TOLNAY, et al. 1996. Pick's disease: hyperphosphorylated tau protein segregates to the somatoaxonal compartment. Acta Neuropathol. **92**: 588–596.
46. ROSE, M. 1935. Cytoarchitektonik und Myeloarchitektonik der Grosshirnrinde. In Handbuch der Neurologie, Vol. 1. O. Bumke & O. Foerster, Eds.: 588–778. Springer. Berlin.
47. SOLODKIN, A. & G.W. VAN HOESEN. 1996. Entorhinal cortex modules of the human brain. J. Comp. Neurol. **365**: 610–627.
48. SPILLANTINI, M.G., M.L. SCHMIDT, et al. 1997. α-Synuclein in Lewy bodies. Nature **388**: 839–840.
49. TOLNAY, M., M.G. SPILLANTINI, et al. 1997. Argyrophilic grain disease: widespread hyperphosphorylation of tau protein in limbic neurons. Acta Neuropathol. **93**: 477–484.
50. TOLNAY, M., C. MISTL, et al. 1998. Argyrophilic grains of Braak: occurrence in dendrites of neurons containing hyper-phosphorylated tau protein. Neuropathol. Appl. Neurobiol. **24**: 53–59.
51. TOLNAY, M. & A. PROBST. 1999. Review: tau protein pathology in Alzheimer's disease and related disorders. Neuropathol. Appl. Neurobiol. **25**: 171–187
52. TROJANOWSKI, J.Q. & V.M.Y. LEE. 1998. Aggregation of neurofilament and α-synuclein proteins in Lewy bodies—implications for the pathogenesis of Parkinson disease and Lewy body dementia. Arch. Neurol. **55**: 151–152.
53. VAN HOESEN, G.W. & B.T. HYMAN. 1990. Hippocampal formation: anatomy and the patterns of pathology in Alzheimer's disease. Prog. Brain Res. **83**: 445–457.
54. VAN HOESEN, G.W., B.T. HYMAN, et al. 1991. Entorhinal cortex pathology in Alzheimer's disease. Hippocampus **1**: 1–8.

55. VONSATTEL, J.P.G., G. BINETTI, *et al.* 1997. Pick's disease. *In* Molecular Mechanisms of Dementia. W. Wasco & R.E. Tanzi, Eds.: 253–269. Humana Press. Toronto.
56. VONSATTEL, J.P.G. & M. DIFIGLIA. 1998. Huntington's disease. J. Neuropathol. Exp. Neurol. **57:** 369–384.
57. WITTER, M.P. 1993. Organization of the entorhinal-hippocampal system: a review of current anatomical data. Hippocampus **3:** 33–44.
58. ZILLES, K. 1990. Cortex. *In* The Human Nervous System. G. Paxinos, Ed.: 757–802. Academic Press. San Diego, CA.
59. ZOLA-MORGAN, S. & L.R. SQUIRE. 1993. Neuroanatomy of memory. Annu. Rev. Neurosci. **16:** 547–563.

From Healthy Aging to Early Alzheimer's Disease: *In Vivo* Detection of Entorhinal Cortex Atrophy

LEYLA DE TOLEDO-MORRELL,[a,b,c,f] IRINA GONCHAROVA,[a,d]
BRADFORD DICKERSON,[a,e] ROBERT S. WILSON,[a,b,c] AND
DAVID A. BENNETT[a,c]

Departments of [a]Neurological Sciences and [b]Psychology, and [c]Rush Alzheimer's Disease Center, Rush-Presbyterian-St. Luke's Medical Center, Chicago, Illinois 60612

ABSTRACT: Using quantitative structural MRI protocols, we examined the effects of age on alterations in entorhinal cortex (EC) volume. The left EC was found to be smaller than the right in both young and healthy aged subjects. More importantly, the right EC, but not the left, was significantly *smaller* in elderly participants compared to young controls. In an attempt to determine the earliest sites of involvement in mild and incipient Alzheimer's disease (AD), we compared entorhinal and hippocampal volume in (1) healthy elderly controls, (2) patients with very mild AD, and (3) elderly patients who were evaluated for cognitive complaints, but did not meet criteria for dementia. Both patient groups differed from controls in EC volume, but not from each other. In contrast, the two patient groups differed in hippocampal volume from controls, as well as from each other, with the mild AD cases showing the greatest atrophy. These results suggest that degeneration of the EC and hippocampal formation occurs before the onset of overt dementia. In fact, follow-up clinical evaluations available on 23 of 28 nondemented patients indicated that 12 of 23 had converted to AD. Converters could be best differentiated from nonconverters on the basis of entorhinal volume.

INTRODUCTION

High-resolution magnetic resonance imaging (MRI) techniques provide a unique tool for examining alterations in brain anatomy *in vivo* during healthy aging as well as in various age-related disease processes. In addition, such techniques make it possible to (a) relate alterations in given brain regions to the sequential development of behavioral symptoms in degenerative diseases and (b) examine the specific role of certain brain structures in human memory function because of the age or disease-related occurrence of "lesions" in these structures.

[d]Current address: Wadsworth Center, New York State Department of Health, Albany, NY.
[e] Current address: Brigham and Women's Hospital, Harvard University, Boston, MA.
[f]Address for correspondence: Leyla deToledo-Morrell, Department of Neurological Sciences, Rush-Presbyterian-St. Luke's Medical Center, 1653 W. Congress Parkway, Chicago, IL 60612. Tel.: (312) 942-5399; fax: (312) 942-2238.
e-mail: leylat@neuro.rush.edu

The entorhinal cortex (EC) and the hippocampal formation (HF) are part of the mesial temporal lobe memory system; the EC connects the neocortex with the HF, thereby providing the latter with multimodal sensory information. Postmortem pathological studies have implicated the EC as one of the early sites of involvement in Alzheimer's disease (AD).[5,6,20,34,39] Although hippocampal atrophy has been well documented in AD and in preclinical cases using quantitative volumetric MRI techniques,[8,9,11-13,22,23,26-29,36,41] such protocols have only recently been developed for the EC.[21,25]

In this paper, we review work from our laboratory on alterations in entorhinal volume detected *in vivo* using quantitative structural MRI in various elderly cohorts, contrasting entorhinal atrophy to that seen in the HF, where appropriate. At the end of the paper, we present some preliminary data suggesting that the EC and HF play different roles in human memory function. Since the MRI techniques used in all the experiments to be described were similar, they will be detailed first.

ACQUISITION AND QUANTITATION OF MRI DATA

All MR images were acquired on a 1.5 Tesla General Electric Signa scanner. Gapless, 5 mm coronal slices were taken perpendicular to the long axis of the HF with the following parameters: matrix = 256×256, field of view = 16 cm, eight acquisitions, TR = 400, TE = 13. In addition, gapless, 5 mm sagittal slices were taken spanning the entire brain with the following parameters: matrix = 256×128, field of view = 24 cm, one acquisition, TR = 200, TE = 12.[g]

Manual segmentation with a PC-based 3-D image analysis program (Amersham Image Analysis System with software by Loates Associates) was used to compute volumes of regions of interest. To correct for normal individual differences in brain size, entorhinal and hippocampal volumes were normalized by dividing with intracranial volume derived from sagittal slices. To compute intracranial volume, the inner table of the cranium was traced in consecutive sagittal sections spanning the entire brain. At the level of the foramen magnum, a straight line was drawn from the inner surface of the clivus to the most anterior extension of the occipital bone.

EC volume was quantified with the use of a new protocol developed and validated in our laboratory, technical details of which will be published elsewhere.[17] The advantage of this protocol is that EC volume is measured from the same oblique coronal sections most commonly used for hippocampal volumetry to avoid overestimation of one of these two adjacent structures at the expense of the other.

Briefly, both entorhinal and hippocampal volumes were computed separately for the right and left hemispheres from coronal slices taken perpendicular to the long axis of the HF. For the EC, tracing began with the first section in which the gyrus ambiens, amygdala, and the white matter of the parahippocampal gyrus first appeared visible. The dorsomedial border in rostral sections was the sulcus semiannularis and in caudal sections the subiculum. The shoulder of the collateral sulcus was

---

[g]We now use a new protocol that acquires 1.6 mm coronal images of the entire head with an SPGR pulse sequence. For purposes of consistency and to have large enough group sizes, the investigations described herein were restricted to those patients and controls scanned with our old protocol.

used as the ventrolateral border. The latter is somewhat of a conservative criterion that allowed consistency in tracings and avoided the use of different ventrolateral borders depending on individual differences in the depth of the collateral sulcus (see protocol by Insausti et al.[21]). The last section measured was the one immediately preceding the image in which the lateral geniculate nucleus first appeared. In the majority of cases, tracings were carried out on 4–5 sections.

The protocol and validation procedures used for quantifying hippocampal volume have been described previously.[11,41] Tracings of the HF started with the first section caudal to the amygdala, where the dentate gyrus could be clearly identified, and included the fimbria, dentate gyrus, the hippocampus proper, and the subiculum. All sections in which the hippocampus could be clearly seen without partial volume averaging were included (usually 6–7 slices).

EFFECTS OF AGE ON ATROPHY OF THE ENTORHINAL CORTEX

The effects of age on hippocampal atrophy determined from sructural MR images have now been well documented.[8–10,16,23] With the recent development of MRI protocols for the quantitation of the EC, similar studies are beginning to be reported.[21]

In our laboratory, we compared EC volume in the following two groups of subjects: (1) 34 healthy elderly individuals (mean age, 70.3; range, 61–84 years) and (2) 30 young controls (mean age, 26.6; range, 21–34 years). Young subjects included medical students, technicians working at the Rush Medical Center and their friends. Healthy elderly subjects were recruited from friends and family members of patients and the Rush Alzheimer's Disease Center staff, as well as from hospital volunteers. Each elderly participant had a standard evaluation including a medical history, neurological examination, and abbreviated neuropsychological testing. Selection as an aged control subject required a Mini Mental State Examination (MMSE)[15] score of ≥ 28, Consortium to Establish a Registry for Alzheimer's Disease (CERAD)[33] delayed list recall of ≥ 6 and absence of evidence of neurologic, systemic or psychiatric disorders. In this and the studies reported below, informed consent was obtained from all participants acording to the rules of the Human Investigation Committee of Rush Medical College.

Mean normalized entorhinal volume is plotted in FIGURE 1 as a function of age and hemisphere. The right entorhinal volume was found to be slightly (by 12%), but significantly, larger than the left in young individuals [t(29) = 3.92, $p = 0.0005$), a finding consistent with that reported by Insausti and colleagues.[21] The effects of age on EC volume were assessed with a two-way repeated measures analysis of variance (ANOVA) with groups (young vs. old) and hemispheres as the two factors. The only signifiicant effect was that for hemisphere [F(1,62) = 20.65, $p < 0.0001$], indicating that in both young and aged subjects, the right EC was larger than the left. Although the group × hemisphere interaction did not reach significance (as was the case in the Insauisti et al.[21] study), we examined the difference between young and old participants in *right* entorhinal volume using a t test, because it seemed smaller in the elderly subjects (see FIG.1). The result showed a significant difference between the age groups (t = 2.47, df = 62, $p = 0.016$), indicating that the right EC may be more vulnerable to the aging process than the left. These results are similar to those previous-

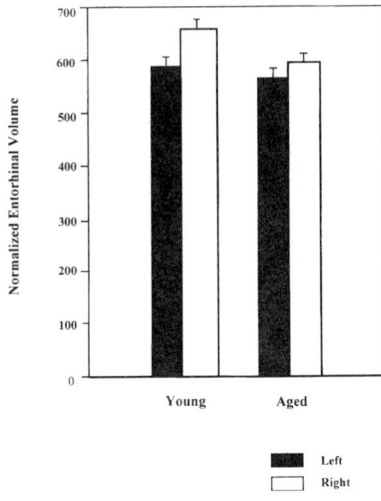

FIGURE 1. Mean normalized entorhinal volume in young and healthy elderly control subjects plotted as a function of hemisphere. Vertical bars represent the standard error of the mean.

ly reported by us for the HF.[10] In that study, compared to their young counterparts, elderly males showed greater *right hippocampal* atrophy than females, but neither had significant *left hippocampal* atrophy.

ENTORHINAL AND HIPPOCAMPAL ATROPHY IN ELDERLY PATIENTS WITHOUT DEMENTIA AND IN THOSE WITH MILD AD

Two studies that measured the entire parahippocampal gyrus failed to detect significant atrophy in this structure in *very mild* AD cases compared to aged controls.[11,23] In these very mild cases, however, there was significant hippocampal atrophy. These results were somewhat surprising at first sight, given postmortem evidence indicating the early pathological involvement of the entorhinal and transentorhinal cortices in the disease process.[5,6,20,34,39] In the two studies cited above, the volume of the parahippocampal gyrus included both white and gray matter and, in the case of the report from our laboratory,[11] measurements continued beyond the anatomical boundaries of the entorhinal and perirhinal cortices. As a result, any changes in the EC itself in patients with very mild AD may have been overshadowed. Therefore, it was important for us to develop a protocol for the quantitation of the EC *in vivo* in order to re-examine its involvement in patients with very mild or incipient AD.

In an attempt to determine the earliest sites of involvement in mild and incipient AD, we quantified and compared entorhinal and hippocampal volume in healthy elderly controls, patients with extremely mild AD, as well as in elderly patients who were evaluated for cognitive complaints, but did not meet criteria for dementia (nondemented participants).[13] All evaluations were performed at the Rush Alzheimer's Disease Center as previously described.[11,41] Briefly, the evaluation incorporated CERAD[33] procedures and included a medical history, a neurological examination,

TABLE 1. Demographic characteristics of participants

	Elderly Controls	Patients with Very Mild AD	Nondemented Patients
	(n = 34)	(n = 16)	(n = 28)
Age	70.3 ± 6.6 (61–84)	71.4 ± 9.1 (49–82)	68.6 ± 8.6 (51–82)
Education (years)	13.6 ± 2.7	14.5 ± 2.9	15.2 ± 3.1
Female/male	20/14	12/4	9/19
MMSE score	29.2 ± 0.7	27.3 ± 1.1*	27.0 ± 2.2*

*Significantly different from controls ($p < 0.05$).

neuropsychological testing, an informant interview, and blood tests. The clinical diagnosis of probable AD followed NINCDS/ADRDA guidelines;[31] it required a history of cognitive decline and neuropsychological test evidence of impairment in at least two cognitive domains, one of which had to be memory. In this study, we only included those patients with a diagnosis of probable AD whose MMSE scores were ≥ 26. Exclusion criteria for both patient groups (i.e., AD and nondemented) were evidence of other neurologic, psychiatric or systemic conditions that could cause cognitive impairment (e.g., stroke, alcoholism, major depression). Inclusion and exclusion criteria for elderly control subjects were described above.

Demograhic data for the three groups are presented in TABLE 1. A one-way ANOVA on MMSE scores showed a significant group effect [$F(2,75) = 18.0$, $p < 0.0001$]. Bonferroni corrected t tests indicated that both the nondemented patients and those with a clinical diagnosis of AD differed significantly from controls in MMSE scores ($p < 0.05$, at least), but not from each other. The three groups did not differ in age or level of education.

Mean normalized entorhinal and hippocampal volume for the three groups of participants are shown in FIGURE 2 as a function of hemisphere. Group differences in the volumes of the two regions of interest were assessed with separate two-way repeated measures ANOVAs with groups and hemispheres as the two factors. The analysis on entorhinal volume showed significant group [$F(2,75) = 15.73$, $p < 0.0001$] and hemisphere [$F(1,75) = 13.11$, $p < 0.0005$] effects, but no significant interaction between them. The hemisphere effect can be accounted for by a larger right EC in all three groups. Bonferroni-corrected t tests showed that both the nondemented and mild AD patients differed significantly from controls ($p < 0.05$, at least) in total (right + left) EC volume, but not from each other. Compared to controls, the extent of EC atrophy in nondemented and mild AD patients was 17.9% and 32.0%, respectively.

The analysis on hippocampal volume also showed significant group [$F(2,75) = 16.65$, $p < 0.0001$] and hemisphere [$F(1,75) = 14.02$, $p < 0.0005$] effects, without a significant interaction between them. However, in this case, Bonferroni-corrected t tests indicated that the two patient groups differed from controls, as well as from each other ($p < 0.05$, at least) in total hippocampal volume, with nondemented cases showing 9.2% atrophy and mild AD cases 25% atrophy.

In addition, logistic regression analyses were performed to determine how well hippocampal and entorhinal volume could predict group membership. These analyses demonstrated that EC volume was better than hippocampal volume at predicting

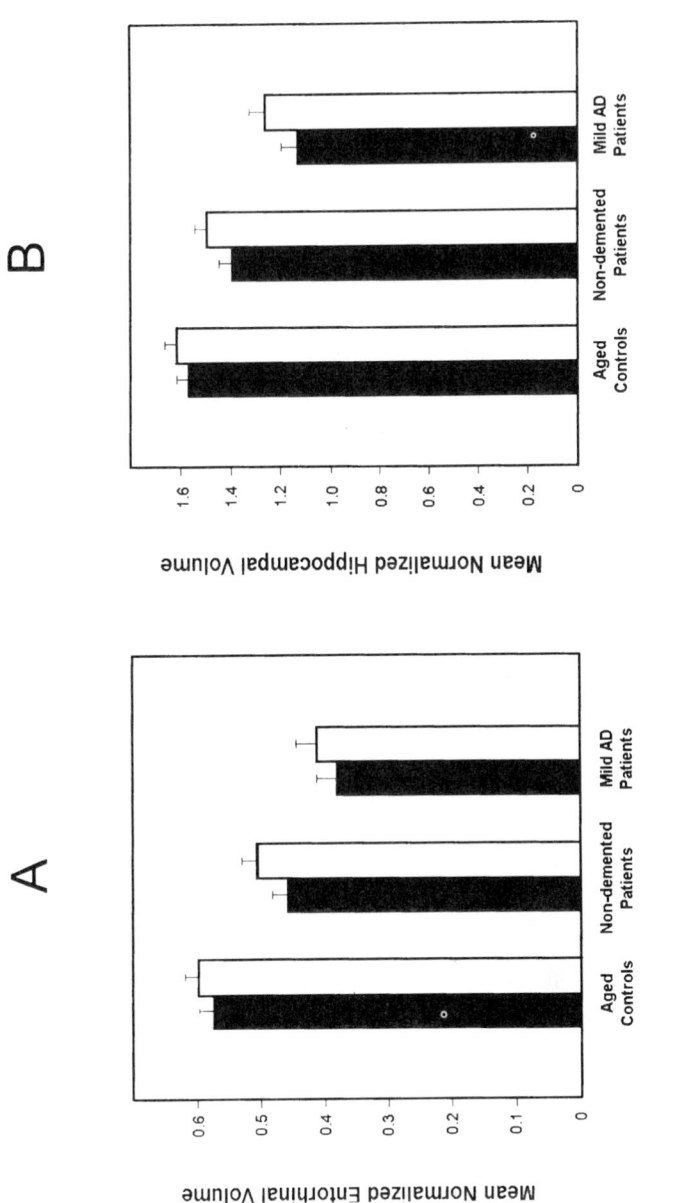

FIGURE 2. Mean normalized entorhinal (**A**) and hippocampal (**B**) volume in elderly control participants, patients with very mild AD, and those who did not meet criteria for dementia. Volumes are shown for each hemisphere separately. Vertical bars represent the standard error of the mean.

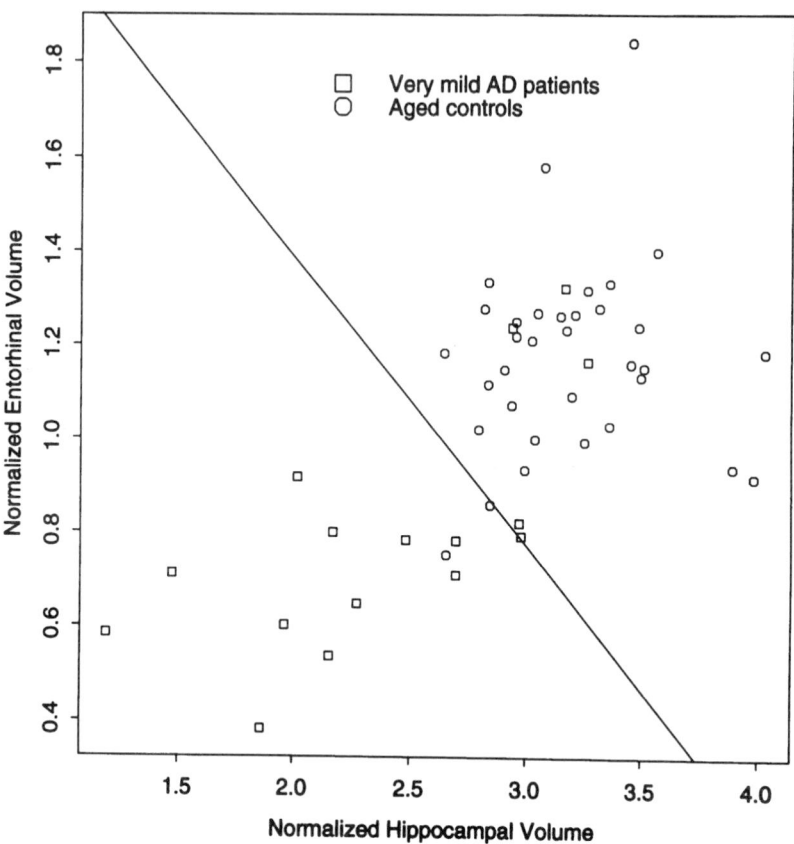

FIGURE 3. Scatterplot showing normalized total (*right + left*) entorhinal and hippocampal volume in elderly control subjects and patients with very mild AD. The two groups could be best differentiated by a combination of entorhinal and hippocampal volume as indicated by the regression line (see text).

membership in the nondemented and control groups, correctly classifying 75% of subjects. In contrast, membership in the two patient groups was best predicted by hippocampal volume which correctly classified 74% of subjects. Finally, entorhinal and hippocampal volumes *both* contributed to predicting group membership for the mild AD and aged control groups, correctly classifying 88 and 82% of subjects, respectively. FIGURE 3 is a scatterplot showing the degree of differentiation of very mild AD cases from controls on the basis of a combination of hippocampal and entorhinal volume.

These *in vivo* results showing the early involvement of the EC in AD are in agreement with other reports in the literature.[4,26] An important contribution of our study was the inclusion of extremely mild cases of AD and a comparison of these mild cases with those at risk for AD. The fact that the two patient groups did not significantly

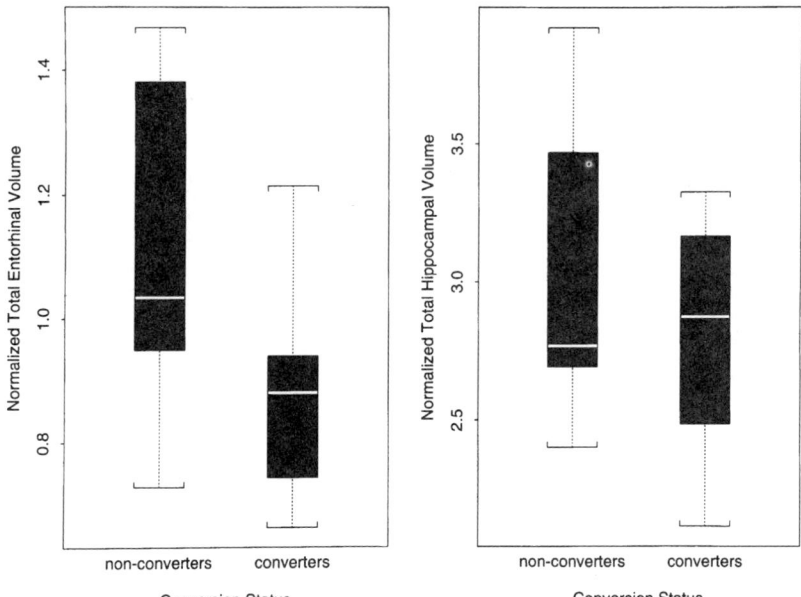

FIGURE 4. Box plot comparing MRI-derived entorhinal (*left*) and hippocampal (*right*) volume in nondemented participants who converted to a diagnosis of Alzheimer's disease, in contrast to those who did not. The central box shows the data between the upper and lower quartiles, with the median represented by the line. The height of the box is the interquartile range (IQR); the "whiskers" extend from the upper and lower quartiles to a distance of 1.5 IQR away or to the most extreme data point within that range, whichever is closer.

differ from each other in EC volume suggests that the EC becomes pathologically involved even in preclinical cases. Thus, MRI-derived entorhinal atrophy may provide an *in vivo* anatomical marker of incipient AD (see below for further evidence).

MRI-DERIVED ENTORHINAL CORTEX VOLUME IDENTIFIES THOSE AT RISK FOR ALZHEIMER'S DISEASE

Our findings thus far indicate that both hippocampal and entorhinal atrophy can be detected in very mild AD cases. Having sensitive *in vivo* anatomical markers of mild AD is important, but of greater interest is whether such markers can be developed for incipient AD. The present study was carried out to address this question and to evaluate whether entorhinal and hippocampal volumes derived from high-resolution MRI scans could differentiate those at risk for developing AD.

The participants in this study consisted of the 28 elderly patients described above who presented at the Rush Alzheimer's Disease Center with cognitive complaints; they were evaluated, but did not meet criteria for dementia. All 28 patients were scanned with our high-resolution protocol at the time of their first evaluation.

Follow-up clinical evaluations available on 23 of the 28 patients initially scanned indicated that 12 of the 23 had converted and received a diagnosis of probable AD. The follow-up period varied from 12–77 months (mean, 39 months) and was equivalent for converters and nonconverters [t(21) = 0.63, p >0.05]. The converters differed significantly from nonconverters in total (right + left) EC volume [t(21) = 2.94, p <0.008], but not hippocampal volume (see FIG. 4).

Furthermore, in logistic regressions using total hippocampal and entorhinal volume as predictors, only EC volume was found to be a significant predictor of the likelihood of conversion (odds ratio = 0.993 per normalized unit volume, p = 0.046). Thus, for every 10-unit decrease in EC volume, the chances of converting to AD increased by 7%. Results were not changed by adjustment for age or follow-up interval. When entorhinal volume alone was used as a predictor, 83.3% of converters, and 72.7% of nonconverters were correctly classified. These *in vivo* results underscore the early involvement of the EC in AD and provide a sensitive anatomical marker for incipient AD.

DIFFERENTIAL ROLES OF THE ENTORHINAL CORTEX AND HIPPOCAMPAL FORMATION IN HUMAN MEMORY FUNCTION

Evidence indicating the involvement of the entorhinal and perirhinal cortices in memory function in animals is accumulating (see chapter by Suzuki and Eichenbaum, this volume). However, the contribution of these cortical regions to human memory is not clear, partly due to the fact that imaging protocols for defining and measuring these regions *in vivo* were developed only recently.[4,17,21] In this study, we investigated the differential contribution of the HF and EC to human memory by examining the relationship between the extent of entorhinal and hippocampal atrophy and performance in the "controlled learning" task developed by Buschke and Grober.[7,18] These authors have argued that it may be difficult to distinguish between "apparent" and "genuine" memory deficits in elderly individuals because they may have impaired attention or may use inefficient strategies in acquiring information. By controlling the type of processing carried out, they were able to identify "genuine" memory deficits in aged subjects and in patients in the early stages of AD. Other laboratories have also reported on the utility of the task for differentiating mild AD cases from controls.[35]

Lesion and imaging experiments have demonstrated that in humans who are left-hemisphere dominant for language, generally the left HF is involved in verbal information processing, whereas the right processes nonverbal or spatial information.[1,24,30,37] Using the "controlled learning" task, we recently reported that in mild AD cases, left hippocampal volume is the best predictor of verbal recall,[12] a finding in agreement with the lesion and functional imaging results.

The subjects in this study were 13 elderly individuals who were evaluated at the Rush Alzheimer's Disease Center for cognitive complaints, but who did not meet criteria for dementia (see above). They were studied with our high-resolution MRI protocol and the Buschke controlled learning task.

For the Buschke task, participants were asked to learn a list of 16 items presented four at a time. Items were shown as line drawings, one picture in each quadrant of a large card (see FIG. 5 for an example). The pictures were from different, easily rec-

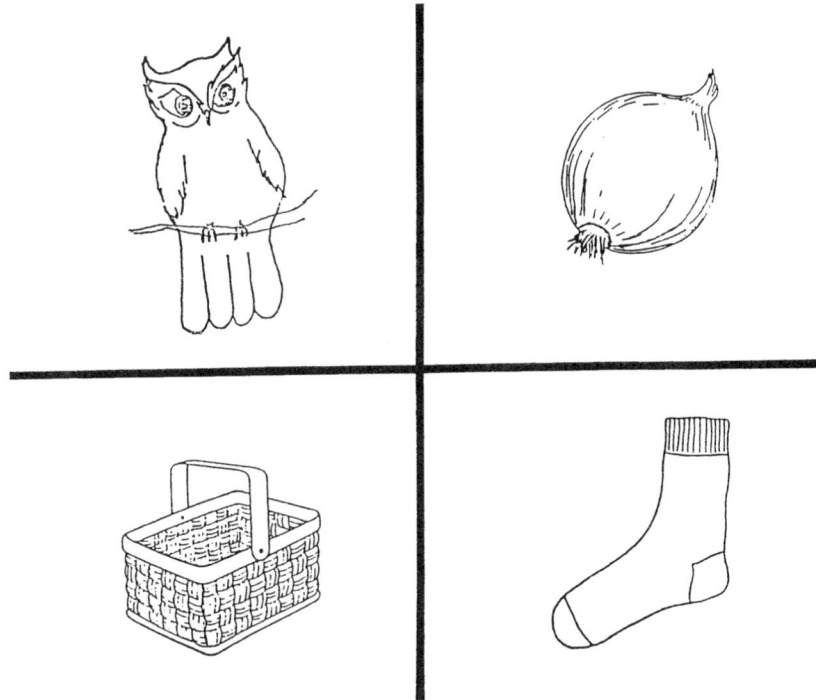

FIGURE 5. An example of four items from the Buschke controlled learning task that subjects had to learn and remember.

ognizable, semantic categories. When the experimenter gave a category cue verbally (e.g., bird), the subject had to search the display, point to and name the object from the category (e.g., owl). After this procedure was completed for all four items, immediate cued recall of the four items was tested by presenting each category cue to the subject. If she or he failed to recall an item in response to its cue, the item was shown again, the search performed, and so on, until immediate cued recall was correct for all four items. Then, the next set of items was presented as described above until all 16 items were identified and retrieved correctly during immediate cued recall. The search and naming procedure ensured that all individuals were using the same strategy in processing information, while immediate cued recall of each item ensured that it had been correctly encoded.

The search phase was followed by three trials of free recall, each trial being preceded by 20 seconds of interference. On each such trial, subjects were allowed a maximum of 2 minutes to name as many of the previously memorized items as they could. Next, a category cue was provided by the examiner for each item missed on that trial. If the subject still failed to recall the item with the cue, the examiner reminded the participant of the missed item which he or she then repeated. An additional trial of free recall was administered 45–60 minutes later to examine delayed recall. Recall following a delay has been demonstrated to be sensitive to hippocam-

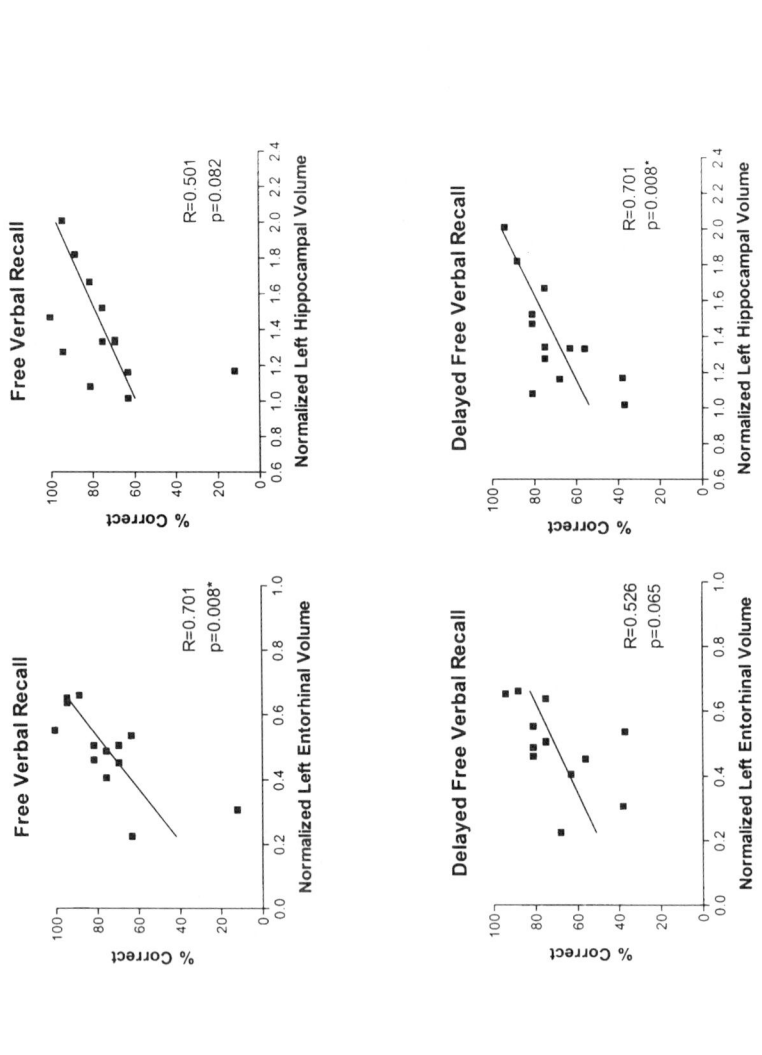

FIGURE 6. The relation between normalized left entorhinal (*left side*) or left hippocampal (*right side*) volume and the recall of verbal informa-tion. The asterisks indicate significant relations.

pal dysfunction[32,38] and to be one of the best discriminators of very mild AD cases.[2,3,40] Scoring consisted of the percentage of correctly recalled items. Data reported here are based on scores for the *third* trial of free recall and for delayed free recall.

The relationship between normalized entorhinal or hippocampal volume and the recall of verbal information was examined using linear regression analyses. The results, which are shown in FIGURE 6, demonstrated the following double dissociation. Left EC volume was significantly related to free verbal recall immediately following the third trial of acquisition ($R = 0.701$, $p = 0.008$), but not delayed recall ($R = 0.501$, $p = 0.082$). In contrast, left hippocampal volume was more strongly associated with delayed recall $R = 0.701$, $p = 0.008$), compared to immediate free recall following the third trial ($R = 0.526$, $p = 0.065$). Essentially the same pattern was observed when total entorhinal or hippocampal volume was considered in that there was a stronger association between immediate recall and entorhinal volume than delayed recall, whereas the opposite held true for the hippocampus.

These preliminary findings suggest that both the EC and HF play an important role in memory function in humans, but their respective contribution seems to be temporally different. Our results showing that atrophy of the EC is more strongly associated with performance at short delays following acquisition are similar to those reported by Hampson *et al.*[19] in rats. Using a delayed matching and nonmatching to sample task, these authors demonstrated that animals with selective ibotenate lesions limited to the hippocampus performed poorly at long delays, but not short ones. However, when lesions encroached on the entorhinal cortex in addition to involving the hippocampus, performance deficits were observed at short and long delays. Our results are also in agreement with a recent report[14] demonstrating temporal differences in the activation of the human rhinal cortex and hippocampus in memory formation.

In summary, data described in this paper demonstrate that, in addition to the hippocampal formation, the entorhinal cortex can be easily and reliably quantified *in vivo* from high-resolution structural images. Although both entorhinal and hippocampal atrophy occur early in the course of AD, the extent of entorhinal atrophy seems to provide a better anatomical marker for identifying those at risk for developing AD.

ACKNOWLEDGMENT

This work was supported by grants P01 AG09466 and P30 AG10161 from the National Institute on Aging, National Institutes of Health.

REFERENCES

1. ABRAHAMS, S., A. PICKERING, C.E. POLKEY & R.G. MORRIS. 1997. Spatial memory deficits in patients with unilateral damage to the right hippocampal formation. Neuropsychologia **35:** 11–24.
2. ALBERT, M.S. 1997. Cognitive and neurobiological markers of early Alzheimer's disease. Proc. Natl. Acad. Sci. USA **93:** 13547–13551.
3. ALBERT, M.S. 1998. Normal and abnormal memory: Aging and Alzheimer's disease. *In* Handbook on the Aging Brain. E. Wang & D.S. Snyder, Eds.: 1–17. Academic Press. San Diego, CA.

4. BOBINSKI, M., M. J. DE LEON, A. CONVIT, S. DE SANTI, J. WEGIEL, C.Y. TARSHISH, L.A.S. LOUIS & H. M. WISNIEWSKI. 1999. MRI of entorhinal cortex in mild Alzheimer's disease. Lancet **353:** 38–40.
5. BRAAK, H. & E. BRAAK. 1991. Neuropathological staging of Alzheimer-related changes. Acta Neuropathol. **82:** 239–259.
6. BRAAK, H. & E. BRAAK. 1995. Staging of Alzheimer's disease-related neurofibrillary changes. Neurobiol. Aging **16:** 271–288.
7. BUSCHKE, H. & E. GROBER. 1986. Genuine memory deficits in age-associated memory impairment. Dev. Neuropsychol. **2:** 287–307.
8. DE LEON, M.J., A. CONVIT, A.E. GEORGE, J. GOLOMB, S. DE SANTI, C. TARSHISH, H. RUSINEK, M. BOBINSKI, C. INCE & D. MILLER. 1996. *In vivo* structural studies of the hippocampus in normal aging and in incipient Alzheimer's disease. Ann. N.Y. Acad. Sci. **777:** 1–13.
9. DE LEON, M.J., A.E. GEORGE, J. GOLOMB, C. TARSHISH, A. CONVIT, A. KLUGER, S. DE SANTI, T. MCRAE, S.H. FERRIS, B. REISBERG, C. INCE, H. RUSINEK, M. BOBINSKI, B. QUINN, D.C. MILLER, & H.M. WISNIEWSKI. 1997. Frequency of hippocampal formation atrophy in normal aging and Alzheimer's disease. Neurobiol. Aging **18:** 1–11.
10. DETOLEDO-MORRELL, L., M.P. SULLIVAN, F. MORRELL, C. SPANOVIC & S. SPENCER. 1995. Gender differences in the vulnerability of the hippocampal formation during aging. Soc. Neurosci. Abstr. **21:** 1708.
11. DETOLEDO-MORRELL, L., M.P. SULLIVAN, F. MORRELL, R.S. WILSON, D.A. BENNETT & S. SPENCER. 1997. Alzheimer's disease: *In vivo* detection of differential vulnerability of brain regions. Neurobiol. Aging **18:** 463–468.
12. DETOLEDO-MORRELL, L., B. DICKERSON, M.P. SULLIVAN, C. SPANOVIC, R.S. WILSON & D.A. BENNETT. 2000. Hemispheric diffferences in hippocampal volume predict verbal and spatial memory performance in patients with Alzheimer's disease. Hippocampus **10:** 136–142.
13. DICKERSON, B.C., I. GONCHAROVA, R.S. SULLIVAN, C. FORCHETTI, R.S. WILSON, D.A. BENNETT, L. BECKETT & L. DETOLEDO-MORRELL. 2000. Entorhinal and hippocampal atrophy in patients with very mild Alzheimer's disease. Submitted.
14. FERNÁNDEZ, G., A. EFFERN, T. GRUNWALD, N. PEZER, K. LEHNERTZ, M. DÜMPLEMANN, D. VAN ROOST & C.E. ELGER. 1999. Real-time tracking of memory formation in the human rhinal cortex and hippocampus. Science **285:** 1582–1585.
15. FOLSTEIN, M.F., S.E. FOLSTEIN & P.R. MCHUGH. 1975. Mini-mental state: a practical method for grading the mental status of patients for the clinician. J. Psychiatr. Res. **12:** 189–198.
16. GOLOMB, J., M.J. DE LEON, A. KLUGER, A.E. GEORGE, C. TARSHISH & S.H. FERRIS. 1993. Hippocampal atrophy in normal aging: an association with recent memory impairment. Arch. Neurol. **50:** 967–973.
17. GONCHAROVA, I.I., B.C. DICKERSON & L. DETOLEDO-MORRELL. 2000. MRI of human entorhinal cortex: a reliable protocol for volumetric measurement. Submitted.
18. GROBER, E. & H. BUSCHKE. 1987. Genuine memory deficits in dementia. Dev. Neuropsychol. **3:** 13–36.
19. HAMPSON, R.E., L.E. JARRARD & S.A. DEADWYLER. 1999. Effects of ibotinate hippocampal destruction on delayed matching and nonmatching to sample behavior in rats. J. Neurosci. **19:** 1492–1507.
20. HYMAN, B.T., G.W. VAN HOESEN, A.R. DAMASIO & C.L. BARNES. 1984. Alzheimer's disease: cell specific pathology isolated the hippocampal formation. 1984. Science **222:** 1168–1170.
21. INSAUSTI, R., K. JUOTTONEN, H. SOININEN, A.M. INSAUSTI, K. PARTANEN, P. VAINIO, M. LAAKSO & A. PITKANEN. 1998. MR volumertric analysis of human entorhinal, perirhinal, and temporopolar cortices. Am. J. Neuroradiol. **19:** 659–671.
22. JACK, C.R., R.C. PETERSEN, P.C. O'BRIAN & E.G. TANGALOS. 1992. MR-based hippocampal volumetry in the diagnosis of Alzheimer's disease. Neurology **42:** 183–188.
23. JACK, C.R., R.C. PETERSEN, Y.C. XU, S.C. WARING, P.C. O'BRIEN, E.G. TANGALOS, G.E. SMITH, R.J. IVNIK & E. KOKMEN. 1997. Medial temporal atrophy on MRI in normal aging and very mild Alzheimer's disease. Neurology **49:** 786–794.

24. JONES-GOTMAN, M. 1986. Right hippocampal excision impairs learning and recall of a list of abstract designs. Neuropsychologia **24:** 659–670.
25. JUOTTONEN, K., M.P. LAAKSO, R. INSAUSTI, M. LEHTOVIRTA, A. PITKANEN, K. PARTANEN & H. SOININEN. 1998. Volumes of the entorhinal and perirhinal cortices in Alzheimer's disease. Neurobiol. Aging **19:** 15–22.
26. JUOTTONEN, K., M.P. LAAKSO, K. PARTANEN & H. SOININEN. 1999. Comparative MR analysis of the entorhinal cortex and hippocampus in diagnosing Alzheimer's disease. Am. J. Neuroradiol. **20:** 139–144.
27. KESSLAK, J.P., O. NALCIOGLU & C.W. COTMAN. 1991. Quantification of magnetic scans for hippocampal and parahippocampal atrophy in Alzheimer's disease. Neurology **41:** 51–54.
28. KILLIANY, R.J., B.M. MOSS, M.S. ALBERT, T. SANDOR, J. TIEMAN & F. JOLESZ. 1993. Temporal lobe regions on magnetic resonance imaging identify patients with early Alzheimer's disease. Arch. Neurol. **50:** 949–954.
29. LAAKSO, M.P., H. SOININEN, K. PARTANEN, M. LEHTOVIRTA, M. HALLIKAINEN, T. HANNINEN, E.L. HELKALA, P. VAINIO & P.J. RIEKKINEN. 1998. MRI of the hippocampus in Alzheimer's disease: sensitivity, specificity and analysis of the incorrectly classified subjects. Neurobiol. Aging **19:** 23–31.
30. MAGUIRE, E.A., R.S.J. FRAKOWIAK & C.D. FRITH. 1997. Recalling routes around London: activation of the right hippocampus in taxi drivers. J. Neurosci. **17:** 7103–7110.
31. MCKHANN, G., D. DRACHMAN, M. FOLSTEIN, R. KATZMAN, D. PRICE & E.M. STADLAN. 1984. Clinical diagnosis of Alzheimer's disease: report of the NINDS/ADRDA work group under the auspices of Department of Health and Human Services Task Force on Alzheimer's disease. Neurology **34:** 939–944.
32. MILLER, L.A., D.G. MUNOZ & M. FINMORE. 1993. Hippocampal sclerosis and human memory. Arch. Neurol. **50:** 391–394.
33. MORRIS, C.J., A. HEYMAN, R.C. MOHS, J.P. HUGHES, G. VAN BELLE, G. FILLENBAUM, E.D. MELLITS, C. CLARK & THE CERAD INVESTIGATORS. 1989. The Consortium to Establish a Registry for Alzheimer's Disease (CERAD). Part I. Clinical and neuropsychological assessment of Alzheimer's disease. Neurology **39:** 1159–1165.
34. MUFSON, E.J., E.Y. CHIN, E.J. COCHRAN, L.A. BECKETT, D.A. BENNETT & J.H. KORDOWER. 1999. Entorhinal cortex beta-amyloid load in individuals with mild cognitive impairment. Exp. Neurol. **158:** 469–490.
35. PETERSEN, R.C., G.E. SMITH, R.J. IVNIK, E. KOKMEN. & E.G. TANGALOS. 1994. Memory function in very early Alzheimer's disease. Neurology **44:** 867–872.
36. SEAB, J.P., W.J. JAGUST, S.T. WONG, M.S. ROOS, B.R. REED & T.F. BUDINGER. 1988. Quantitative NMR measurements of hippocampal atrophy in Alzheimer's disease. Magn. Reson. Med. **8:** 200–208.
37. SMITH, M.L. & B. MILNER. 1981. The role of the right hippocampus in the recall of spatial location. Neuropsychologia **19:** 781–793.
38. SQUIRE, L.R. & S. ZOLA-MORGAN. 1991. The medial temporal lobe memory system. Science **253:** 1380–1386.
39. VAN HOESEN, G.W., B.T. HYMAN & A.R. DAMASIO. 1991. Entorhinal cortex pathology in Alzheimer's disease. Hippocampus **1:** 1–8.
40. WELSH, K., N. BUTTERS, J.P. HUGHES, R.C. MOHS & A. HEYMAN. 1991. Detection of abnormal memory decline in mild cases of Alzheimer's disease using CERAD neuropsychological measures. Arch. Neurol. **48:** 278–281.
41. WILSON, R.S., M.P. SULLIVAN, L. DETOLEDO-MORRELL, G.T. STEBBINS, D.A. BENNETT & F. MORRELL. 1996. Association of memory and cognition in Alzheimer's disease with volumetric estimates of temporal lobe structures. Neuropsychology **10:** 459–463.

The Parahippocampal Gyrus in Alzheimer's Disease

Clinical and Preclinical Neuroanatomical Correlates

GARY W. VAN HOESEN,[a] JEAN C. AUGUSTINACK, JASON DIERKING,
SARAH J. REDMAN, AND RAMASAMY THANGAVEL

*Departments of Anatomy and Cell Biology, and Neurology, The University of Iowa,
Iowa City, Iowa 52242, USA*

ABSTRACT: The human parahippocampal gyrus forms a large part of the limbic lobe along the ventromedial part of the temporal cortical mantle. It is a variable and complicated cortex in terms of structure, and the latter is aggravated further by interfaces with the anterior insula anteriorly and the cingulate gyrus and occipital lobe posteriorly. Additional complications relate to its lateral border with the temporal cortex and especially the sulcal configurations that define this junction. The rhinal sulcus, which separates parahippocampal and temporal cortices in other species, including the anthropoid apes, is either lacking or rudimentary in the human brain. Thus, defining this junction requires cytoarchitectural examination and precludes the use of mere inspection of sulcal existing patterns. The cortical areas that form the parahippocampal gyrus are vulnerable to pathological changes in Alzheimer's disease (AD), and its entorhinal and perirhinal subdivisions are both the most heavily damaged cortical areas and the focus for disease onset. The neurons that acquire neurofibrillary tangles (NFTs) occupy the junction of the isocortical mantle with the limbic cortical mantle, but share, or partially share, a vulnerability phenotype with large neurons in both domains. The differential expression of this phenotype across time creates the false impression of NFT spread in cross-sectional comparisons of AD brains. The questions of what this phenotype is and why it is expressed first in the perirhinal and entorhinal cortices of the parahippocampal gyrus are the central molecular biological/neuroanatomical questions in understanding the etiology of AD.

INTRODUCTION

The human parahippocampal gyrus is an expansive area of cortex that forms the ventral portion of the limbic lobe, or that component of the limbic annulus between the retrosplenial part of the cingulate gyrus and the anterior insular cortex (FIG. 1). In addition to its expansiveness, the parahippocampal gyrus is also a highly diverse part of the cortical mantle formed by unique fields of allocortex, periallocortex, proisocortex, and isocortex.[1,17,25,38,41,56,65,66] Olfaction and some forms of memory are the most clear-cut functional attributes of the parahippocampal gyrus,[61] although

[a]Address for correspondence: Dr. Gary W. Van Hoesen, Department of Anatomy and Cell Biology, The University of Iowa, Iowa City, IA 52242. Tel.: (319) 335-7741; fax: (319) 335-7198.
e-mail: gary-van-hoesen@uiowa.edu

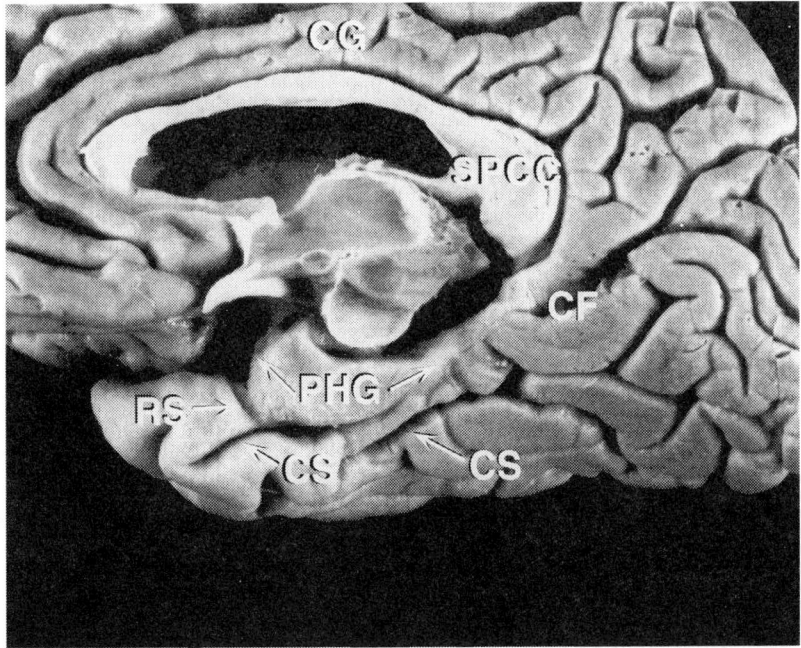

FIGURE 1. Photograph of the medial surface of the human brain, showing the cingulate gyrus (CG) and the parahippocampal gyrus (PHG), the two major components of the limbic lobe. Note the continuity of the cortex around the splenium of the corpus callosum (SPCC) and the manner in which the calcarine fissure (CF) notches it. The collateral (CS) and rhinal (RS) sulci form the lateral border of the PHG.

many of its constituent areas and neural systems are uninvestigated in functional terms. Indeed, abnormalities in the parahippocampal gyrus have been noted in many neurological and psychiatric illnesses, ranging from schizophrenia[4,6,7,8,14,26,43] to temporal lobe epilepsy,[12,23,24] and while memory and/or olfactory dysfunction may be present clinically, other behavioral changes can be equally manifest.[67,68]

Our aim is to focus on only one of these illnesses, namely, Alzheimer's disease (AD), where parahippocampal pathology is extensive, but neuroanatomically selective. Additionally, we consider only the largely non-olfactory parts of the parahippocampal gyrus and do not include the primary olfactory cortex and the cortical nuclei of the amygdala. These areas are damaged in AD, but their treatment here expands this effort beyond its required scope.

HUMAN PARAHIPPOCAMPAL TOPOGRAPHY

General Subdivisions

The anterior and anteromedial parts of the human parahippocampal gyrus are formed by allocortical areas that constitute the primary olfactory cortex and those parts of the amygdala that have a pial surface and a molecular layer. Immediately posterior and ventral to these, the parahippocampal gyrus is dominated by the expansive entorhinal periallocortex, the largest of its cortical fields. The lateral cortical areas of the parahippocampal gyrus are formed by two belts of perirhinal cortex, the medialmost being periallocortex and the lateralmost proisocortex. The former lacks a granular layer IV, whereas the latter has variable granularity in this layer often characterized as incipient. The medialmost cortex of the parahippocampal gyrus is formed by two periallocortical areas known, respectively, as the parasubiculum and presubiculum. These occur along the posterior two thirds of the parahippocampal gyrus, posterior to the amygdala and in alignment with the hippocampal fissure. The posterior cortex of the parahippocampal gyrus, known as the ectorhinal cortex, is isocortical, having well differentiated layers including a granular layer IV.[1,17,25,38,41,56,65,66] This cortex posteriorly abuts the ventral association cortices of the occipital lobe, whereas anteriorly and laterally it deviates away from the parahippocampal gyrus and becomes incorporated into the inferior temporal gyrus (FIG. 2). Brodmann assigned numbers 51 to the olfactory and periamygdaloid cortices, 28 and 34 to the entorhinal cortex, 35 to the perirhinal cortex, 49 to the parasubiculum, 27 to the presubiculum, and 36 to the ectorhinal cortex, respectively (FIG. 3).

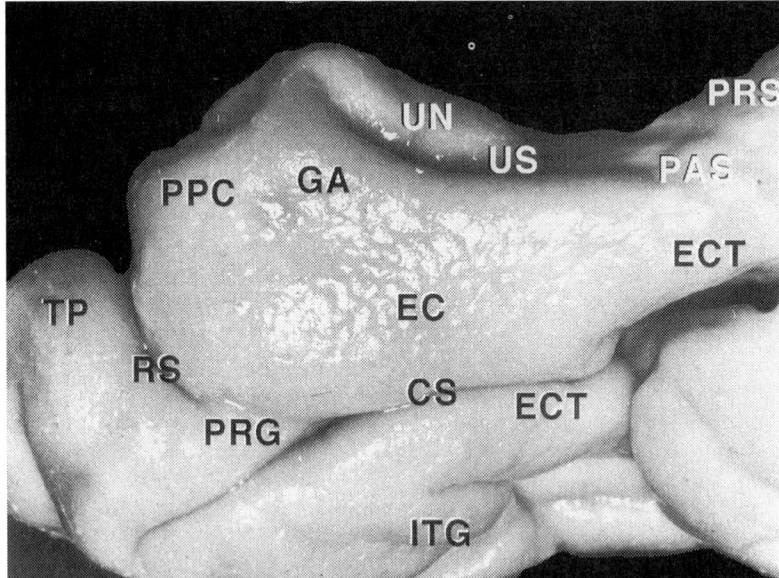

FIGURE 2. Photograph of the human parahippocampal gyrus, inferior temporal gyrus (ITG), and temporal pole (TP) showing the approximate location of cortical fields and other landmarks. CS, collateral sulcus; EC, entorhinal cortex; ECT, ectorhinal cortex; GA, gyrus ambiens; PAS, parasubiculum; PPC, prepyriform or primary olfactory cortex; PRS, presubiculum; RS, rhinal sulcus; UN, uncus; and US, uncal sulcus. Note the location of the perirhinal gyrus (PRG) marking the point at which the perirhinal cortex moves from a position lateral to the rhinal sulcus into the collateral sulcus.

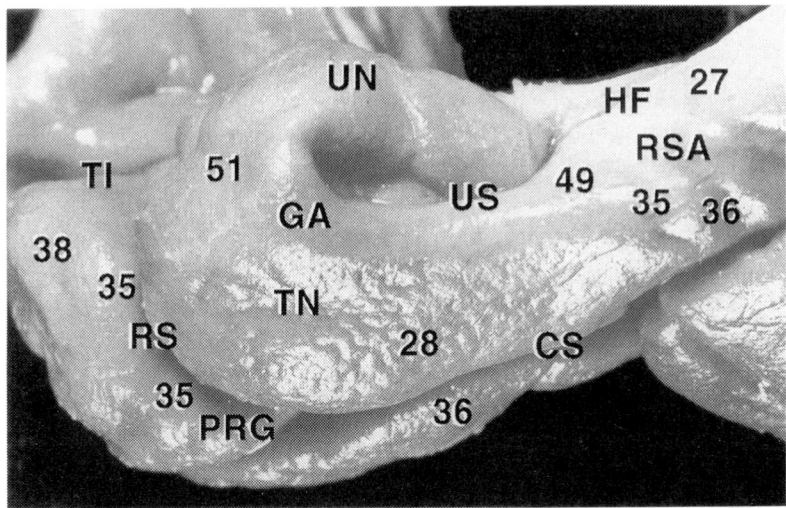

FIGURE 3. Photograph of the human parahippocampal gyrus showing the approximate location of Brodmann's cortical fields (see text) and other key landmarks. Note the unusual texture of the cortex above and below the tentorial notch (TN) that demarcates the location of the entorhinal cortex. Note also the shiny white appearance of the parahippocampal gyrus posteriorly caused by myelinated axons that form the reticular substance of Arnold (RSA). Finally, as in FIGURE 2, note the location of the perirhinal gyrus (PRG) where Brodmann's area 35, the perirhinal cortex, moves from a position lateral to the rhinal sulcus (RS) into the collateral sulcus (CS). Other abbreviations: GA, gyrus ambiens; HF, hippocampal fissure; TI, temporal incisura; UN, uncus; and US, uncal sulcus.

Sulcal Boundaries of the Parahippocampal Gyrus

The sulcal patterns that help to delimit the parahippocampal gyrus are a combination of invariant and variant enfoldings of the cortex that can cause substantial confusion in identification. Anteriorly, the temporal incisura formed by the abutment of the frontal and temporal lobes with the insula is an invariant landmark from brain to brain and a good approximation for anteriormost parahippocampal cortices (FIG. 3). The equally invariant hippocampal fissure is a consistent medial landmark, with the parasubiculum lying immediately ventral to it on its exposed lip and the presubiculum on its lower bank (FIG. 3). Posterior sulcal landmarks are seldom present in the human brain, but the point at which the anterior part of the calcarine fissure cuts the parahippocampal gyrus approximates the point at which medial temporal areas give way to cortical areas belonging to the occipital lobe.[25,56] This also approximates the point where medial posterior parahippocampal areas dovetail, with the presubiculum sweeping dorsally to join the retrosplenial cortex, as it does in other non-human primates,[11] and the parasubiculum, along with the prostriate cortex, forming the cortex that occupies the mouth of calcarine fissure anterior to the primary visual cortex.[33,50]

The lateral margin of the parahippocampal gyrus is defined by the often variant collateral and rhinal fissures. In some specimens, identifying these is not problematic, with the former forming a long deep sulcus whose anteriormost tip deviates laterally as the temporal pole is approximated (FIGS. 2 and 3). In other specimens the anterior one third of the collateral fissure may be separated from its posterior stem (FIG. 1). Still in others, the collateral fissure appears to join the rhinal fissure. In the absence of cytoarchitectural study, it is critical to consider three relationships when defining the lateral border of the parahippocampal gyrus in the human brain. First is a reminder from classical neuroanatomy that the rhinal fissure separates the "olfactory brain" from the "non-olfactory brain." In its absence, which is the case in over 50% of human brains, the perirhinal cortex intervenes at this juncture and always demarcates the lateral boundary of the parahippocampal gyrus.[1,38,56,66] Secondly, the perirhinal cortex continues posteriorly into the collateral sulcus, whether a rhinal sulcus is present or not. When a rhinal sulcus is present, the perirhinal cortex is located in its fundus and lateral bank, as is the case for nonhuman primates and all other mammals. Thirdly, when the rhinal sulcus is present and ends, a small, but conspicuous, perirhinal gyrus can be seen in many brains marking the point where perirhinal cortex moves from a position lateral to the rhinal sulcus to a position into the collateral fissure (FIGS. 2 and 3). Microscopic cytoarchitectural study confirms these relationships, making it unnecessary to use guesswork and label what is collateral fissure as rhinal fissure, a practice that was started by Retzius[54] over a century ago and continues in modern times.[29,51] The key point is that perirhinal cortex forms the lateral margin of the parahippocampal gyrus, separating both the olfactory and the entorhinal cortex from the temporal neocortex. Sometimes it is associated with a rhinal sulcus or groove and located in its fundus and lateral bank. When a rhinal sulcus is absent, the perirhinal cortex simply aligns itself with the collateral sulcus and continues posteriorly. Its position in the collateral fissure can vary from brain to brain, but typically, its location favors the medial bank and fundus (FIG. 8). However, if the collateral sulcus is shallow, the perirhinal cortex may occupy parts of both its medial and lateral banks (FIG. 9). Whichever, it maintains its anatomical position of separating olfactory and entorhinal cortex from temporal isocortex.

Lastly, some authors label a small groove in the entorhinal cortex, found in approximately 70% of human brains, the inferior rhinal sulcus or intrarhinal sulcus.[1,41,54] As pointed out by ourselves and others, this is not a sulcus, but merely the point where the free edge of the tentorium cerebelli contacts and grooves the entorhinal cortex before its attachment to the clinoid process. The bulge of cortex medial to it corresponds roughly to Brodmann's area 34 and the gyrus ambiens (FIG. 2), and it lies in the tentorial aperture unprotected by dura. Uncal notch[25] or tentorial notch[66–68] are more appropriate names for this indentation (FIG. 3). Although this may seem like anatomical minutia, it is important to realize that the entorhinal cortex that forms the gyrus ambiens leads all degrees of uncal herniation into the space of Bichat due to increased intracranial pressure in the supratentorial space. And likewise, in head trauma, it is the entorhinal cortex of the parahippocampal gyrus that is forced onto and damaged by the free edge of the tentorium cerebelli.[67,68] This has important implications for the memory impairment observed clinically that nearly always accompanies these forms of injury.

Unique Surface Features of the Human Parahippocampal Gyrus

While it is unusual to draw attention to the usually homogeneous surface of the cortical gray matter, except in pathological conditions, the human parahippocampal gyrus is unique in the gross brain and deserves special mention. For example, the anterior parts of the gyrus, at levels coincident with the entorhinal cortex, have a corrugated appearance with distinct elevations or bumps visible to the naked eye (FIGS. 2 and 3). Retzius[54] commented on the resemblance of this phenomenon to the skin of certain amphibians and named the elevations verrucae. As implied by this name, the verrucae resemble certain viral skin diseases characterized by mosaic-like non-erupted epidermal elevations. Klingler[47] illustrated the verrucae of the entorhinal cortex in a dramatic and detailed illustration of the parahippocampal gyrus that summarized many of Retzius' classic observations. The entorhinal verrucae mark the location of the islands or nests of large multipolar and pyramidal neurons that form its layer II. These islands are cytochrome oxidase[30] and parvalbumin rich[49,58,60] and give rise to the entorhinodentate part of the perforant pathway. As described later, neurons that form the verrucae are ravaged by neurofibrillary tangles in AD.

Another conspicuous feature of the parahippocampal gyrus in both the fixed and the unfixed brain is its unusually white and shiny appearance (FIGS. 2 and 3). This was first described by Arnold[3] in 1851, and its matrix-like organization was illustrated by Reichert[53] in 1859 (FIG. 4). It is a prominent feature in myelin-stained cross-sections of the parahippocampal gyrus that ends abruptly at the junction of the perirhinal cortex with the temporal isocortex anteriorly, and at the junction of the presubiculum with the occipitotemporal isocortices posteriorly. Intermeshed and reticulated axons literally pack layer I and the superficial parts of layer II, contribut-

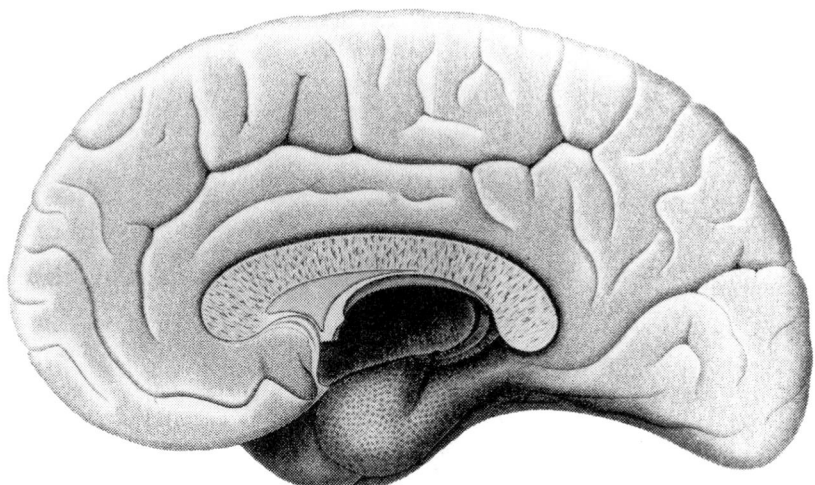

FIGURE 4. Reichert's[53] depiction of the medial surface of the human brain from his classic embryological study. Note the texturing he used on the parahippocampal gyrus and uncus. He refers to Arnold's reticular substance in his text but uses the general term "matrix" in the legend for this figure. In this sense, it is difficult to know exactly what he was illustrating, but it could have been a combination of the reticular white appearance of the parahippocampal gyrus, the verrucae of the entorhinal cortex, and possibly, even the mosaic-like pigmentation seen occasionally in the cortex of the ventromedial temporal area.

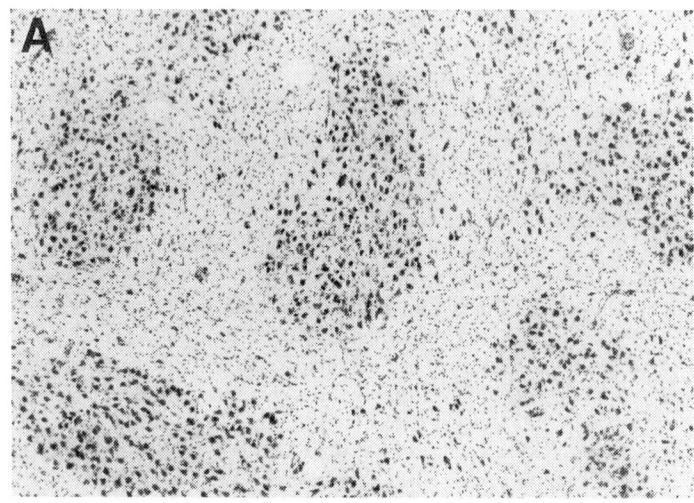

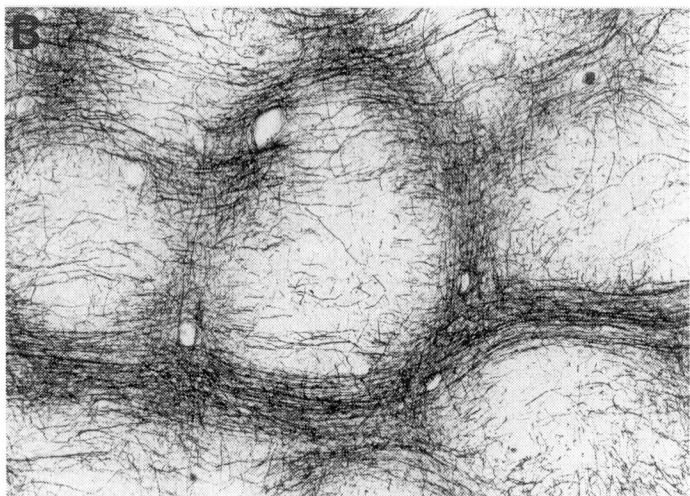

FIGURE 5. (**A**) Photomicrograph of a tangential section through entorhinal cortex layer II of the human brain stained for Nissl substance with cresyl violet. Note the islands of large neurons that correspond to the location of verrucae in the gross brain. (**B**) Photomicrograph of the adjacent section shown in **A**, stained for axons using the Gallyas method. Note the complex matrix of axons that surround the cell islands and its reticular appearance. Note also the satellite arterioles that position themselves in the surrounding fibers. These never penetrate a cell island, but give rise to a dense meshwork of capillaries that invade the cell island.

ing to the white appearance. Appropriately, this feature is named the reticular substance of Arnold. In general, it is most conspicuous posteriorly and medially where there is a dense myelin-stained axon plexus filling the superficial layers of the presubiculum. However, it is seen anteriorly in the entorhinal cortex as well, where the plexus surrounds the nests of layer II neurons that form the verrucae (FIG. 5A and 5B). Little has been learned about this unusual parahippocampal plexus in the century and a half since Arnold's description, but it is likely that it is formed, at least in part, by the massive convergence of cortical association axons to the entorhinal and presubicular cortices from other parts of the cortical mantle.[20,39,65,72,73] Overlapping axons from diverse sources and axonal branching patterns may account for its intermeshed and reticular appearance.

Parahippocampal Gyrus Nomenclature

Although used periodically in the early literature, the term or concept of parahippocampal gyrus is relatively new, sanctioned as an annotation at the Sixth International Congress of Anatomists in Paris and listed in *Nomina Anatomica*, 1955. It replaced the classical but confusing term hippocampal gyrus from the *Basle Nomina Anatomica* of 1895. Hippocampal gyrus left doubt as to whether one was referring to the hippocampal allocortex or to the cortical gyrus that lies medial to the inferior temporal gyrus on the ventral surface of the temporal lobe. If it were interpreted to mean hippocampus, it meant that the medialmost temporal gyrus had no name. If it meant the medialmost exposed temporal gyrus, which was the intent of early anatomists, it could be interpreted that there were two hippocampal gyri. Coining the term parahippocampal gyrus ameliorated the confusion and established this gyrus as the fifth temporal convolution, in line with the superior, middle, inferior, and occipitotemporal gyri, respectively. The rolled up allocortex in the inferior horn of the lateral ventricle became the hippocampal formation alone, or the true hippocampal gyrus.

Although the foregoing designation has been respected during the last five decades, some authors include periallocortical parts of the parahippocampal gyrus, such as the presubicular, parasubicular, and entorhinal cortices, in a broader hippocampal formation concept.[1,2,62,63] This is predicated on the rich anatomical interconnectivity of these structures among themselves and with the hippocampus and dentate gyrus, and it is a matter of preference. However, as more is learned about these cortical areas neuroanatomically, it is clear that they connect strongly with many parts of the cortex, and we favor no retreat from the views expressed in *Nomina Anatomica*, 1955. Indeed, the entorhinal cortex is a sizeable part of the parahippocampal area in all species. Including it along with the presubiculum and parasubiculum, as parts of the hippocampal formation, strips the parahippocampal gyrus concept of meaning.

PARAHIPPOCAMPAL GYRUS IN ALZHEIMER'S DISEASE

Entorhinal Cortex

Parahippocampal gyrus involvement in AD has been recognized for many years, but this forms a confusing history because of the terminology used or combinations of the terminology with different meanings. The general lack of neuroanatomical understanding of the parahippocampal gyrus also contributed to the difficulty of early neuropathologists. For example, the first mention of neurofibrillary tangles (NFTs) in the parahippocampal gyrus can be found in a footnote in a chapter by Bielschowsky[13] published in the *Handbuch der Mikroskopischen Anatomie des Menschen* in 1928. After describing the histopathological characteristics of NFTs, Bielschowsky states, "The islands of Cajal in the outer layer of the subiculum represent sites of predilection for these changes." It seems appropriate to infer that Bielschowsky was using a somewhat broad definition of the subiculum, and granting him to mean entorhinal cortex is very generous in neuroanatomical terms. However, Cajal described entorhinal cell islands in the human brain, and it is likely that Bielschowsky was describing them. Goodman[28] in 1953 had similar difficulties. For example, he states, "it will be seen that, while argentophilic plaques are scanty in the substantia reticulata of Arnoldi (in presubiculum), the nerve cells of this area exhibit a greater vulnerability to Alzheimer type neurofibrillary degeneration than those of any other area of the brain examined." As will be discussed, the presubiculum seldom contains substantial NFTs in AD, and as discussed earlier, the reticular substance of Arnold refers to white matter and not cortical gray matter. Nevertheless, despite these difficulties in terminology, one has to infer that Goodman "meant," or was referring to, the islands of neurons that form layer II of the entorhinal cortex. In fact, in his tables he uses the term "glomeruli substantia reticulata Arnoldi," and his photomicrographs show clearly NFT-affected entorhinal layer II neurons. Hirano and Zimmerman[31] in 1962 also refer to and illustrate what they term the "glomerular formations of the hippocampal gyrus" and, like Goodman, indicate that these neurons are the most vulnerable for NFTs in AD. They also note that the earliest changes in AD occur in these neurons, although throughout their report, they refer to them as pyramidal neurons. Hooper and Vogel[34] in 1976, using more modern terminology, also reported similar observations, but implied that NFTs had a uniform distribution in presubiculum, parasubiculum, and entorhinal cortex.

More contemporary investigations of the entorhinal cortex in AD confirm these earlier observations and inferences just reviewed.[5,9,15–18,27,35–37,69] Indeed, in the gross brain of endstage AD, the entorhinal cortex is typically visibly altered by a flattening and narrowing of the cortex and by discoloration. Associated with this is the disappearance of the verrucae (FIG. 6). Microscopic examination of the entorhinal cortex confirms the presence of pathology, with NFTs in nearly all layer II islands of neurons[15,27,36,59] (FIG. 7). Layer III of this cortex can be more variably affected, but in nearly every instance, when layer II contains heavy NFTs, at least the superficial parts of layer III contain them as well. The layer of large pyramids that forms layer IV, immediately deep to the lamina dessicans, is also heavily affected by NFTs at endstage. Like layer III, layers V and VI can be more variably affected in AD, but it is not unusual to see dense NFTs in these layers after a long duration of illness.

By any measure, the entorhinal cortex is devastated in AD, and all cell layers can be affected at endstage. In general, however, there is a laminar predilection that correlates with duration of illness, with layers II and III affected earlier than layer IV, and this layer affected earlier than layers V and VI. Mediolateral differences are commonly observed as well, with lateral areas affected earlier than medial areas. Histopathologically, the more lateral areas of entorhinal cortex contain NFTs in both

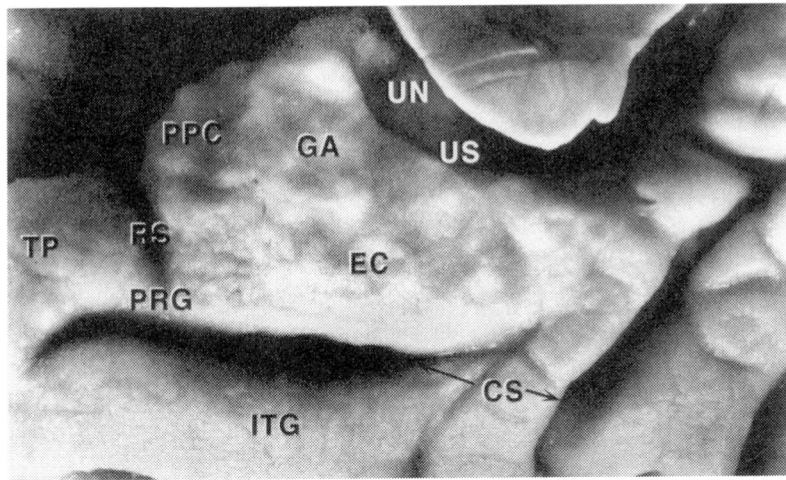

FIGURE 6. Photograph of the parahippocampal gyrus from a brain donor with endstage AD. Note the narrowing of the parahippocampal gyrus, its flat appearance, and the absence of entorhinal cortex (EC) verrucae. Other abbreviations are defined in FIGURES 2 and 3.

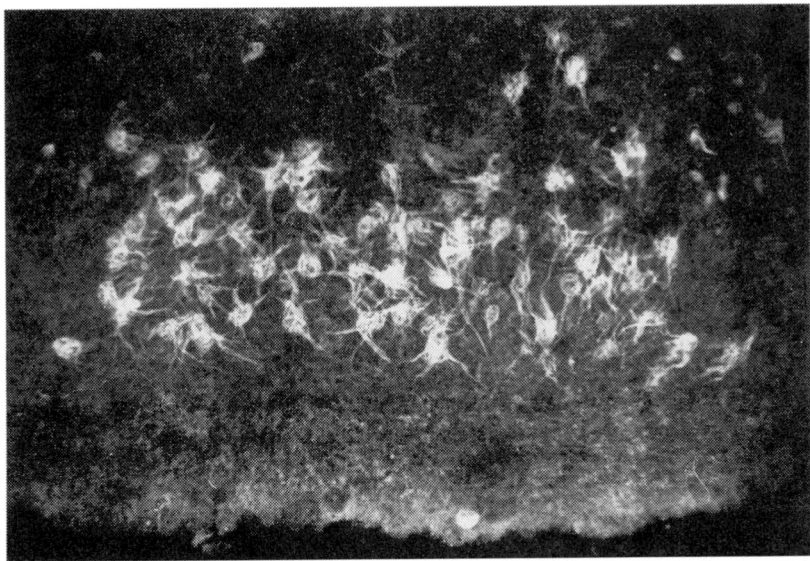

FIGURE 7. Photomicrograph of an entorhinal cortex layer II island of neurons in endstage AD stained with the fluorochrome Thioflavin S and photographed with mercury vapor illumination to reveal NFTs. Note the mixture of large stellate and pyramidal neurons with NFTs. Note also that the pial surface is flat, corresponding with the disappearance of the verrucae in the gross brain.

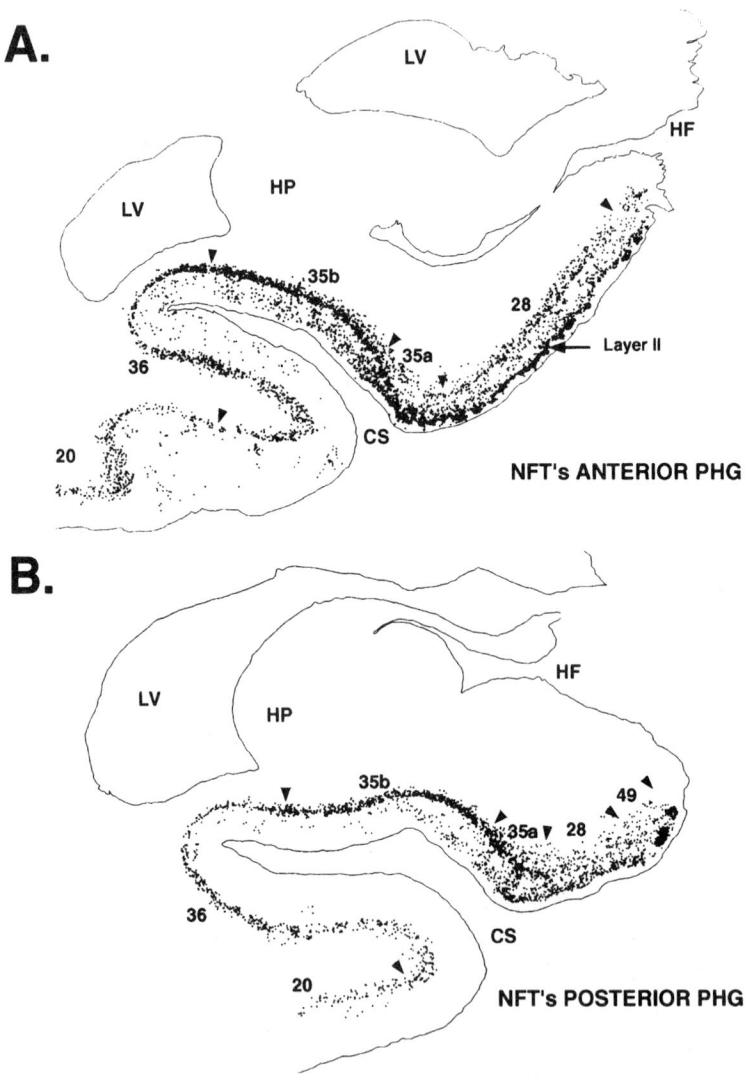

FIGURE 8A and B. Neurolucida chartings of the distribution of NFTs at two levels of the parahippocampal gyrus (PHG) in AD, showing the topography of cellular pathology in several parahippocampal subdivisions. Note in **A** the heavy involvement of area 28 layers II and IV and the deep parts of layer III in areas 35a and b in both anterior (**A**) and posterior (**B**) parts of the parahippocampal gyrus. Also note that in this brain, area 35 is confined to the medial bank of the deep collateral sulcus. Abbreviations: CS, collateral sulcus; HF, hippocampal fissure; HP, hippocampus; LV, inferior horn of lateral ventricle.

the classical multipolar stellate neurons and the medium and large pyramidal neurons that invade layer II from the laterally adjacent perirhinal and ectorhinal cortex.

Perirhinal Cortex

Brodmann's area 35, the perirhinal cortex, is a bipartite area composed of periallocortices medially, where it adjoins the olfactory and entorhinal cortex, and proisocortex laterally where it adjoins the temporal isocortex. As already discussed, it is the lateralmost part of the parahippocampal gyrus. Like Brodmann's area 28, the en-

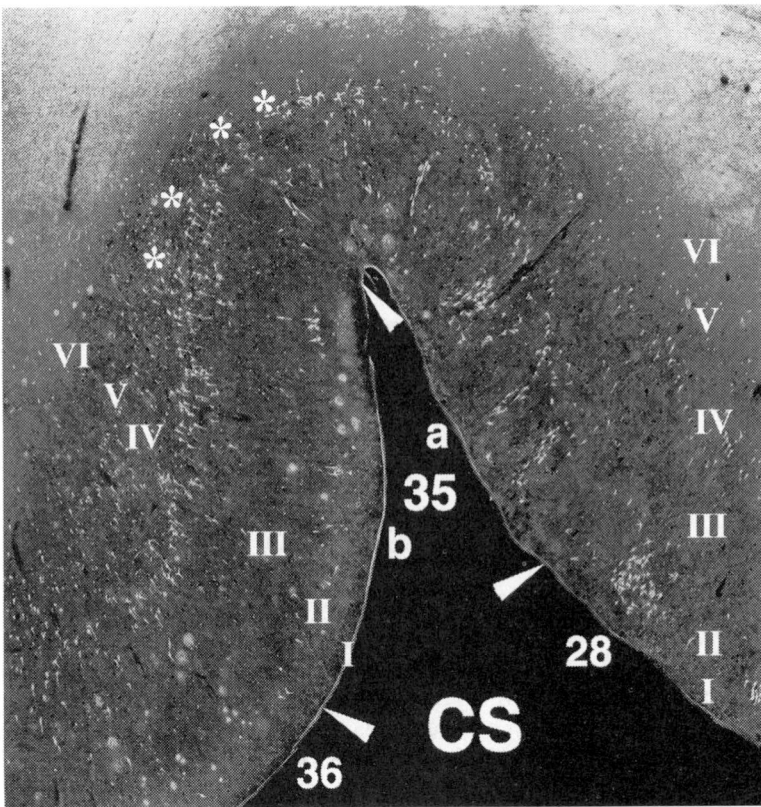

FIGURE 9. Photomontage of Thioflavin S stained NFTs in AD on both banks of a shallow collateral sulcus (CS) where area 35 is distributed on both banks of the sulcus. Note the angular abutment of area 28, the entorhinal cortex with area 35, the perirhinal cortex. Note also that NFTs of layers III and V of 35b coalesce (*asterisks*) into a single band of pyramidal neurons when layer IV ends. These arch medially into area 35a and form columns of pyramidal neurons that descend towards the pia and invade layer II of area 28, the entorhinal cortex. Area 35 NFTs represent the earliest cortical changes in aging.

torhinal cortex, the perirhinal cortex is heavily affected in AD and represents the first cortical area where NFTs occur.[5,15,46] Its medialmost belt, area 35a, is a complex zone composed of large and small pyramidal neurons that invade layer II of the entorhinal cortex laterally. In their descent into the latter, they align vertically, and in early AD, they form conspicuous columns of NFTs (FIGS. 8 and 9). These columns aid in defining the anteroposterior topography of the perirhinal cortex and faithfully follow sulcal variation around the lateral parahippocampal gyrus. For example, in cases without a rhinal sulcus, perirhinal columns separate olfactory cortex from temporal neocortex anteriorly, then entorhinal cortex from temporal neocortex more posteriorly along the medial bank of the collateral sulcus. In cases with a rhinal sulcus, NFT columns occur in its fundus and lateral bank, then assume a position on the medial bank of the collateral sulcus when the rhinal sulcus ends. The deviation of the perirhinal cortex from the fundus and lateral bank of the rhinal sulcus onto the medial bank of the collateral sulcus forms a small, but characteristic gyrus that we name the perirhinal gyrus (FIGS. 2 and 3).

Parasubiculum

Brodmann's area 49, the parasubicular cortex, lies along the lower exposed lip of the hippocampal fissure and is damaged heavily in AD. Like the laterally adjacent entorhinal cortex, with which it shares many similarities, NFTs occur in its superficial and deep layers at endstage AD when there is a long duration of illness. Layer II neurons of this cortex form one or two large islands of neurons, and NFTs in these provide a histopathologic feature that sets the parasubiculum apart from the entorhinal cortex, where layer II NFTs affect multiple, but smaller islands of neurons (FIG. 8B). Similar to the medial parts of the entorhinal cortex, the parasubiculum appears to be affected later in the illness, after pathology in the lateral entorhinal cortex and the perirhinal cortex is well established and extensive.

Presubiculum

Brodmann's area 27, the presubicular cortex, is a multilayered periallocortex that is continuous posteriorly with the retrosplenial cortex of the posterior cingulate gyrus. As implied by its name, it lies adjacent to the subiculum of the hippocampal formation. Its most conspicuous histologic feature in cell stains is large, somewhat concentric islands of small pyramidal neurons in layer II that are segregated from its deeper layers by a prominent lamina dessicans. In myelin stains, layer I and the islands of layer II pyramids are engulfed by a dense and complicated plexus of axons forming the posteromedial part of the reticular substance of Arnold. In our experience and that of others, NFTs are seldom observed in the islands of small pyramids that form the lamina principalis externa of the presubiculum, but they can be observed occasionally in its deep layers which form the lamina principalis interna. Some of these neurons are in direct continuity with the subicular part of the hippocampal formation where NFTs are typically abundant throughout much of the course of AD. Diffuse clouds of amyloid β peptide often fill the layer II islands and form a conspicuous feature of the AD brain.[45,71]

Ectorhinal Cortex

Brodmann's area 36 forms the lateral boundary of area 35 and has a variable relationship with the parahippocampal gyrus. At anterior levels it frequently lies lateral to the parahippocampal gyrus, but it is not unusual in some cases for it to invade the fundus of the collateral fissure and extend onto its medial bank for a short distance. Posteriorly, when the entorhinal cortex narrows, it parallels the course of the perirhinal cortex and forms the posterior part of the gyrus. The ectorhinal cortex is damaged heavily throughout its long anteroposterior course in AD, with NFTs in layers III and V in cases of long duration.[32] In cases of shorter or moderate duration, layer III contains the major portion of NFTs and large pyramids form a band between the perirhinal cortex and Brodmann's area 20 of the inferior temporal gyrus (FIGS. 8 and 9). The ectorhinal pyramids of layers III and V, along with their counterparts in the perirhinal cortex, coalesce into a band medially when layer IV ends in medial perirhinal cortex. They descend towards the pia in stepwise columns across the medial perirhinal cortex and invade the lateralmost islands of entorhinal cortex layer II. This is conspicuous in AD where the pyramidal neuron phenotype is often enhanced by the presence of NFTs. Inspection of the lateralmost islands of the entorhinal cortex always reveals a mixture of cellular phenotypes, and pyramidal neurons with NFTs often outnumber multipolar stellate neurons so affected. Braak and Braak[15] label this interface the transentorhinal cortex and assert that entorhinal layer II stellate neurons progressively alter their morphological phenotype laterally, until they assume a pyramidal shape and insert into the deep part of layer III. We agree that recognition of layer IIIc of the perirhinal cortex is a key element in understanding this neocortical-limbic cortical interface, but find little reason to believe that any of the neurons involved undergo changes in their shapes and/or neuronal classification. Instead, the pyramidal neurons of the perirhinal layers III and V simply merge and invade entorhinal layer II, as discussed above.

In summary, the parahippocampal gyrus is heavily damaged in AD. Quantitatively, the entorhinal cortex has the greatest changes, followed closely by the perirhinal cortex.[5] The latter, however, has the distinction of being the cortical area where NFTs occur first with advancing age. These changes in AD would seem of necessity to greatly alter the normal flow of neural activity into and out of the hippocampal formation. For example, it is well documented in several species that the perirhinal, parasubicular, and ectorhinal cortices are major contributors of input to the entorhinal cortex[39,56,62,63,65,72,73] with secondary projections, in the case of the perirhinal and ectorhinal cortices, to the subicular/CA1 zone of the hippocampal formation.[64] The entorhinal cortex itself is the origin for the perforant pathway, which provides the largest source of input to the hippocampal formation and its major cortical input[74,75] (FIG. 10). The exact neurons that give rise to the perforant pathway contain NFTs in AD.[36] Concomitantly, layer IV of the entorhinal cortex is also damaged heavily by NFTs in AD, and this layer of neurons receives a powerful hippocampal formation output that is relayed to many limbic and distal association cortices.[48,55] Thus, all told, AD pathology alone greatly alters the neurons that give rise to neural systems that underlie the reciprocal relationship between the cortex and the hippocampal formation. Such changes would certainly be strong candidates for the histopathological basis of the clinical observations of memory impairment in AD.

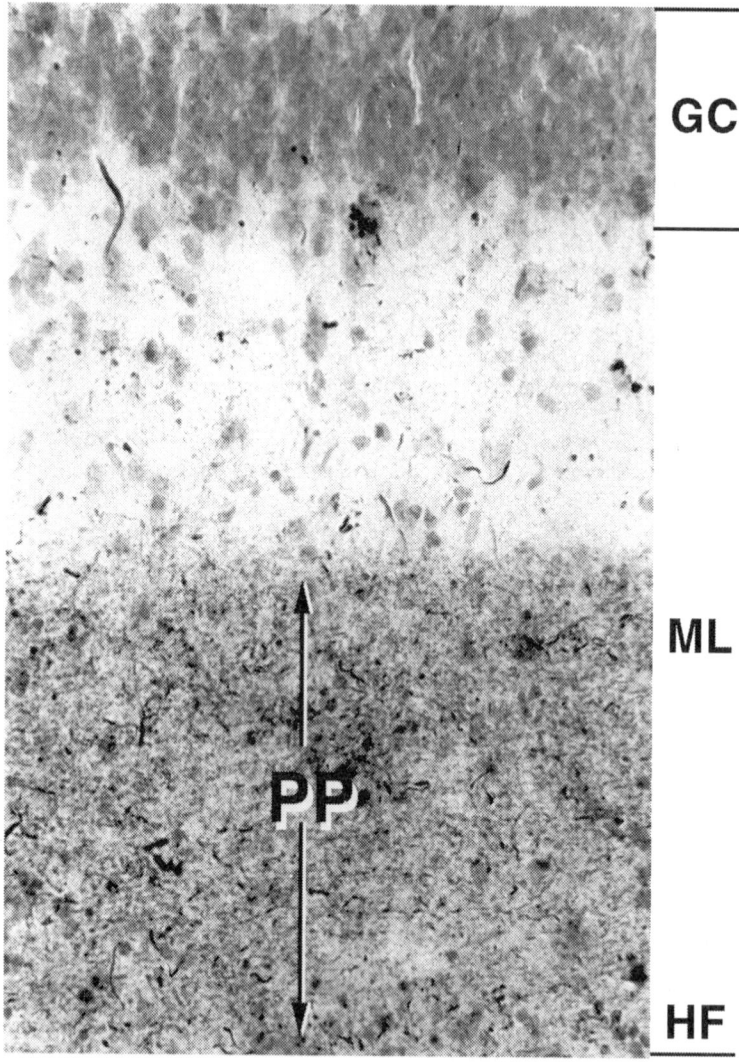

FIGURE 10. Photomicrograph of the dentate gyrus in AD, showing the granule cell (GC) layer and its molecular layer (ML) where granule cell dendrites are distributed. The entorhinal cortex was damaged heavily by NFTs in this donor. The tissue was immunostained with Alz-50 to label the abnormally phosphorylated tau protein A68 found in AD and then overstained with methylene blue to reveal Nissl substance and cell somas. Note the dense immunostaining of the outer molecular layer proximal to the hippocampal fissure (HF) where the perforant pathway (PP) ends. This pathway arises from entorhinal layer II neurons.

PARAHIPPOCAMPAL GYRUS AND PRECLINICAL
ALZHEIMER'S DISEASE

The pathological descriptions summarized above apply to well established end-stage Alzheimer's disease, where premorbid clinical observations and postmorbid neuropathological autopsy observations confirm this illness. They highlight pathological changes in cortical areas that form the parahippocampal gyrus, and particularly, those in the entorhinal and perirhinal cortices which are invariant in AD and where quantitative estimates reveal that the greatest destruction in cortex has occurred.[5] Several investigators have made the important observation that NFTs can occur in these cortical areas many years before the clinical and behavioral signs that characterize the disease. These "silent changes" in the parahippocampal gyrus and hippocampal formation have been observed in imaging research,[22,40,42,44] autopsy surveys,[19,21,76] and closely monitored aging studies with clinical study before death and pathological analyses after death.[10,52,57] They all raise the ominous red flag that neuropathologically, AD may have a remarkably early onset and progress insidiously for many years in otherwise healthy and productive individuals before the pathological changes reach a threshold and the expression of the stereotypical clinical signs of AD become manifest.[19] They also reshape the playing field of disease prevention, such that AD research has to have a dual focus not only of defining the elusive etiology of the disorder, but also of identifying its victims premorbidly, well in advance of irreversible destructive pathology. In this sense, AD loses its status as a disease of the elderly and becomes instead a disease that simply "manifests" itself in some elderly, not unlike many other diseases in other organ systems. The optimistic goal of arresting the disease in a symptomatic senior citizen is desirable, but undershoots the magnitude of the problem.

If one asserts that the preclinical lesion for AD is the formation of NFTs in the perirhinal and entorhinal cortices, it raises many questions about the affected neurons. For example, why are they vulnerable, how are they different from the other large neurons in the cortex, and why don't humans share AD with other mammals if these "limbic cortices" are old in a phylogenetic sense? Obviously, these are complicated questions to answer, but some deductions can be made. Foremost would be the fact that perirhinal and entorhinal cortex neurons must be phenotypically unique and that this phenotype is shared with other pyramidal neurons in AD victims and only partially so or not at all in elderly individuals who acquire the preclinical lesion but never progress beyond it. Also, it could be deduced that expression of the NFT phenotype underlies what others have described as the "spread of pathology or disease," the scourge of cross-sectional comparisons.[16] In this sense, what appears to be spread is nothing more than the differential expression of a phenotype. Variable rates of disease progression would be related to phenotype dose, the presence of other catalytic factors, or both.

Whatever the mechanisms of AD may be, the neuroanatomical question of why the disease begins in the parahippocampal gyrus will have to be addressed, because affected neurons in the perirhinal and entorhinal cortices harbor the molecular clues as to why they develop NFTs and why other large pyramids develop these changes as the disease progresses.

CONCLUDING REMARKS

In the foregoing sections, we highlighted the major neuroanatomical features of the normal human parahippocampal gyrus and commented on neuroanatomical variations that have hindered the understanding of this part of the cortical mantle. In particular, we addressed the issue of the rhinal sulcus in the human brain and commented on its historical and present-day misidentification. Against this background we reviewed the major changes in the parahippocampal gyrus in AD and how NFT pathology leads to the neuroanatomical uncoupling of the hippocampal formation and the association cortices. This disconnection forms the histopathological correlate of the early memory changes in AD. We then reviewed the nature of early pathological changes in aging and the preclinical lesion of the parahippocampal gyrus. We commented on how this forces us to alter our view of AD from a disease of aging to a disease that starts earlier in life, but is manifested in aging. Finally, we examined the issue of the NFT phenotype in the entorhinal and perirhinal cortices. It was concluded that neighboring pyramidal neurons must share or, at least, partially share a phenotype first expressed in the perirhinal cortex and that the differential expression of it, and not its spread, accounts for the elaboration of the disease in other cortical areas over time. In this sense, understanding the etiology of AD is both a sharply focused neuroanatomical question that is equally coupled with molecular biological questions aimed at dissecting the unique phenotype of the first vulnerable perirhinal pyramids and other cortical pyramidal neurons affected in AD.

ACKNOWLEDGMENTS

This work was supported by National Institutes of Health grants NS 14944 and PO NS 19632. We thank Sherry Lohman for library research and typing the manuscript, Paul Reiman for photography, and Darrell Wilkins and Patrick Elbert for brain acquisitions through The University of Iowa Deeded Body Program.

REFERENCES

1. AMARAL, D.G. & R. INSAUSTI. 1990. Hippocampal formation. *In* The Human Nervous System. G. Paxinos, Ed. : 711–755. Academic Press, Inc. San Diego.
2. AMARAL, D.G., R. INSAUSTI & W.M. COWAN. 1987. The entorhinal cortex of the monkey: I. Cytoarchitectonic organization. J. Comp. Neurol. **264:** 326–355.
3. ARNOLD, J.C. 1851. Handbuch der Anatomie des Menschen, 2 Bd. Herder. Freiburg i. Br.
4. ARNOLD, S.E., B.R. FRANZ, R.C. GUR, R.E. GUR, R.M. SHAPIRO, P.J. MOBERG & J.Q. TROJANOWSKI. 1995. Smaller neuron size in schizophrenia in hippocampal subfields that mediate cortical-hippocampal interactions. Am. J. Psychiatry **152:** 738–748.
5. ARNOLD, S.E., B.T. HYMAN, J. FLORY, A.R. DAMASIO & G.W. VAN HOESEN. 1991. The topographical and neuroanatomical distribution of neurofibrillary tangles and neuritic plaques in the cerebral cortex of patients with Alzheimer's disease. Cerebr. Cortex **1:** 103–116.
6. ARNOLD, S.E., V.M.Y. LEE, R.E. GUR & J.Q. TROJANOWSKI. 1991. Abnormal expression of two microtubule-associated proteins (MAP2 and MAP5) in specific subfields of the hippocampal formation in schizophrenia. Proc. Natl. Acad. Sci. USA **88:** 10850–10854.

7. ARNOLD, S.E., D.D. RUSCHEINSKY & L.-Y. HAN. 1997. Further evidence of abnormal cytoarchitecture of the entorhinal cortex in schizophrenia using spatial point pattern analyses. Biol. Psychiatry **42:** 639–647.

8. ARNOLD, S.E. & J.Q. TROJANOWSKI. 1996. Recent advances in defining the neuropathology of schizophrenia. Acta Neuropathol. **92:** 217–231.

9. ARRIAGADA, P.V., K. MARZLOFF & B.T. HYMAN. 1992. Distribution of Alzheimer-type pathologic changes in nondemented elderly individuals matches the pattern in Alzheimer's disease. Neurology **42:** 1681–1688.

10. BERG, L., D.W. MCKEEL, JR., J.P. MILLER, M. STORANDT, E.H. RUBIN, J.C. MORRIS, J. BATY, M. COATS, J. NORTON, A.M. GOATE, J.L. PRICE, M. GEARING, S.S. MIRRA & A.M. SAUNDERS. 1998. Clinicopathologic studies in cognitively healthy aging and Alzheimer disease. Arch. Neurol. **55:** 326–335.

11. BERGER, B., C. ALVAREZ & D. PELAPRAT. 1997. Retrosplenial/presubicular continuum in primates: a developmental approach in fetal macaques using neurotensin and parvalbumin as markers. Dev. Brain Res. **101:** 207–224.

12. BERNASCONI, N., A. BERNASCONI, F. ANDERMANN, F. DUBEAU, W. FEINDEL & D.C. REUTENS. 1999. Entorhinal cortex in temporal lobe epilepsy: a quantitative MRI study. Neurology **52:** 1870–1876.

13. BIELSCHOWSKY, M. 1928. Morphologie der Ganglienzelle. *In* Handbuch de Mikroskopischen Anatomie de Menschen. W. von Mölendorff, Ed. : 8–96. Springer-Verlag. Berlin.

14. BOGERTS, B., M. ASHTARI, G. DEGREEF, J.M. ALVIR, R.M. BILDER & J.A. LIEBERMAN. 1990. Reduced temporal limbic structure volumes on magnetic resonance images in first episode schizophrenia. Psychiatry Res. Neuroimaging **35:** 1–13.

15. BRAAK, H. & E. BRAAK. 1985. On areas of transition between entorhinal allocortex and temporal isocortex in the human brain. Normal morphology and lamina-specific pathology in Alzheimer's disease. Acta Neuropathol. **68:** 325–332.

16. BRAAK, H. & E. BRAAK. 1991. Neuropathological staging of Alzheimer-related changes. Acta Neuropathol. **82:** 239–259.

17. BRAAK, H. & E. BRAAK. 1992. The human entorhinal cortex: normal morphology and lamina-specific pathology in various diseases. Neurosci. Res. **15:** 6–31.

18. BRAAK, H. & E. BRAAK. 1996. Evolution of the neuropathology of Alzheimer's disease. Acta Neuropathol. Scand. Suppl. **165:** 3–12.

19. BRAAK, H. & E. BRAAK. 1997. Frequency of stages of Alzheimer-related lesions in different age categories. Neurobiol. Aging **18:** 351–357.

20. BURWELL, R.D., M.P. WITTER & D.G. AMARAL. 1995. Perirhinal and postrhinal cortices of the rat: a review of the neuroanatomical literature and comparison with findings from the monkey brain. Hippocampus **5:** 390–408.

21. DAVIS, D.G., F.A. SCHMITT, D.R. WEKSTEIN & W.R. MARKESBERY. 1999. Alzheimer neuropathologic alterations in aged cognitively normal subjects. J. Neuropathol. Exp. Neurol. **58:** 376–388.

22. DE LEON, M.J., A. CONVIT, S. DE SANTI & M. BOBINSKI. 1999. Structural neuroimaging: early diagnosis and staging of Alzheimer's disease. *In* Alzheimer's Disease and Related Disorders. K. Iqbal, D.F. Swaab, B. Winblad & H.M. Wisniewski, Eds. : 105–126. John Wiley & Sons Ltd. Chichester, UK.

23. DU, F., T. EID, E.W. LOTHMAN, C. KOHLER & R. SCHWARCZ. 1995. Preferential neuronal loss in layer III of the medial entorhinal cortex in rat models of temporal lobe epilepsy. J. Neurosci. **15:** 6301–6313.

24. DU, F., R. SCHWARCZ & C.A. TAMMINGA. 1995. Entorhinal cortex in temporal lobe epilepsy. Am. J. Psychiatry **152:** 826.

25. DUVERNOY, H.M. 1988. The Human Hippocampus: An Atlas of Applied Anatomy. Bergmann. Munich.

26. FALKAI, P., B. BOGERTS & M. ROZUMEK. 1988. Limbic pathology in schizophrenia: the entorhinal region. A morphometric study. Biol. Psychiatry **24:** 515–521.

27. GÓMEZ-ISLA, T., J.L. PRICE, D.W. MCKEEL, JR., J.C. MORRIS, J.H. GROWDON & B.T. HYMAN. 1996. Profound loss of layer II entorhinal cortex neurons occurs in very mild Alzheimer's disease. J. Neurosci. **16:** 4491–5000.

28. GOODMAN, L. 1953. Alzheimer's disease. J. Nerv. Mental Dis. **117:** 97–130.

29. HANKE, J. 1997. Sulcal pattern of the anterior parahippocampal gyrus in the human adult. Ann. Anat. **179:** 335–339.
30. HEVNER, R.F. & M.T.T. WONG-RILEY. 1992. Entorhinal cortex of the human, monkey, and rat:metabolic map as revealed by cytochrome oxidase. J. Comp. Neurol. **326:** 451–469.
31. HIRANO, A. & H.M. ZIMMERMAN. 1962. Alzheimer's neurofibrillary changes. Arch. Neurol. **7:** 73–88.
32. HOF, P.R., K. COX & J.H. MORRISON. 1990. Quantitative analysis of a vulnerable subset of pyramidal neurons in Alzheimer's disease. I. Superior frontal and inferior temporal cortex. J. Comp. Neurol. **301:** 44–54.
33. HOF, P.R. & J.H. MORRISON. 1995. Neurofilament protein defines regional patterns of cortical organization in the Macaque monkey visual system: a quantitative immunohistochemical analysis. J.Comp. Neurol. **352:** 161–186.
34. HOOPER, M.W. & F.S. VOGEL. 1976. The limbic system in Alzheimer's disease. Am. J. Pathol. **85:** 1–13.
35. HYMAN, B.T., L.J. KROMER & G.W. VAN HOESEN. 1988. A direct demonstration of the perforant pathway terminal zone in Alzheimer's disease using the monoclonal antibody Alz-50. Brain Res. **450:** 392–397.
36. HYMAN, B.T., G.W. VAN HOESEN, A.R. DAMASIO & C.L. BARNES. 1984. Alzheimer's disease:cell-specific pathology isolates the hippocampal formation. Science **225:** 1168–1170.
37. HYMAN, B.T., G.W. VAN HOESEN, L.J. KROMER & A.R. DAMASIO. 1986. Perforant pathway changes and the memory impairment of Alzheimer's disease. Ann. Neurol. **20:** 472–481.
38. INSAUSTI, R. 1993. Comparative anatomy of the entorhinal cortex and hippocampus in mammals. Hippocampus **3:** 19–26.
39. INSAUSTI, R., D.G. AMARAL & W.M. COWAN. 1987. The entorhinal cortex of the monkey: II. Cortical afferents. J. Comp. Neurol. **264:** 356–395.
40. INSAUSTI, R., K. JUOTTONEN, H. SOININEN, A.M. INSAUSTI, K. PARTANEN, P. VAINIO, M.P. LAAKSO & A. PITKÄNEN. 1998. MR volumetric analysis of the human entorhinal, perirhinal, and temporopolar cortices. Am. J. Neuroradiol. **19:** 659–671.
41. INSAUSTI, R., T. TUÑÓN, T. SOBREVIELA, A.M. INSAUSTI & L.M. GONZALO. 1995. The human entorhinal cortex: a cytoarchitectonic analysis. J. Comp. Neurol. **355:** 171–198.
42. JACK, C.R., JR., R.C. PETERSEN, Y.C. XU, S.C. WARING, P.C. O'BRIEN, E.G. TANGALOS, G.E. SMITH & R.J. IVNIK & E. KOKMEN. 1997. Medial temporal atrophy on MRI in normal aging and very mild Alzheimer's disease. Neurology **49:** 786–794.
43. JAKOB, H. & H. BECKMANN. 1994. Circumscribed malformation and nerve cell alterations in the entorhinal cortex of schizophrenics. J. Neural Transm. **98:** 83–106.
44. JUOTTONEN, K., M.P. LAAKSO, R. INSAUSTI, M. LEHTOVIRTA, A. PITKÄNEN, K. PARTANEN & H. SOININEN. 1998. Volumes of the entorhinal and perirhinal cortices in Alzheimer's disease. Neurobiol. Aging **19:** 15–22.
45. KALUS, P., H. BRAAK, E. BRAAK & J. BOHL. 1989. The presubicular region in Alzheimer's disease: topography of amyloid deposits and neurofibrillary changes. Brain Res. **494:** 198–203.
46. KEMPER, T.L. 1978. Senile dementia: a focal disease in the temporal lobe. *In* Senile Dementia: A Biomedical Approach. K. Nandy, Ed. :105–113. Elsevier North-Holland Biomedical Press.
47. KLINGLER, J. 1948. Die makroskopische Anatomie der Ammonsformation. Denkschr. schweiz. naturforsch. 78.
48. KOSEL, K.C., G.W. VAN HOESEN & D.L. ROSENE. 1982. Non-hippocampal cortical projections from the entorhinal cortex in the rat and rhesus monkey. Brain Res. **244:** 210–213.
49. MIKKONEN, M., H. SOININEN & A. PITKANEN. 1997. Distribution of parvalbumin-, calretinin-, and calbindin-D28k-immunoreactive neurons and fibers in the human entorhinal cortex. J. Comp. Neurol. **388:** 64–88.

50. MORECRAFT, R.J., K.S. ROCKLAND & G.W. VAN HOESEN. 2000. Localization of area prostriata and its projection to the cingulate motor cortex in the rhesus monkey. Cerebral Cortex. In press.
51. ONO, M., S. KUBIK & C.D. ABERNATHEY. 1990. Atlas of the Cerebral Sulci. George Thieme. Stuttgart.
52. PRICE, J.L. & J.C. MORRIS. 1999. Tangles and plaques in nondemented aging and "preclinical" Alzheimer's disease. Ann. Neurol. **45:** 358–368.
53. REICHERT, C.B. 1859. Der Bau des menschlichen Gehirns. Engelmann. Leipzig.
54. RETZIUS, G. 1896. Das menschenhirn. Studien in der makroskopischen Morphologie. Norstedt & Sohne. Stockholm.
55. ROSENE, D.L. & G.W. VAN HOESEN. 1977. Hippocampal efferents reach widespread areas of cerebral cortex and amygdala in the rhesus monkey. Science **198:** 315–317.
56. ROSENE, D.L. & G.W. VAN HOESEN. 1987. The hippocampal formation of the primate brain: a review of some comparative aspects of cytoarchitecture and connections. *In* Cerebral Cortex. Vol. 6. E. G. Jones & A. Peters, Eds. : 345–456. Plenum Press. New York.
57. RUBIN, E.H., J.C. MORRIS, E.A. GRANT & T. VENDEGNA. 1989. Very mild senile dementia of the Alzheimer type. I. Clinical assessment. Arch. Neurol. **46:** 379–382.
58. SCHMIDT, S., E. BRAAK & H. BRAAK. 1993. Parvalbumin-immunoreactive structures of the adult human entorhinal and transentorhinal region. Hippocampus **3:** 459–470.
59. SOLODKIN, A. & G.W. VAN HOESEN. 1996. Entorhinal cortex modules of the human brain. J. Comp. Neurol. **365:** 610–627.
60. SOLODKIN, A., S.D. VELDHUIZEN & G.W. VAN HOESEN. 1996. Contingent vulnerability of entorhinal parvalbumin-containing neurons in Alzheimer's disease. J. Neurosci. **16:** 3311–3321.
61. SQUIRE, L.R. & S. ZOLA-MORGAN. 1991. The medial temporal lobe memory system. Science **253:** 1380–1386.
62. SUZUKI, W.A. & D.G. AMARAL. 1994. Perirhinal and parahippocampal cortices of the macaque monkey: cortical afferents. J. Comp. Neurol. **350:** 497–533.
63. SUZUKI, W.A. & D.G. AMARAL. 1994. Topographic organization of the reciprocal connections between the monkey entorhinal cortex and the perirhinal and parahippocampal cortices. J. Neurosci. **14:** 1856–1877.
64. VAN HOESEN, G.W., D.L. ROSENE & M.-M. MESULAM. 1979. Subicular input from the temporal cortex in the rhesus monkey. Science **205:** 608–610.
65. VAN HOESEN, G.W. 1982. The parahippocampal gyrus: new observations regarding its cortical connections in the monkey. Trends Neurosci. **5:** 345–350.
66. VAN HOESEN, G.W. 1995. Anatomy of the medial temporal lobe. Magnetic Resonance Imaging **13:** 1047–1055.
67. VAN HOESEN, G.W. 1997. Ventromedial temporal lobe anatomy, with comments on Alzheimer's disease and temporal injury. J. Neuropsychiatry Clin. Neurosci. **9:** 331–341.
68. VAN HOESEN, G.W., J. AUGUSTINACK & S.J. REDMAN. 1999. Ventromedial temporal lobe pathology in dementia, brain trauma, and schizophrenia. Ann. N.Y. Acad. Sci. **877:** 575–594.
69. VAN HOESEN, G.W. & A. SOLODKIN. 1993. Some modular features of temporal cortex in humans as revealed by pathological changes in Alzheimer's disease. Cerebr. Cortex **3:** 465–475.
70. VAN HOESEN, G.W. & A. SOLODKIN. 1994. Cellular and systems neuroanatomical changes in Alzheimer's disease. Ann. N.Y. Acad. Sci. **747:** 12–35.
71. WISNIEWSKI, H.M., M. SADOWSKI, K. JAKUBOWSKA-SADOWSKA, M. TARNAWSKI & J. WEGIEL. 1998. Diffuse, lake-like amyloid-β deposits in the parvopyramidal layer of the presubiculum in Alzheimer disease. J. Neuropathol. Exp. Neurol. **57:** 674–683.
72. WITTER, M., H.J. GROENEWEGEN, F.H. LOPES DA SILVA & A.H.M. LOHMAN. 1989. Functional organization of the extrinsic and intrinsic circuitry of the parahippocampal region. Prog. Neurobiol. **33:** 161–254.
73. WITTER, M.P. 1993. Organization of the entorhinal-hippocampal system: a review of current anatomical data. Hippocampus **3:** 33–44.

74. WITTER, M.P. & D.G. AMARAL. 1991. Entorhinal cortex of the monkey: V. Projections to the dentate gyrus, hippocampus, and subicular complex. J. Comp. Neurol. **307:** 437–459.
75. WITTER, M.P., G.W. VAN HOESEN & D.G. AMARAL. 1989. Topographical organization of the entorhinal projection to the dentate gyrus of the monkey. J. Neurosci. **9:** 216–228.
76. YILMAZER-HANKE, D. & J. HANKE. 1999. Progression of Alzheimer-related neuritic plaque pathology in the entorhinal region, perirhinal cortex and hippocampal formation. Dementia & Geriatric Cognit. Disord. **10:** 70–76.

Cellular and Molecular Neuropathology of the Parahippocampal Region in Schizophrenia

STEVEN E. ARNOLD[a]

Center for Neurobiology and Behavior, Department of Psychiatry,
University of Pennsylvania, Philadelphia, Pennsylvania 19104, USA

ABSTRACT: The entorhinal cortex, subiculum, and hippocampus have been regions of great interest in both clinical and neuropathological investigations of schizophrenia. Postmortem studies have identified numerous abnormalities, although many remain controversial or unconfirmed. Among the cellular and molecular neuropathological findings are (1) abnormal cytoarchitecture of the entorhinal cortex characterized by poorly formed layer II neuron clusters and laminar disorganization; (2) normal neuron density but smaller neuron size in the superficial lamina of the entorhinal cortex and subiculum; (3) abnormal expression of the microtubule-associated protein MAP2 in the entorhinal cortex and subiculum; (4) aberrant glutamatergic and catecholaminergic innervation of the entorhinal cortex; (5) abnormal mRNA expression of various transcription factors, ion channels, and neurosecretory pathway-related proteins in entorhinal stellate neurons; and (6) an absence of any neurodegeneration. Altogether, these findings suggest that aberrant neurodevelopmental processes play a key role in the pathobiology of schizophrenia and provide a neuroanatomic basis for understanding many of the clinical and neuropsychological abnormalities in the disorder.

INTRODUCTION

Schizophrenia is a severe mental illness affecting approximately 1% of the world's population. It is characterized by deterioration in personality, hallucinations and delusions, and cognitive impairments. For investigators of schizophrenia, the hippocampus and parahippocampal region have been regions of special interest. Indeed, the ventromedial temporal lobe has been perhaps the most frequently studied brain region of any in both clinical and postmortem neurobiological studies.[1-3] Clinicians have long noted similarities between the symptoms of schizophrenia and those of the schizophrenia-like organic psychoses associated with temporal lobe lesions such as epileptic foci, temporal lobe tumors and cerebrovascular lesions,

[a]Address for correspondence: Steven E. Arnold, M.D., Center for Neurobiology and Behavior, University of Pennsylvania, 142 Clinical Research Building, 415 Curie Boulevard, Philadelphia, PA 19104. Tel.: (215) 573-3258; fax: (215) 573-2041.
e-mail: alveus@mail.med.upenn.edu

herpes encephalitis, and neurodegenerative diseases (e.g., Alzheimer's disease) that have particular predilections for the region.[4] Furthermore, early clinical neurobiological investigators described enlarged temporal horns in schizophrenia using pneumoencepholgraphy,[5] while electroencephalographers frequently reported abnormal recordings from temporal electrodes.[6]

Contemporary neuropsychological studies have found that within the context of widespread cognitive impairments there also are differential deficits in both verbal and visual declarative memory which have been attributed to hippocampal dysfunction.[7,8] Longitudinal studies find that these deficits persist even after the more florid psychotic symptoms improve or resolve with treatment.[9] This stability of memory deficit suggests a static, perhaps neuroanatomically-based abnormality in the ventromedial temporal lobe.

Structural neuroimaging studies with magnetic resonance imaging have reported selective volume deficits in the amygdalo-hippocampal region and parahippocampal gyrus in schizophrenia,[10–12] although findings are controversial as some investigators find that the smaller volumes are not regionally selective.[13–16] It is also interesting that while magnetic resonance imaging (MRI) studies consistently report smaller hippocampal and parahippocampal volumes, the postmortem findings are less consistent. Investigators have reported decreases in the cross-sectional area as well as the volume of the hippocampus[17–19] and decreased parahippocampal area, volume,[17,20] and parahippocampal cortical thickness.[21–23] However, a number of studies failed to find any differences in hippocampus size in schizophrenia compared to normals,[22–25] while one stereological study found no differences in either hippocampus of parahippocampal gyrus size.[26] There are a number of methodological variables that might explain these inconsistencies such as the limited sample sizes of most postmortem studies, the methods of sampling cross-sectional profiles for area determination, or varying methods for determining the boundaries of the hippocampus.

Some neuroimaging researchers have tried to more specifically elucidate the importance of neuroanatomic abnormalities of the hippocampal formation in schizophrenia by correlating volumetric measures with the disease's symptoms and signs. For instance, poor performance on tests of verbal memory, abstraction, and categorization as well as positive symptoms have been reported to correlate with reduced size of ventromedial temporal lobe structures.[27–29] Similarly, functional neuroimaging studies employing positron emission tomography (PET) and functional MRI have reported abnormal blood flow or metabolic activity in the hippocampal region, and these also have been found to correlate with psychiatric measures.[30–33] Here, too, findings have been diverse and controversial.

Remaining controversies notwithstanding, these findings from clinical research all together provide ample justification for the attention that has been paid to the parahippocampal/hippocampal region in postmortem studies. Finally, these brain areas are especially attractive regions for neuropathological study, because the normal neuroanatomy and connectivity are so well characterized. It is an excellent model system in which to identify subtle cytoarchitectural, cellular, and molecular differences. This paper will review the microscopic neuropathological findings in the ventromedial temporal lobe in schizophrenia with an emphasis on the entorhinal cortex and subiculum, highlighted by work from our own studies. We have taken a "top down" approach, starting with diagnostic neuropathology and then describing cytoarchitecture, neuronal morphometry, cytoskeletal protein expression and, most recently, single cell mRNA profiling in the entorhinal cortex.

ABSENCE OF NEURODEGENERATIVE LESIONS
OR OTHER EVIDENCE OF NEURAL INJURY

The possibility of premature and/or progressive dementia and neurodegeneration in patients with schizophrenia is an historically important hypothesis, first described by Morel[34] and later by Kraepelin,[35] who marked *dementia praecox* as a brain disorder. Kraepelin emphasized a chronic, deteriorating course over time with only a minority of patients showing recovery or remission. The possibility of a neurodegenerative process recently has been supported by a few longitudinal volumetric MRI studies which found progressive brain atrophy in some patients.[36] In addition, recent lifespan studies focusing on schizophrenia in late life have revealed a high frequency and severity of cognitive and functional impairments among some elderly, very chronic patients.[37,38] Psychometric testing in this population revealed a neuropsychological profile with similarities to that of Alzheimer's disease.[39,40]

Diagnostic neuropathologic examinations have failed to find any consistent explanations for the dementia in these deteriorated, elderly patients. The frequency of various abnormal neuropathologic findings (e.g., lacunar infarcts, Alzheimer's disease, Parkinson's disease, meningiomas, etc.) is perhaps only slightly greater than that seen among a general, community-based elderly population.[24,38,41] However, the particular lesions are highly miscellaneous and most patients, even with severe dementia, still are without apparent abnormalities.

To assess the possibility of even subtle neurodegeneration or neural injury in schizophrenia, there have been a number of investigations quantifying various histopathologic markers in schizophrenia. These include specific disease-related lesions such as neurofibrillary tangles, amyloid plaques, and Lewy bodies, as well as more general responses to a large number of degenerative, infectious, traumatic, or other causes, including astrocytosis, microglial proliferation, and excessive ubiquitin expression. Beyond its purported role in schizophrenia, the hippocampal formation has been of special interest for these studies because of its selective vulnerability for these lesions in a number of neurodegenerative disorders.[42,43]

Almost without controversy, quantitative neuropathological studies have found no evidence of ongoing neurodegeneration and neural injury in schizophrenia, even among the most severely ill, elderly, and deteriorated. No abnormalities have been reported in the quantity of neurofibrillary tangles and senile plaques in the hippocampal formation,[44–48] nor for other disease-specific neurodegeneration markers such as Lewy bodies, Pick bodies, or protease-resistant prions.[49,50] Similarly, studies have not identified any excess astrocytosis using either traditional histological staining or modern immunohistochemical methods examining glial fibrillary acidic protein (GFAP) expression.[20,46,51–53]

We recently approached the issue of neurodegeneration in schizophrenia in a fairly comprehensive manner by quantifying markers of neurodegenerative disease and neural injury in the parahippocampal region, hippocampus, and other cortical regions in a sample of 23 elderly individuals with schizophrenia.[49] The patients had been prospectively accrued, diagnosed by consensus according to standard criteria, and clinically characterized with a battery of assessment scales. All had been chronically hospitalized and 2/3 had been found to have sufficient cognitive and functional impairment to warrant an additional diagnosis of dementia. This sample was particularly well suited for studies of neurodegeneration because of the severity, chronicity, advanced age, and poor outcome of the schizophrenia. Thus, if accumulated degenerative pathology were an aspect of the disease, it should be more evident in this sample than in a younger or better functioning group.[5]

Six common neurodegeneration markers were immunohistochemically labeled, including neurofibrillary tangles, senile plaques, Lewy bodies, GFAP-positive astrocytes, as well as resting and reactive microglia and dystrophic neurites (identified by their immunoreactivity for ubiquitin). The densities of these markers were quantified using nonbiased stereological counting methods in the entorhinal cortex, subiculum, and CA1 of the hippocampal formation, as well as mid-frontal cortex, orbitofrontal cortex, and calcarine cortex. There were no statistically significant differences between the schizophrenics and matched nonneuropsychiatric controls for the densities of any of the neurodegenerative markers in the hippocampal subfields or other neocortical regions, while both groups exhibited far fewer lesions than an Alzheimer's disease "positive" control group. Furthermore, clinicopathological correlation analyses within the schizophrenia sample failed to identify any significant correlations between cognitive and psychiatric ratings and densities of any of the neuropathological markers. We concluded that there was no significant histologic evidence of neurodegeneration or ongoing neural injury in the cerebral cortex in schizophrenia beyond that seen in a normal control group and that common age-related degenerative lesions could not account for the dementia observed.

Without evidence of conventional neurodegenerative pathology in schizophrenia, other factors must be considered in order to explain the deterioration and dementia that occurs in at least some patients. It remains a possibility that the effects of other normal age-related changes are amplified in the setting of presumably abnormal neural circuitry in schizophrenia. Thus, neurodevelopmental abnormalities may represent a state of decreased cerebral reserve with commensurately increased vulnerability to the cognitive toxicity of even small amounts of neural injury or neurodegenerative lesions that accompany aging. Accordingly, patients may demonstrate neuropsychological deficits prior to their first psychotic episode and relatively static deficits in short-term follow-up studies, but a very slow decline over decades, in a manner as described by Davidson et al.[37]

In considering this decreased cerebral reserve hypothesis, it is especially interesting to note the topographical similarities between the brain regions with reported cytoarchitectural and neuronal morphometric abnormalities in schizophrenia (as described below) and those that are most vulnerable in aging and the common neurodegenerative diseases, such as the entorhinal cortex. Given that initial studies found no correlations between the quantity of neurodegenerative markers in the hippocampus and neocortex and cognitive impairment, it is possible there is a correlation between the "baseline" severity of developmentally based abnormalities and clinical features, including dementia. The task remains to better delineate the nature of such abnormalities.

TABLE 1. Cytoarchitectural findings in entorhinal cortex

Study	Sample Size (SCZ / Control)	Findings
Positive Findings		
Jakob & Beckmann, 1986 [54]	64 / 10	Two-thirds of the schizophrenics exhibit abnormalities, esp., layer II (pre-α) with heterotopic neurons and neuron clusters
Falkai et al., 1988 [20]	13 / 11	Decreased volume and estimated total number of neurons
Jakob & Beckmann, 1989 [112]	76 / 16	52% exhibit cytoarchitectural abnormalities
Arnold et al., 1991 [57]	6 / 16	Abnormal invaginations of surface, disorganized laminar appearance, heterotopy of layer II-type neurons, paucity of neurons
Arnold et al., 1995 [71]	14 / 10	Smaller size of layer II neurons, normal neuron density
Arnold et al., 1997 [64]	8 / 8	Spatial point pattern analysis showed increased effective radius ("dead space") around neurons in layer II and increased clustering of neurons in layer III
Falkai et al., 1999 [65]	19 / 21	Displacement of layer II neuron clusters deeper within cortical thickness and smaller clusters (males only)
Negative Findings		
Heinsen et al., 1996 [60]	109 / 136	No abnormalities in sulcal patterning in parahippocampal region
Krimer et al., 1997 [63]	14 / 14	No abnormalities in neuron number, density, or layer volumes
Akil et al., 1997 [62]	10 / 10	No qualitative differences in cytoarchitectural appearance
Bernstein et al., 1998 [61]	31 / 45	No differences in counts of heterotopic clusters per section

CYTOARCHITECTURE AND NEURONAL MORPHOMETRY

Cytoarchitectural Studies

Reports of cytoarchitectural abnormalities in the entorhinal cortex and hippocampus in schizophrenia have been among the more prominent and controversial in the field (TABLE 1). Because cytoarchitecture is largely determined during fetal brain development, descriptions of cytoarchitectural abnormalities of the entorhinal cortex and hippocampus have played important roles in discussions of schizophrenia as a neurodevelopmental disorder.

In the first description, Jakob and Beckmann[54] reported "definite" cytoarchitectural abnormalities in superficial layers of the rostral entorhinal cortex in 20 of 64 patients with schizophrenia, and "equivocal" changes in another 22. These abnormalities consisted of poor development of layers II and III (also known as layers pre-α, pre-β, and pre-γ in the nomenclature of Braak[55]) with atypically ordered neurons of differing size in layer II (pre-α) instead of the characteristic clustering of neurons into islands, a reduced number of neurons in the superficial portion of layer III (pre-β), and heterotopic groups of neurons belonging to layer II that instead appeared to be formed in layer III. In addition, they reported that many of the neurons appeared smaller and that there was poor development and a reduction in neuron numbers in layer IV (pri-α). Glial cell number and distribution appeared normal. The authors suggested that the findings were most consistent with an abnormality of neuronal migration occurring in the second trimester of gestation when the laminar pattern of the entorhinal cortex is set.[54,56]

Stimulated by this report, we examined the entorhinal cortex in a small sample of 6 patients (all postleukotomy) and 16 controls (including 3 postleukotomy and 2 postthalamotomy for nonschizophrenic conditions) from the archival Yakovlev Collection.[57] Case selection was determined by rigorous application of diagnostic criteria to chart review. Blind to diagnosis, raters identified various abnormalities in the rostral and intermediate portions of the entorhinal cortex in each of the schizophrenia individuals. These included bizarre invaginations of the normally smooth entorhinal surface with disruption of superficial cortical layers, poorly formed layer II neuron clusters with apparent heterotopic displacement of neurons typical of layer II deep into layer III, paucity of neurons in superficial layers, and attenuation of deeper layers (FIG. 1). Similar to Jakob and Beckmann, we concluded that such abnormalities were most consistent with disturbed cortical development. Furthermore, because of the pivotal role that the entorhinal cortex plays in cortical-hippocampal connectivity, we suggested that disturbance of these extensive connections could have far-reaching neuropsychological consequences typical of those seen in schizophrenia.

These findings and conclusions have been influential for neurodevelopmental theorists of schizophrenia and have even helped spawn animal models which explore the effects of fetal or neonatal lesions of the entorhinal and hippocampal regions on later behavior in rats.[58,59] However, some groups have not been able to confirm the initial findings. One of the chief criticisms is that the described abnormalities in schizophrenia just reflect the normal variability of cytoarchitectural appearance of the entorhinal cortex.[60,61] Indeed, the cytoarchitecture of the entorhinal cortex is quite heterogeneous along its rostral-caudal axis and individual variability may be most prominent in the rostral subfields where the purported abnormalities in schizophrenia were described. With an eye to such considerations, Akil and Lewis[62] and Krimer et al.[63] both recently reported no qualitative differences between schizophrenic and control subjects in entorhinal cytoarchitecture.

Another criticism of all of these studies is that they are qualitative descriptions and thus vulnerable to substantial subjectivity on the part of the investigators. In addition to some quantitative studies of neuron density and size in the entorhinal cortex (described below), there have been only two studies attempting to quantify cytoarchitecture or spatial arrangement of neurons per se. Krimer et al.[63] measured the volumes and positioning of individual layers of the entorhinal cortex and found no differences for these variables between schizophrenics and controls. Bernstein et al.[61] found no differences in the numbers of layer II cluster-like heterotopias between

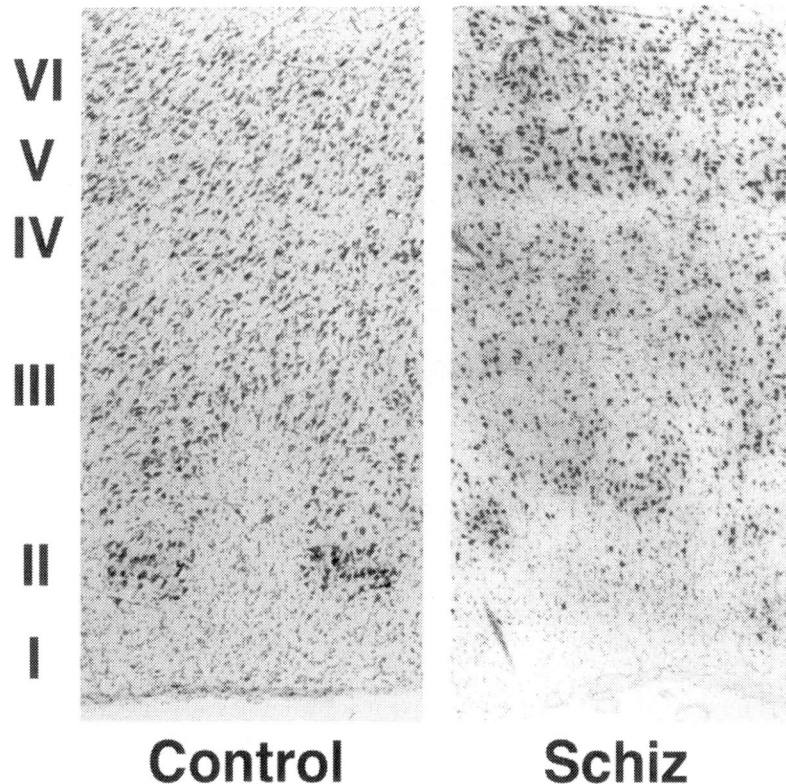

FIGURE 1. Control and schizophrenic entorhinal cortex. Compared to the control, the entorhinal cortex from this schizophrenic shows disorganization of superficial lamina with poorly formed and disorganized neuron clusters in layer II, a patchy appearance in layer III, and smaller neurons in layers II and III. (100×)

schizophrenics and normals. In contrast, we[64] mapped the coordinates of neurons in layers II, III, and V of the rostral entorhinal cortex and used spatial point pattern analyses to compare their distributions in 8 schizophrenics and 8 matched controls. We found subtle but statistically significant between group differences, with schizophrenics having an abnormally clustered dispersion of neurons and a reduced mean effective radius ("dead space") around neurons in layer III, increased mean effective radius in layer II, and no changes in layer V. Although they were not as obvious and dramatic to the naked eye, these findings were interpreted as roughly concordant with our previous qualitative findings in the Yakovlev Collection. Finally and most recently, Falkai et al.[65] measured the vertical distance of layer II-type neuron clusters relative to the entorhinal cortical thickness and found that these clusters were more deeply placed in schizophrenia than in control tissues and also smaller in size (in males only).

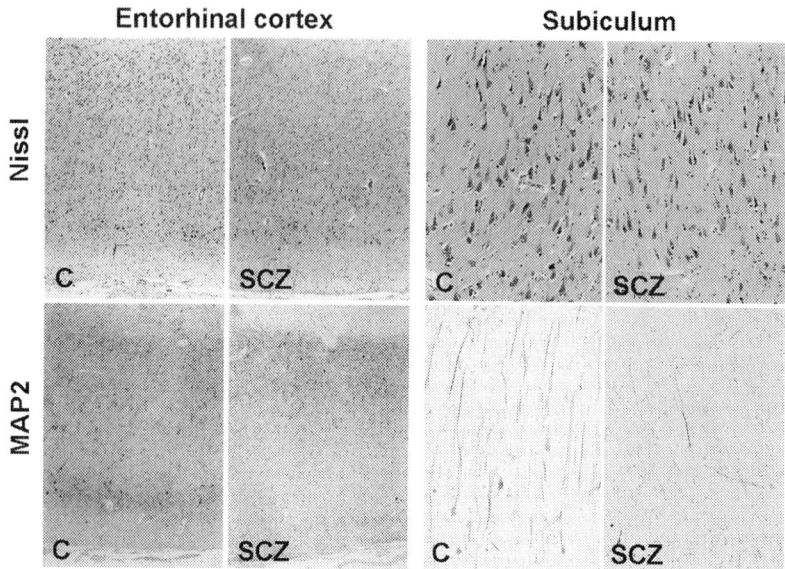

FIGURE 2. Entorhinal cortex (40×) and subiculum (100×) stained with cresyl violet for Nissl substance and immunolableled with AP14 for MAP2. Note the decrease in MAP2 expression confined to superficial layers of the entorhinal cortex in one schizophrenia subject and the nearly absent MAP2 expression in the subiculum in another.

If there are subtle cytoarchitectural abnormalities of the entorhinal cortex in schizophrenia, the neurobiological basis for them remains uncertain. Aberrant migration of nascent neurons from the ventricular zone to the cortex during fetal development has been the mechanism most heralded as the basis for the disturbed cytoarchitectural appearance. However, cytoarchitecture is determined by a complex orchestration of a host of developmental and degenerative processes,[66–68] and a defect in any of these could affect the final neuronal arrangement. Migration, neuron enlargement and differentiation under the influence of intrinsic and extrinsic growth factors, programmed cell death during brain maturation, cell death with normal aging and intercurrent diseases, and the amounts and arrangements of innervating nerve fibers, as well as other components of the neuropil space separating neurons, all contribute to the ultimate cytoarchitectural appearance of the entorhinal cortex at the time of postmortem examination. Which of these determinants might be responsible for the abnormalities that have been observed in at least some patients with schizophrenia is not yet known.

Neuron Density and Number

Quantifying the number of neurons within the hippocampal region also has been of great interest. Here, too, results are controversial. Given the nature of schizophrenia as a disease with remote or very protracted pathoetiologies and no obvious histopathologic abnormalities to the eye in most cases, the methodology used to discern subtle differences in cell density or number is especially critical. Most studies of schizophrenia have assessed neuron *density* on a per unit area basis rather than the total number of neurons. This is problematic in that neuron loss may or may not be reflected in decreased neuron density. Commensurate shrinkage of the neuropil space as a component of the reference volume for the density measurement would tend to hide any true reduction in overall neuron number. Furthermore, most studies have used cell-counting methods that do not account for under- or overcounting due to size, orientation, shape, or splitting of cells. Failure to account for these variables may introduce substantial variances.[69] More modern nonbiased methods help address these limitations and are beginning to be used by schizophrenia researchers.

Several qualitative reports described decreased neuron densities in the entorhinal cortex.[54,57,70] For quantitative studies, only one reported decreased neuron density,[63] whereas three others reported no differences.[20,71,72] Only one study estimated total neuron number and reported a decrease that was primarily due to a decrease in the estimated volume of the entorhinal cortex.[20] This finding awaits confirmation.

Most studies have found no abnormalities in neuron density in the ammonic subfields of the hippocampus either,[25,71,73,74] although one reported decreased density in CA3 and CA4,[18] and one recent study found a lateralized *increase* in neuron density in the right CA3 and CA1 subfields.[75] Two studies have estimated total neuron numbers in the hippocampus. While Falkai and Bogerts[73] found no differences between schizophrenics and controls for neuron densities, total neuron numbers were decreased in all ammonic subfields in schizophrenia because of the decreased volumes of the hippocampus. In contrast, using stereological methods, Heckers *et al.*[72] found no differences between schizophrenics and controls for either neuron density or total neuron estimates.

More recently, Benes *et al.* used a spatial counting approach to measure the densities and total numbers of pyramidal and nonpyramidal neurons in the ammonic subfields in schizophrenia.[76] Compared to matched controls, they found a selective reduction in density and total number of nonpyramidal neurons in CA2 in the schizophrenia group.

The weight of the evidence at this time indicates no substantial abnormality in overall neuron density in the the parahippocampal region or hippocampus in schizophrenia, although the possibility of selective decreases in neuronal subpopulations is intriguing. Whether or not individuals with schizophrenia have abnormally few neurons overall in the hippocampal formation thus hinges on the reference volume for the region. MRI volumetric studies suggest that hippocampal and parahippocampal volumes are indeed decreased in schizophrenia, albeit modestly.

Neuron Size and Cytoskeletal Protein Expression

Several studies have reported decreased neuron size in the parahippocampal/hippocampal region, and findings have been relatively consistent. Benes *et al.*[25] measured pyramidal neuron size in the posterior hippocampus and found 13–18% reductions in CA1–CA4 in schizophrenia compared to controls. We similarly reported smaller neurons in the ammonic subfields, but also in the subiculum (21%) and layer II of the entorhinal cortex (14%).[71] We further measured neurons in primary motor and primary visual cortices to examine the regional specificity of findings for the hippocampal formation and noted no size differences between control and schizophrenia groups for these nonlimbic regions. Most recently, Zaidel et al.[77] examined size and shape of neurons in the ammonic subfields with an additional eye to possible asymmetries. They found significantly decreased neuron size in the left CA1 and CA2 subfields and the right CA3 subfields, without a significant reduction in subicular neuron size on either side. Shape was also measured, and they found a significant elongation of neurons in the left subiculum and CA1, and right CA3.

The above findings from several independent groups indicate cellular dystrophy in schizophrenia. The nature of this is not yet clear. The size of a neuron soma generally corresponds to the extent of neuronal processes (axons and dendritic arbors) that need to be supported by it. Whether neuronal processes are attenuated in the hippocampal formation in schizophrenia is not known. One recent Golgi study found abnormal dendritic arborization in the subiculum, while other studies in neocortex have described decreased dendritic spine density[78–81] in the setting of otherwise normal-appearing dendritic morphology.[78]

At the molecular level, neuron size and shape are determined by several families of cytoskeletal proteins including neurofilament proteins, actins, tubulins, and microtubule-associated proteins.[82] Multiple proteins from these families interact to construct the scaffolding of the cell body, dendritic diameter and branch diameter, axonal diameter, and spine morphology. The neuronal cytoskeleton has been probed in schizophrenia. In a small qualitative immunohistochemical study, we used a panel of well-characterized antibodies to assess the expression of variously phosphorylated neurofilament triplet proteins, α- and β-tubulins, and microtubule-associated proteins MAP2, MAP5 (also known as MAP1B), and tau.[83] We observed relatively specific deficits in the expression of MAP2 and MAP5 in the subiculum in 5 of 6 individuals with schizophrenia compared to controls and a deficit in MAP2 in the entorhinal cortex in 4 of 6, particularly in superficial layers (see FIG. 2). We have confirmed these earlier findings in a separate, larger sample of 21 patients with schizophrenia where we found a significant decrease in the proportion of MAP2 immunoreactive neurons in the subiculum and, to a somewhat lesser extent, entorhinal cortex compared to controls.[84] It is noteworthy that these are the same regions where decreased neuron size has been reported.[71]

Rosoklija et al.[85] later independently examined subicular MAP2 immunohistochemical optical density in a much larger series of patients and showed the deficit in approximately 1/3 of their sample, but not in normal controls. However, they questioned the disease specificity in that some patients with other neuropsychiatric conditions also showed decreased subicular MAP2. Finally, Cotter et al. examined phosphorylated and nonphosphorylated MAP2 expression in schizophrenia and found an increase in left-sided, nonphosphorylated MAP2 immunodensity in subiculum and CA1, whereas MAP2 immunoreactive neuron counts were similar to those of controls, and there were no associated alterations in interneuronal distance or neuron orientation.[86]

The point at which MAP2 or other as yet undefined cytoskeletal abnormalities may fit in the neurobiologic pathways that ultimately lead to schizophrenia is unclear.

A direct relationship between MAP2 expression and neuronal morphology has not been demonstrated yet. Furthermore, MAP2 expression itself is regulated by a number of neurotransmitters and neurotrophic factors such as glutamate via NMDA receptors, serotonin, nerve growth factor, gangliosides, and both cyclic AMP and phosphoinositol second messenger systems.[87–89] It is possible that abnormalities in these or other mechanisms are the primary culprits. Nonetheless, while still young, these neuronal cytoskeletal studies represent an important effort toward elucidating the molecular neuropathological pathways that might culminate in neuronal morphologic abnormalities in schizophrenia.

STUDIES OF PARAHIPPOCAMPAL CONNECTIVITY

"Miswiring" of the brain is an important hypothetical construct for schizophrenia that holds that the unusual sensory and thought processes and cognitive deficits of schizophrenia arise from aberrant patterns or fidelity of neuroanatomic connections.[90–93] Studies of axons, dendrites, and synapses represent investigational avenues relevant to this hypothesis, but only a few studies have been conducted in the parahippocampal/hippocampal region in schizophrenia. In a Golgi study with Scholl analysis, Rosoklija et al. reported decreases in dendritic spine density and apical dendrite arborization in the subiculum in schizophrenia compared to nonpsychiatric controls.[94] In a small study of the entorhinal cortex in four individuals with schizophrenia, Longson et al.[95] reported that the density of small caliber glutamatergic vertical axons was increased compared to controls. Based on analogy to the known connectional neuroanatomic circuits in nonhuman species, they proposed that this was due to increased extrinsic innervation from the amygdala. In another preliminary study, Akil and Lewis[96] reported a decrease in tyrosine-hydroxylase containing axons to the entorhinal cortex.

Two studies have examined the zinc-rich mossy fiber pathway in the hippocampus in schizophrenia, with conflicting findings. These investigations were prompted by the relationship between hippocampal zinc and learning and memory[97,98] and the possibility that the purported abnormalities in the entorhinal cortex in schizophrenia alter the innervation of the dentate gyrus granule cells, which in turn would lead to alterations of the mossy fiber pathway connecting the dentate gyrus with CA3 and CA4. Such phenomena have been described in experimental animals.[99] Goldsmith and Joyce[100] reported that the optical density of Timm's stained mossy fibers was significantly decreased in the hilus of the dentate gyrus, CA4 and CA3, in their elderly schizophrenia sample compared to both normal elderly and Alzheimer's disease control cases. In contrast, Adams et al.[101] found no differences between schizophrenia, normal control and psychiatric control groups. The basis for the discrepancy is unclear. Adams et al.'s cases were somewhat younger, but otherwise the sample sizes, staining methods, and optical densitometric methods were almost identical.

There have been a number of studies of synapse-related proteins in the parahippocampal/hippocampal region which indicate abnormal synaptic fidelity in various subregions. Immunohistochemical and Western blot studies have found alterations in the expression of synapsin[102] and SNAP-25,[103] while abnormalities in the expression of synaptophysin have been more controversial.[103–105] In situ hybridization studies have found reduced synaptophysin mRNA levels in the hippocampus, subiculum, and entorhinal cortex,[105] as well as reduced growth associated protein-43 (GAP-43)[106] and complexin II.[107]

Regional and Single-Cell mRNA Expression Profiling in the Entorhinal Cortex

Given the various neuroanatomic, neuropsychological, and clinical abnormalities relevant to the entorhinal cortex in schizophrenia, this may be an excellent region in which to screen for abnormalities in multiple molecular pathways. However, the cellular composition of the entorhinal cortex is complex, containing diverse types of neurons, astrocytes, other glia, various innervations, etc. Furthermore, the proportion of the genome that is expressed in a cell-selective manner is large (~70%). Most molecular analysis methods (e.g., Northern blotting, cDNA library construction, etc.) rely on large amounts of tissue, and interpretation of findings derived from such experiments is difficult because the diversity of cells within the tissue dilutes the mRNA from the cells of interest. *In situ* hybridization is useful because of its single-cell resolution; however, it can only examine one or a few mRNAs at a time.

To begin to establish a molecular "fingerprint" for schizophrenia and to identify novel candidate molecular pathways for further in-depth investigation, we recently employed novel single-cell mRNA recovery, aRNA amplification, and cDNA microchip array technology in the entorhinal cortex.[108] After immunohistochemical and morphological identification in paraffin-embedded sections from subjects with schizophrenia and matched controls, mRNA from individual stellate neurons in layer II as well as microdissected layer II/III of the entorhinal cortex was extracted, linearly amplified, and relative abundances determined using several cDNA microchip arrays. Over 25,000 genes were assessed. Forced clustering of the data revealed at least twofold differences between schizophrenics and controls in mRNA expression of various transcription factors (e.g., fos, junB, PML-1, Brg, and Brm), receptors (GABA-A, α-7 nicotinic, interleukin-2, retinoic acid), ion channels (Na^+, K^+, Cl^-), synaptic proteins (syntaxin, synaptotagmins, synaptic vesicle amine transporter, SNAP-25, and γ-adaptin), as well as other known mRNAs and a number of expressed sequence tags. These data provide a preliminary expression profile of schizophrenia, suggesting the involvement of novel genes and pathways in the expression of the disease. Further investigation of candidate genes and pathways identified by this technique will include *in situ* hybridization and immunohistochemistry to confirm and extend the findings.

CONCLUDING REMARKS

While controversies remain, the principal morphologic and molecular neuroanatomic findings in the hippocampal/parahippocampal region in schizophrenia have been entorhinal cytoarchitectural disorganization, smaller neuron size, abnormal cytoskeletal protein expression, aberrant axonal innervation, alterations in synapse-related proteins, and an absence of evidence for neurodegeneration and neural injury. Furthermore, new methods, such as single-cell mRNA profiling are emerging that greatly expand the scope of investigations to encompass simultaneous analysis of multiple genetic pathways. Increased understanding of the coordinated involvement of multiple genes in human disease will provide insight into the molecular basis of the disease and offer new targets for pharmacotherapeutic intervention.

It is difficult at this point to know the extent to which the abnormalities described above are more or less selective for the parahippocampal region. Considerably more work needs to be done. The neuropsychological profile of schizophrenia indicates widespread impairment, but with some special involvement of limbic, temporal, and frontal neural systems. Much attention from neurobiological researchers has rightfully focused on the neuroanatomy, neurochemistry, and functioning of regions within these systems. However, there are also numerous data indicating neurobiological abnormalities elsewhere in the central nervous system.[109–111] Thus, it is possible that some as yet undefined neurobiological abnormalities associated with schizophrenia are present throughout the nervous system. The reason why the predominant symptoms of schizophrenia may preferentially involve higher cognitive, emotional, and social domains could be that the cellular/molecular abnormalities of schizophrenia become most eloquent in brain regions that are of high connectional complexity, high plasticity, or prolonged maturation, like the entorhinal cortex and hippocampus.

ACKNOWLEDGMENTS

Research from our laboratory described here was supported by the National Institutes of Health, the Theodore and Vada Stanley Foundation, and the National Alliance for Research on Schizophrenia and Depression.

REFERENCES

1. ARNOLD, S.E. & J.Q. TROJANOWSKI. 1996. Recent advances in defining the neuropathology of schizophrenia. Acta Neuropathol. **92:** 217–231.
2. ARNOLD, S.E. 1997. The medial temporal lobe in schizophrenia. J. Neurosychiatry Clin. Neurosci. **9:** 460–470.
3. HARRISON, P.J. 1999. The neuropathology of schizophrenia. A critical review of the data and their interpretation. Brain **112:** 593–624.
4. DAVISON, K. 1983. Schizophrenia-like psychoses associated with organic cerebral disorders: a review. Psychiatr. Dev. **1:** 1–34.
5. JACOBI, W. & H. WINKLER. 1929. Untersuchungen des Liquor Cerebrospinalis mit dem Zeisschen Spektographen für Chemiker. Deutsche Z. Nervenheilkunde **111:** 5–18.
6. ELLINGSON, R.J. 1954. The incidence of EEG abnormality among patients with mental disorders of apparaently nonorganic origin: a critical review. Am. J. Psychiatry **111:** 263–285.
7. SAYKIN, A.J., R.C. GUR, R.E. GUR, D. MOZLEY, L.H. MOZLEY, S.M. RESNICK, B. KESTER & P. STAFINIAK. 1991. Neuropsychological function in schizophrenia: selective impairment in memory and learning. Arch. Gen. Psychiatry **48:** 618–624.
8. GRUZELIER, J., K. SEYMOUR & J. WILSON. 1988. Impairments on neuropsychological tests of temporohippocampal and frontohippocampal functions and word fluency in remitting schizophrenic and affective disorders. Arch. Gen. Psychiatry **45:** 623–629.
9. GUR, R.E., P. COWELL, B.I. TURETSKY, F. GALLACHER, T. CANNON, W. BILKER & R.C. GUR. 1998. A follow-up MRI study of schizophrenia: relationship of neuroanatomic changes with clinical and neurobehavioral measures. Arch. Gen. Psychiatry. **55:** 145–152.
10. KELSOE, J.R., J.L. CADET, D. PICKAR & D.R. WEINBERGER. 1988. Quantitative neuroanatomy in schizophrenia: a controlled magnetic resonance imaging study. Arch. Gen. Psychiatry **45:** 533–541.
11. PEARLSON, G.D., W.S. KIM, K.L. KUBOS, P.J. MOBERG, G. JAYARAM, M.J. BASCOM, G.A. CHASE, A.D. GOLDFINGER & L.E. TUNE. 1989. Ventricle-brain ratio, computed tomographic density, and brain area in 50 schizophrenics. Arch. Gen. Psychiatry **46:** 690–697.
12. BECKER, T., K. ELMER, F. SCHNEIDER, M. SCHNEIDER, W. GRODD, M. BARTELS, S. HECKERS & H. BECKMANN. 1996. Confirmation of reduced temporal limbic structure

volume on magnetic resonance imaging in male patients with schizophrenia. Psychiatry Res. **67:** 135–143.

13. SUDDATH, R.L., M.F. CASANOVA, T.E. GOLDBERG, D.G. DANIEL, J.R. KELSOE, JR. & D.R. WEINBERGER. 1989. Temporal lobe pathology in schizophrenia: a quantitative magnetic resonance imaging study. Am. J. Psychiatry **146:** 464–472.

14. SUDDATH, R.L., G.W. CHRISTISON, E.F. TORREY & D.R. WEINBERGER. 1990. Cerebral anatomic abnormalities in monozygotic twins discordant for schizophrenia. N. Engl. J. Med. **322:** 789–794.

15. BOGERTS, B., M. ASHTARI, G. DEGREEF, J. ALVIR, R.M. BILDER & J.A. LIEBERMAN. 1990. Reduced temporal limbic structure volumes on magnetic resonance images in first episode schizophrenia. Psychiatry Res. Neuroimaging **35:** 1–13.

16. BREIER, A., R.W. BUCHANAN, A. ELKASHEF, R.C. MUNSON, B. KIRKPATRICK & F. GELLAD. 1992. Brain morphology and schizophrenia. A magnetic resonance imaging study of limbic, prefrontal cortex, and caudate structures. Arch. Gen. Psychiatry **49:** 921–926.

17. BOGERTS, B., E. MEERTZ & R. SCHONFELDT-BAUSCH. 1985. Basal ganglia and limbic system pathology in schizophrenia. Arch. Gen. Psychiatry **42:** 784–791.

18. JESTE, D.V. & J.B. LOHR. 1989. Hippocampal pathologic findings in schizophrenia: a morphometric study. Arch. Gen. Psychiatry **46:** 1019–1024.

19. BOGERTS, B., P. FALKAI, M. HAUPTS, B. GREVE, S. ERNST, U. TAPERNON-FRANZ & U. HEINZMANN. 1990. Post-mortem volume measurements of limbic system and basal ganglia structures in chronic schizophrenics. Initial results from a new brain collection. Schizophr. Res. **3:** 295–301.

20. FALKAI, P., B. BOGERTS & M. ROZUMEK. 1988. Limbic pathology in schizophrenia: the entorhinal region—a morphometric study. Biol. Psychiatry **24:** 515–521.

21. BROWN, R., N. COLTER, J.A.N. CORSELLIS, T.J. CROW, C.D. FRITH, R. JAGOE, E.C. JOHNSTONE & L. MARSH. 1986. Postmortem evidence of structural brain changes in schizophrenia. Arch. Gen. Psychiatry **43:** 36–42.

22. COLTER, N., S. BATTAL, T.J. CROW, E.C. JOHNSTONE, R. BROWN & C. BRUTON. 1987. White matter reduction in the parahippocampal gyrus of patients with schizophrenia. Arch. Gen. Psychiatry **44:** 1023.

23. ALTSHULER, L.L., M.F. CASANOVA, T.E. GOLDBERG & J.E. KLEINMAN. 1990. The hippocampus and parahippocampus in schizophrenic, suicide, and control brains. Arch. Gen. Psychiatry **44:** 1094–1098.

24. BRUTON, C.J., T.J. CROW, C.D. FRITH, E.C. JOHNSTONE, D.G.C. OWENS & G.W. ROBERTS. 1990. Schizophrenia and the brain: a prospective clinico-neuropathological study. Psychol. Med. **20:** 285–304.

25. BENES, F.M., I. SORENSEN & E.D. BIRD. 1991. Reduced neuronal size in posterior hippocampus of schizophrenic patients. Schizophr. Bull. **17:** 597–608.

26. HECKERS, S., H. HEINSEN, Y.C. HEINSEN & H. BECKMANN. 1990. Limbic structures and lateral ventricle in schizophrenia: a quantitative postmortem study. Arch. Gen. Psychiatry **47:** 1016–1022.

27. SHENTON, M.E., R. KIKINIS & F.A. JOLESZ. 1992. Abnormalities of the left temporal lobe and thought disorder in schizophrenia: a quantitative magnetic resonance imaging study. N. Engl. J. Med. **327:** 604–612.

28. NESTOR, P.G., M.E. SHENTON, R.W. MCCARLEY, J. HAIMSON, R.S. SMITH, B. O'DONNELL, M. KIMBLE, R. KIKINIS & F.A. JOLESZ. 1993. Neuropsychological correlates of MRI temporal lobe abnormalities in schizophrenia. Am. J. Psychiatry **150:** 1849–1855.

29. BOGERTS, B., J.A. LIEBERMAN, M. ASHTARI, R.M. BILDER, G. DEGREEF, G. LERNER, C. JOHNS & S. MASIAR. 1993. Hippocampus-amygdala volumes and psychopathology in chronic schizophrenia. Biol. Psychiatry **33:** 236–246.

30. FRISTON, K.J., P.F. LIDDLE, C.D. FRITH, S.R. HIRSCH & R.S. FRACKOWIAK. 1992. The left medial temporal region and schizophrenia. A PET study. Brain **115:** 367–382.

31. SCHROEDER, J., M.S. BUCHSBAUM, B.V. SIEGEL, F.J. GEIDER & R. NIETHAMMER. 1995. Structural and functional correlates of subsyndromes in chronic schizophrenia. Psychopathology **28:** 38–45.

32. SILBERSWEIG, D.A., E. STERN, C. FRITH, C. CAHILL, A. HOLMES, S. GROOTOONK, J. SEEAWARD, P. MCKENNA, S.E. CHUA, L. SCHNORR, *et al.* 1995. A functional neuroanatomy of hallucinations in schizophrenia. Nature **378:** 176–179.

33. SAYKIN, A.J., H.J. RIORDAN, J.B. WEAVER, T.C. MASCHRECK, L.A. FLASHMAN, E.M. KAHN, K.A. FLANNERY, A. MAMOURIAN & T.W. MCALLISTER. 1995. Memory activation in schizophrenia—preliminary observations using functional magnetic resonance imaging (FMRI). Schizophr. Res. **15:** 97.

34. MOREL, B.A. 1860. Maladies Mentales. Masson. Paris.

35. KRAEPELIN, E. 1919. Dementia Praecox and Paraphrenia. Livingstone. Edinburgh.

36. DELISI, L.E., W. TEW, S.H. XIE, A.L. HOFF, M. SAKUMA, M. KUSHNER, G. LEE, K. SHEDLACK, A. M. SMITH & R. GRIMSON. 1995. A prospective follow-up study of brain morphology and cognition in first-episode schizophrenic patients—preliminary findings. Biol. Psychiatry **38:** 349–360.

37. DAVIDSON, M., P.D. HARVEY, P. POWCHIK, M. PARELLA, L. WHITE, H.Y. KNOBLER, M.F. LOSONCZY, R.S.E. KEEFE, S. KATZ & E. FRECSKA. 1995. Severity of symptoms in chronically institutionalized geriatric schizophrenic patients. Am. J. Psychiatry **152:** 197–207.

38. ARNOLD, S.E., R.E. GUR, R.M. SHAPIRO, K.R. FISHER, P.J. MOBERG, M.R. GIBNEY, R.C. GUR, P. BLACKWELL & J.Q. TROJANOWSKI. 1995. Prospective clinicopathological studies of schizophrenia: accrual and assessment. Am. J. Psychiatry **152:** 731–737.

39. MOBERG, P.J., R. MAHR, M. GIBNEY, S.E. ARNOLD, R. SHAPIRO, A. KUMAR, G. GOTTLIEB & R.E. GUR. 1995. Neuropsychological functioning in elderly patients with schizophrenia and Alzheimer's disease. J. Int. Neuropsychol. Soc. **1:** 132.

40. KURTZ, M.M., P.J. MOBERG, L. HARPER-MOZLEY, T. HICKEY, S.E. ARNOLD & R.E. GUR. 2000. The relationship of neuropsychological impairment to functional outcome in elderly patients with schizophrenia. Submitted.

41. GOLIER, J.A., M. DAVIDSON, V. HAROUTUNIAN, P. POWCHIK, D. PUROHIT, D. PERL & K.L. DAVIS. 1995. Neuropathological study of 101 elderly schizophrenics: preliminary findings. Schizophr. Res. **15:** 120.

42. BRAAK, H. & E. BRAAK. 1991. Neuropathological staging of Alzheimer-related changes. Acta Neuropathol. **82:** 239–259.

43. ARNOLD, S.E., B.T. HYMAN, J. FLORY, A.R. DAMASIO & G.W.V. HOESEN. 1991. The topographical and neuroanatomical distribution of neurofibrillary tangles and neuritic plaques in the cerebral cortex of patients with Alzheimer's disease. Cereb. Cortex **1:** 103–116.

44. CASANOVA, M.F., N.W. CAROSELLA, J.M. GOLD, J.E. KLEINMAN, D.R. WEINBERGER & R.E. POWERS. 1993. A topographical study of senile plaques and neurofibrillary tangles in the hippocampi of patients with Alzheimer's disease and cognitively impaired patients with schizophrenia. Psychiatry Res. **49:** 41–62.

45. ARNOLD, S.E., B.R. FRANZ & J.Q. TROJANOWSKI. 1994. Elderly patients with schizophrenia exhibit infrequent neurodegenerative lesions. Neurobiol. Aging **15:** 299–303.

46. ARNOLD, S.E., B.R. FRANZ, J.Q. TROJANOWSKI, P.J. MOBERG & R.E. GUR. 1996. Glial fibrillary acidic protein immunoreactive astrocytosis in elderly patients with schizophrenia and dementia. Acta Neuropathol. **91:** 269–277.

47. POWCHIK, P., M. DAVIDSON, C.B. NEMEROFF, V. HAROUTUNIAN, D.P. PUROHIT, M. LOSONCZY, G. BISSETTE, D. PERL, H. GHANBARI, B. MILLER & K. DAVIS. 1993. Alzheimer's-disease-related protein in geriatric schizophrenic patients with cognitive impairment. Am. J. Psychiatry **150:** 1726–1727.

48. PUROHIT, D.P., D.P. PERL, V. HAROUTUNIAN, P. POWCHIK, M. DAVIDSON & K.L. DAVIS. 1998. Alzheimer disease and related neurodegenerative diseases in elderly patients with schizophrenia: a postmortem neuropathologic study of 100 cases. Arch. Gen. Psychiatry **55:** 205–211.

49. ARNOLD, S.E., J.Q. TROJANOWSKI, R.E. GUR, L.-Y. HAN & C. CHOI. 1998. Absence of neurodegeneration and neural injury in the cerebral cortex in a sample of elderly patients with schizophrenia. Arch. Gen. Psychiatry **55:** 225–232.

50. ARNOLD, S.E., J.Q. TROJANOWSKI & P. PARCHI. 1999. Protease resistant prion proteins are not present in sporadic "poor outcome" schizophrenia. J. Neurol. Neurosurg. Psychiatry **66:** 90–92.

51. CROW, T.J., J. BALL, S.R. BLOOM, R. BROWN, C.J. BRUTON, N. COLTER, C.D. FRITH, E.C. JOHNSTONE, D.G. OWENS & G.W. ROBERTS. 1989. Schizophrenia as an anomaly of development of cerebral asymmetry. A postmortem study and a proposal concerning the genetic basis of the disease. Arch. Gen. Psychiatry **46:** 1145–1150.

52. FALKAI, P., B. BOGERTS, B. GREVE, U. PFEIFFER, B. MACHUS, B. FOLSCH-REETZ, C. MAJTENYI & I. OVARY. 1992. Loss of sylvian fissure assymmetry in schizophrenia. A quantitative post mortem study. Schizophr. Res. **7**: 23–32.
53. ROBERTS, G.W., N. COLTER, R. LOFTHOUSE, E.C. JOHNSTONE & T.J. CROW. 1987. Is there gliosis in schizophrenia? Investigation of the temporal lobe. Biol. Psychiatry **22**: 1459–1468.
54. JAKOB, H. & H. BECKMANN. 1986. Prenatal developmental disturbances in the limbic allocortex in schizophrenics. J. Neural Transm. **65**: 303–326.
55. BRAAK, H. 1980. Architectonics of the Human Telencephalic Cortex. Springer. Berlin.
56. JAKOB, H. & H. BECKMANN. 1994. Cicumscribed malformation and nerve cell alterations in the entorhinal cortex of schizophrenics. Pathogenetic and clinical aspects. J. Neural Transm. **98**: 83–106.
57. ARNOLD, S.E., B.T. HYMAN, G.W.V. HOESEN & A.R. DAMASIO. 1991. Some cytoarchitectural abnormalities of the entorhinal cortex in schizophrenia. Arch. Gen. Psychiatry **48**: 625–632.
58. LIPSKA, B.K., G.E. JASKIW & D.R. WEINBERGER. 1993. Postpubertal emergence of hyperresponsiveness to stress and to amphetamine after neonatal excitotoxic hippocampal damage: a potential animal model of schizophrenia. Neuropsychopharmacology **9**: 67–75.
59. TALAMINI, L.M., T. KOCH, G.J. TER HORST & J. KORF. 1998. Methylazoxymethanol acetate-induced abnormalities in the entorhinal cortex of the rat; parallels with morphological findings in schizophrenia. Brain Res. **789**: 293–306.
60. HEINSEN, H., E. GROSSMAN, U. RUB, W. EISENMENGER, M. BAUER, G. ULMAR, B. BETHKE, M. SCHULER, H.-P. SCHMITT, M. GOTZ, U. LOCKEMANN & K. PUSCHEL. 1996. Variability in the human entorhinal region may confound neuropsychiatric diagnoses. Acta Anatomica **157**: 226–237.
61. BERNSTEIN, H.G., D. KRELL, B. BAUMANN, P. DANOS, P. FALKAI, S. DIEKMANN, H. HENNING & B. BOGERTS. 1998. Morphometric studies of the entorhinal cortex in neuropsychiatric patients and controls: clusters of heterotopically displaced lamina II neurons are not indicative of schizophrenia. Schizophr. Res. **33**: 125–132.
62. AKIL, M. & D.A. LEWIS. 1997. Cytoarchitecture of the entorhinal cortex in schizophrenia. Am. J. Psychiatry **154**: 1010–1012.
63. KRIMER, L.S., M.M. HERMAN, R.C. SAUNDERS, J.C. BOYD, T.M. HYDE, J.M. CARTER, J.E. KLEINMAN & D.R. WEINBERGER. 1997. A qualitative and quantitative analysis of the entorhinal cortex in schizophrenia. Cereb. Cortex **7**: 732–739.
64. ARNOLD, S.E., L.-Y. HAN & D.D. RUSCHEINSKY. 1997. Further evidence of cytoarchitectural abnormalities of the entorhinal cortex in schizophrenia using spatial point pattern analyses. Biol. Psychiatry **42**: 639–647.
65. FALKAI, P., T. SCHNEIDER-AXMANN & W.G. HONER. 2000. Entorhinal cortex pre-alpha cell clusters in schizophrenia: quantitative evidence of a developmental abnormality. Submitted.
66. ARNOLD, S.E. & J.Q. TROJANOWSKI. 1996. Human fetal hippocampal development. I. Cytoarchitecture, myeloarchitecture and neuronal morphology. J. Comp. Neurol. **367**: 274–292.
67. MATTSON, M.P. 1989. Cellular signaling mechanisms common to the development and degeneration of neuroarchitecture. A review. Mech. Ageing Dev. **50**: 103–157.
68. NOWAKOWSKI, R.S. & P. RAKIC. 1981. The site of origin and route and rate of migration of neurons to the hippocmapal region in the rhesus monkey. J. Comp. Neurol. **196**: 129–154.
69. WEST, M.J. 1993. New stereological methods for counting neurons. Neurobiol. Aging **14**: 287–293.
70. CASANOVA, M.F., N. CAROSELLA & J.E. KLEINMAN. 1990. Neuropathological findings in a suspected case of childhood schizophrenia. J. Neuropsychiatry Clin. Neurosci. **2**: 313–319.
71. ARNOLD, S.E., B.R. FRANZ, R.C. GUR, R.E. GUR, R.M. SHAPIRO, P.J. MOBERG & J.Q. TROJANOWSKI. 1995. Smaller neuron size in schizophrenia in hippocampal subfields that mediate cortical-hippocampal interactions. Am. J. Psychiatry **152**: 738–748.

72. HECKERS, S., H. HEINSEN, B. GEIGER & H. BECKMANN. 1991. Hippocampal neuron number in schizophrenia. A stereological study. Arch. Gen. Psychiatry **48:** 1002–1008.
73. FALKAI, P. & B. BOGERTS. 1986. Cell loss in the hippocampus of schizophrenics. Eur. Arch. Psychiatry Neurol. Sci. **236:** 154–161.
74. KOVELMAN, J.A. & A.B. SCHEIBEL. 1984. A neurohistological correlate of schizophrenia. Biol. Psychiatry **19:** 1601–1621.
75. ZAIDEL, D.W., M.M. ESIRI & P.J. HARRISON. 1997. The hippocampus in schizophrenia: lateralized increase in neuronal density and altered cytoarchitectural asymmetry. Psychol. Med. **27:** 703–713.
76. BENES, F.M., E.W. KWOK, S.L. VINCENT & M.S. TODTENKOPF. 1998. A reduction of nonpyramidal cells in sector CA2 of schizophrenics and manic depressives. Biol. Psychiatry **44:** 88–97.
77. ZAIDEL, D.W., M.M. ESIRI & P.J. HARRISON. 1997. Size, shape, and orientation of neurons in the left and right hippocampus: Investigations of normal asymmetries and alterations in schizophrenia. Am. J. Psychiatry **154:** 812–818.
78. GLANTZ, L.A. & D.A. LEWIS. 1995. Assessment of spine density on layer III pyramidal cells in the prefrontal cortex of schizophrenic subjects. Soc. Neurosci. Abstr. **21:** 239.
79. LEWIS, D.A. & L.A. GLANTZ. 1997. Specificity of decreased spine density on layer III pyramidal cells in schizophrenia. Schizophr. Res. **24:** 39.
80. AGANOVA, E.A. & N.A. URANOVA. 1992. Morphometric analysis of synaptic contacts in the anterior limbic cortex in the endogenous psychoses. Neurosci. Behav. Physiol. **22:** 59–65.
81. GAREY, L.J., W.Y. ONG, T.S. PATEL, M. KANANI, A. DAVIS, C. HORNSTEIN & M. BAUER. 1995. Reduction in dendritic spine number on cortical pyramidal neurons in schizophrenia. Soc. Neurosci. Abstr. **21:** 237.
82. BURGOYNE, R.D., Ed.. 1991. The Neuronal Cytoskeleton. Wiley-Liss. New York.
83. ARNOLD, S.E., V.M.Y. LEE, R.E. GUR & J.Q. TROJANOWSKI. 1991. Abnormal expression of two microtubule-associated proteins (MAP2 and MAP5) in specific subfields of the hippocampal formation in schizophrenia. Proc. Natl. Acad. Sci. USA **88:** 10850–10854.
84. ARNOLD, S.E., L.-Y. HAN, L. RIOUX & E. FALKE. 1999. Abnormal MAP2 neuron representation in subiculum and entorhinal cortex in poor-outcome schizophrenia. Soc. Neurosci. Abstr. **25:** 575.
85. ROSOKLIJA, G., M.A. KAUFMAN, D. LIU, A.P. HAYS, N. LATOV, C. WANIEK, J.G. KEILP, A. WU, S.A. SADIQ, J. GORMAN, I. PROHOVNIK & A.J. DWORK. 1995. Subicular MAP-2 immunoreactivity in schizophrenia. Soc. Neurosci. Abstr. **21:** 2126.
86. COTTER, D., R. KERWIN, B. DOSHI, C.S. MARTIN & I.P. EVERALL. 1997. Alterations in hippocampal non-phosphorylated MAP2 protein expression in schizophrenia. Brain Res. **765:** 238–246.
87. HALPAIN, S. 1996. Dynamic regulation of MAP2 in living neurons. J. Neurochem. **66:** S33.
88. PEREZ, J., S. MORI, M. CAIVANO, M. POPOLI, R. ZANARDI, E. SMERALDI & G. RACAGNI. 1995. Effects of fluvoxamine on the protein phosphorylation system associated with rat neuronal microtubules. Eur. Neuropsychopharmacol. Suppl.: S65–69.
89. SANO, M., R. KATOH-SEMBA, S. KITAJIMA & C. SATO. 1990. Changes in levels of microtubule-associated proteins in relation to the outgrowth of neurites form PC12D cells, a forskolin- and nerve growth factor-responsive subline of PC12 pheochromocytoma cells. Brain Res. **510:** 269–276.
90. FRITH, C.D. & D.J. DONE. 1988. Towards a neuropsychology of schizophrenia. Br. J. Psychiatry **153:** 437–443.
91. GRAY, J.A., J. FELDON, J.N.P. RAWLINS, D.R. HELMSLEY & A.D. SMITH. 1991. The neuropsychology of schizophrenia. Behav. Brain Sci. **14:** 1–84.
92. BENES, F.M. 1993. Neurobiological investigations in cingulate cortex of schizophrenic brain. Schizophr. Bull. **19:** 537–549.
93. STEVENS, J.R., M. CASANOVA, M. POLTORAK, L. GERMAIN & G.C. BUCHAN. 1992. Comparison of immunocytochemical and Holzer's methods for detection of acute chronic gliosis in human postmortem material. J. Neuropsychiatry Clin. Neurosci. **4:** 168–173.

94. ROSOKLIJA, G., G. TOOMAYAN & A.J. DWORK. 1999. Golgi studies of the subiculum in severe psychiatric illness. J. Neuropathol. Exp. Neurol. **58:** 549.
95. LONGSON, D., J.F.W. DEAKIN & F.M. BENES. 1996. Increased density of entorhinal glutamate-immunoreactive vertical fibers in schizophrenia. J. Neural Transm. **103:** 503–507.
96. AKIL, M. & D.A. LEWIS. 1995. The catecholaminergic innervation of the human entorhinal cortex: alterations in schizophrenia. Soc. Neurosci. Abstr. **21:** 238.
97. FREDERICKSON, R.E., C.J. FREDERICKSON & G. DANSCHER. 1990. *In situ* binding of bouton zinc reversibly disrupts performance on a spatial memory task. Behav. Brain Res. **38:** 25–33.
98. GUIDOLIN, D., P. POLATO, G. VENTURIN, A. ZANOTTI, E. MOCCHEGIANI, N. FABRIS & M.G. NUNZI. 1992. Correlation between zinc level in mossy fibers and spatial memory in aged rats. Ann. N.Y. Acad. Sci. **673:** 187–193.
99. STEWARD, O. 1992. Lesion-induced synapse reorganization in the hippocampus of cats: Sprouting of entorhinal, commisural/associational, and mossy fiber projections after unilateral entorhinal cortex lesions, with comments on the normal organization of these pathways. Hippocampus **2:** 247–268.
100. GOLDSMITH, S.K. & J.N. JOYCE. 1995. Alterations in hippocampal mossy fiber pathway in schizophrenia and Alzheimer's disease. Biol. Psychiatry **37:** 122–126.
101. ADAMS, C.E., B K. DEMASTERS & R. FREEDMAN. 1995. Regional zinc staining in postmortem hippocampus form schizophrenic patients. Schizophr. Res. **18:** 71–77.
102. BROWNING, M.D., E.M. DUDEK, J.L. RAPIER, S. LEONARD & R. FREEDMAN. 1993. Significant reductions in synapsin but not synaptophysin-specific activity in the brains of some schizophrenics. Biol. Psychiatry **34:** 529–535.
103. YOUNG, C.E., K. ARIMA, J. XIE, L. HU, T.G. BEACH, P. FALKAI & W.G. HONER. 1998. SNAP-25 deficit and hippocampal connectivity in schizophrenia. Cereb. Cortex **8:** 261–268.
104. EASTWOOD, S.L. & P.J. HARRISON. 1995. Decreased synaptophysin in the medial temporal lobe in schizophrenia demonstrated using immunoautoradiography. Neuroscience **69:** 339–343.
105. EASTWOOD, S.L., P.W.J. BURNET & P.J. HARRISON. 1995. Altered synaptophysin expression as a marker of synaptic pathology in schizophrenia. Neuroscience **66:** 309–319.
106. EASTWOOD, S.L. & P.J. HARRISON. 1998. Hippocampal and cortical growth-associated protein-43 messenger RNA in schizophrenia. Neuroscience **86:** 437–448.
107. HARRISON, P.J. & S.L. EASTWOOD. 1998. Preferential involvement of excitatory neurons in medial temporal lobe in schizophrenia [see comments] [published erratum in Lancet 1999 Jan. 9; **353**(9147): 154]. Lancet **352:** 1669–1673.
108. HEMBY, S.E., S.D. GINSBURG, K. BECKER, B. BRUNK, S.E. ARNOLD, C. OVERTON, J.Q. TROJANOWSKI & J.J. EBERWINE. 2000. A mRNA expression profile for schizophrenia: single-neuron transcription patterns from the entorhinal cortex. Submitted.
109. GREEN, M. & E. WALKER. 1986. Symptom correlates of vulnerability to backward masking in schizophrenia. Am. J. Psychiatry **143:** 181–186.
110. PURI, B.K., N.J. DAVEY, P.H. ELLAWAY & S.W. LEWIS. 1996. An investigation of motor function in schizophrenia using transcranial magnetic stimulation of the motor cortex. Br. J. Psychiatry **169:** 690–695.
111. SCHRODER, J., M.S. BUCHSBAUM, B.V. SIEGEL, F.J. GEIDER, J. LOHR, C. TANG, J. WU & S.G. POTKIN. 1996. Cerebral metabolic activity correlates of subsyndromes in chronic schizophrenia. Schizophr. Res. **19:** 41–53.
112. JAKOB, H. & H. BECKMANN. 1989. Gross and histological criteria for deveopmental disorders in brains of schizophrenics. J. R. Soc. Med. **82:** 466–46.

Amygdalo-Entorhinal Inputs to the Hippocampal Formation in Relation to Schizophrenia

FRANCINE M. BENES[a] AND SABINA BERRETTA

Laboratory for Structural Neuroscience, McLean Hospital, Belmont, Massachusetts, USA, and Program in Neuroscience and Department of Psychiatry, Harvard Medical School, Boston, Massachusetts, USA

ABSTRACT: This chapter reviews recent postmortem studies of schizophrenic brain and discusses the potential role of the amygdala in the induction of hippocampal abnormalities in this disorder. Based on available evidence, sectors CA4, CA3, and CA2, but not CA1, show preferential changes in schizophrenic subjects, although the most pronounced changes have been found in CA3 and CA2. It seems likely that the amygdala would contribute in some way to the induction of abnormalities along the trisynaptic pathway via its direct input to sectors CA3 and CA2, as well as an indirect one that involves the entorhinal cortex and its perforant path projection to the area dentata. The postmortem findings reported to date have been integrated into a working model in which decreases of inhibitory GABAergic modulation are invoked to explain the observation from a recent PET scan study (Heckers *et al.*, 1999) that baseline metabolic activity in the hippocampus of schizophrenics is increased. In addition, however, the apparent inability of schizophrenics to increase metabolic activity in the hippocampus when challenged with a memory retrieval task may reflect a disturbance of disinhibitory modulation postulated herein to occur in sector CA3, a key relay point along the trisynaptic pathway. Overall, it seems plausible that an increase of excitatory activity entering the hippocampus from the basolateral complex via both direct and indirect pathways may make a significant contribution to the pathophysiology of schizophrenia.

INTRODUCTION

Many investigators conducting postmortem studies on schizophrenic brain have focused their attention on the hippocampus because of its strategic location within the corticolimbic system and the likelihood that it may contribute to the cognitive and emotional disturbances commonly seen in this disorder.[1] Consistent with this idea, several histopathologic studies have reported significant structural alterations in this region in schizophrenics, including shrinkage[2] and pyramidal cell loss.[3,4] Although more recent studies have failed to replicate the finding of neuronal loss,[5–7] one recent report has detected a highly selective decrease of nonpyramidal neurons (NPs) in sector CA2 of schizophrenic brain.[8] Since evidence for a gliotic reaction is

[a]Address for correspondence: Francine M. Benes, M.D., Ph.D., McLean Hospital, 115 Mill Street, Belmont, MA 02478. Tel.: (617) 855-2401; fax: (617) 855-3199.
e-mail: benesf@mclean.harvard.edu

lacking, these changes are believed to be related to a neurodevelopmental disturbance,[9] although an excitotoxic mechanism could nevertheless play a contributory role in the pathophysiology of schizophrenia.[10]

ALTERATIONS OF THE HIPPOCAMPAL GLUTAMATE AND GABA SYSTEMS IN SCHIZOPHRENIA

There is evidence that schizophrenia may involve abnormalities of the glutamate and GABA neurotransmitter systems that are known to play a role in excitotoxic injury. In the hippocampal formation, a reduction of non-NMDA glutamate receptors, particularly those that are sensitive to kainate, and associated mRNA has been observed in sectors CA2, CA3, and CA4 of patients with this disorder,[11–13] while little change in NMDA or AMPA receptors was observed.[11] More recently, a significant reduction of immunoreactivity for the $GluR_{5,6,7}$ subunits of the kainate receptor has been found on apical dendrites of pyramidal neurons in the stratum radiatum and stratum pyramidale of sectors CA3, CA2, and proximal portions of CA1, although the greatest absolute change occurred in CA2.[14] Although it is possible that the reduction of kainate receptors is the result of a primary genetic anomaly, it is equally plausible that a reduction of kainate-sensitive glutamate binding may represent a compensatory downregulation in response to increased incoming excitatory activity. If this latter hypothesis were correct, it would be consistent with the idea that an excitotoxic mechanism mediated through the kainate receptor might play a role in the changes seen in the hippocampus of schizophrenics. This idea is appealing because some believe that GABAergic cells in the hippocampus are particularly sensitive to kainate receptor-mediated injury.[15–20] In any case, it seems plausible that an increase of glutamatergic activity mediated by this receptor could potentially contribute to disturbances in the relay of impulses along the trisynaptic pathway.

Other evidence for disturbances of neurotransmission in the hippocampus of schizophrenics has pointed to the GABA system. For example, recent studies have demonstrated a reduction of high-affinity GABA uptake[21] and increased $GABA_A$ receptor binding activity[22,23] in schizophrenics. In the case of the latter study, the findings were most strikingly present in sectors CA4, CA3, and CA2, whereas CA1 showed only a small difference (FIG. 1). Interestingly, using a high-resolution autoradiographic approach, a preferential increase of $GABA_A$ receptor binding has been detected on NPs of sector CA3, a pattern suggestive of reduced disinhibitory activity in this subregion of schizophrenic brain. In sector CA1, however, the only significant difference was a modest 15% increase of $GABA_A$ receptor binding activity that was found selectively on pyramidal neurons. The cellular distribution in CA1 was similar to that seen previously in both the anterior cingulate[24] and prefrontal[22] cortices and was interpreted as reflecting a compensatory upregulation of this receptor in response to a decrease of GABAergic inhibition of projection neurons. It is noteworthy that an analysis of puncta immunoreactive for the 65 kDa isoform of glutamate decarboxylase (GAD_{65}) has demonstrated no overall differences in the density of GABAergic terminals. Notably, however, neuroleptic-free schizophrenics had the lowest density, whereas those treated with these drugs showed a dose-related increase of GAD_{65} terminals.[25] It is possible that antipsychotic medications may be capable of acting, at least in part, by inducing an increase of GABAergic terminals in the hippocampus of the schizophrenic brain. This conclusion is consistent with findings in rat medial prefrontal cortex where chronic haloperidol administration was associated with a marked increase in the numerical density of GABA-immunoreactive terminals forming axosomatic contacts with pyramidal neurons.[26] Thus, it appears that neuroleptic drugs may be capable of inducing neuroplastic changes in GABAergic terminals that could help compensate for a decrease in the activity of this system.

Taken together, the above changes in schizophrenics have suggested that alterations of the corticolimbic system may involve both the glutamate and GABA systems. Furthermore, the changes noted at the local circuitry level seem to vary on a region-by-region and perhaps even subregional basis and may reflect the unique aspects of connectivity found within this complex system.[27] Clearly, a better understanding of how the connections between the major components of the corticolimbic system may be altered can help provide us with a better understanding of the pathophysiology of schizophrenia.

POTENTIAL INVOLVEMENT OF THE AMYGDALA IN SCHIZOPHRENIA

The amygdala is a component of the limbic system that plays a pivotal role in the integration of emotional experience and the stress response.[28] The hypothesis that this region may play a role in the pathophysiology of schizophrenia has been suggested, in part, by the fact that this region sends a massive projection to layer II of the anterior cingulate cortex where several microscopic anomalies have been observed in schizophrenia.[29,30,6,31,24,25] More direct evidence, however, comes from the report of a decrease of high-affinity GABA uptake in the amygdala of the postmortem schizophrenic brain.[21] It is relevant, therefore, to consider more closely the specific ways in which this region interacts with the hippocampal formation, particularly because both of these regions have been found to show volume reduction in brain imaging studies of schizophrenia (for a detailed review, see Lawrie and Abukmeil[32]).

The basolateral subdivision of the amygdala comprises a frontotemporal system that innervates several key components of the corticolimbic system, including the hippocampal formation.[34] The projections of the amygdala to the hippocampus are rather complex and include the perforant pathway terminations in the stratum moleculare of the area dentata, as well as various other fiber systems that enter the CA subfields either through the stratum oriens (i.e., to CA3) or the stratum moleculare.[34] The direct projections of the basolateral complex to the CA subfields, together with its indirect influences exerted via the entorhinal region, constitute a compelling network to consider in relation to schizophrenia. Interestingly, blockade of the $GABA_A$ receptor results in marked changes in the regulation of emotional responses mediated by this region.[35–37] Because a dysfunction of the GABA system is believed to occur in the amygdala in schizophrenia (see above), an increased outflow of activity from this latter region to the entorhinal region and hippocampus could contribute to the disturbances in affective experience and the heightened response to stress that are observed in this disorder.

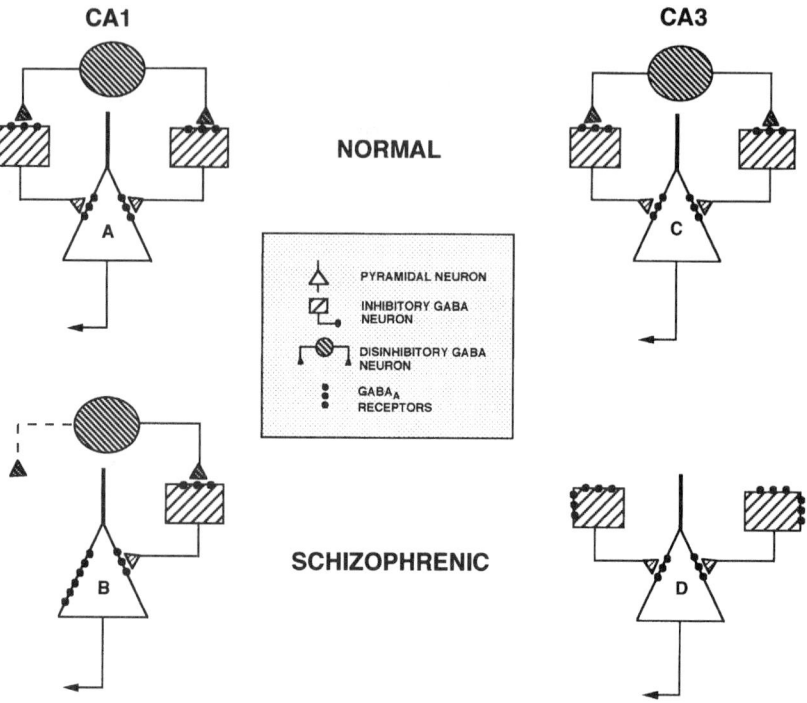

FIGURE 1. Depiction of changes in GABA$_A$ receptor binding activity (*black circles*) on pyramidal (**A, B, C,** and **D**) and nonpyramidal neurons in sectors CA1 and CA3 of the hippocampus in normal control and schizophrenic brain. **Sector CA1:** Pyramidal neuron A shows three GABA$_A$ receptors in relation to each inhibitory GABA input. Pyramidal neuron B in the schizophrenic circuit also shows three GABA$_A$ receptors near the intact GABA cell, but six receptors on the opposite side of the cell where the inhibitory GABA input is missing. The disinhibitory neuron is present in both the normal and schizophrenic circuit and the inhibitory GABA cells in both cases show three GABA receptors. **Sector CA3:** Pyramidal neuron C in normal controls shows a similar set of inhibitory and disinhibitory inputs and GABA$_A$ receptors as depicted in CA1. Pyramidal neuron D in the schizophrenic group also shows normal, i.e., three, GABA$_A$ receptors in relation to the two intact inhibitory GABA inputs; however, a decrease of disinhibitory GABAergic activity results in a compensatory upregulation of GABA$_A$ receptors (six) on the two inhibitory GABA cells.

As a general rule, it is not possible to study connectivity of corticolimbic networks in human brain because traditional tract-tracing techniques cannot be employed. One approach that is currently feasible, however, is the use of immunocytochemistry to localize fiber systems within various components of this system. Although such a strategy can be relatively specific for projections that emerge from discrete nuclei and employ a characteristic transmitter system (e.g., dopamine and serotonin), it can also provide nonspecific data from which meaningful inferences can be drawn. For example, using antibodies against a neurofilament 200K subunit of the axon cytoskeleton in the anterior cingulate cortex, an excessive number of vertical axons were found in superficial layers of schizophrenics.[30] Subsequently, this finding was replicated and extended using a monoclonal antibody against a glutamate-glutaraldehyde conjugate.[31] In both studies, an increased density of vertical axons in schizophrenics was not observed in the prefrontal cortex.[39,24] Initially, it was thought that the vertical fibers showing this increase in the anterior cingulate cortex might be associative afferents from other cortical regions because such fibers pass through layer II toward layer I, where they travel horizontally for considerable distances (for a review, see Benes[38]). It is noteworthy, however, that the superficial laminae of the anterior cingulate region also receive a "massive" input from the amygdala,[39] whereas the dorsolateral prefrontal area does not.[40] Since this latter region did not show an increase of vertical fibers in schizophrenics, it seemed possible that those fibers showing an increase in the anterior cingulate area might originate in a region that projects to the latter, but not the former. Accordingly, the basolateral nuclear complex of the amygdala presented an intriguing candidate. To test this hypothesis, a subsequent study evaluated the density of glutamate-immunoreactive axons in superficial layers of the entorhinal cortex, another cortical region receiving a substantial projection from the basolateral complex.[41] Once again, the results revealed a significant increase in the density of vertical axons in the superficial layers of this region.[42] Taken together with the prior results from the anterior cingulate, these findings provided compelling, albeit inferential, support for the possibility that the amygdala might send a superabundant projection to at least two key corticolimbic regions in the schizophrenic brain.

A MODEL FOR TRISYNAPTIC DYSFUNCTION IN SCHIZOPHRENIA

It is useful to consider how the postmortem findings concerning the circuitry within the hippocampus (for a detailed review, see Benes[43]) might be related to the entorhinal cortex and the basolateral nucleus of the amygdala. As shown in FIGURE 2, the trisynaptic pathway consists of (1) perforant fibers from the entorhinal cortex that project to the area dentata; (2) mossy fibers from the granule cells of the area dentata that project to the stratum radiatum of CA3; (3) Schaffer collaterals of pyramidal cells in CA3 that project to the stratum radiatum of CA1. There are intrinsic GABAergic interneurons throughout the hippocampal formation (FIG. 2) that provide inhibitory modulation of the pyramidal cells. Many of these GABA neurons also send collateral branches that form disinhibitory connections with other GABA cells.

The neuropathological and clinical observations described in the previous section are consistent with a model that predicts that an impairment of GABAergic function would be associated with an overall increase of excitation in the hippocampus (FIG. 2, lower panel). This model is noteworthy because it suggests that schizophrenics might show a deficit of not only inhibitory, but also disinhibitory integration in CA3.[27] If this assumption were correct, an overall increase in the level of hippocampal activation, like that observed in schizophrenic subjects by Heckers et al.,[44] would be predicted. As suggested in FIGURE 2, these changes would likely bear some relationship to increased excitatory activity generated in the amygdala and entering the hippocampus either directly via the CA3 or indirectly from the amygdala via the entorhinal cortex. It might therefore be expected that the increased activation from the amygdala and, by inference, the entorhinal cortex could increase further the overall level of activation detected in the hippocampus using PET scanning, and perhaps even be the primary cause of it.

An exception to the pattern of decreased inhibitory tone was suggested by the selective upregulation of this receptor on nonpyramidal neurons that was detected in the stratum pyramidale of sector CA3. This observation suggests that there is a decrease in GABA–GABA interactions in this sector and that such a selective deficiency of disinhibitory modulation could play a partial role in the pathophysiology of schizophrenia.[9] Disinhibitory GABAergic fibers in the hippocampus can arise from either extrinsic or intrinsic sources. For example, neurons in the septal nuclei form GABA–GABA interactions with intrinsic hippocampal interneurons[45] and may contribute to the generation of rapid gamma oscillations.[46,47] There are also slow theta rhythms[48,49] that require GABA–GABA interactions, but these are probably intrinsic to the hippocampus.[50]

A recent study has demonstrated that the ratio of pyramidal neurons to interneurons in human hippocampus is approximately 10:1.[8] In contrast, the analogous figure in human cortex is approximately 1:1.[5,51] It can be concluded from these data that the hippocampus has a strong tendency to generate an excitatory output, because there appears to be a relatively small number of inhibitory neurons. In addition, the hippocampus has a much higher packing density of projection cells in the granule cell layer and in the stratum pyramidale than is seen in the cortex. The net effect of this cytoarchitectonic arrangement is that the network formed is capable of acting as an amplifier for stimuli transmitted from the entorhinal cortex to the hippocampus. Each stimulus conducted along a perforant path axon entering the area dentata has the capability of inducing a response that is progressively increased in magnitude as it is conducted along this dense band of excitatory projection cells placed along the trisynaptic pathway. There are several subcortical components of the limbic system, such as the amygdala, septal nuclei, and hypothalamus, which are also capable of further amplifying this relay of activity along the trisynaptic pathway. Some of those coming from the septal nuclei, however, are GABAergic (inhibitory) in nature and are believed to play an important role in the generation of oscillatory rhythms.[45]

As discussed above, postmortem evidence from the study on schizophrenia has suggested that there may be a decreased number of interneurons in sector CA2[8] and those present in CA3 may be receiving a diminished GABA–GABA input.[22] The net effect of such a change would be a set of GABA cells in stratum pyramidale of CA3 with an unfettered ability to inhibit the pyramidal cells of CA3. Such an effect could hypothetically result in a decreased flow of activity along the Schaffer collaterals projecting to CA1. It is noteworthy, however, that this proposed defect could potentially be compensated for in the stratum oriens where the basal dendrites of pyramidal neurons receive a significantly decreased inhibitory modulation by GABAergic neurons in schizophrenics. Although the effect of GABA inputs directly to the neuronal cell bodies in the stratum pyramidale would tend to be more potent than that received via the basal dendrites in the stratum oriens, it is difficult to predict with certainty what pattern (i.e., disinhibitory vs. inhibitory) might prevail in this sector. More precise information regarding the relative distribution of these changes in schizophrenia is needed. In CA1, on the other hand, there is no decrease of interneurons, and a modest upregulation of the $GABA_A$ receptor was observed only on pyramidal cells. This latter arrangement suggests that there may be a small decrease in inhibitory modulation flowing from interneurons to projection cells in CA1.

Normal Control

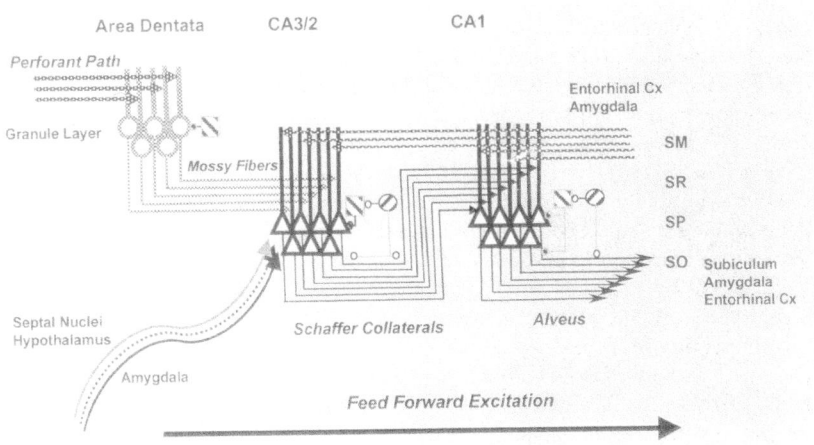

Schizophrenic

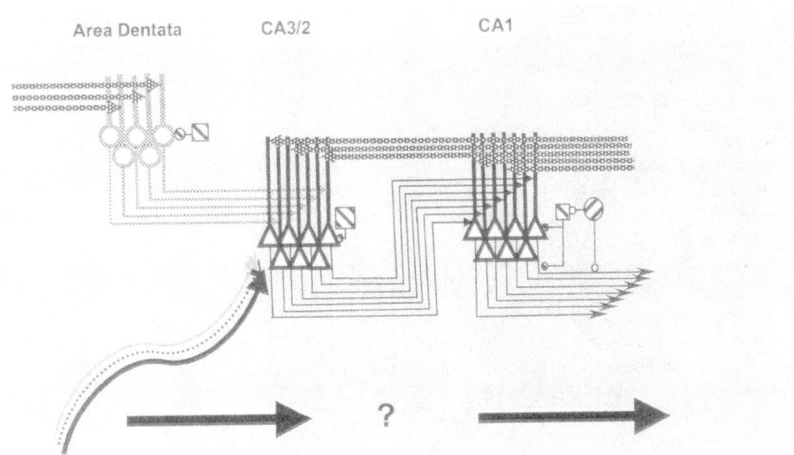

FIGURE 2. Depiction of a model for conduction along the trisynaptic pathway in normal controls and schizophrenics. **Normal Controls:** The trisynaptic pathway consists of three components: (1) Perforant path fibers providing an excitatory input to the molecular layer in the area dentata; (2) mossy fibers providing an excitatory input to the stratum radiatum of CA3; and (3) Schaffer collaterals that provide an excitatory input to the stratum radiatum of CA1. The activity relayed along the trisynaptic pathway is funneled toward pyramidal cells in CA1, which sends an efferent output to the subiculum, amygdala, and entorhinal region. The latter two regions also project back into the CA subfields along the stratum moleculare (see text for details). Sector CA3 of the hippocampus also receives direct afferents from the septal nuclei (*gray arrow*), hypothalamus (*hatched arrow*), and basolateral complex (*solid arrow*). The progressive shading toward the right-hand side of the diagram indicates the direction (*arrow*) of a "feed forward" excitation that probably results in

An important component of the model shown in FIGURE 2 is the implication that there might be an increase of activity flowing into the hippocampus from the amygdala and entorhinal region. As discussed above, a direct projection exists from the caudal portion of the parvocellular subdivision of the basolateral nuclear complex of the amygdala to sector CA3 via the stratum oriens.[34] A recent series of studies has demonstrated that infusion of a specific $GABA_A$ antagonist, picrotoxin, into this locus results in a rapid decrease in the density of GAD_{65}- and GAD_{67}-immunoreactive terminals in sectors CA3 and CA2, but not CA1.[52] Since this same subdivision of the basolateral complex also sends an abundant projection to layer II of the anterior cingulate cortex (unpublished observation), it seems plausible that this hippocampal input could play a pivotal role in the pathophysiology of schizophrenia.

As noted above, an increase of glutamate-immunoreactive vertical fibers was observed in superficial layers of the entorhinal cortex. Presumably, such fibers might have the ability to increase the level of excitation within the entorhinal region and then secondarily the flow of stimuli along the perforant path to the area dentata (see FIG. 2, lower panel). Another component to the model shown in FIGURE 2 that should be considered is the suggestion that there may be an increase of excitatory activity traveling in the stratum moleculare of the dentate gyrus and the CA subfields.

Projection neurons in layer II of the medial and lateral entorhinal areas project preferentially to CA3 and the subiculum, whereas those located in layer III project primarily to the dentate gyrus and CA1 (see Witter in this volume). It is conceivable

---

an amplified signal leaving sector CA1 (see text for details). Inhibitory interneurons (*square cells with hatched filling*) provide GABAergic input to pyramidal cells in CA3 and CA1 and to the stratum oriens. Some GABA cells are disinhibitory interneurons (*circular cells with hatched filling*) that decrease the ability of the GABAergic cell to fire. **Schizophrenics:** There is increased excitatory activity (*thickened arrows*) entering the trisynaptic pathway from three routes: (1) basolateral nucleus of the amygdala, (2) entorhinal projections to the stratum moleculare of the dentate gyrus, and (3) entorhinal projections to CA1 and CA3 from layers III and II, respectively, that travel along the stratum moleculare of these subfields (see text for details). In addition, a defect of GABAergic modulation is found at various points along the trisynaptic pathway. First, inhibitory GABAergic activity appears to be decreased in sectors CA4, CA3, and CA2, but not CA1. There is also a subtle decrease of disinhibitory modulation in the stratum pyramidale of CA3 that would result in an increased inhibition of pyramidal cell firing in this sector. Although it is difficult to understand how a dual defect in inhibitory *and* disinhibitory modulation in CA3 might impact on the final output, it seems likely that an overall increase of excitatory activity would occur along most of the trisynaptic pathway. The latter is indicated as an intensification of the dark shading occurring uniformly from the area dentata through sector CA1. In the area dentata, the feed forward excitatory drive progressively increases as the conduction of impulses passes toward CA1. Since the changes in GABAergic integration in CA3 are complex, and the increase of disinhibitory activity may have the ability to offset some of this excitation, the arrow is missing in this sector and is replaced by a question mark (**?**). In CA1, the excitatory drive attains its highest level of activity, particularly since a decrease of inhibitory modulation appears to be minimally present in this sector. Taken together, these hypothesized changes would be capable of generating an overall increase of basal metabolism in this region, but an impaired ability to selectively retrieve information when challenged with a specific task.

that the indirect pathway from the amygdala via the entorhinal inputs to the dentate gyrus, on the one hand, and the CA subfields, on the other, could potentially exert a preferential effect on sector CA3 by virtue of a convergence of activity from two opposite ends of the trisynaptic pathway. Such an effect emanating from the superficial layers of the entorhinal area seems plausible, because studies of other cortical regions have implicated layer II as being preferentially involved in the pathophysiology of schizophrenia (for a review, see Benes[38]). Thus, the notion that the changes in the GABA system in the hippocampus of schizophrenics are most pronounced in CA3/2 could be explained by a convergence of three excitatory influences: (1) a direct one from the basolateral nuclear complex to the stratum oriens, stratum pyramidale, and stratum radiatum of CA3/2; (2) an indirect one from layer II of the entorhinal cortex projecting to the stratum moleculare of CA3; and (3) another indirect one involving a relay through layer III of the entorhinal region to the dentate gyrus and the stratum moleculare of CA1. Overall, such changes in the glutamate and GABA systems would likely result in potentially significant disruptions of the integration of activity along the trisynaptic pathway within the hippocampal formation. Because sector CA1 is the largest sector containing the greatest number of pyramidal neurons, the feeding forward of excitatory activity via CA3 into this sector would be expected to result in a significant increase of activity in CA1 as well, particularly since this subregion also receives an entorhinal input.

FUNCTIONAL IMPLICATIONS OF HIPPOCAMPAL PATHOLOGY IN SCHIZOPHRENIA

Retrieval of information from memory storage is an important function associated with the hippocampus.[53–56] A recent PET-scanning study examined the response of the hippocampus to episodic memory retrieval[44] and demonstrated that basal metabolic activity is increased in the hippocampus at rest. The schizophrenic subjects in this study showed a significantly higher basal metabolic rate in the hippocampal formation. Under the conditions of low recall, however, no change in cerebral blood flow to the hippocampus was found, whereas under high-recall conditions there was a slight decrease. The fact that the baseline was much higher than in normal subjects suggests the possibility that a "ceiling effect" might have occurred in the subjects included in this study. An alternative possibility, however, is that the hippocampus of schizophrenics may have disturbances in the relay of information along the trisynaptic pathway, ones that belie the overall increase of activity that is detected under baseline conditions. Based on the above discussion, it also seems plausible that a complex impairment of GABAergic integration within CA3/2, where it would be interposed between the increased afferent excitatory activity in the molecular layer of both the area dentata and CA1, could result in a disturbance of normal information processing in this region. In the setting of excessive activity, perhaps generated in the basolateral complex, the efficiency of the system would nevertheless be compromised due to the complex changes noted in the GABAergic integration within sector CA3. Taken together, these changes would be expected to result in a paradoxical failure to show an activation in response to a behavioral challenge like that recently reported in schizophrenic subjects.[44]

CONCLUSIONS

Significant progress is being made toward identifying the ways in which neural circuitry is altered within the corticolimbic system of schizophrenic brain. Future work will be directed toward understanding the specific ways by which alterations of the connectivity among the amygdala, entorhinal cortex, and hippocampal formation may contribute to the occurrence of cognitive impairments in schizophrenia. While it is clear that this work is in a relatively early phase, it is notable that there is remarkable consistency between the findings obtained with PET imaging and those detected in postmortem investigations.

ACKNOWLEDGMENTS

This work was supported by grants from the National Institutes of Health (MH00423, MH42261, MH31862, and MH31154) and the Stanley Foundation.

REFERENCES

1. BENES, F.M. 1996. A neurodevelopmental approach to the understanding of schizophrenia and other mental disorders. *In* Developmental Psychopathology. Vol. 1. Theory and Methods. D. Cicchetti & D.J. Cohen, Eds.: 227–253. John Wiley & Sons, Inc. New York.
2. BOGERTS, B., E. MEERTZ & R. SCHONFELDT-BAUSCH. 1985. Basal ganglia and limbic system pathology in schizophrenia: a morphometric study of brain volume and shrinkage. Arch. Gen. Psychiatry **42:** 784–791.
3. FALKAI, P. & B. BOGERTS. 1986. Cell loss in the hippocampus of schizophrenics. Eur. Arch. Psychiatry Neurol. Sci. **236:** 154–161.
4. JESTE, D. & J.B. LOHR. 1989. Hippocampus pathologic findings in schizophrenia. Arch. Gen. Psychiatry **46:** 1019–1024.
5. BENES, F.M., J. MCSPARREN, E.D. BIRD, S.L. VINCENT & J.-P. SANGIOVANNI. 1991. Deficits in small interneurons in prefrontal and anterior cingulate cortex of schizophrenic and schizoaffective patients. Arch. Gen. Psychiatry **48:** 996–1001.
6. HECKERS, S., H. HEINSEN, B. GEIGER & H. BECKMANN. 1991. Hippocampal neuron number in schizophrenia. Arch. Gen. Psychiatry **48:** 1002–1008.
7. ARNOLD, S.E., B.R. FRANZ, R.C. GUR, R.E. GUR, R.M. SHAPIRO, P.J. MOBERG & J.Q. TROJANOWSKI. 1995. Smaller neuron size in schizophrenia in hippocampus subfields that mediate cortical-HIPP interactions. Am. J. Psychiatry **152:** 738–748.
8. BENES, F.M., E.W. KWOK, S.L. VINCENT & M.S. TODTENKOPF. 1998. A reduction of nonpyramidal cells in sector CA2 of schizophrenics and manic depressives. Biol. Psychiatry **44:** 88–97.
9. BENES, F.M. 1995. Is there a neuroanatomic basis for schizophrenia? The Neuroscientist **1:** 104–115.
10. COYLE, J.T. & P. PUTTFARCKEN. 1993. Oxidative stress, glutamate and neurodegenerative disorders. Science **262:** 689–695.
11. KERWIN, R.W., S. PATEL, B.S. MELDRUM, C. CZUDEK & G.P. REYNOLDS. 1988. Asymmetrical loss of glutamate receptor subtype in left hippocampus in schizophrenia. Lancet **1:** 583–584.
12. KERWIN, R., S. PATEL & B. MELDRUM. 1990. Quantitative autoradiographic analysis of glutamate binding sites in the hippocampus formation in normal and schizophrenic brain post mortem. Neuroscience **39:** 25–32.
13. HARRISON, P.J., D. MCLAUGHLIN & R.W. KERWIN. 1991. Decreased hippocampus expression of a glutamate receptor gene in schizophrenia. Lancet **337:** 450–452.

14. BENES, F.M., M.S. TODTENKOPF & P. KOSTOULAKOS. 2000. Decreased kainate receptor immunoreactivity in hippocampus of schizophrenics, but not manic depressives. Hippocampus. In press.
15. SCHWARCZ, R., R. ZACZEK & J.T. COYLE. 1978. Microinjection of kainic acid into the rat hippocampus. Eur. J. Pharmacol. **50:** 209–220.
16. SPERK, G., H. LASSMANN, H. BARAN, S.J. KISH, F. SEITELBERGER & O. HORNYKIEWICZ. 1983. Kainic acid induced seizures: neurochemical and histopathological changes. Neuroscience **10:** 1301–1315.
17. BEN-ARI, Y. 1985. Limbic seizure and brain damage produced by kainic acid: mechanisms and relevance to human temporal lobe epilepsy. Neuroscience **14:** 375–403.
18. ZHANG, W.Q., B.C. ROGERS, P. TANDON, P.M. HUDSON, T.J. SOBOTKA, J.S. HONG & H.A. TILSON. 1990. Systemic administration of kainic acid increases GABA levels in perfusate from the hippocampus of rats *in vivo*. Neurotoxicology **11:** 593–600.
19. BEST, N., J. MITCHELL, K.G. BAIMBRIDGE & H.V. WHEAL. 1993. Changes in parvalbumin-immunoreactive neurons in the rat hippocampus following a kainic acid lesion. Neurosci. Lett. **155:** 1–6.
20. MORIN, F., C. BEAULIEU & J. LACAILLE. 1998. Selective loss of GABA neurons in area CA1 of the rat hippocampus after intraventricular kainate. Epilepsy Res. **32:** 363–369.
21. REYNOLDS, G.P., C. CZUDEK & H. ANDREWS. 1990. Deficit and hemispheric asymmetry of GABA uptake sites in the hippocampus in schizophrenia. Biol. Psychiatry **27:** 1038–1044.
22. BENES, F.M., Y. KHAN, S.L. VINCENT & R. WICKRAMASINGHE.1996. Differences in the subregional and cellular distribution of GABA$_A$ receptor binding in the hippocampal formation of schizophrenic brain. Synapse **22:** 338–349.
23. BENES, F.M., R. WICKRAMASINGHE, S.L. VINCENT, Y. KHAN & M.S. TODTENKOPF. 1997. Uncoupling of GABA$_A$ and benzodiazepine receptor binding activity in the hippocampal formation of schizophrenic brain. Brain Res. **755:** 121–129.
24. BENES, F.M., S.L. VINCENT, G. ALSTERBERG, E.D. BIRD & J.P. SANGIOVANNI. 1992. Increased GABA-A receptor binding in superficial layers of cingulate cortex in schizophrenics. J. Neurosci. **12:** 924–929.
25. TODTENKOPF, M.S. & F.M. BENES. 1998. Distribution of glutamate decarboxylase$_{65}$ immunoreactive puncta on pyradmidal and nonpyramidal neurons in hippocampus of schizophrenic brain. Synapse **29:** 323–332.
26. VINCENT, S.L., E. ADAMEC, I. SORENSEN & F. M. BENES.1994. The effects of chronic haloperidol administration on GABA-immunoreactive axon terminals in rat medial prefrontal cortex. Synapse **17:** 26–35.
27. BENES, F.M. 2000. Emerging principles of altered neural circuitry in schizophrenia. Brain Res. Interact. (Nobel Symposium No.111). Brain Res. Rev. **31:** 251–269.
28. MACDONALD, A.J. 1992. Cell types and intrinsic connections of the amygdala. *In* The Amygdala: Neurobiological Aspects of Emotion, Memory, and Mental Dysfunction. J.P. Aggleton, Ed.: 67–96. John Wiley & Sons, Inc. New York.
29. BENES, F.M. & E.D. BIRD. 1987. An analysis of the arrangement of neurons in the cingulate cortex of schizophrenic patients. Arch. Gen. Psychiatry **44:** 608–616.
30. BENES, F.M., R. MAJOCHA, E.D. BIRD & C.A. MARROTTA.1987. Increased vertical axon numbers in cingulate cortex of schizophrenics. Arch. Gen. Psychiatry **44:** 1017–1021.
31. BENES, F.M., I. SORENSEN, S.L. VINCENT, E.D. BIRD & M. SATHI. 1992a. Increased density of glutamate-immunoreactive vertical processes in superficial laminae in cingulate cortex of schizophrenic brain. Cereb. Cortex **2:** 502–512.
32. LAWRIE, S.M. & S.S. ABUKMEIL.1998. Brain abnormality in schizophrenia. A systematic and quantitative review of volumetric magnetic resonance imaging studies. Br. J. Psychiatry **172:** 110–120.
33. SWANSON, L.W. & G.D. PETROVICH.1998. What is the amygdala? Trends Neurosci. **21:** 323–331.
34. PIKKARAINEN, M., S. RONKKO, V. SAVANDER, R. INSAUSTI & A. PITKÄNEN. 1999. Projections from the lateral, basal, and accessory basal nuclei of the amygdala to the hippocampal formation in rat. J. Comp. Neurol. **403:** 229–260.

35. DAVIS, M., D. RAINNIE & M. CASSELL. 1994. Neurotranmission in the rat amygdala related to fear and anxiety. Trends Neurosci. **17:** 208–214.
36. SANDERS, S.K. & A. SHEKHAR. 1995. Regulation of anxiety by GABA$_A$ receptors in the rat amygdala. Pharmacol. Biochem. Behav. **52:** 701–706.
37. SANDERS, S.K., S.L. MORZORATI & A. SHEKHAR.1995. Priming of experimental anxiety by repeated subthreshold GABA blockade in the rat amygdala. Brain Res. **699:** 250–259.
38. BENES, F.M. 1993. The relationship of cingulate cortex to schizophrenia. In Neurobiology of Cingulate Cortex and Limbic Thalamus. B.A. Vogt & M. Gabriel, Eds.: 581–605. Birkhäuser, Inc. Boston, MA.
39. VOGT, B.A., D.N. PANDYA & D.L. ROSENE. 1987. Cingulate cortex of the rhesus monkey. I. Cytoarchitecture and thalamic afferents. J. Comp. Neurol. **262:** 256–270.
40. VAN HOESEN, G.W., R.J. MORECRAFT & B.A. VOGT.1993. Connections of the monkey cingulate cortex. In Neurobiology of Cingulate Cortex and Limbic Thalamus. B.A. Vogt & M. Gabriel, Eds.: 249–284. Birkhäuser. Boston, MA.
41. AMARAL, D.G., J.L. PRICE, A. PITKÄNEN & S.T. CARMICHAEL.1992. Anatomical organization of the primate amygdaloid complex. In Amygdala. J.P. Aggleton, Ed.: 1–66. Wiley-Liss. New York.
42. LONGSON, D., J.W.F. DEAKIN & F.M. BENES. 1996. Increased density of entorhinal glutamate-immunoreactive vertical fibers in schizophrenia. J. Neural Transm. **103**(4)**:** 503–507.
43. BENES, F.M. 1999. Evidence for altered trisynaptic circuitry in schizophrenic hippocampus. Biol. Psychiatry **46:** 589–599.
44. HECKERS, S., H. HEINSEN, B. GEIGER, S. HECKERS, S.L. RAUSCH, D. GOFF, C.R. SAVAGE, D.L. SCHACTER, A.J. FISCHMAN & M.M. ALPERT. 1998. Impaired recruitment of the hippocampus during conscious recollection in schizophrenia. Nature Neurosci. **1:** 318–323.
45. FREUND, T.F. & M. ANTAL. 1988. GABA-containing neurons in the septum control inhibitory interneurons in the hippocampus. Nature **336:** 170–173.
46. WHITTINGTON, M.A., R.D. TRAUB & J.G.R. JEFFERYS. 1995. Metabotropic receptor activation drives synchronized 40 Hz oscillations in networks of inhibitory interneurons. Nature **373:** 612–615.
47. TRAUB, R.D., J.G.R. JEFFERYS & M.A. WHITTINGTON. 1997. Simulation of gamma rhythms in networks of interneurons and pyramidal cells. J. Comp. Neurosci. **4:** 141–150.
48. BUZSÁKI, G., Z. HORVÁTH, R. URIOSTE, J. HETKE & K. WISE. 1992. High-frequency network oscillation in the hippocampus. Science **256:** 1025–1027.
49. YLINEN, A., I. SOLTÉSZ, A. BRAGIN, M.PENTTONEN, A. SIK & G. BUZSÁKI. 1995. Intracellular correlates of hippocampal theta rhythm in identified pyramidal cells, granule cells, and basket cells. Hippocampus **5:** 78–90.
50. SIK, A., M. PENTTONEN, A. YLINEN & G. BUZSÁKI. 1995. Hippocampal CA1 interneurons: an in vivo intracellular labeling study. J. Neurosci. **15:** 6651–6665.
51. SELEMON, L.D., G. RAJKOWSKA & P.S. GOLDMAN-RAKIC. 1995. Abnormally high neuronal density in the schizophrenic cortex: A morphometric analysis of prefrontal area 9 and occipital area 17. Arch. Gen. Psychiatry **52:** 805–818.
52. BERRETTA, S., D.W. MUNNO & F.M. BENES. 1999. Does the amygdala contribute to hippocampal abnormalities in schizophrenia? A study on the effects of amygdala stimulation on the GABAergic system of the hippocampus in rat. Schizophrenia Res. **36:** 61.
53. DETOLEDO-MORRELL, L., Y. GEINISMAN & F. MORRELL. 1988. Age-dependent alterations in hippocampus synaptic plasticity: relation to memory disorders. Neurobiol. Aging **9:** 581–590.
54. SQUIRE, L.R., B. KNOWLTON & G. MUSEN. 1993. The structure and organization of memory. Annu. Rev. Psychol. **44:** 453–495.
55. EICHENBAUM, H. 1997. Declarative memory: insights from cognitive neurobiology. Annu. Rev. Psychol. **48:** 547–572.
56. EICHENBAUM, H., P. DUDCHENCKO, E. WOOD, M. SHAPIRO & H. TANILA. 1999. The hippocampus, memory, and place cells: Is it spatial memory or a memory space? Neuron **23:** 209–226.

Epileptogenesis in the Parahippocampal Region

Parallels with the Dentate Gyrus

HELEN E. SCHARFMAN

Neurology Research Center, Helen Hayes Hospital, West Haverstraw, New York 10993-1195, USA, and Departments of Pharmacology and Neurology, Columbia University, College of Physicians and Surgeons, New York, New York 10032, USA

ABSTRACT: Limbic seizures have often been attributed to pathology in the hippocampus, such as the well described condition termed Ammon's Horn sclerosis, in which many of the hippocampal principal cells have degenerated. However, several studies in both the clinical and basic literature indicate that the parahippocampal region may also play an important role. This region sustains a characteristic pattern of damage in most animal models of epilepsy that is similar to that identified in humans with intractable temporal lobe epilepsy. Perhaps the most striking aspect of parahippocampal pathology is the marked loss of neurons in layer III of the entorhinal cortex. The similarity of cell loss in layer III and cell loss in the hilus of the dentate gyrus is compared, as is the characteristic resistance of layer II neurons and dentate granule cells. Cellular electrophysiological results are used as a basis for the hypothesis that synaptic inhibition plays a role in the relative vulnerability of these neurons. Studies of neurogenesis in both areas is also discussed. It is proposed that this may be an additional factor that influences vulnerability in these areas.

INTRODUCTION

Importance of the Parahippocampal Region

The importance of the parahippocampal region in epilepsy has been noted often, highlighted by Morin and Gastaut[66] (see also Refs. 7, 11, 25, 32, 68, and 77). Although many discussions of the role of the parahippocampal region refer to it together with the hippocampus, a specific role of the parahippocampal region alone in the pathology and etiology of temporal lobe epilepsy (TLE) was also considered. More recently, the role of the parahippocampal region in epilepsy, and specifically the entorhinal cortex (EC), has been the focus of many animal studies. The results document the sensitivity of the entorhinal cortex to epileptogenic treatment, such as electrolytic lesions of the EC,[20] chemoconvulsants (kainic acid, muscarinic agonists, 4-aminopyridine, etc.[21,54,64,67,78,92]), repetitive afferent stimulation,[5,14,56,59,72–74] or manipulations of Krebs-Ringer buffer (low magnesium, high potassium).[6,58,109,116,118] It is perhaps fair to say, however, that the precise role of the entorhinal cortex in epileptogenesis remains unclear.

Cell Loss in the Superficial Layers of the Medial Entorhinal Cortex in Temporal Lobe Epilepsy

One reason for the interest in the entorhinal cortex in the context of epileptogenesis is that pathology in this area is a hallmark of TLE. One of the most common and easily recognizable areas of cell loss in TLE are the superficial layers of the EC, particularly layer III of the medial EC. This was originally demonstrated in early studies of tissue from patients with TLE[121] and has been examined more recently in humans as well.[25] Layer III cell loss is also evident in animal models of epilepsy.[24] Du and colleagues[24,25] showed preferential layer III neuronal loss in the pilocarpine model of epilepsy, after kainic acid treatment, and also in the self-sustaining limbic status epilepticus (SSLSE) and amino-oxyacetic acid (AOAA) models. In the pilocarpine and kainic acid models, drug is administered systemically, followed by several hours of continuous seizures (status epilepticus). After status ends, which occurs naturally after several hours (or is induced by anticonvulsant administration), several days or weeks pass with few or no behavioral seizures, and subsequently spontaneous behavioral seizures occur intermittently.[41] In the AOAA model, drug is microinjected into the EC in an anesthetized rat using stereotaxic methods.[26,61] SSLSE occurs after a period of continuous hippocampal stimulation in the anesthetized rat *in vivo*.[5,56,59,74] Layer III cell loss has also been shown in monkeys after alumina gel treatment.[76] In all cases, layer III cell loss occurs throughout the medial EC and sometimes the lateral EC. GABAergic parvalbumin-immunoreactive neurons as well as most neurons in layers II, V, and VI survive.[23]

To gain insight into the mechanisms for layer III vulnerability and, in particular, the reasons why damage to the superficial layers might be linked to epileptogenesis, other vulnerable areas were examined.

COMPARISON OF LAYER III OF THE MEDIAL ENTORHINAL CORTEX AND DENTATE GYRUS HILUS

One of the vulnerable areas of the brain is the hilus of the dentate gyrus, which has long been noted as an area of cell loss, gliosis, and shrinkage in both epileptics and animal models of epilepsy.[60,62,94] In their 1966 study of 55 epileptics, Margerison and Corsellis[60] noted that the hilar region was one of the most common areas of all surveyed that demonstrated pathology. In animal models, hilar cell loss and shrinkage have been demonstrated after kainic acid, pilocarpine, prolonged perforant path stimulation, kindling, and also ischemia and traumatic brain injury.[12,17,41,43,52,57,100,102] Vulnerable hilar neurons include, for example, somatostatin-immunoreactive neurons that project to the outer molecular layer, as well as glutamatergic mossy cells.[42,45,82,83,100]

In the rest of the chapter, the characteristics of the medial EC and dentate gyrus hilus are compared in order to shed light on mechanisms underlying cell death in each area.

Parallels in Normal Conditions and after Seizures

Several parallels between the medial EC and the dentate gyrus can be appreciated independent of a discussion of epileptogenesis. For example, both structures are substantially expanded in primates relative to rodents. From these changes with phylogeny, we can predict that the function as well as the dysfunction of these areas could be very important in man.

Both regions are an example of relatively simple cortex, meaning that there is no six-layer scheme as in neocortex, but lamina similar to neocortex do exist. For the medial EC, the distinguishing features from neocortex include the presence of a relatively cell-free lamina dissecans and the lack of clear borders between layers 5 and 6. The dentate gyrus, like the hippocampus, has a much simpler laminar organization. Nevertheless, there are clear parallels. In both the EC and the dentate gyrus, circuits are based on glutamatergic principal cells and a diverse array of GABAergic interneurons.[55,85,94] There is more than one type of principal cell in each area; in the EC there are multiple pyramidal and stellate neurons; in the dentate gyrus there are both granule cells and mossy cells. Depending on the perspective, one could include CA3c pyramidal cells with granule cells and mossy cells in listing the principal cells of the dentate gyrus, because CA3 neurons are interconnected with dentate neurons and have strong, synaptically mediated effects.[51,89,90]

For the present discussion, principal cells are defined by an axon that projects out of the local circuit. For example, layer II/III axons innervate the hippocampus via the perforant path, granule cells project to CA3, and mossy cells project to the ipsilateral and contralateral dentate gyrus. "Nonprincipal cells" refer to neurons with axons that arborize in the local circuit, such as GABAergic neurons. Although there are GABAergic dentate neurons that have contralateral projections, these are thought to be relatively small in number.[4,36,97]

The GABAergic interneurons in both areas are diverse. They have distinct target sites,[39] morphologies,[3] and physiology[9] and colocalize a variety of peptides.[28,101] The range of morphologies and peptides that are expressed in the dentate interneurons are, by and large, similar to those expressed in the medial EC interneurons. For example, basket cells, chandelier cells, and bipolar neurons are found in each area. Neurons expressing neuropeptide Y and somatostatin are in each region. The calcium binding proteins parvalbumin, calretinin, and calbindin also are localized to neurons in both areas.[13,31,63,65,69,96,110,119] Many of these neurons form distinct axonal arbors around the principal cell layers, particularly layer II of the EC and the granule cell layer of the dentate gyrus. Interestingly, calbindin is also expressed in a principal cell in each region (layer II projection cells and granule cells), and in each area this is a relatively resistant type of cell in terms of excitotoxicity. As has been proposed in other contexts, calbindin may confer neuroprotection to granule cells[81,99] and, analogously, layer II neurons (but see Ref. 29).

The comparison of the medial EC and dentate gyrus hilus is particularly apt in the context of epilepsy. For example, peptide expression is increased after seizures in both areas. A particularly good example of a peptide that increases its expression after seizures is neuropeptide Y (NPY). Induction of NPY in these areas occurs after a wide range of seizure-inducing protocols, including convulsant treatment, stimulation, and kindling.[107,112,113,115] This is evident in stronger immunoreactivity in individual neurons in the vulnerable regions (non-principal cells) as well as fibers. After seizures, a fiber plexus becomes apparent as a band of dense fibers at the approximate location of lamina dissecans. Moreover, the fibers that innervate the vulnerable zones in the medial EC and hilus both increase expression of NPY after seizures. Thus, NPY is induced in the mossy fiber axons of the granule cells after seizures, which target hilar neurons, and NPY is also induced in parasubicular fibers, which innervate the superficial layers.[107,112,113,115] Thus, there is an interesting parallel of NPY induction in afferents to the vulnerable areas (hilus, superficial layers of the medial EC). However, this parallel is not perfect, because the parasubicular fibers appear to innervate the relatively resistant layer II neurons preferentially. Hence, increased NPY expression after seizures and its functional consequences per se are unlikely to completely explain vulnerability of hilar and layer III neurons.

Another similarity is the innervation of superficial neurons in the medial EC and the hilus by BDNF-immunoreactive fibers. In the hilus, the mossy fibers contain BDNF, whereas the origin of the fibers in the superficial region is not presently clear.[16,120] In both areas, BDNF is induced after seizures.[44,95,114] The pattern of NPY and BDNF induction is similar, including an increase in non-principal neurons as well as an increase in fiber staining within each region.[114] Similar to NPY, the parasubicular region is more intensely BDNF-immunoreactive after seizures.[114] Because increased BDNF could actually lead to changes in NPY,[18] this may have physiological consequences, such as influencing vulnerability of the neurons contacted, because BDNF bath application can increase excitability in the dentate gyrus/CA3 and medial EC networks.[93] Indeed, it has been proposed that BDNF increases glutamate release by a presynaptic action.[37,48,53,93,108] This could be a mechanism underlying increased excitability.[19,93]

Zinc is also common in the two regions. For example, zinc is contained in afferent fibers that innervate layers II/III of the medial EC, and zinc is present in abundance in the mossy fibers that innervate hilar neurons.[40,98] Although the physiological actions of zinc are currently unclear, zinc may have actions that influence excitability.[27,117]

In summary, several parallels exist between the hilus and medial EC, some of which might bear on the epileptogenic susceptibility of the neurons in these two areas: (1) its disproportional expansion in primates relative to rodents; (2) its general cortical organization; (3) the normal and seizure-associated expression of NPY and BDNF; and (4) the expression of zinc in fibers that innervate the areas where vulnerable neurons are located.

Characteristics of Vulnerable and Resistant Neurons and Their Local Circuit Properties

The parallels between the medial EC and hilus are perhaps best exemplified upon further analysis of the cell types that are vulnerable and resistant.

After seizures, cell loss of a specific type of principal neuron occurs in both the medial EC and the hilus: layer III pyramidal cells of the medial EC and mossy cells of the hilus. Also in both areas, there is relative cell preservation of specific types of principal cells, and in each area they are the principal neurons that lie immediately adjacent to the vulnerable cells. In the medial EC, these are the stellate and pyramidal cells of layer II, and in the dentate gyrus, these are the granule cells.

Furthermore, there are a group of GABA neurons containing parvalbumin that are relatively resistant in both the medial EC and the dentate gyrus. In the hilus are other types of GABA neurons, for example, those that contain somatostatin, that are relatively vulnerable as well. However, in the medial EC, loss of somatostatin neurons does not appear to occur after seizures.[113]

Layer III Pyramidal Cells and Hilar Mossy Cells

A parallel exists between many of the characteristics of layer III pyramidal cells and mossy cells, and also layer II and granule cells have characteristics in common. Discussion of these similarities raises possible reasons for their vulnerability and resistance, respectively.

Morphology

Layer III pyramidal cells and hilar mossy cells are similar in several ways, as shown in TABLE 1. Both types of neurons use an excitatory amino acid as a neurotransmitter, probably glutamate.[55,94,106] In addition, there is a small degree of zinc, inferred from the light Timm staining of their terminal zones (area CA3 stratum lacunosum/moleculare for layer III and the inner molecular layer for hilar mossy cells[40,98]). Peptides have not been identified in these neurons, except for calcitonin gene-related peptide (CGRP), which is present in mossy cells.[30] They are both extremely spiny, although it can be argued that the mossy cells have more complex spine clusters (thorny excrescences).[3]

Each type of neuron is a principal cell with a long projection out of the local region and out of the hippocampal lamella where the soma is located. There is also a local axon that arborizes around the soma and a contralateral projection.[55,85]

In layer III pyramidal cells, the projection to area CA1 innervates neurons in stratum lacunosum-moleculare, where controversy exists regarding the particular net effect on CA1 neurons.[104] For hilar mossy cells, the functional effect of the projection to the inner molecular layer has also been debated, somewhat analogous to the debate concerning layer III effects.[94] In both the case of the layer III input to CA1 and the mossy cell input to granule cells, the net effect appears to be a combination of direct excitatory effects (i.e., innervation of CA1 pyramidal cell or granule cell dendrites) as well as indirect inhibitory effects (by excitation of interneurons that in turn innervate CA1 pyramidal cells or granule cells).[94,104]

Intrinsic Physiological Properties

A number of groups have now described the intrinsic properties of layer III neurons and mossy cells based on intracellular recordings.[10,22,34,80,103,111] The characteristics are similar to those of mossy cells in several ways (TABLE 1). For example, both are "regular spiking" neurons in that they have long duration action potentials compared to many of the GABA neurons (so-called "fast spiking" interneurons). There is little evidence of intrinsic burst activity; for this discussion, "burst" refers to the discharges of area CA3c neurons[88] or some cortical neurons[15] in which three to five action potentials of decreasing amplitude occur on a depolarization that can be evoked by intracellular current.[88] Responses to a range of intracellularly injected rectangular current pulses demonstrate rectification in both types of neurons, although there is little of the "sag" that has been described for other cell types, such as layer II neurons.[1,50]

TABLE 1. Comparison of "vulnerable" cell types[a]

	Layer III Pyramidal	Hilar Mossy Cells
Neurotransmitter	Glutamate	Glutamate
Other	?	CGRP
Afferents	Glutamatergic (layer V)	Glutamatergic (granule, PC)
	Diverse neuromodulators	Diverse neuromodulators
	BDNF, zinc?	BDNF, zinc
Efferents	Local and distant	Local and distant
	Innervates principal cell which is involved in trisynaptic pathway (layer II)	Innervates principal cell which is involved in trisynaptic pathway (granule cell)
	Innervates GABA neurons	Innervates GABA neurons
Spines	Many	Many; some complex (thorns)
Intrinsic properties	Regular spiking; no bursts; no sag	Regular spiking; no bursts; no sag

[a]Characteristics of layer III pyramidal cells and hilar mossy cells are compared. Afferents, input to the cell type; efferents, projections of the cell type; ?, unknown; PC, pyramidal cell; regular spiking, relatively long duration axon; burst, intrinsic bursts (see text); sag, inward rectification in response to hyperpolarizing current (see Refs. 1 and 50); parv, parvalbumin.

Synaptic Physiology

Gloveli *et al.*[34,35] reported that two types of layer III pyramidal neurons can be distinguished on the basis of morphology and synaptic responses to deep layer stimulation or other inputs. Their "type I" pyramidal neuron has a wide basal dendritic tree that stretches for relatively long distances horizontally (i.e., staying mostly within layer III). The first branch point of the apical dendrite is relatively far from the soma compared to type II pyramidal neurons. In tests of single stimuli, the response to stimulation shows more evidence of an excitatory postsynaptic potential (EPSP) than type II cells (i.e., FIG. 1 of Ref. 35). Type II neurons have a more confined basal dendritic tree, with dendrites radiating in multiple directions. Type II neurons appear to have more inhibition in their synaptic response to a single stimulus. However, at high stimulus strengths or after repetitive stimuli, both type I and type II neurons can demonstrate hyperpolarizing synaptic responses.[34,35]

Studies of mossy cell synaptic responses to dentate molecular layer stimulation show similarities to layer III neurons. For example, at low stimulus strengths, excitation dominates, but as stimulus strength increases, inhibition appears to be recruited.[87] There usually is little inhibitory postsynaptic potential (IPSP) in response to a single afferent stimulus to the major afferent (the perforant path), unless inhibition is blocked by GABA antagonists.[84,105] However, there are also reports of mossy cells with stronger inhibition.[9,103] Upon examination specifically of mossy cells near and far from the granule cell layer, we found that mossy cells that were adjacent to the granule cell layer had the least evidence of IPSPs under normal recording conditions (to be discussed). Mossy cells located adjacent to CA3c had IPSPs as well as EPSPs in several cases (to be discussed). Heterogeneity of mossy cells is further supported by reports that some mossy cells have sag in response to hyperpolarizing

TABLE 2. Comparison of layer III and mossy cell subtypes[a]

	Layer III Pyramidal		Hilar Mossy Cell	
	Type I	Type II	Type I	Type II
Morphology	Lateral basal dendrites	Radial basal dendrites	Near GCL	Near CA3c
	Late branch of apical dendrite	Early branch of apical dendrite	Molecular layer dendrites[b]	No dendrites in molecular layer
Synaptic physiology				
Single stimulation	EPSP>IPSP	IPSP>EPSP	EPSP	EPSP or EPSP and IPSP
AOAA	Sensitive	Less sensitive		
Repetitive stimulation			Sensitive	Less sensitive

[a]Characteristics of layer III pyramidal cells and mossy cells are listed according to a division into subtypes. Layer III nomenclature and morphological characteristics are from Gloveli *et al.*[34,35] "Late branch" or "early branch" refers to the distance from the soma of the first branch of the apical dendrite. "Single stimulation" refers to evoked responses to white matter or deep layer stimulation (layer III) or molecular layer stimulation (mossy cells) in normal buffer. >, larger amplitude (i.e., EPSP larger in amplitude than IPSP) or only an EPSP was evoked; comparisons were made at similar membrane potentials; AOAA, effect of focal or bath-application of amino oxyacetic acid; repetitive stimulation, effect of prolonged intermittent stimulation of the perforant path.[82,83]
[b] See Ref. 86.

pulses,[10] but others do not.[80] Our recent studies comparing mossy cells near (soma < 250 μm from the granule cell layer/hilar border, $n = 21$) and far (< 200 μm from end of the pyramidal layer, $n = 19$) indicated that cells near the layer did not exhibit sag and did not have subthreshold IPSPs to outer molecular layer stimulation, whereas 9 of 19 near CA3c had sag and 7 of 19 had subthreshold EPSPs followed by IPSPs. In these studies, sag and subthreshold PSPs were examined at a variety of holding potentials (−50 to −80 mV) and tests of sag were made with various current steps (−0.1 to 1.0 nA). Sag was defined as > 1 mV change in potential between the instantaneous and steady-state response to a hyperpolarizing current pulse (150-ms duration). Mossy cells near the granule cell layer also showed a higher frequency and amplitude of spontaneous depolarizations, which are likely to represent EPSPs generated by afferents, such as mossy fiber axons. However, the large spontaneous, presumed EPSPs in cells near the granule cell layer could simply be due to an increased chance that the granule cell-to-mossy cell afferents are sliced as the distance from the granule cell layer is increased.

Thus, from the intrinsic properties, synaptic responses, and locations of mossy cells relative to the granule cell layer, it appears that the mossy cells can be subdivided like layer III neurons into two groups, those that are more excitatory (layer III type I, mossy cells near the granule cell layer) and those that are more inhibited (layer III type II, mossy cells near CA3c; TABLE 2). In both the EC and hilus, those that are more excitable appear to be the ones that are more vulnerable (to be discussed).

Vulnerability of Layer III Neurons and Mossy Cells in Slices

To determine the possible relation between physiological properties, synaptic inhibition, and vulnerability, layer III neurons were tested for their sensitivity to the indirect excitotoxin AOAA. As described in the review by Schwarcz *et al.* (this volume and elsewhere[24,26,61]), AOAA is a potent tool to damage layer III neurons when microinjected *in vivo*. AOAA appears to act, at least in part, by increasing NMDA receptor-mediated depolarizations in medial EC neurons.[26,61,92]

In intracellular studies of layer III neurons in slices, most layer III neurons were affected by AOAA (*n* = 13/14). These effects, when they occur, include an increase in the late portion of the stimulus-evoked EPSP.[92] This result can follow either focal application using a microdrop of 10 mM AOAA[92] or bath application of 5–100 µM AOAA.[92] Of the six cells that were stained in the recent experiments, the five that had morphology similar to that of type I neurons were affected by AOAA, and the one with type II morphology was not. In our sample, the general morphology of the basal dendrites was used to distinguish type I and type II cells. Type I cells had long basal dendrites that extended in a horizontal direction, perpendicular to the apical dendrite, whereas type II neurons had basal dendrites that radiated in many directions and formed a more circular, smaller basal dendritic tree.[34] Gloveli *et al.*[34] also reported a difference between type I and type II neurons that was based on the distance from the soma to the first branchpoint of the apical dendrite, but all of the neurons sampled in our experiments were similar in this regard. Thus, this criterion was not used.

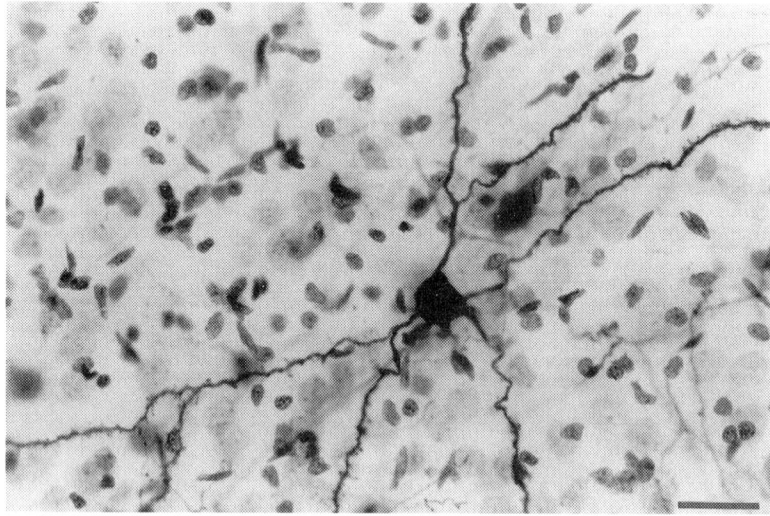

FIGURE 1. An intracellularly labeled neurobiotin-stained layer III pyramidal neuron. This neuron was recorded in the medial entorhinal cortex of a horizontally cut slice as previously described.[92] It has some of the characteristics of type I cells,[34] such as long basal dendrites that extended for relatively long distances laterally. Only some of the dendrites are shown. The apical dendrite at the top extended to the pial surface. Recordings from this neuron are shown in FIGURE 2. Calibration = 50 µm. Counterstained with cresyl violet.

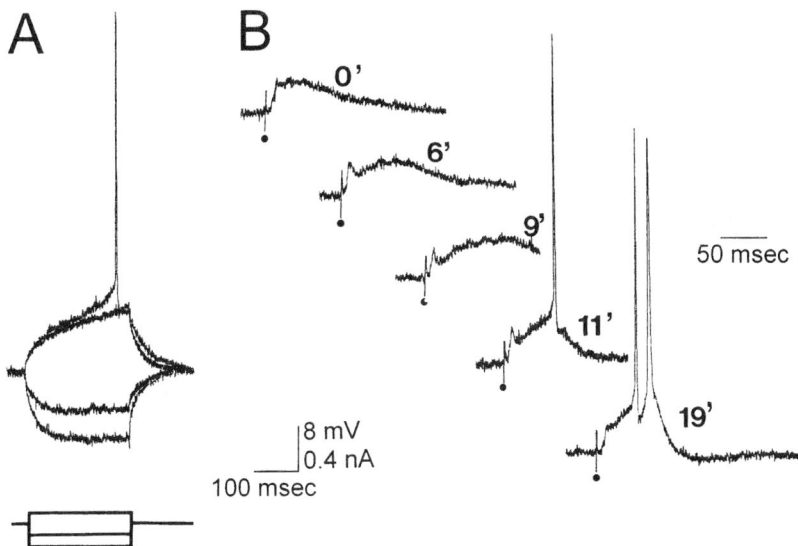

FIGURE 2. Physiological responses of the layer III pyramidal cell shown in FIGURE 1. (**A**) Responses to intracellular current injection (rectangular current pulses, schematized at the bottom) illustrate that little anomalous rectification or "sag" (see FIG. 5 for definition) was present, as is typical of layer III neurons. (**B**) Responses to white matter stimulation (at the dot; stimulus artifacts are truncated) evoked a depolarizing potential, presumably an EPSP, because if depolarized with DC current, it evoked discharge (not shown). This is a typical response of type I neurons.[34] The same stimulus was triggered at various times after the addition of AOAA to the buffer (bath application; 10 μM). This cell responded to bath-applied AOAA in a typical fashion of type I cells: a late component was increased in the synaptic response and led to discharges.

FIGURE 1 shows a type I pyramidal cell from layer III that was clearly affected by AOAA (FIG. 2). This is consistent with previous studies in which labeled pyramidal neurons with basal dendrites similar to those of type I neurons demonstrated effects of AOAA.[92] In contrast, FIGURE 3 illustrates a type II pyramidal neuron of layer III that was not affected by AOAA. Thus, the subtype with the weakest inhibition was more sensitive to AOAA, and conversely, cells with the strongest synaptically evoked inhibition (type II) were less sensitive to AOAA. This correlation indicates a possible relationship between synaptic inhibition and sensitivity to excitotoxins.

Analogous results were obtained in studies of mossy cells after prolonged, intermittent repetitive stimulation of the perforant path, originally developed as an *in vivo* paradigm to selectively kill hilar neurons.[81,82,83,101] Similar to layer III pyramidal cells, those mossy cells with the least synaptically evoked inhibition (i.e., those closest to the granule cell layer) were also the ones that were most affected by the treatment. Mossy cells that were affected depolarized rapidly and irreversibly, and deteriorated in other electrophysiological parameters also.[82,83] Neurons that were at the border with CA3c and the hilus became less depolarized, required longer periods

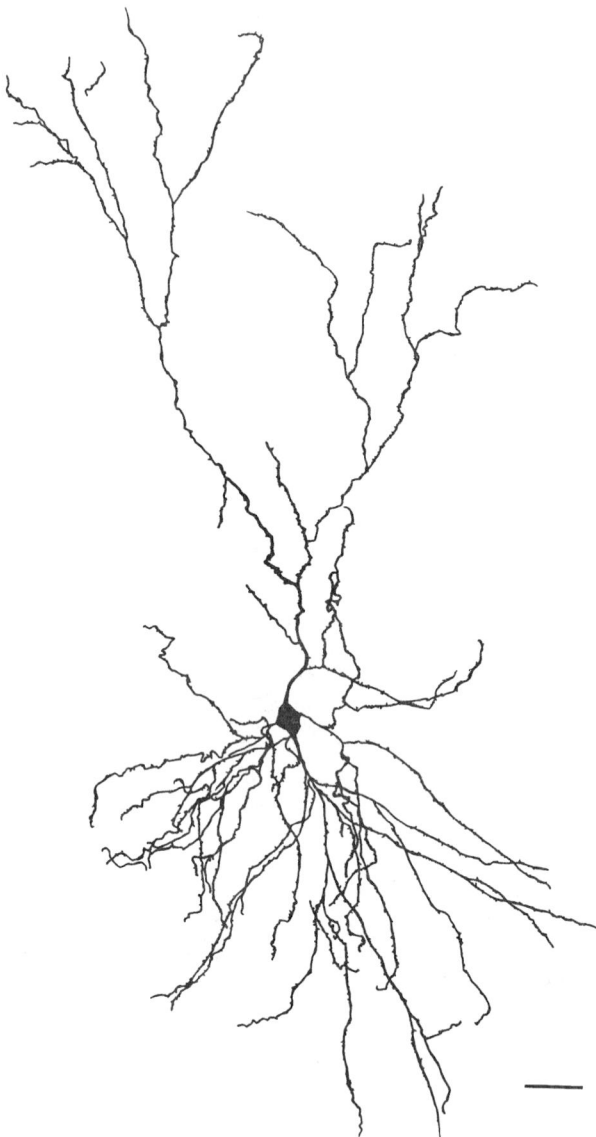

FIGURE 3. A neurobiotin-stained layer III pyramidal neuron is shown. This neuron has morphological features consistent with the type II cells described by Gloveli *et al.*[34] in that its basal dendrites were more radial than elongated, and the basal dendritic tree was more confined. This neuron's synaptic response did not changed after exposure to 10 μM bath-applied AOAA.

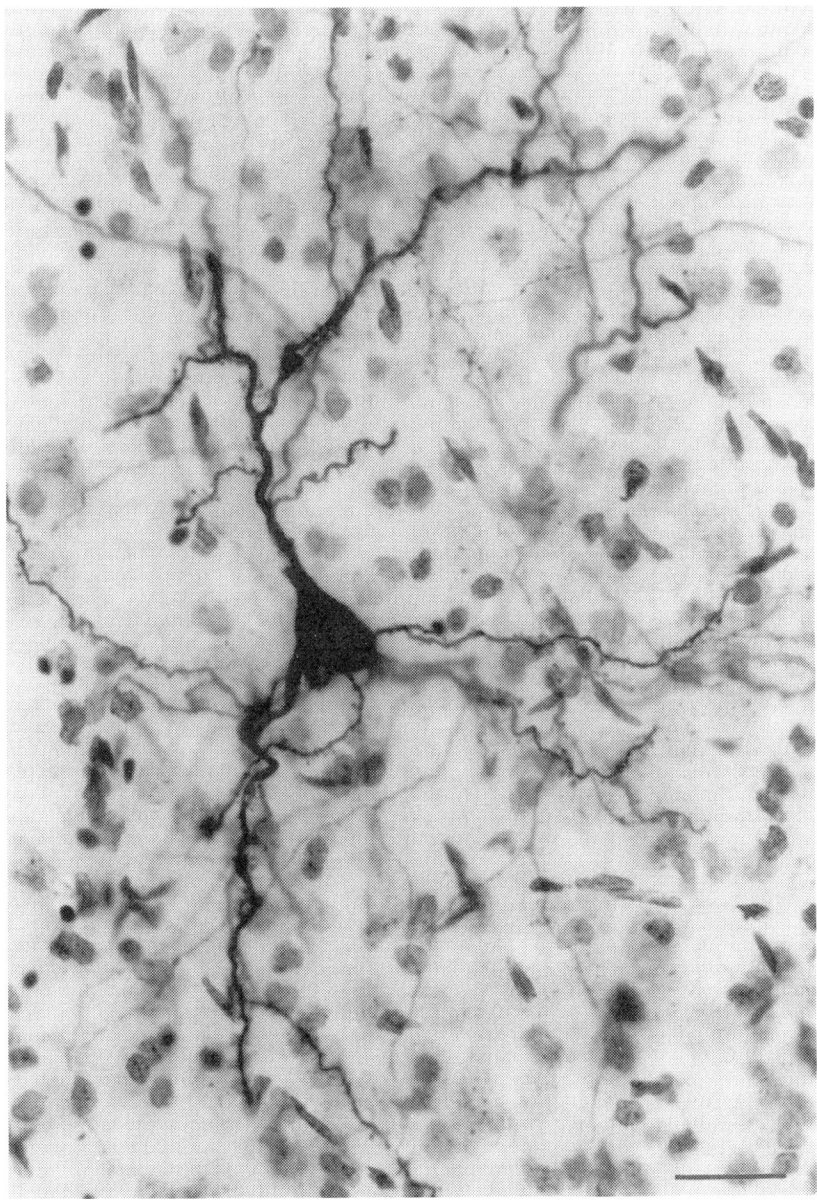

FIGURE 4. A layer II pyramidal neuron is shown. Recordings from this neuron are shown in FIGURE 5. Calibration = 35 μm. Counterstained with cresyl violet. The pial surface is above the top of the figure.

of stimulation to become depolarized, and the depolarization was not necessarily permanent if stimulation stopped.

Thus, in examining the vulnerability of these different types of neurons, the ones with the weaker synaptic inhibition were more vulnerable, that is, type I layer III neurons or the mossy cells closest to the granule cell layer.

Characteristics of Relatively Resistant Neurons

Studies of relatively resistant neurons, that is, layer II neurons and granule cells, indicated certain characteristics that might prevent vulnerability. For example, the resistant neurons appeared to have intrinsic mechanisms to resist depolarization, such as anomalous rectification in response to depolarizing current injection (layer II cells), or simply a very high resting potential (granule cells). However, it can certainly be argued that some of their other intrinsic properties might encourage depolarization, such as the multiple types of sodium current,[2,117] including persistent sodium current.[50]

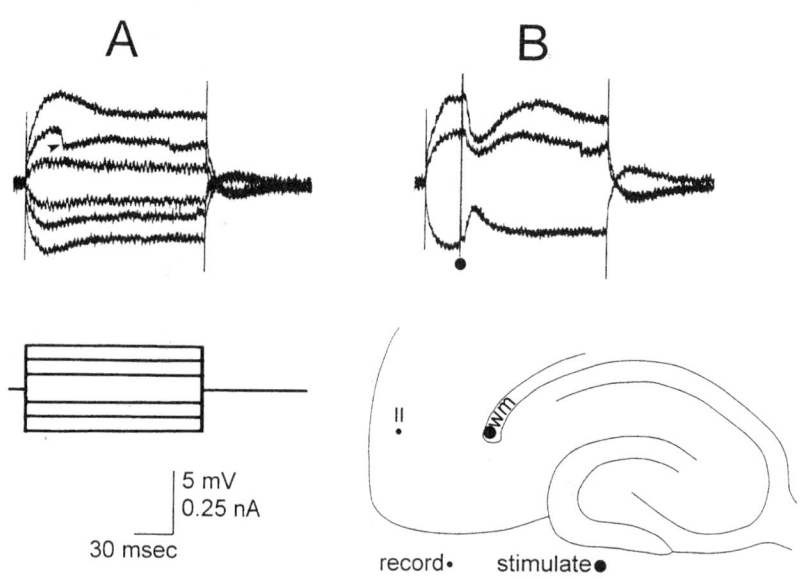

FIGURE 5. Evoked responses from the layer II pyramidal neuron shown in FIGURE 4. (**A**) Responses to intracellular current injection (*diagrammed at the bottom*) demonstrate anomalous rectification or "sag," defined as a decrease in the voltage response at steady-state relative to the initial voltage response. Spontaneous hyperpolarizing events were present (*arrow*) in this and other layer II neurons. (**B**) *Top*: Stimulation of the white matter (at the dot) evoked an IPSP that was reversed when a stimulus was triggered during a hyper-polarizing current pulse. *Bottom*: Schematic of the slice that was used to record the cell, and the location of the stimulating electrode tip. II, layer II; wm, white matter; record, location of recording electrode; stimulate, location of stimulating electrode.

TABLE 3. Comparison of "resistant" cell types[a]

	Layer II Neurons	Granule Cells
Neurotransmitter	Glutamate	Glutamate
Modulator	Zinc, calbindin, BDNF	Zinc, calbindin, BDNF
Afferents	Strong glutamatergic input (deeper layers)	Strong glutamatergic input (perforant path, mossy cells)
	GABAergic/parv/calretinin plexus	GABAergic/parv/calretinin plexus
Efferents	Local and projection neuron	Local and projection neuron
	Innervates principal cells involved in trisynaptic pathway (granule cells)	Innervates principal cells involved in trisynaptic pathway (CA3)
	GABA neurons	GABA neurons
Spines	Many	Many
Intrinsic properties	Regular spiking; no bursts; sag	Regular spiking; no bursts; no sag

[a]For legend, see TABLE 1.

Studies of synaptic responses demonstrated similarities between layer II and granule cells also, that is, IPSPs rather than EPSPs were dominant[33,46] (FIGS. 4 and 5). Layer II neurons also exhibited spontaneous IPSPs; in fact, some layer II neurons only demonstrated spontaneous IPSPs like granule cells (FIG. 5). The large and frequent spontaneous IPSPs of granule cells have been well documented.[70] Thus, analogous to the correlation between weak inhibition and vulnerability just discussed, resistant neurons appear to have strong synaptic inhibition.

Consistent with the hypothesis that AOAA sensitivity is stronger in neurons with a predilection for synaptic excitation, sensitivity to AOAA was not detected in layer II neurons with prominent IPSPs (FIGS. 4 and 5; $n = 8/9$). In the one exception, when a layer II cell was affected, the cell's initial response to stimulation included a prominent EPSP component, which was rare for layer II cells that were tested. These data support the hypothesis that vulnerability is associated with weaker synaptic inhibition and, conversely, that resistance is associated with relatively strong inhibition. These data also may explain why some layer II neurons are damaged after excitotoxic insults;[23] the small fraction of layer II neurons that are damaged may be those with a prominent excitatory component to synaptic responses. The striking similarity in characteristics of layer II neurons and granule cells just described are summarized in TABLE 3.

There are other resistant neurons in both regions, such as parvalbumin-immunoreactive interneurons. Consistent with the hypothesis that resistance is related to synaptic inhibition, some of these resistant interneurons are indeed strongly inhibited. This is known from anatomical studies showing mutual innervation of GABA neurons[38] and dual recordings showing the same phenomenon physiologically.[79] In addition, the pyramidal-shaped neurons at the granule cell layer/hilar border, many of which are thought to contain parvalbumin[75] and are relatively resistant,[99] often have limited responses to afferent stimulation, frequent spontaneous IPSPs, and high sensitivity to bicuculline,[91] a GABA receptor antagonist.

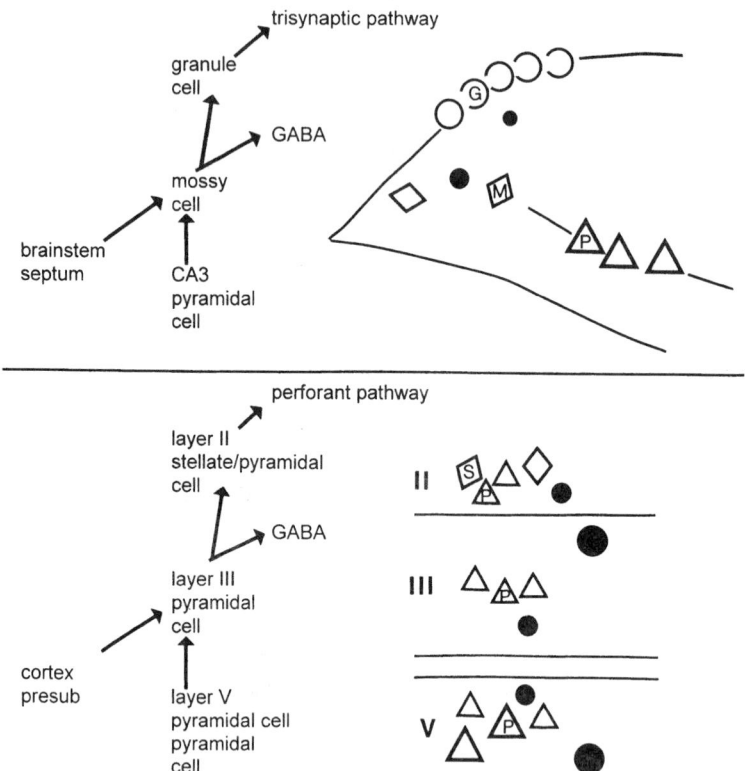

FIGURE 6. Schematic comparing the characteristics of layer III pyramidal neurons and hilar mossy cells. *Arrows* indicate the direction of afferent fibers. GABA, GABAergic neurons; presub, presubiculum; S, stellate; P, pyramidal; M, mossy cells; G, granule cell.

Summary

A summary of several of the comparisons just described is illustrated in FIGURE 6. The focus of this schematic is a comparison of vulnerable neurons, either a mossy cell or a layer III pyramidal cell, and resistant neurons, either granule cells or layer II cells. For the vulnerable cells, both have a local and projecting axon that leaves the lamella of the hippocampus. Both are placed in an intermediary position, between principal cells as well as interneurons. Both receive major input from a glutamatergic principal cell, and they form a major input to a glutamatergic principal cell also. The glutamatergic principal cells they project to are relatively resistant cells that contain calbindin. The entire area in which the vulnerable cell is located (hilus or layer III) is the endpoint of a diverse array of modulatory inputs. In the case of the hilus these arise from the brainstem, septum, or other areas.[85] Potential modulatory input to layer III arises from, for example, the presubiculum or parasubiculum, amygdala, septum, and thalamus.[55]

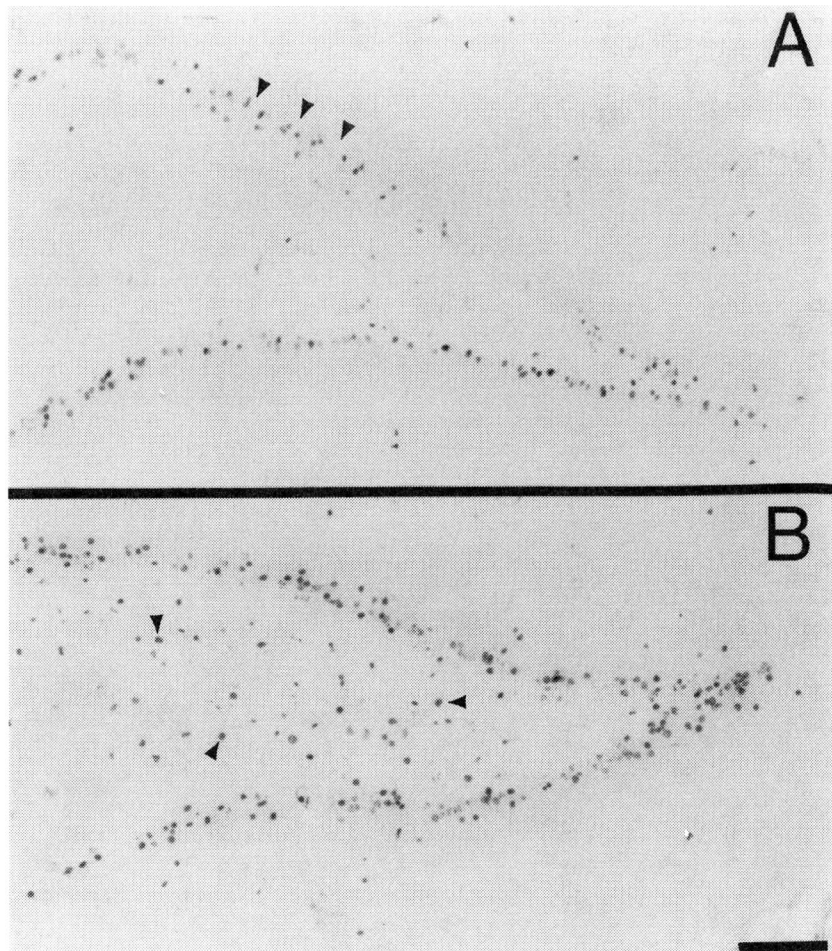

FIGURE 7. Newly-born cells in the hilar region of the dentate gyrus after pilocarpine-induced status epilepticus. (**A**) BrdU-labeled neurons in the dentate gyrus of a rat that was injected with saline and 7–11 days later injected with BrdU once/day to label newly born cells. Many labeled neurons are located in the area just below the granule cell layer (*arrowheads*). (**B**) BrdU-labeled neurons of a rat treated the same as the one in **A**, but instead of saline, pilocarpine was injected systemically and status epilepticus occurred. Diazepam was used to terminate status after 1 hour. Note that many labeled neurons appear in the hilar region (*arrowheads*). Calibration = 125 µm.

Review of the characteristics of vulnerable and resistant cells suggests possible reasons for vulnerability. Vulnerable neurons appear to be in a prime position for excitotoxicity, because synaptic excitation is strong relative to synaptic inhibition. In resistant cells, the converse appears to be the case. In relation to this, calcium entry may be a key factor in synaptic excitation of vulnerable cells, because calcium chelation in mossy cells protects them from prolonged perforant path stimulation.[81] NMDA receptors may also contribute, given the striking demonstration of NMDA receptor-mediated activation of medial EC neurons upon repetitive stimulation[47] and the effects of AOAA.[26,61,92]

NEUROGENESIS

Another parallel between the medial EC and the hilus is that seizure-induced cell birth occurs in both areas. This is particularly interesting to discuss, because it may shed light on the role of these areas in epilepsy.

The subgranular layer in the dentate gyrus has long been known to normally contain newly-born cells, and this has set the dentate gyrus granule cells apart because it is such an unusual characteristic. Over the last few years it has become apparent that an increased number of newly-born granule cells occurs after a variety of manipulations, such as learning, exercise, stress, and seizures (for review, see Ref. 49). Parent et al.[71] noted that some of these newly-born neurons enter the hilar region, as we have found in our pilocarpine-treated rats in which status epilepticus was trun-

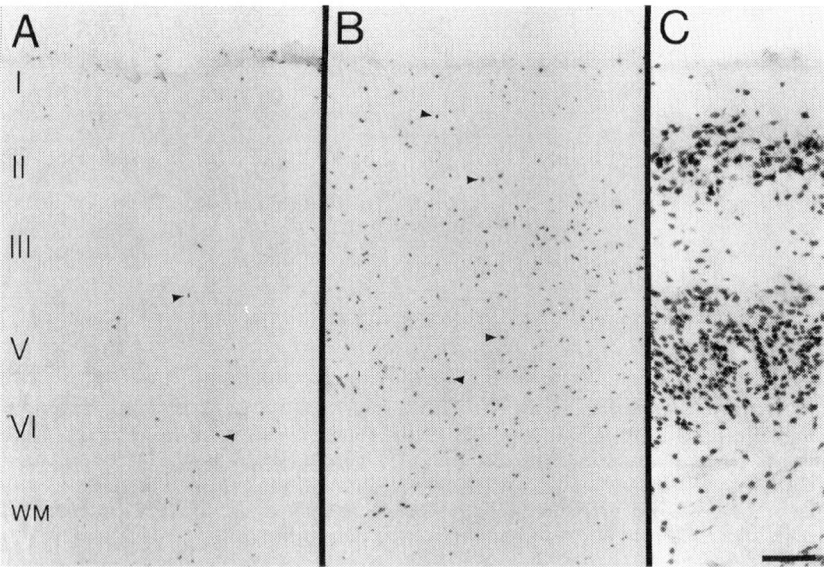

FIGURE 8. Newly-born cells in the medial entorhinal cortex after seizures. (**A**) BrdU-labeled cells (*arrowheads*) in the same rat as in FIGURE 7A. The layers are marked at the left and apply to A–C (I = layer I, II = layer II, III = layer III, V = layer V, VI = layer VI, wm = white matter). (**B**) BrdU-labeled cells in the same rat as in FIGURE 7B. Numerous newly born cells are labeled throughout the layers of the cortex (*arrowheads*). (**C**) An adjacent section to the one in **B** was stained using an antibody to a neuronal nuclear protein (NeuN) to demonstrate the location of neurons. Note that many newly-born cells are located in areas where neurons are located and also in areas where neurons are sparse. Therefore, the newly born cells could be both neurons and non-neuronal cells. Calibration (A–C) = 100 μm.

cated at 1 hour by diazepam injection[71,78A] (FIG. 7). We found in the same animals an unusual number of newly-born cells in the medial EC. FIGURE 8 shows that the medial EC superficial layer contains numerous dividing cells. In these experiments, bromodeoxyuridine (BrdU) is used to label dividing cells by injecting BrdU several days after pilocarpine-induced status epilepticus.[49,71] Immunocytochemistry using an antibody to BrdU is then used to stain the nucleus of dividing neurons. It is possible that the new cells are neurons, because neurons are located in the area of the BrdU-labeled cells (FIG. 8). However, it is also possible that some of the newly born cells are glia or other types of non-neuronal cells. Caution is necessary before assuming that the newly born cells are neurons.

SUMMARY

There is a historical precedent for consideration of the parahippocampal region in epilepsy, and this is borne out in more recent studies of animal models of epilepsy. One of the most striking aspects of the EC in TLE or animal models of epilepsy is the vulnerability of the superficial layers of the medial EC. Based on the parallels of this area with those of the dentate gyrus in terms of both overall circuitry and analysis of cellular properties of vulnerable and resistant neurons, it is hypothesized that synaptic inhibition is a predictor of vulnerability (weak inhibition) and resistance (strong inhibition). There may also be a contribution of seizure-induced newly-born cells in the hilus and medial EC in the epileptogenicity of these two areas. The new circuitry that newly-born cells could lead to might be an important, previously unrecognized aspect of epileptic pathology and epileptogenesis. Manipulations of new excitatory circuits and preservation of new inhibitory connections could be a way of tailoring future therapies to optimize outcome of patients with TLE.

REFERENCES

1. ALONSO, A. & R. KLINK. 1993. Differential electroresponsiveness of stellate and pyramidal-like cells of medial entorhinal cortex layer II. J. Neurophysiol. **70:** 128–143.
2. ALONSO, A. & R.R. LLINÁS. 1989. Subthreshold Na$^+$-dependent theta-like rhythmicity in stellate cells of entorhinal cortex layer II. Nature **342:** 175–177.
3. AMARAL, D.G. 1978. Golgi study of cell types in the hilar region of the hippocampus. J. Comp. Neurol. **182:** 851–914.
4. BAKST, I., C. AVENDANO, J.H. MORRISON & D.G. AMARAL. 1986. An experimental analysis of origins of somatostatin-like immunoreactivity in dentate gyrus of rat. J. Neurosci. **6:** 1452–1462.
5. BEAR, J., N.B. FOUNTAIN & E.W. LOTHMAN. 1996. Responses of the superficial entorhinal cortex in slices from naive and chronically epileptic rats. J. Neurophysiol. **76:** 2928–2950.
6. BEAR, J. & E.W. LOTHMAN. 1993. An *in vitro* study of focal epileptogenesis in combined hippocampal-parahippocampal slices. Epilepsy Res. **14:** 183–193.
7. BRAGIN, A., J. ENGEL, JR., C.L. WILSON, I. FRIED & G.W. MATHERN. 1999. Hippocampal and entorhinal cortex high-frequency oscillations (100-500 Hz) in human epileptic brain and in kainic acid-treated rats with chronic seizures. Epilepsia **40:** 127–137.
8. BUCKMASTER, P.S. & P.A. SCHWARTZKROIN. 1995. Interneurons and inhibition in the dentate gyrus of the rat *in vivo*. J. Neurosci. **15:** 774–789.

9. BUCKMASTER, P.S. & P.A. SCHWARTZKROIN. 1995. Physiological and morphological heterogeneity of dentate gyrus-hilus interneurons in the gerbil hippocampus. Eur. J. Neurosci. **7:** 1393–1402.
10. BUCKMASTER, P.S., B.W. STROWBRIDGE & P.A. SCHWARTZKROIN. 1993. A comparison of rat hippocampal mossy cells and CA3c pyramidal cells. J. Neurophysiol. **70:** 1281–1299.
11. CAVANAUGH, J.B. & A. MEYER. 1956. Aetiological aspects of Ammon's horn sclerosis associated with temporal lobe epilepsy. Br. Med. J. **2:** 1403–1407.
12. CAVAZOS, J.E. & T. SUTULA. 1990. Progressive neuronal loss induced by kindling: a possible mechanism for mossy fiber synaptic reorganization and hippocampal sclerosis. Brain Res. **527:** 1–6.
13. CELIO, M.R. 1990. Calbindin D-28k and parvalbumin in the rat nervous system. Neuroscience **35:** 375–475.
14. COLLINS, R., R.G. TEARSE & E.W. LOTHMAN. 1983. Functional anatomy of limbic seizures: focal discharges from medial entorhinal cortex in rat. Brain Res. **280:** 25–40.
15. CONNORS, B.W. & M.J. GUTNICK. 1990. Intrinsic firing patterns of diverse neocortical neurons. Trends Neurosci. **13:** 99–104.
16. CONNOR, J.M., J.C. LAUTERBORN, Q. YAN, C.M. GALL & S. VARON. 1997. Distribution of brain-derived neurotrophic factor (BDNF) protein and mRNA in the normal adult rat CNS: evidence for anterograde axonal transport. J. Neurosci. **17:** 2295–2313.
17. CRAIN, B.J., W.D. WESTERKAM, A.H. HARRISON & J.V. NADLER. 1988. Selective neuronal death after transient forebrain ischemia in the mongolian gerbil: a silver impregnation study. Neuroscience **27:** 387–402.
18. CROLL, S.D., S.J. WIEGAND, K.D. ANDERSON, R.M. LINDSAY & H. NAWA. 1994. Regulation of neuropeptides in adult rat forebrain by the neurotrophins BDNF and NGF. Eur. J. Neurosci. **6:** 1343–1353.
19. CROLL, S.D., C. SURI, D.L. COMPTON, M.V. SIMMONS, G.D. YANCOPOULOS, R.M. LINDSAY, S.J. WIEGAND, J.S. RUDGE & H.E. SCHARFMAN. 1999. Brain-derived neurotrophic factor transgenic mice exhibit passive avoidance deficits, increased seizure severity and *in vitro* hyperexcitability in the hippocampus and entorhinal cortex. Neuroscience **93:** 1491–1506.
20. DASHEIFF, R.M. & J.O. MCNAMARA. 1982. Electrolytic entorhinal lesions cause seizures. Brain Res. **231:** 444–450.
21. DICKSON, C.T. & A. ALONSO. 1997. Muscarinic induction of synchronous population activity in the entorhinal cortex. J. Neurosci. **17:** 6729–6744.
22. DICKSON, C.T., A.R. MENA & A. ALONSO. 1997. Electroresponsiveness of medial entorhinal cortex layer III neurons *in vitro*. Neuroscience **81:** 937–950.
23. DU, F., T. EID, E.W. LOTHMAN, C. KÖHLER & R. SCHWARCZ. 1995. Preferential neuronal loss in layer III of the medial entorhinal cortex in rat models of temporal lobe epilepsy. J. Neurosci. **15:** 6301–6313.
24. DU, F. & R. SCHWARCZ. 1992. Aminooxyacetic acid causes selective neuronal loss in layer III of the rat medial entorhinal cortex. Neurosci. Lett. **147:** 185–188.
25. DU, F., W.O. WHETSELL, JR., B. ABOU-KHALIL, B. BLUMENKOPF, E.W. LOTHMAN & R. SCHWARCZ. 1993. Preferential neuronal loss in layer III of the entorhinal cortex in patients with temporal lobe epilepsy. Epilepsy Res. **16:** 223–233.
26. EID, T., F. DU & R. SCHWARCZ. 1995. Differential neuronal vulnerability to aminooxyacetate and quinolinate in the rat parahippocampal region. Neuroscience **68:** 645–656.
27. FREDERICKSON, C.J. 1989. Neurobiology of zinc and zinc-containing neurons. Int. Rev. Neurobiol. **31:** 145–238.
28. FREUND, T.F. & G. BUSZÁKI. 1996. Interneurons of the hippocampus. Hippocampus **6:** 347–470.
29. FREUND, T.F., G. BUZSÁKI, A. LEON, K.G. BAIMBRIDGE & P. SOMOGYI. 1990. Relationship of neuronal vulnerability and calcium binding protein immunoreactivity in ischemia. Exp. Brain Res. **83:** 55–66.
30. FREUND, T.F., N. HÁJOS, L. ACSÁDY, T.J. GÖRCS & I. KATONA. 1997. Mossy cells of the rat dentate gyrus are immunoreactive for calcitonin gene-related peptide (CGRP). Eur. J. Neurosci. **9:** 1815–1830.

31. FUJIMARU, Y. & T. KOSAKA. 1996. The distribution of two calcium binding proteins, calbindin D-28K and parvalbumin, in the entorhinal cortex of the adult mouse. Neurosci. Res. **24:** 329–343.
32. GASTAUT, H., M. TOGA, J. ROGER & W.C. GIBSON. 1959. A correlation of clinical, electroencephalographic and anatomical findings in nine autopsied cases of "temporal lobe epilepsy." Epilepsia **1:** 56–81.
33. GLOVELI, T., D. SCHMITZ, R.M. EMPSON & U. HEINEMANN. 1997. Frequency-dependent information flow from the entorhinal cortex to the hippocampus. J. Neurophysiol. **78:** 3444–3449.
34. GLOVELI, T., D. SCHMITZ, R.M. EMPSON, T. DUGLADZE & U. HEINEMANN. 1997. Morphological and electrophysiological characterization of layer III cells of the medial entorhinal cortex of the rat. Neuroscience **77:** 629–648.
35. GLOVELI, T., D. SCHMITZ & U. HEINEMANN. 1997. Prolonged inhibitory potentials in layer III projection cells of the rat medial entorhinal cortex induced by synaptic stimulation *in vitro*. Neuroscience **80:** 119–131.
36. GOODMAN, J.H. & R. SLOVITER. 1992. Evidence for commissurally projecting parvalbumin-immunoreactive basket cells in the dentate gyrus of the rat. Hippocampus **1:** 13–21.
37. GOTTSCHALK, W., L.D. POZZO-MILLER, A. FIGUROV & B. LU. 1998. Presynaptic modulation of synaptic transmission and plasticity by brain-derived neurotrophic factor in the developing hippocampus. J. Neurosci. **18:** 6330–6836.
38. HÁJOS, N., L. ASCÁDY & T.F. FREUND. 1996. Target selectivity and neurochemical characteristics of VIP-immunoreactive interneurons in the rat dentate gyrus. Eur. J. Neurosci. **8:** 1415–1431.
39. HAN, Z.-S., E.H. BUHL, Z. LÖRINCZI & P. SOMOGYI. 1993. A high degree of spatial selectivity in the axonal and dendritic domains of physiologically-identified local circuit neurons in the dentate gyrus of the rat hippocampus. Eur. J. Neurosci. **5:** 395–410.
40. HAUG, F.-M.S. 1973. Heavy Metals in the Brain. Springer-Verlag. New York.
41. HELLIER, J.L., P.R. PATRYLO, P.S. BUCKMASTER & F.E. DUDEK. 1998. Recurrent spontaneous motor seizures after repeated low-dose systemic treatment with kainate: assessment of a rat model of temporal lobe epilepsy. Epilepsy Res. **31:** 73–84.
42. HOUSER, C.R. & M. ESCLAPEZ. 1996. Vulnerability and plasticity of the GABA system in the pilocarpine model of spontaneous recurrent seizures. Epilepsy Res. **26:** 207–218.
43. HSU, M. & G. BUZSÁKI. 1993. Vulnerability of mossy fiber targets in the rat hippocampus to forebrain ischemia. J. Neurosci. **13:** 3964–3979.
44. ISACKSON, P.J., M.M. HUNTSMAN, K.D. MURRAY & C.M. GALL. 1991. BDNF mRNA expression is increased in adult rat forebrain after limbic seizures: temporal patterns of induction distinct from NGF. Neuron **6:** 937–948.
45. JOHANSEN, F.F., J. ZIMMER & N.H. DIEMER. 1987. Early loss of somatostatin neurons in the dentate hilus after cerebral ischemia in the rat precedes CA-1 pyramidal cell loss. Acta Neuropathol. **73:** 110–114.
46. JONES, R.S.G. 1994. Synaptic and intrinsic properties of neurons of origin of the perforant path in layer II of the rat entorhinal cortex in vitro. Hippocampus **4:** 335–353.
47. JONES, R.S.G. 1995. Frequency-dependent alterations in synaptic transmission in entorhinal-hippocampal pathways. Hippocampus **5:** 125–128.
48. KANG, H. & E.M. SCHUMAN. 1995. Long-lasting neurotrophin-induced enhancement of synaptic transmission in the adult hippocampus. Science **267:** 1658–1662.
49. KEMPERMANN, G. & F. GAGE 1999. New nerve cells for the adult brain. Sci. Am. **5:** 48–53.
50. KLINK, R. & A. ALONSO. 1993. Ionic mechanisms for the subthreshold oscillations and differential electroresponsiveness of medial entorhinal cortex layer II neuron. J. Neurophysiol. **70:** 144–157.
51. LI, X.-G., P. SOMOGYI, A. YLINEN & G. BUZSÁKI. 1994. The hippocampal CA3 network: an *in vivo* intracellular labeling study. J. Comp. Neurol. **33:** 181–208.
52. LIU A., T. NAGAO, G.C. DESJARDINS, P. GLOOR & M. AVOLI. 1994. Quantitative evaluation of neuronal loss in the dorsal hippocampus in rats with long-term pilocarpine seizures. Epilepsy Res. **17:** 237–247.
53. LOHOF, A.M., N.Y. IP & M.-M. POO. 1993. Potentiation of developing neuromuscular synapses by the neurotrophins NT-3 and BDNF. Nature **363:** 350–353.

54. LOPANTSEV, V. & M. AVOLI. 1996. Reverberation of chloride-dependent synaptic potentials in the rat entorhinal cortex in vitro. Neurosci. Lett. **210:** 5–8.
55. LOPES DA SILVA, F., M.P. WITTER, P.H. BOEIJINGA & A.H.M. LOTHMAN. 1990. Anatomic organization and physiology of the limbic cortex. Physiol. Rev. **70:** 453–511.
56. LOTHMAN, E.W., D.A. REMPE & P.S. MANGAN. 1995. Changes in excitatory neurotransmission in the CA1 region and dentate gyrus in chronic model of temporal lobe epilepsy. J. Neurophysiol. **74:** 841–848.
57. LOWENSTEIN, D.H., M.J. THOMAS, D.H. SMITH & T.K. MCINTOSH. 1992. Selective vulnerability of dentate hilar neurons following traumatic brain injury: a potential mechanistic link between head trauma and disorders of the hippocampus. J. Neurosci. **12:** 4846–4853.
58. LÜCKE, A., N. TAKEKI, R. KÖHLING & M. AVOLI. 1995. Synchronous potentials and elevations in $[K+]_o$ in the adult rat entorhinal cortex maintained in vitro. Neurosci. Lett. **185:** 155–158.
59. MANGAN, P.S., D.A. REMPE & E.W. LOTHMAN. 1995. Changes in inhibitory neurotransmission in the CA1 region and dentate gyrus in a chronic model of temporal lobe epilepsy. J. Neurophysiol. **74:** 829–839.
60. MARGERISON, J.H. & J.A.N. CORSELLIS. 1966. Epilepsy and the temporal lobes: a clinical electroencephalographic and neuropathological study of the brain in epilepsy, with particular reference to the temporal lobes. Brain **89:** 499–530.
61. MCMASTER, O.G., F. DU, E.D. FRENCH & R. SCHWARCZ. 1991. Focal injection of aminooxyacetic acid produces seizures and lesions in rat hippocampus: evidence for mediation by NMDA receptors. Exp. Neurol. **113:** 378–385.
62. MELDRUM, B.S. & C.J. BRUTON. Epilepsy. In Greenfield's Neuropathology. J.H. Adams & L.W. Duchen, Eds. : 1246–1283. Oxford University Press. New York.
63. MIETTINEN, A., A. PITKÄNEN & R. MIETTINEN. 1997. Distribution of calretinin-immunoreactivity in the rat entorhinal cortex: coexistence with GABA. J. Comp. Neurol. **378:** 363–378.
64. MIETTINEN, R., T. KOTTI, J. TUUNANEN, A. TOPPINEN, P. RIEKKINEN, SR. & T. HALONEN. 1998. Hippocampal damage after injection of kainic acid into the rat entorhinal cortex. Brain Res. **813:** 9–17.
65. MIETTINEN, M., E. KOIVISTO, P. RIEKKINEN, SR. & R. MIETTINEN. 1995. Coexistence of parvalbumin and GABA in nonpyramidal neurons of the rat entorhinal cortex. Brain Res. **706:** 113–122.
66. MORIN, G. & H. GASTAUT. 1954. Colloquium concerning normal and pathological anatomical problems raised by epileptic discharges. Acta Med. Belg. Brussels. 140 pp.
67. NAGAO, T., A. ALONSO & M. AVOLI. 1996. Epileptiform activity induced by pilocarpine in the rat hippocampal-entorhinal slice preparation. Neuroscience **72:** 399–408.
68. NAKASATO, N., M.F. LÉVESQUE & T.L. BABB. 1992. Seizure outcome following standard temporal lobectomy: correlation with hippocampal neuron loss and extrahippocampal pathology. J. Neurosurg. **77:** 194–200.
69. NITSCH, R., E. SORIANO & M. FROTSCHER. 1990. The parvalbumin-containing nonpyramidal neurons in the rat hippocampus. Anat. Embryol. **181:** 413–425.
70. OTIS, T.S., K.J. STALEY & I. MODY. 1991. Perpetual inhibitory activity in mammalian brain slices generated by spontaneous GABA release. Brain Res. **545:** 142–150.
71. PARENT, J.M., T.W. YU, R.T. LEIBOWITZ, D.H. GESCHWIND, R.S. SLOVITER & D.H. LOWENSTEIN. 1997. Dentate granule cell neurogenesis is increased by seizures and contributes to aberrant network reorganization in the adult rat hippocampus. J. Neurosci. **17:** 3727–3728.
72. RAFIQ, A., R.J. DELORENZO & D.A. COULTER. 1993. Generation and propagation of epileptiform discharges in a combined entorhinal cortex/hippocampal slice. J. Neurophysiol. **70:** 1962–1972.
73. RAFIQ, A., Y.-U. ZHANG, R.J. DELORENZO & D.A. COULTER. 1995. Long-duration self-sustained epileptiform activity in the hippocampal-parahippocampal slice: a model of status epilepticus. J. Neurophysiol. **74:** 2028–2041.
74. REMPE, D.A., P.S. MANGAN & E.W. LOTHMAN. 1995. Regional heterogeneity of pathophysiological alterations in CA1 and dentate gyrus in a chronic model of temporal lobe epilepsy. J. Neurophysiol. **74:** 816–828.

75. RIBAK, C.E., R. NITSCH & L. SERESS. 1990. Proportion of parvalbumin-positive basket cells in the GABAergic innervation of pyramidal and granule cells of the rat hippocampal formation. J. Comp. Neurol. **300:** 449–461.
76. RIBAK, C.E., L. SERESS, P. WEBER, C.M. EPSTEIN, T.R. HENRY & R.A.E. BAKAY. 1998. Alumina gel injections into the temporal lobe of rhesus monkeys cause complex partial seizures and morphological changes found in human temporal lobe epilepsy. J Comp. Neurol. **401:** 266–290.
77. RUTECKI, P.A., R.G. GROSSMAN, D. ARMSTRONG & S. IRISH-LOEWEN. 1989. Electrophysiological connections between the hippocampus and entorhinal cortex in patients with complex partial seizures. J. Neurosurg. **70:** 667–675.
78. SCHARFMAN, H.E., J.H. GOODMAN, F. DU & R. SCHWARCZ. 1998. Chronic changes in synaptic responses of entorhinal and hippocampal neurons after amino-oxyacetic acid (AOAA)-induced entorhinal cortical neuron loss. J. Neurophysiol. **80:** 3031–3046.
78A. SCHARFMAN, H.E., J.H. GOODMAN & A.L. SOLLAS. 1999. Granule-like hilar neurons in pilocarpine-treated rats and their synchronization with CA3 pyramidal cells. Epilepsia **40(S7):** 156.
79. SCHARFMAN, H.E., D.D. KUNKEL & P.A. SCHWARTZKROIN. 1990. Synaptic connections of dentate granule cells and hilar neurons: results of paired intracellular recordings and intracellular horseradish peroxidase injections. Neuroscience **37:** 693–707.
80. SCHARFMAN, H.E. & P.A. SCHWARTZKROIN. 1988. Electrophysiology of morphologically-identified dentate hilar "mossy" cells in rat hippocampal slices. J. Neurosci. **8:** 3812–3821.
81. SCHARFMAN, H.E. & P.A. SCHWARTZKROIN. 1989. Protection of dentate hilar mossy cells from prolonged stimulation by intracellular calcium chelation. Science **246:** 257–260.
82. SCHARFMAN, H.E. & P.A. SCHWARTZKROIN. 1990. Consequences of prolonged afferent stimulation of the rat fascia dentata: epileptiform activity in area CA3 of hippocampus. Neuroscience **35:** 505–517.
83. SCHARFMAN, H.E. & P.A. SCHWARTZKROIN. 1990. Responses of cells of the fascia dentata to prolonged stimulation of the perforant path: sensitivity of hilar cells and changes in granule cell excitability. Neuroscience **35:** 491–504.
84. SCHARFMAN, H.E. 1992. Blockade of excitation reveals inhibition of dentate spiny hilar neurons recorded in rat hippocampal slices. J. Neurophysiol. **68:** 978–984.
85. SCHARFMAN, H.E. 1992. Differentiation of rat dentate neurons by morphology and electrophysiology in hippocampal slices: granule cells, spiny hilar cells and aspiny, "fast-spiking" cells. Prog. Brain Res. **83:** 93–109.
86. SCHARFMAN, H.E. 1991. Dentate hilar cells with dendrites in the molecular layer have lower thresholds for synaptic activation by perforant path than granule cells. J. Neurosci. **11:** 1660–1673.
87. SCHARFMAN, H.E. 1993. Characteristics of spontaneous and evoked EPSPs recorded from dentate spiny hilar cells in rat hippocampal slices. J. Neurophysiol. **70:** 742–757.
88. SCHARFMAN, H.E. 1993. Spiny neurons of area CA3c in rat hippocampal slices have similar electrophysiological properties and synaptic responses despite morphological variation. Hippocampus **3:** 9–28.
89. SCHARFMAN, H.E. 1994. EPSPs of dentate gyrus granule cells during epileptiform bursts of dentate hilar mossy cells and area CA3 pyramidal cells in disinhibited rat hippocampal slices. J. Neurosci. **14:** 6041–6057.
90. SCHARFMAN, H.E. 1994. Evidence from simultaneous intracellular recordings in rat hippocampal slices that area CA3 pyramidal cells innervate dentate hilar mossy cells. J. Neurophysiol. **72:** 2167–2180.
91. SCHARFMAN, H.E. 1995. Electrophysiological diversity of pyramidal-shaped neurons at the granule cell layer/hilus border of the rat dentate gyrus recorded in vitro. Hippocampus **5:** 287–305.
92. SCHARFMAN, H.E. 1996. Hyperexcitability of entorhinal cortex and hippocampus after application of aminooxyacetic acid (AOAA) to layer III of the rat entorhinal cortex in vitro. J. Neurophysiol. **76:** 2986–3001.
93. SCHARFMAN, H.E. 1997. Hyperexcitability in combined entorhinal/hippocampal slices of adult rat after exposure to brain-derived neurotrophic factor. J. Neurophysiol. **78:** 1082–1095.

94. SCHARFMAN, H.E. 1999. The role of nonprincipal cells in dentate gyrus excitability and its relevance to animal models of epilepsy and temporal lobe epilepsy. *In* Jasper's Basic Mechanisms of the Epilepsies, 3rd Ed. Advances in Neurology, Vol. 79. A.V. Delgado-Escueta, W.A. Wilson, R.W. Olsen & R.J. Porter, Eds. : 805–820. Lippincott Williams & Wilkins. Philadelphia.
95. SCHMIDT-KASTNER R., C. HUMPEL, C. WETMORE & L. OLSON. 1996. Cellular hybridization for BDNF, trkB, and NGF mRNAs and BDNF-immunoreactivity in rat forebrain after pilocarpine-induced status epilepticus. Exp. Brain Res. **107:** 331–347.
96. SERESS, L., R. NITSCH & C. LERANTH. 1993. Calretinin immunoreactivity in the monkey hippocampal formation-1. Light and electron microscopic characteristics and colocalization with other calcium-binding proteins. Neuroscience **55:** 775–796.
97. SERESS, L. & C.E. RIBAK. 1983. GABAergic cells in the dentate gyrus appear to be local circuit and projection neurons. Exp. Brain Res. **50:** 173–182.
98. SLOMIANKA, L. 1992. Neurons of origin of zinc-containing pathways and the distribution of zinc-containing boutons in the hippocampal region of the rat. Neuroscience **48:** 325–352.
99. SLOVITER, R.S. 1989. Calcium-binding protein (calbindin D28k) and parvalbumin immunocytochemistry: localization in the rat hippocampus with specific reference to selective vulnerability of hippocampal neurons to seizure activity. J. Comp. Neurol. **280:** 183–196.
100. SLOVITER, R.S. 1991. Permanently altered hippocampal structure, excitability and inhibition after experimental status epilepticus in the rat: the "dormant basket cell" hypothesis and its possible relevance to temporal lobe epilepsy. Hippocampus **1:** 41–66.
101. SLOVITER, R.S. & G. NILAVER. 1987. Immunocytochemical localization of GABA-, cholecystokinin-, vasoactive intestinal polypeptide-, and somatostatin-like immunoreactivity in the area dentata and hippocampus of the rat. J. Comp. Neurol. **256:** 42–61.
102. SMITH, D.H., D.H. LOWENSTEIN, T.A. GENNARELLI & T.K. MCINTOSH. 1994. Persistent memory dysfunction is associated with bilateral hippocampal damage following experimental brain injury. Neurosci. Lett. **168:** 151–154.
103. SOLTESZ, I., J. BOURASSA & M. DESCHÊNES. 1993. The behavior of mossy cells of the rat dentate gyrus during theta oscillations *in vivo*. Neuroscience **57:** 555–564.
104. SOLTESZ, I. & R.S.G. JONES. 1995. The direct perforant path input to CA1: excitatory or inhibitory? Hippocampus **5:** 101–103.
105. SOLTESZ, I. & I. MODY. 1994. Patch-clamp recordings reveal powerful GABAergic inhibition in dentate hilar neurons. J. Neurosci. **14:** 2365–2376.
106. SORIANO, E. & M. FROTSCHER. 1994. Mossy cells of the rat fascia dentata are glutamate-immunoreactive. Hippocampus **4:** 65–70.
107. SPERK, G., J. MARKSTEINER, B. GRUBER, R. BELLMANN, M. MAHATA, & M. ORTLER. 1992. Functional changes in neuropeptide Y and somatostatin containing neurons induced by limbic seizures in the rat. Neuroscience **50:** 831–846.
108. TAKEI, N., K. SASAOKA, K. INOUE, M. TAKAHASHI, Y. ENDO & H. HATANAKA. 1997. Brain-derived neurotrophic factor increases the stimulation-evoked release of glutamate and the levels of exocytosis-associated proteins in cultured cortical neurons from embryonic rats. J. Neurochem. **68:** 370–375.
109. TANCREDI, V., G.G.C. HWA, C. ZONA, A. BRANCATI & M. AVOLI. 1990. Low magnesium epileptogenesis in the rat hippocampus slice: electrophysiological and pharmacological features. Brain Res. **511:** 280–290.
110. TUÑÓN, T., R. INSAUSTI, I. FERRER, T. SOBREVIELA & E. SORIANO. 1992. Parvalbumin and calbindin D-28K in the human entorhinal cortex. An immunohistochemical study. Brain Res. **589:** 24–32.
111. VAN DER LINDEN, S. & F.H. LOPES DA SILVA. 1998. Comparison of the electrophysiology and morphology of layers III and II neurons of the rat medial entorhinal cortex *in vitro*. Eur. J. Neurosci. **10:** 1479–1489.
112. VEZZANI, A., S. GÜNTHER & W.F. COLMERS. 1999. Neuropeptide Y: emerging evidence for a functional role in seizure modulation. Trends Neurosci. **22:** 25–30.
113. VEZZANI, A, R. MONHEMIUS, P. TUTKA, R. MILANI & R. SAMANIN. 1996. Functional activation of somatostatin and neuropeptide Y containing neurons in the entorhinal cortex of chronically epileptic rats. Neuroscience **75:** 551–557.

114. VEZZANI, A., T. RAVIZZA, D. MONETA, M. CONTI, A. BARONNI, M. RIZZI, R. SAMANIN & R. MAJ. 1999. Brain-derived neurotropic factor immunoreactivity in the limbic system of rats after acute seizures and during spontaneous convulsions: temporal evolution of changes as compared to neuropeptide Y. Neuroscience **90:** 1445–1461.
115. VEZZANI, A., C. SCHWARZER, E.W. LOTHMAN, J. WILLIAMSON & G. SPERK. 1996. Functional changes in somatostatin and neuropeptide Y containing neurons in the rat hippocampus in chronic models of limbic seizures. Epilepsy Res. **26:** 267–279.
116. WALTHER, H., J.D.C. LAMBERT, R.S.G. JONES, U. HEINEMANN & B. HAMON. 1986. Epileptiform activity in combined slices of the hippocampus, subiculum and entorhinal cortex during perfusion with low magnesium medium. Neurosci. Lett. **69:** 156–161.
117. WHITE, J.A., A. ALONSO & A.R. KAY. 1993. A heart-like Na$^+$ current in the medial entorhinal cortex. Neuron **11:** 1037–1047.
118. WILSON, W.A., H.S. SWARTZWELDER, W.W. ANDERSON & D.V. LEWIS. 1988. Seizure activity *in vitro*: a dual focus model. Epilepsy Res. **2:** 289–293.
119. WOUTERLOOD, F.G., W. HÄRTIG, G. BRÜCKNER & M.P. WITTER. 1995. Parvalbumin-immunoreactive neurons in the entorhinal cortex of the rat: localization, morphology, connectivity and ultrastructure. J. Neurocytol. **24:** 135–153.
120. YAN, Q., R.D. ROSENFELD, C.R. MATHESON, N. HAWKINS, O.T. LOZEZ, L. BENNETT & A.A. WELCHER. 1997. Expression of brain-derived neurotrophic factor (BDNF) protein in the adult rat central nervous system. Neuroscience **78:** 431–448.
121. ZIMMERMAN, H.M. 1938. The histopathology of convulsive disorders of children. J. Pediatr. **13:** 839–890.

Neurons in Layer III of the Entorhinal Cortex

A Role in Epileptogenesis and Epilepsy?

ROBERT SCHWARCZ,[a] TORE EID, AND FU DU

Maryland Psychiatric Research Center, University of Maryland School of Medicine, Baltimore, Maryland, USA

ABSTRACT: A preferential lesion of neurons in layer III of the entorhinal cortex (EC) is often observed in patients suffering from temporal lobe epilepsy and in several animal models of the disease. This lesion is duplicated in rats by a focal, intra-entorhinal injection of the "indirect" excitotoxin aminooxyacetic acid (AOAA), providing a model that can be used to study the mechanisms underlying seizure-induced cell death and epilepsy. Doomed neurons in the EC and in several associated limbic structures show pathological changes within hours after the AOAA injection, but GABAergic neurons in layer III of the EC are quite resistant. This pattern of neuron loss eventually results in hippocampal and entorhinal hyperexcitability. Notably, the seizure-induced death of layer III neurons in the EC can be attenuated by eliminating the prominent excitatory input from the presubiculum. Taken together, these results suggest opportunities to target parahippocampal structures for the treatment of temporal lobe epilepsy.

INTRODUCTION

The parahippocampal region has long been known to play a role in the generation and propagation of spontaneously recurring seizures, the major clinical hallmark of temporal lobe epilepsy ("psychomotor epilepsy"). In fact, several of the leading epileptologists of the 19th century had already recognized the importance of "perihippocampal structures" and ascribed to them certain pathophysiological functions (see reference 1 and citations therein). In the first half of the 20th century, this view was continuously refined, and a consensus was reached that prolonged seizure episodes (i.e., status epilepticus), in particular, cause a preferential degeneration of neurons in the "third cortical layer".[2–5] In spite of the idiosyncratic anatomical terminology used at the time, review of the pertinent literature suggests that the structure showing neurodegeneration in several of these publications refers to the rostral portion of the entorhinal cortex (EC).

A precipitous disregard for those earlier findings and concepts coincided with an increasing attention to the hippocampus, which was believed by many to play a primary role in the genesis of epileptic phenomena. Soon, very little consideration was given to a participatory function of the parahippocampal region in epilepsy, to the point that the entorhinal lesion was ignored in the most influential reviews of the

[a]Address for correspondence: Robert Schwarcz, Ph.D., Maryland Psychiatric Research Center, P.O. Box 21247, Baltimore, Maryland 21228. Tel.: (410) 402-7635; fax: (410) 747-2434.
e-mail: rschwarc@umaryland.edu

neuropathology of epilepsy.[6,7] This development was reversed only with the realization of the functional interdependence of the hippocampus and the parahippocampal region in the normal mammalian brain[8,9] and the indication, from neurosurgical and imaging studies, that parahippocampal structures are often critically involved in seizure disorders.[10–13]

Our own interest in the role of the parahippocampal region in the pathophysiology of epilepsy originated from studies with several animal models of temporal lobe epilepsy, which reliably presented with a highly localized, bilateral lesion of layer III of the EC.[14] Analysis of parahippocampal tissue samples from patients undergoing epilepsy surgery led to the evaluation of the previously described pattern of neurodegeneration (see above) in a modern neuroanatomical context.[15] It is noteworthy that, in both epileptic animals and humans, a small number of neurons were found to survive in the otherwise neuron-depleted, gliotic EC tissue. In the animal models, these surviving neurons were identified as parvalbumin-positive, GABAergic cells,[14,16] and it can be reasonably assumed that the same type of neurons survive in the human disease. Thus, epileptic EC damage appears to be readily duplicated in rodents that develop spontaneous seizures after prolonged electrical stimulation[17] or chemoconvulsant treatments.[18,19] Notably, a qualitatively very similar pattern of entorhinal damage also occurs in epileptic nonhuman primates.[20]

FOCAL AMINOOXYACETIC ACID (AOAA) INJECTIONS INTO THE RAT ENTORHINAL CORTEX

The pronounced and preferential vulnerability of neurons in layer III of the EC, along with the discovery that the irreversible neuronal damage in the EC appears to be essentially completed within 48 hours after an extended seizure episode,[14,21] renewed interest in the possibility that EC lesions play an early and critical role in the development of epilepsy. More specifically, since the most seizure-sensitive neurons in layer III of the medial EC give rise to the temporo-ammonic pathway, which projects monosynaptically to the subiculum and area CA1 of the hippocampus,[22] we postulated that entorhinal neurodegeneration may secondarily result in hippocampal hyperexcitability and thus contribute to epilepsy.[14] Ideally, this hypothesis could be tested by examining the short- and long-term consequences of a selective, contained EC lesion. Unfortunately, conventional animal models of epilepsy, induced by continuous stimulation of the ventral hippocampus[17] or by the systemic administration of chemoconvulsants such as kainate[23] or pilocarpine,[19] were not suitable for this purpose because they showed extensive neuronal loss in several limbic brain regions and beyond.

In our search for a methodology to produce animals with a selective neurodegeneration in layer III of the EC, we were guided by reports that seizure-related nerve cell loss occurs by excitotoxic mechanisms. This conclusion was based on the light microscopic appearance of seizure-related damage,[24] on pharmacological studies using excitatory amino acid receptor antagonists,[25,26] and on the ultrastructural analysis of degenerating neurons, which revealed the characteristic "axon-sparing" nature of seizure-induced lesions.[27] However, the qualitative features of the EC lesion could not be duplicated by intra-entorhinal microinjections of widely used excitotoxins such as ibotenate,[28] N-methyl-D-aspartate (NMDA),[29] or quinolinate.[30] Instead, low concentrations of these toxins caused preferential neurodegeneration of layers II or V, and layer III was only affected at higher doses.

In contrast to these classic excitotoxins, which exert their action by direct stimulation of excitatory amino acid receptors, "indirect" excitotoxins promote neurodegeneration by weakening neuronal resistance to normally innocuous concentrations of endogenous excitatory receptor agonists such as glutamate.[31] This may involve interference with cellular energy metabolism,[32,33] a reduction in endogenous defense mechanisms,[31,34–36] or a combination of these factors. During the past decade, several indirect excitotoxins have been introduced as lesioning tools in experimental neurobiology. Two of those agents, aminooxyacetic acid (AOAA) and γ-acetylenic GABA (GAG), also decrease GABA formation at high concentrations[37,38] and were therefore deemed to be particularly useful for modeling seizure-related damage in epilepsy, a putative GABA deficiency disorder.[39]

Intra-entorhinal injections of either AOAA or GAG in adult rats result in a pattern of local neurodegeneration, which closely resembles that seen in patients with temporal lobe epilepsy.[40,41] As illustrated in FIGURE 1 for AOAA, the lesions affect primarily layer III of the EC and are particularly apparent when viewed in horizontal tissue sections. Both toxins cause acute generalized seizures, which can be recorded by EEG between 2 and 4 hours after an AOAA injection and between 3 and 12 hours after a GAG injection. Moreover, the neurodegenerative effects of both agents are characterized by very steep dose-response relationships leading, for example, to massive additional loss of neurons in the hilus of the dentate gyrus when the GAG dose is raised from 4 to 5 μg.[41] Other parallels between AOAA and GAG include the preferential vulnerability of the ventromedial portion of layer III, and the ability of the noncompetitive NMDA receptor antagonist MK-801 to convey neuroprotection (cf. the chapter by Kontkanen et al. for additional effects of MK-801 on layer III neurons).

Most of the experimental studies reported so far have used AOAA to eliminate layer III neurons in the medial EC. Essentially, those studies have begun to explore (a) the qualitative nature of the neuropathological changes over time, (b) the acute and chronic electrophysiological sequelae of an intra-entorhinal AOAA injection, and (c) the mechanisms that underlie the preferential vulnerability of layer III neurons in the EC.

ACUTE AND SUBACUTE CONSEQUENCES OF AN INTRA-ENTORHINAL AOAA INJECTION IN RATS

Various histological methods have been used to assess the nature and temporal characteristics of the structural changes that occur after a focal AOAA injection into the rat EC. The first brief report was limited to the analysis of Nissl-stained sections and emphasized the preferential lesion of layer III neurons in the medial portion of the EC. Neuropathology was noted irrespective of the location of the injection cannula within the EC.[40] More extensive study of the lesioned brains revealed neuronal damage and associated gliosis also in other areas, such as the subiculum, area CA1 of the hippocampus (FIG. 1), and the lateral amygdaloid nuclei. In the EC, neurons

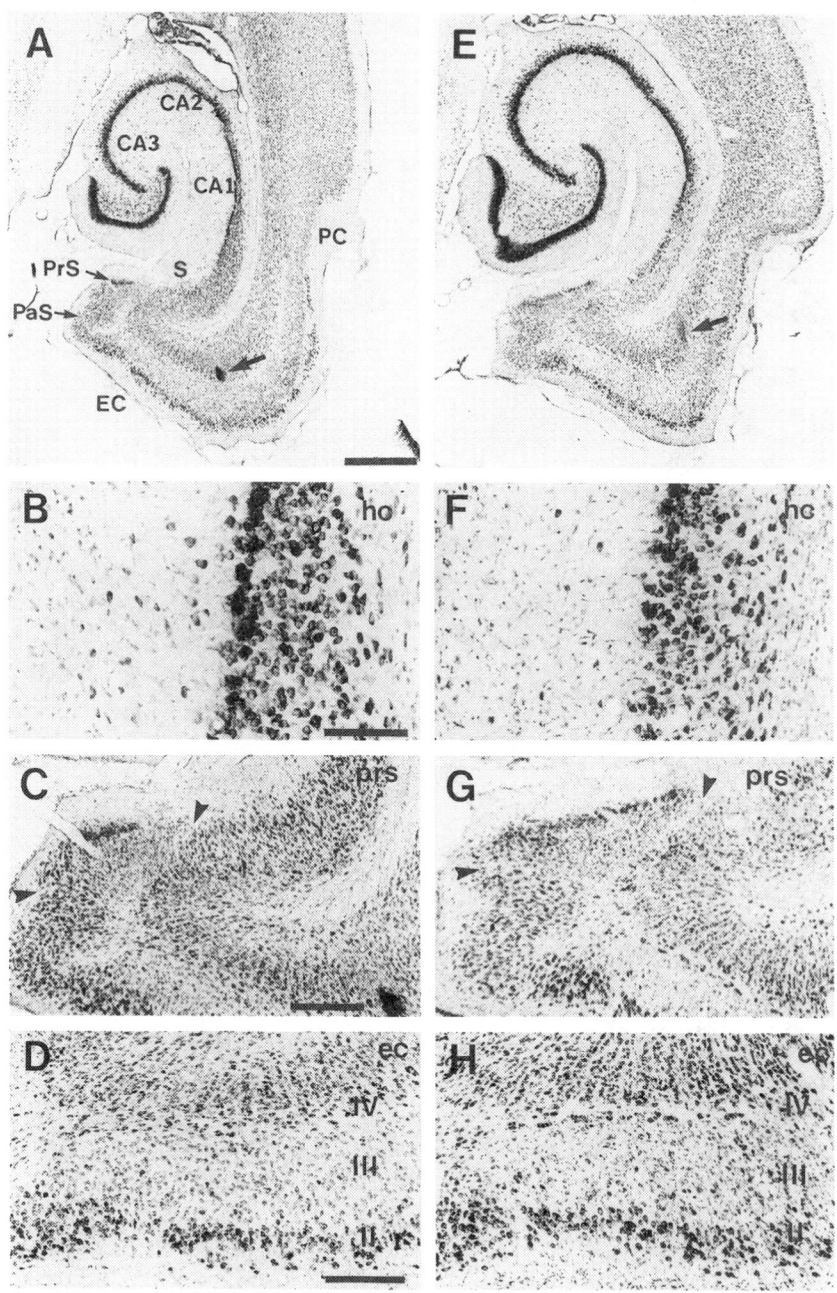

FIGURE 1. *See following page for caption.*

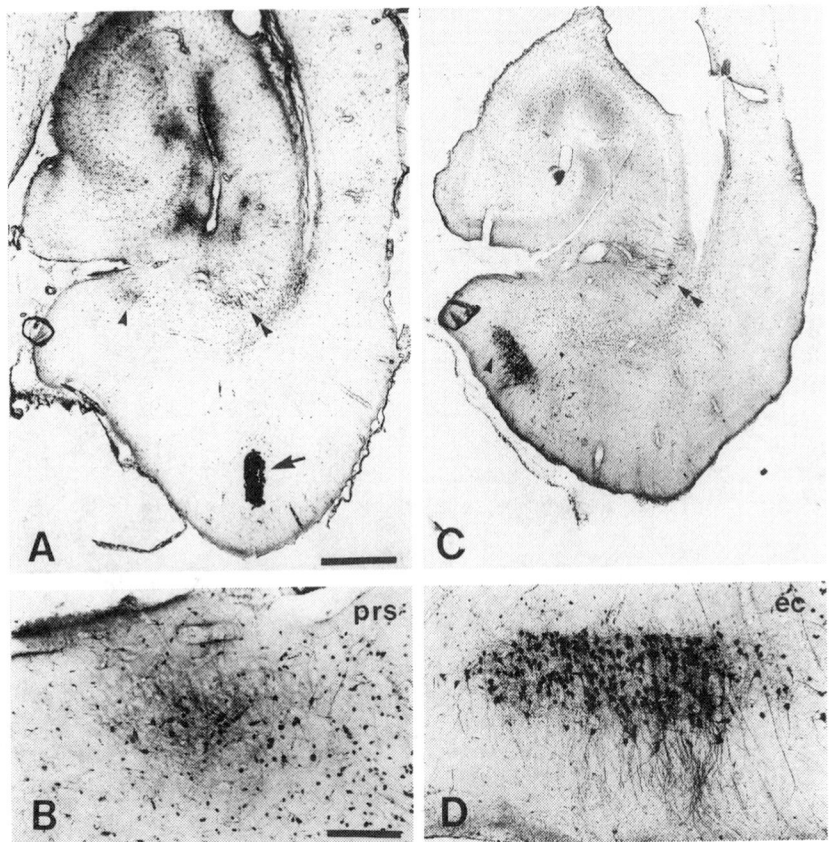

FIGURE 2. Micrographs of silver-stained horizontal sections through the EC of rats receiving an intra-entorhinal injection of AOAA (75 µg/0.75 µL) given 3 hours (**A, B**) or 6 hours (**C, D**) earlier. Note the absence of silver-stained neurons in layer III of the EC in **A**. **B** and **D** are high-power views of the presubiculum (prs) and entorhinal cortex (ec) of the areas indicated by single arrowheads in **A** and **C**, respectively. Double arrowheads mark the subiculum/CA1 transition zone. The arrow in **A** indicates the track of the injection needle. Scale bars—**A, C**: 350 µm; **B, D**: 80 µm. (From reference 21, with permission.)

FIGURE 1. Micrographs of horizontal, Nissl-stained sections through the middle level of the EC from a saline-injected (**A–D**) and an AOAA (75 µg/0.75 µL)–injected (**E–H**) rat, respectively. Animals were killed 5 days after the intra-entorhinal injections. **B–D** and **F–H** are high-power micrographs of the hippocampus (hc), presubiculum (prs), and entorhinal cortex (ec) of the sections depicted in **A** and **E**, respectively. In the AOAA-treated rat, layer III of the medial entorhinal cortex shows a dramatic loss of neurons (**H**). Some neurons have also degenerated in the subiculum/CA1 transition zone (**F**), but a loss of neurons is not immediately apparent in the presubiculum (region between the arrowheads in **G**). PaS: parasubiculum; PrS: presubiculum; S: subiculum; PC: perirhinal cortex; CA1–3: hippocampal subfields. Scale bars—**A, E**: 400 µm; **B, D, F, H**: 80 µm; **C, G**: 200 µm.

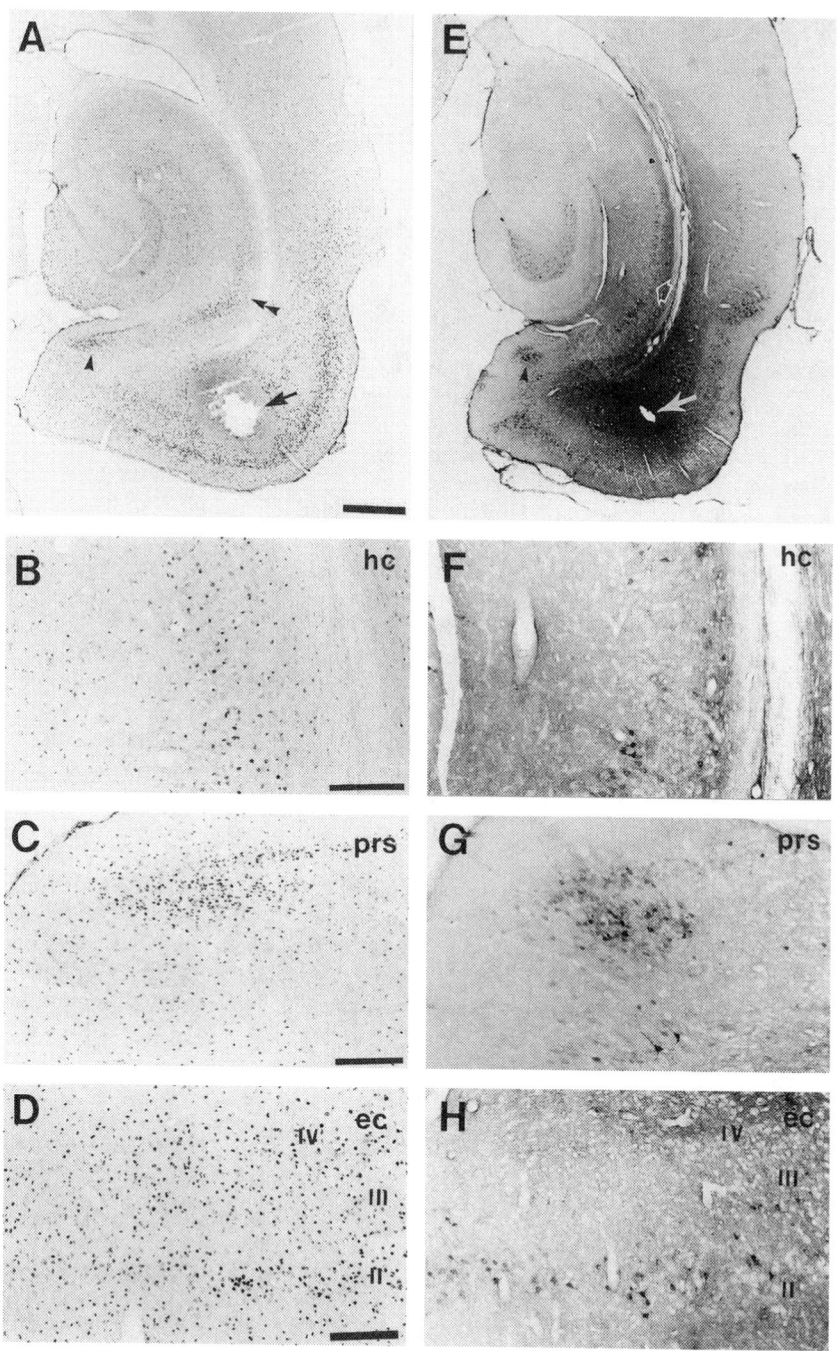

FIGURE 3. *See following page for caption.*

in the lateral part of layer III were clearly less susceptible to degeneration than in the medial segment, and there was also a pronounced dorso-ventral gradient of vulnerability.[40] Taken together, this pattern of neurodegeneration suggested a close relationship between the damage in the EC and in areas with known anatomical connections to or from the degenerated entorhinal neurons[42] (also see Witter *et al.*, this volume).

A silver stain study conducted on tissue from animals killed between 3 hours and 5 days after an intra-entorhinal AOAA injection indicated the involvement of the subiculum/CA1, and also the presubiculum, in the neurodegenerative process.[21] As illustrated in FIGURE 2, silver-impregnated cells were readily detectable in both of these areas 3 hours after AOAA, that is, at a time when silver-positive cells were conspicuously absent from the EC. Three hours later, at the 6-hour time point, a large number of neurons in the medial portion of layer III of the EC and their processes were heavily labeled, but only relatively sporadic cellular silver grains were seen in brain regions distant from the injection site. Notably, the staining technique used in this study does not necessarily identify irreversibly damaged cells, but indicates cellular impairment that *might* result in cell death.[43] The silver impregnation study therefore demonstrated that highly localized cellular abnormalities at discrete distant sites precede the death of entorhinal neurons after a focal AOAA injection.

The recruitment of both the presubiculum and the subiculum/CA1 transition zone after intra-entorhinal AOAA was further substantiated in immunohistochemical studies of animals killed 15 hours after an entorhinal AOAA injection. In these experiments, cells were visualized with two established markers of excessive neuronal activation, c-fos and 72-kDa heat-shock protein (HSP 72).[44,45] In both cases, antibodies also labeled cells in the EC, namely doomed neurons in the medial portion of layer III, and cells throughout the entire extent of layer II (FIG. 3). Taken together with the results of the silver stain study, these data demonstrated that an intra-entorhinal AOAA injection activates a series of chronologically and topographically distinct processes, which may jointly determine the viability of the affected nerve cells.

There is reason to assume that these acute cytoarchitectonic and chemical changes are directly related to the seizure activity that reliably accompanies intra-entorhinal AOAA injections *in vivo.*[30,40] Thus, electrophysiological studies in tissue slices showed that focal application of AOAA to the medial EC results in a progressive increase in field potentials evoked by afferent stimulation and that these poten-

---

FIGURE 3. Micrographs of horizontal sections through the middle level of the EC from AOAA (75 µg/0.75 µL)-injected rats killed 15 hours after the intra-entorhinal injections. The sections were immunostained with antibodies against c-fos (**A–D**) and the 72-kDa heat-shock protein (HSP72) (**E–H**). B–D and F–H are high-power micrographs of the hippocampus (hc), presubiculum (prs), and entorhinal cortex (ec) of the sections depicted in **A** and **E**, respectively. A large number of neurons are c-fos-immunoreactive in the subiculum/CA1 transition zone, the presubiculum, and layer II of the EC. Fewer neurons are immunostained in layer III of the medial EC. HSP72-immunoreactive neurons are present in the presubiculum, in layer II of the EC, and to a lesser degree in the subiculum/CA1 transition zone. Very few immunoreactive neurons are seen in layer III of the EC. Arrow: needle track. Single arrowhead: presubiculum. Double arrowhead/open arrow: subiculum/CA1 transition zone. Scale bars—**A, E**: 300 µm; **B–D, F–H**: 80 µm.

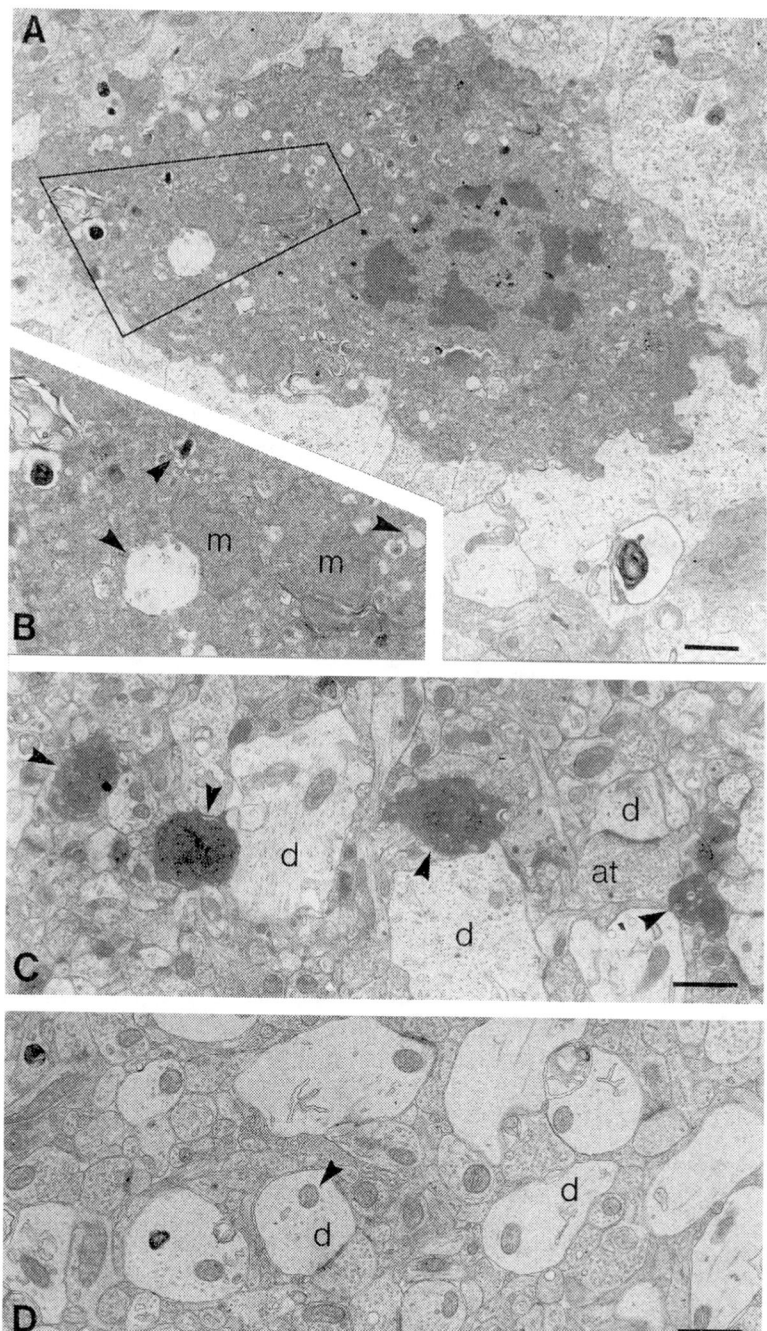

FIGURE 4. *See following page for caption.*

tials are usually largest in layer III. Moreover, repetitive stimulation produced changes that led to spontaneous synchronous discharges, which persisted even after the termination of the afferent stimulation[46] (also see elsewhere in this volume). The fact that these excitatory effects of AOAA in the EC were prevented by an NMDA receptor antagonist provided a conceptual link between AOAA-induced seizures and NMDA receptor–mediated excitotoxicity. In other words, these findings suggested that the morphological and pathological changes seen after an intra-entorhinal AOAA injection *in vivo* might be triggered by an overstimulation of NMDA receptors.[46] This interpretation is in agreement with several reports describing a rapid increase in c-fos- and HSP 72–immunoreactivity in association with NMDA receptor–mediated neurotoxicity.[45,47] Notably, as in the present case, these phenomena are often observed not only at the site of the primary insult, but also in distant brain areas, presumably mediated by excessive transmitter release from glutamatergic projection neurons.

Electron microscopic analysis of the medial portion of EC layer III was performed 5 days after a focal AOAA injection in order to examine evidence for ongoing degenerative events, perhaps similar to those that were recently described to occur days and weeks after cerebral hypoxia/ischemia.[48–50] In contrast to Nissl-stained tissue sections, which had indicated that cell loss was essentially completed by 48 hours after AOAA,[21] the ultrastructural study revealed enduring swollen dendritic profiles and perturbed cytoskeletons scattered throughout the neuropil (FIG. 4). This indicates persistent neurodegeneration in the subacute phase following AOAA-induced seizure activity.

CHRONIC CONSEQUENCES OF AN INTRA-ENTORHINAL AOAA INJECTION IN RATS

As a consequence of AOAA-induced neuronal loss, layer III of the EC eventually undergoes substantial shrinkage, resulting in a pathological appearance that is similar to that seen in human temporal lobe epilepsy.[15] Electrophysiological studies in chronically AOAA-lesioned animals revealed long-lasting increases in evoked and spontaneous activity in parts of the EC and its major projection area, the hippocampus.[51,52] Studies in tissue slices from these animals suggested that the hyperexcitability in the EC might be caused by axonal sprouting of layer V neurons onto layer II neurons and/or residual neurons in layer III. It is also conceivable that presubicular fibers, which normally project to neurons in layer III of the medial EC[53–56] and also contact axons of layer V neurons (cf. Witter *et al.*, this volume) rearrange in response to the loss of their postsynaptic targets to form new excitatory

FIGURE 4. Ultrastructure of the medial EC at 5 days after an intra-entorhinal AOAA injection (75 µg/0.75 µL). **A:** Degenerating layer III neuron. Note budding of the plasma membrane, condensed cytoplasm, and clumping and margination of the chromatin. **B:** High-power field of **A**, showing large, dense mitochondria (m) with intact membranes. Arrowheads point at dilated cisternae of Golgi apparatus and endoplasmic reticulum. **C:** Neuropil of layer III with condensed neuronal profiles (arrowheads) and normal dendrites (d) and axon terminals (at). **D:** Neuropil of layer I with slightly swollen dendrites (d) harboring normal mitochondria (arrowhead). Scale bars: 1 µm.

circuits. An alternative explanation for entorhinal hyperexcitability was suggested by a recent immunohistochemical study, conducted 28 days after a focal AOAA injection. As demonstrated by electron microscopy, GABAergic neurons in layer III, which are remarkably resistant to seizure-induced damage,[14] appeared disconnected from their normal excitatory afferents, possibly rendering their putative target neurons in EC layer II "disinhibited".[16] These speculative scenarios are clearly not mutually exclusive and may, in fact, jointly cause chronic hyperexcitability in the lesioned EC. Together with the upregulation of NMDA receptors in area CA1 of the hippocampus[57] and the associated chronic hippocampal hyperexcitability, these mechanisms have been suggested to play an important role in the occurrence of spontaneously recurring seizures.[52]

ROLE OF PRESUBICULAR AFFERENTS IN SEIZURE-INDUCED ENTORHINAL DAMAGE

The potential importance of neurons in layer III of the medial EC in epileptogenesis and epilepsy stimulated research into the cause of their pronounced vulnerability to seizures. As mentioned earlier, both the neuropathological features of

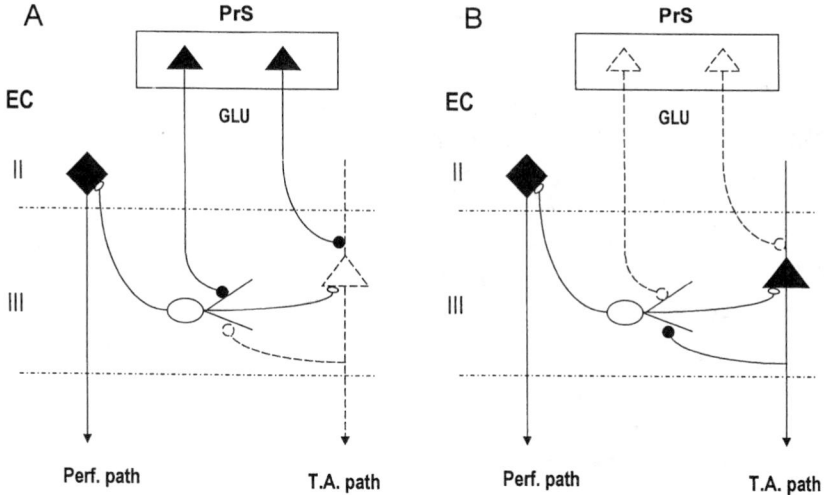

FIGURE 5. Schematic representation of the experimental paradigm used to examine the effect of a presubicular lesion on seizure-related neuronal death in layer III of the entorhinal cortex (EC). **A:** In the normal brain, glutamatergic fibers (GLU) from the presubiculum (PrS) terminate on dendrites of putative excitatory pyramidal cells (triangular cell body) or inhibitory interneurons (oval cell body) in layer III of the EC. The pyramidal cells give rise to the "temporo-ammonic" (T.A.) path to areas CA1 and the subiculum, whereas the interneurons are assumed to terminate on layer III pyramidal cells and on stellate cells in EC layer II (diamond-shaped cell body), the cells of origin of the perforant path. In the presence of intact presubicular afferents, EC layer III pyramidal cells degenerate (dotted lines) following prolonged seizures. **B:** After a lesion of the PrS, EC layer III pyramidal cells do not succumb to prolonged seizure activity.

seizure-induced layer III lesions and the neuroprotection by NMDA receptor blockade[30] suggested that excitotoxic mechanisms were involved. Since deafferentation is known to prevent excitotoxic damage to target neurons,[58,59] the excitotoxic nature of the entorhinal lesion was tested further by eliminating the major excitatory input to the vulnerable neurons prior to a convulsive insult (see FIG. 5 for schematic illustration). The presubiculum constitutes an optimal target for such an intervention. First, it sends a massive projection to the seizure-susceptible neurons in layer III of the EC[53,55] (also see Witter *et al.*, this volume). Second, although both excitatory and inhibitory neurons are present in the dorsal portion of the structure, ventral

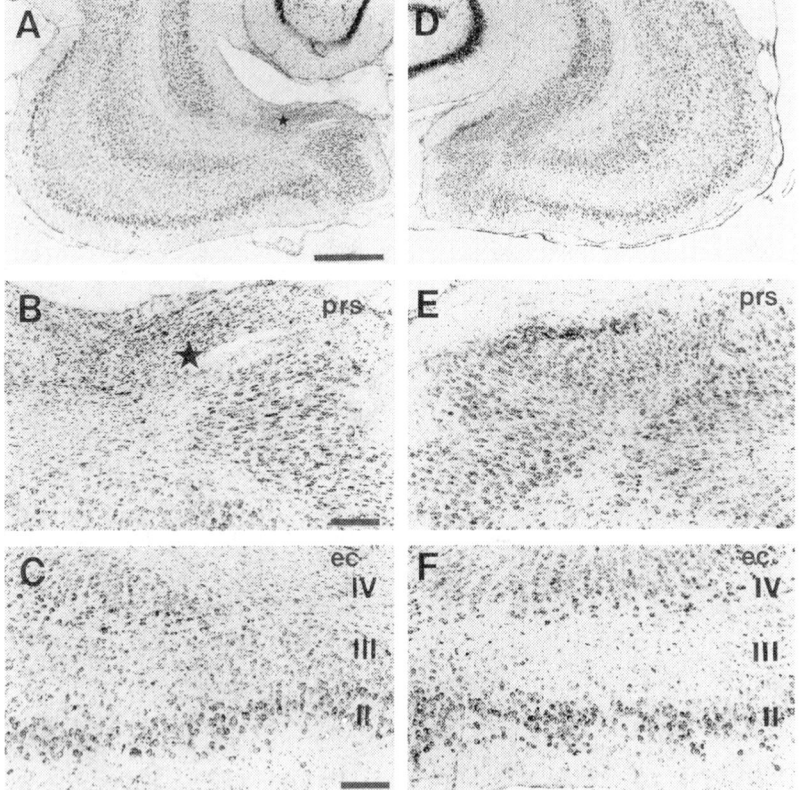

FIGURE 6. Nissl-stained horizontal section through the ventral level of the EC. This rat received an injection of ibotenate (3 µg/0.75 µL, injected in equal aliquots at three dorsoventral levels) into the presubiculum (prs), followed by a subcutaneous kainate injection 5 days later (10 mg/kg). The rat was killed 24 hours after the kainate administration. **A–C:** Hemisphere receiving an ibotenate injection into the presubiculum (star). **D–F:** Contralateral hemisphere. **B,C** and **E,F:** High magnifications of the presubiculum and the medial entorhinal cortex (ec) shown in **A** and **D**, respectively. Note lesion of the presubiculum and neuroprotection in the entorhinal cortex ipsilateral to the ibotenate injection (**A–C**). Scale bars—**A, D:** 450 µm; **B, C, E, F:** 50 µm.

presubicular fibers, which project to the ventral, exquisitely vulnerable EC neurons, are exclusively excitatory in nature.[56] Finally, as shown in FIGURES 2 and 3, the presubiculum is involved in the very early phases of entorhinal degeneration and may therefore occupy a key position in controlling reverberating seizure activity and excitotoxic neuron loss in the EC.

In spite of the methodological difficulties of selectively destroying the presubiculum, which is positioned close to the midline and extends in a narrow band along the dorso-ventral axis, the structure was successfully lesioned by the focal application of ibotenate (injected at three dorso-ventral levels; FIG. 6B). Five days later, the animals received a systemic injection of a dose of kainate that reliably causes acute status epilepticus[23] and bilateral lesions of neurons in layer III of the medial EC.[14] As shown in FIGURE 6 (A, C), a prior ablation of the presubiculum attenuated the kainate-induced neuron loss on the side of the lesion, but not in the contralateral EC (FIG. 6D and F).

These results have several implications. In neurobiological terms, the data provide another example of neuroprotection by deafferentation, suggesting that seizure-susceptible neurons in layer III of the medial EC die by an excitotoxic mechanism. Further, the experiment highlights the functional significance of presubicular afferents to the EC and indicates that the presubiculum ought to be regarded as an integral component of the reverberating limbic seizure circuit.[60] This realization, in turn, should provoke further studies on the connectivity and physiological significance of the presubiculum in normal and abnormal brains[9] (cf. also van Hoesen, this volume). Finally, the demonstration of entorhinal neuroprotection following the experimental removal of the presubiculum, together with the potential role of the EC in epileptogenesis and epilepsy elaborated above, may have ramifications for the treatment of epilepsy. Thus, it is conceivable that targeting the presubiculum for surgical removal or for specific pharmacological intervention will provide benefits to patients with temporal lobe epilepsy.

CONCLUSIONS

The question if the preferential lesion of layer III of the EC is of functional significance in temporal lobe epilepsy can now be addressed in rats receiving an intra-entorhinal injection of the indirect excitotoxins AOAA or GAG. Studies in these animal models have so far indicated that entorhinal abnormalities may play a critical role in both epileptogenesis and epilepsy. These studies have also revealed that the presubiculum, which provides the most prominent excitatory input to the seizure-susceptible neurons in layer III of the medial EC, may constitute an important, and previously underestimated, component of the limbic seizure circuit. These new findings may eventually lead to the targeting of parahippocampal structures and mechanisms for the treatment of temporal lobe epilepsy.

ACKNOWLEDGMENTS

We thank Joyce Burgess for excellent secretarial assistance. This work was supported by USPHS Grant No. NS 16102.

REFERENCES

1. SOMMER, W. 1880. Erkrankung des Ammonshorns als aetiologisches Moment der Epilepsie. Arch. Psychiatr. Nervenkr. **10**: 631–675.
2. CLARK, L.P. & T.P. PROUT. 1903. Status epilepticus: a clinical and pathological study in epilepsy. Am. J. Insanity **60**: 291–306.
3. ZIMMERMAN, H.M. 1938. The histopathology of convulsive disorders of children. J. Pediatr. **13**: 839–890.
4. EARLE, K.M., M. BALDWIN & W. PENFIELD. 1953. Incisural sclerosis and temporal lobe seizures produced by hippocampal herniation at birth. Arch. Neurol. Psychiatry **69**: 27–42.
5. CAVANAGH, J.B. & A. MEYER. 1956. Aetiological aspects of Ammon's horn sclerosis associated with temporal lobe epilepsy. Br. Med. J. **2**: 1403–1407.
6. CORSELLIS, J.A.N. & C.J. BRUTON. 1983. Neuropathology of status epilepticus in humans. In Status Epilepticus: Mechanisms of Brain Damage and Treatment, pp. 129–139. Raven Press. New York.
7. MELDRUM, B.S. & C.J. BRUTON. 1992. Epilepsy. In Greenfield's Neuropathology. Fifth edition, pp. 1246–1283. Oxford University Press. London/New York.
8. WITTER, M.P. & D.G. AMARAL. 1991. Entorhinal cortex of the monkey: V. Projections to the dentate gyrus, hippocampus, and subicular complex. J. Comp. Neurol. **307**: 437–459.
9. INSAUSTI, R., M.T. HERRERO & M.P. WITTER. 1997. Entorhinal cortex of the rat: cytoarchitectonic subdivisions and the origin and distribution of cortical efferents. Hippocampus **7**: 146–183.
10. RUTECKI, P.A., R.G. GROSSMAN, D. ARMSTRONG & S. IRISH-LOEWEN. 1989. Electrophysiological connections between the hippocampus and entorhinal cortex in patients with complex partial seizures. J. Neurosurg. **70**: 667–675.
11. PLATE, K.H., H-G. WIESER, M.G. YASARGIL & O.D. WIESTLER. 1993. Neuropathological findings in 224 patients with temporal lobe epilepsy. Acta Neuropathol. **86**: 433–438.
12. SPENCER, S.S. & D.D. SPENCER. 1994. Entorhinal-hippocampal interactions in medial temporal lobe epilepsy. Epilepsia **35**: 721–727.
13. BERNASCONI, N., A. BERNASCONI, F. ANDERMANN, F. DUBEAU, W. FEINDEL & D.C. REUTENS. 1999. Entorhinal cortex in temporal lobe epilepsy: a quantitative MRI study. Neurology **52**: 1870–1876.
14. DU, F., T. EID, E.W. LOTHMAN, C. KÖHLER & R. SCHWARCZ. 1995. Preferential neuronal loss in layer III of the medial entorhinal cortex in rat models of temporal lobe epilepsy. J. Neurosci. **15**: 6301–6313.
15. DU, F., W.O. WHETSELL, JR., B. ABOU-KHALIL, B. BLUMENKOPF, E.W. LOTHMAN & R. SCHWARCZ. 1993. Preferential neuronal loss in layer III of the entorhinal cortex in patients with temporal lobe epilepsy. Epilepsy Res. **16**: 223–233.
16. EID, T., R. SCHWARCZ & O.P. OTTERSEN. 1999. Ultrastructure and immunocytochemical distribution of GABA in layer III of the rat medial entorhinal cortex following aminooxyacetic acid–induced seizures. Exp. Brain Res. **125**: 463–475.
17. LOTHMAN, E.W., E.H. BERTRAM, J.W. BEKENSTEIN & J.B. PERLIN. 1989. Self-sustaining limbic status epilepticus induced by "continuous" hippocampal stimulation: electrographic and behavioral characteristics. Epilepsy Res. **3**: 107–119.
18. SPERK, G., H. LASSMANN, H. BARAN, S.J. KISH, F. SEITELBERGER & O. HORNYKIEWICZ. 1983. Kainic acid induced seizures: neurochemical and histopathological changes. Neuroscience **10**: 1301–1315.
19. TURSKI, W.A., E.A. CAVALHEIRO, C. COIMBRA, M. DA PENHA BERZAGHI, C. IKONOMIDOU-TURSKI & L. TURSKI. 1987. Only certain antiepileptic drugs prevent seizures induced by pilocarpine. Brain Res. Rev. **12**: 281–305.
20. RIBAK, C.E., L. SERESS, P. WEBER, C.M. EPSTEIN, T.R. HENRY & R.A.E. BAKAY. 1998. Alumina gel injections into the temporal lobe of rhesus monkeys cause complex partial seizures and morphological changes found in human temporal lobe epilepsy. J. Comp. Neurol. **401**: 266–290.
21. DU, F., T. EID & R. SCHWARCZ. 1998. Neuronal damage after the injection of aminooxyacetic acid into the rat entorhinal cortex: a silver impregnation study. Neuroscience **82**: 1165–1178.

22. WITTER, M.P., A.W. GRIFFIOEN, B. JORRITSMA-BYHAM & J.L.M. KRIJNEN. 1988. Entorhinal projections to the hippocampal CA1 region in the rat: an underestimated pathway. Neurosci. Lett. **85:** 193–198.
23. SPERK, G. 1994. Kainic acid seizures in the rat. Prog. Neurobiol. **42:** 1–32.
24. SLOVITER, R.S. 1983. "Epileptic" brain damage in rats induced by sustained electrical stimulation of the perforant path. I. Acute electrophysiological and light microscopic studies. Brain Res. Bull. **10:** 675–697.
25. CLIFFORD, D.B., C.F. ZORUMSKI & J.W. OLNEY. 1989. Ketamine and MK-801 prevent degeneration of thalamic neurons induced by focal cortical seizures. Exp. Neurol. **105:** 272–279.
26. FUJIKAWA, D.G., A.H. DANIELS & J.S. KIM. 1994. The competitive NMDA receptor antagonist CGP 40116 protects against status epilepticus–induced neuronal damage. Epilepsy Res. **17:** 207–219.
27. OLNEY, J.W., T. DEGUBAREFF & R.S. SLOVITER. 1983. "Epileptic" brain damage in rats induced by sustained electrical stimulation of the perforant path. II. Ultrastructural analysis of acute hippocampal pathology. Brain Res. Bull. **10:** 699–712.
28. UEKI, A., C. MIWA, K. OOHARA & K. MIYOSHI. 1996. Histological evidence for cholinergic alteration in the hippocampus following entorhinal cortex lesion. J. Neurol. Sci. **142:** 7–11.
29. LEVISOHN, L.F. & O. ISACSON. 1991. Excitotoxic lesions of the rat entorhinal cortex: effects of selective neuronal damage on acquisition and retention of a non-spatial reference memory task. Brain Res. **564:** 230–244.
30. EID, T., F. DU & R. SCHWARCZ. 1995. Differential neuronal vulnerability to aminooxyacetic acid and quinolinic acid in the rat parahippocampal region. Neuroscience **68:** 645–656.
31. MCMASTER, O.G., F. DU, E.D. FRENCH & R. SCHWARCZ. 1991. Focal injection of aminooxyacetic acid produces seizures and lesions in rat hippocampus: evidence for mediation by NMDA receptors. Exp. Neurol. **113:** 367–374.
32. BEAL, M.F., K.J. SWARTZ, B.T. HYMAN, E. STOREY, S.F. FINN & W. KOROSHETZ. 1991. Aminooxyacetic acid results in excitotoxin lesions by a novel indirect mechanism. J. Neurochem. **57:** 1068–1073.
33. GREENE, J.G. & J.T. GREENAMYRE. 1996. Bioenergetics and glutamate excitotoxicity. Prog. Neurobiol. **48:** 613–634.
34. MCMASTER, O.G., H. BARAN, H-Q. WU, F. DU, E.D. FRENCH & R. SCHWARCZ. 1993. Gamma acetylenic GABA produces axon-sparing neurodegeneration after focal injection into the rat hippocampus. Exp. Neurol. **124:** 184–191.
35. TATTER, S.B., W.R. GALPERN & O. ISACSON. 1995. Neurotrophic factor protection against excitotoxic neuronal death. Neuroscientist **1:** 286–297.
36. ZEEVALK, G.D. & W.J. NICKLAS. 1996. Attenuation of excitotoxic cell swelling and GABA release by the GABA transport inhibitor SKF 89976A. Mol. Chem. Neuropathol. **29:** 27–36.
37. JUNG, M.J., B. LIPPERT, B.W. METCALF, P.J. SCHECHTER, P. BÖHLEN & A. SJOERDSMA. 1977. The effect of 4-amino hex-5-ynoic acid (gamma-acetylenic GABA, gammaethynyl GABA), a catalytic inhibitor of GABA transaminase, on brain GABA metabolism *in vivo*. J. Neurochem. **28:** 717–723.
38. LÖSCHER, W. 1980. Effect of inhibitors of GABA transaminase on the synthesis, binding, uptake, and metabolism of GABA. J. Neurochem. **34:** 1603–1608.
39. ROBERTS, E. 1984. GABA-related phenomena, models of nervous system function, and seizures. Ann. Neurol. **16:** S77–S89.
40. DU, F. & R. SCHWARCZ. 1992. Aminooxyacetic acid causes selective neuronal loss in layer III of the rat medial entorhinal cortex. Neurosci. Lett. **147:** 185–188.
41. WU, H-Q. & R. SCHWARCZ. 1998. Focal microinjection of γ-acetylenic GABA into the rat entorhinal cortex: behavioral and electroencephalographic abnormalities, and preferential neuronal loss in layer III. Exp. Neurol. **153:** 203–213.
42. BEHR, J., T. GLOVELI & U. HEINEMANN. 1998. The perforant path projection from the medial entorhinal cortex layer III to the subiculum in the rat combined hippocampal–entorhinal cortex slice. Eur. J. Neurosci. **10:** 1011–1018.

43. GALLYAS, F., F.H. GÜLDNER, G. ZOLTAY & J.R. WOLFF. 1990. Golgi-like demonstration of "dark" neurons with an argyrophil III method for experimental neuropathology. Acta Neuropathol. **79:** 620–628.
44. MORGAN, J.I. & T. CURRAN. 1991. Proto-oncogene transcription factors and epilepsy. Trends Pharmacol. Sci. **12:** 343–349.
45. SLOVITER, R.S. & D.H. LOWENSTEIN. 1992. Heat shock protein expression in vulnerable cells of the rat hippocampus as an indicator of excitation-induced neuronal stress. J. Neurosci. **12:** 3004–3009.
46. SCHARFMAN, H.E. 1996. Hyperexcitability of entorhinal cortex and hippocampus after application of aminooxyacetic acid (AOAA) to layer III of the rat medial entorhinal cortex *in vitro*. J. Neurophysiol. **76:** 2986–3001.
47. KINOUCHI, H., F.R. SHARP, P.H. CHAN, J. KOISTINAHO, S.M. SAGAR & T. YOSHIMOTO. 1994. Induction of c-fos, junB, c-jun, and hsp70 mRNA in cortex, thalamus, basal ganglia, and hippocampus following middle cerebral artery occlusion. J. Cereb. Blood Flow Metab. **14:** 808–817.
48. DELL'ANNA, E., Y. CHEN, E. ENGIDAWORK, K. ANDERSSON, G. LUBEC, J. LUTHMAN & M. HERRERA-MARSCHITZ. 1997. Delayed neuronal death following perinatal asphyxia in rat. Exp. Brain Res. **115:** 105–115.
49. LEHRMANN, E., T. CHRISTENSEN, J. ZIMMER, N.H. DIEMER & B. FINSEN. 1997. Microglial and macrophage reactions mark progressive changes and define the penumbra in the rat neocortex and striatum after transient middle cerebral artery occlusion. J. Comp. Neurol. **386:** 461–476.
50. YAMAMOTO, T., S. YUKI, T. WATANABE, M. MITSUKA, K-I. SAITO & K. KOGURE. 1997. Delayed neuronal death prevented by inhibition of increased hydroxyl radical formation in transient cerebral ischemia. Brain Res. **762:** 240–242.
51. DENSLOW, M.J., E.W. LOTHMAN, T. EID, F. DU & R. SCHWARCZ. 1995. Hyperexcitability in area CA1 after selective lesions of layer III of the entorhinal cortex [abstract]. Soc. Neurosci. **21:** 181.16.
52. SCHARFMAN, H.E., J.H. GOODMAN, F. DU & R. SCHWARCZ. 1998. Chronic changes in synaptic responses of entorhinal and hippocampal neurons after entorhinal cortical cell loss produced by intracortical aminooxyacetic acid (AOAA) injection: an *in vitro* and *in vivo* study in the rat. J. Neurophysiol. **80:** 3031–3046.
53. KÖHLER, C. 1986. Intrinsic connections of the retrohippocampal region in the rat brain. II. The medial entorhinal area. J. Comp. Neurol. **246:** 149–169.
54. CABALLERO-BLEDA, M. & M.P. WITTER. 1993. Regional and laminar organization of projections from the presubiculum and parasubiculum to the entorhinal cortex: an anterograde tracing study in the rat. J. Comp. Neurol. **328:** 115–129.
55. EID, T., B. JORRITSMA-BYHAM, R. SCHWARCZ & M.P. WITTER. 1996. Afferents to the seizure-sensitive neurons in layer III of the medial entorhinal area: a tracing study in the rat. Exp. Brain Res. **109:** 209–218.
56. VAN HAEFTEN, T., F.G. WOUTERLOOD, B. JORRITSMA-BYHAM & M.P. WITTER. 1997. GABAergic presubicular projections to the medial entorhinal cortex of the rat. J. Neurosci. **17:** 862–874.
57. TAMMINGA, C.A., X.M. GAO, F. DU & R. SCHWARCZ. 1994. "Indirect excitotoxin" lesion of layer III in rat entorhinal cortex produces glutamate receptor changes in hippocampus [abstract]. Soc. Neurosci. **20:** 213.20.
58. BIZIERE, K. & J.T. COYLE. 1978. Influence of cortico-striatal afferents on striatal kainic acid neurotoxicity. Neurosci. Lett. **8:** 303–310.
59. KÖHLER, C., R. SCHWARCZ & K. FUXE. 1978. Perforant path transactions protect hippocampal granule cells from kainate lesion. Neurosci. Lett. **10:** 241–246.
60. LOTHMAN, E.W. & E.H. BERTRAM III. 1993. Epileptogenic effects of status epilepticus. Epilepsia **34:** S59–S70.

The Parahippocampal Cortices and Kindling

DAN C. McINTYRE[a] AND MARY ELLEN KELLY

Department of Psychology, Institute for Neuroscience, Carleton University, Ottawa, Ontario, Canada

ABSTRACT: The piriform and perirhinal cortices are parahippocampal structures with strong connections to limbic structures, including the amygdala and hippocampus, as well as other parahippocampal structures such as the entorhinal cortex. In this paper, we present results, based on anatomical, physiological, and kindling studies, that suggest that the perirhinal and piriform cortices might be very important in the secondary generalization of limbic seizures, particularly those with convulsive expression. These kindling data further suggest that the progressive lowering of afterdischarge thresholds in the parahippocampal structures, due to insult and/or genetic predisposition, might provide the neural basis for the clinical presentation of temporal lobe epilepsy.

INTRODUCTION

Despite greater understanding and improved management, epilepsy continues to be the most common neurological disorder in humans, with a reported incidence of ~2%.[1] Of the many forms in which epilepsy presents, the most common and insidious appear as the partial or complex partial seizures characteristic of temporal lobe epilepsy (TLE).[2] Equally important, and unfortunate, TLE is often pharmacologically unresponsive and can readily become intractable. For patients experiencing such intractability, neurosurgery frequently becomes their last hope (e.g., Ref. 3). Surgical removal of tissue believed to be responsible for the manifestations of TLE usually includes the anterior hippocampus and/or amygdala.[4] Inherent to this approach, however, is the removal of structures adjacent to the targeted region, which involve parahippocampal structures such as the piriform, perirhinal, and entorhinal cortices. Not surprisingly, therefore, it is the raison d'être of this conference to establish a better understanding of those parahippocampal structures and their involvement in various normal and abnormal behaviors, including TLE and the experimental models used to study this disorder.

Our interest in parahippocampal structures, such as the piriform and perirhinal cortices, arose because of their apparent involvement in the development of kindled seizures. Kindling, the most commonly used model of TLE,[5] is characterized by the progressive development of electrographic and behavioral seizure activity following the spaced, repeated application of low-intensity electrical stimulation to one of many different limbic structures such as the amygdala.[6] The behavioral and electrophysiological changes observed during kindling indicate that the neural circuits both

[a]Address for correspondence: Dan C. McIntyre, Carleton University, Psychology, Neuroscience Institute, Colonel By Drive, Ottawa, Ontario, Canada. Tel.: (613) 520-2646; fax: (613) 520-4052.

e-mail: dmcintyr@ccs.carleton.ca

within the kindled site and connected to the kindled site undergo modifications that render them hyperexcitable and more easily recruited into propagating and convulsive seizures. The structures and pathways critical to such kindling development and convulsive recruitment have remained largely unknown.

Historically, the speed of convulsive seizure development during kindling, often measured by *kindling rate* or number of stimulations to the first behavioral expression of convulsive activity, has suggested how important such a structure might be to the seizure generalization process. In our original determinations, the amygdala was the fastest kindling structure in the forebrain, so we hypothesized that the closer the anatomical proximity of a structure to the amygdala, the more critical that structure might be for recruitment and seizure generalization.[6] In later experiments, however, the olfactory or piriform cortex was shown to be even faster kindling than the amygdala.[7] Based on these and other findings,[8–10] the piriform cortex soon became an important candidate for a critical role in limbic seizure generalization.[11] As evidenced in these conference proceedings, it remains so today.

PIRIFORM/PERIRHINAL CORTICES *IN VITRO*

To investigate piriform cortex circuitry at a cellular level, we developed a novel coronal slice preparation that maintained communication between the amygdala and the piriform cortex[12,13] (FIG. 1). The results of that work indicated that the neural networks in the piriform cortex had the capacity to show strong recruitment and epileptiform behavior involving both ictal and interictal events and that previous kindling resulted in significant enhancement of that excitability compared to that of control tissue.[12,13]

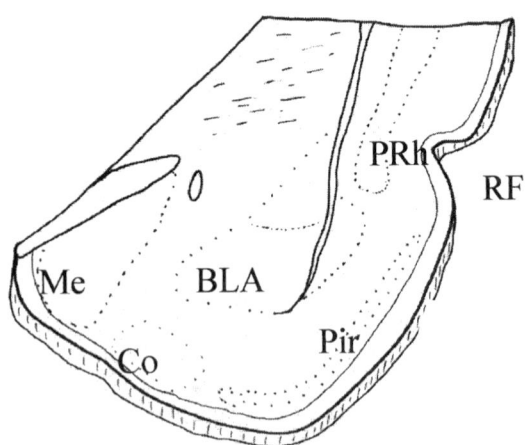

FIGURE 1. Schematic diagram of the combined amygdala-piriform-perirhinal cortex slice preparation. Abbreviations: BLA = basolateral amygdala nucleus; Co = cortical amygdala nucleus; Me = medial amygdala nucleus; Pir = piriform cortex; PRh = perirhinal cortex; RF = rhinal fissure.

In additional *in vitro* explorations of the amygdala-piriform slice preparation, we increased the excitability of the slices by removing Mg^{2+} from the bath perfusate.[14] This, of course, provoked considerable burst discharging with ictal activity, the origins of which we sought. Surprisingly, the burst events began in an area dorsal to the piriform cortex called the anterior perirhinal cortex (FIG. 1). This area emitted large and long-lasting paroxysmal deplorization shifts that looked remarkably similar to those reported previously in the entorhinal cortex (e.g., Refs. 15 and 16).

Intrigued by this *in vitro* observation, we questioned the excitability of the perirhinal area in intact rats using the kindling procedure. Consistent with the *in vitro* experiments, the perirhinal cortex kindled faster than did the two fastest known kindling sites, the amygdala and the piriform cortex.[17] Perhaps more important, the latency from the stimulus onset to the beginning of the forelimb clonus in the perirhinal kindled rats was extremely fast (~1–2 s) and much faster than that of other sites, including the amygdala and the dorsal hippocampus. This observation suggested that the perirhinal area must be strongly connected to motor structures that support clonic convulsive behavior. Yet no anatomical basis for this behavior was apparent in the literature.

PERIRHINOFRONTAL CONNECTION

Because the convulsion latencies in perirhinal kindled rats were so brief and similar to those triggered from the frontal motor cortices,[18] we anticipated a possible perirhinofrontal connection and explored this possibility with both anterograde and retrograde tract tracing techniques.[19] Such a connection was determined. Indeed, the anterograde projections of the anterior perirhinal cortex, determined using *Phaseolus vulgaris* leucoagglutinin (PhAL), indicated extensive divergent connections from the perirhinal injection sites to the frontal motor cortices. The most dense projections arose from layer V perirhinal cells, the axons of which extensively branched with numerous varicosites in frontal area Fr2 (FIG. 2). On the other hand, the retrograde tracer fluorogold, injected into different frontal areas (Fr1, 2, and 3), indicated at each different injection site a substantial convergence of perirhinal projections onto those sites. Thus, perirhinal afferents to the frontal cortex showed both extensive divergence and convergence and appeared well postured to impact significantly on frontal cortex activity.

If amygdala kindling alters excitability in parahippocampal networks such as the piriform and the perirhinal cortices,[14,20] facilitating recruitment of the frontal cortex, presumably manipulations of frontal cortex activity *before* the triggering of an amygdala-kindled seizure might alter the electrographic and/or behavioral profiles of the elicited response. To assess such a possibility, we induced cortical spreading depression (CSD) over *one* hemisphere (frontal cortex) using cannulated potassium chloride either contralateral or ipsilateral to the kindled amygdala.[21] Three minutes following induction of unilateral CSD, the kindled amygdala was stimulated at its previous afterdischarge threshold. In cases of CSD *contralateral* to the kindled amygdala, the ensuing electrographic discharge in the kindled amygdala was normal and indistinguishable from trials in which either saline or no treatment had been applied to the cortex.[21] However, the convulsive response associated with that 'normal'

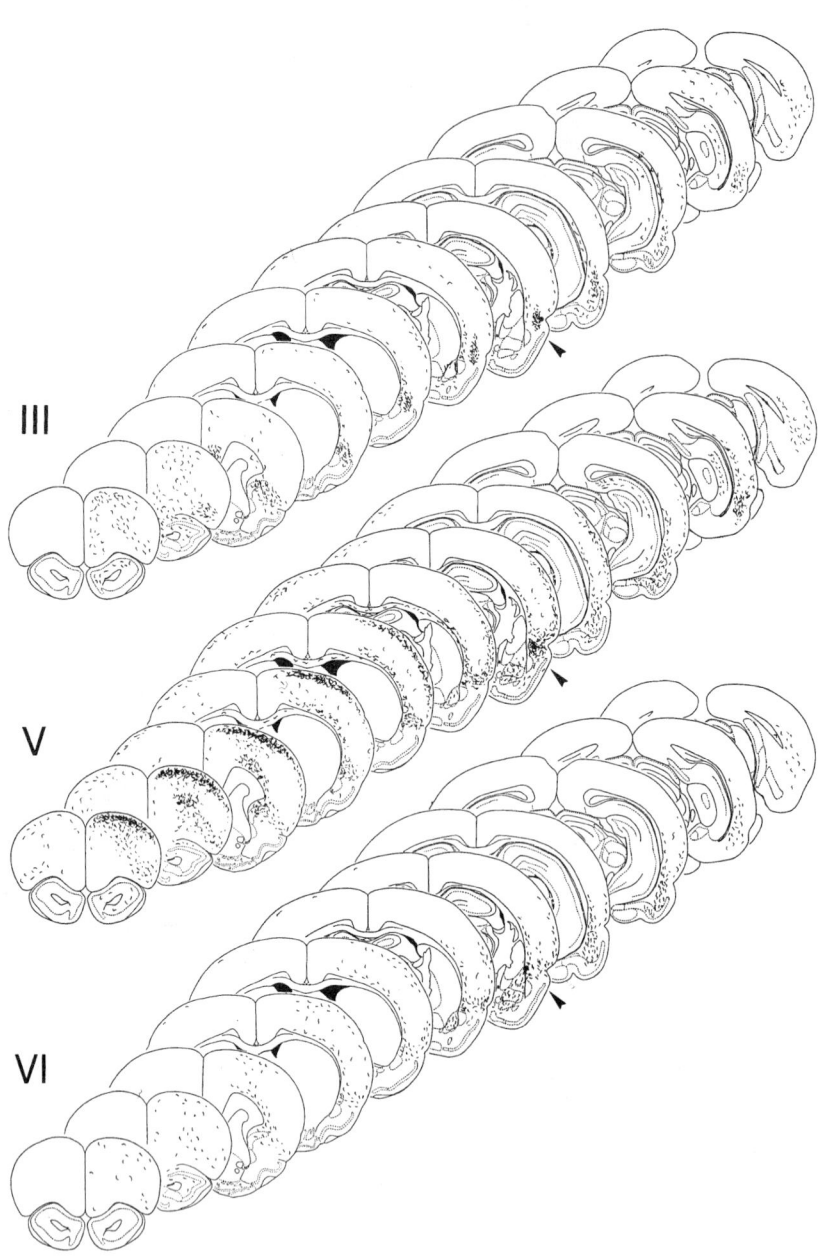

FIGURE 2. Summary schematic diagrams showing the distribution of PhAL-labeled fibers in cortices both anterior and posterior to the three different perirhinal cortex injection sites (indicated by *arrowheads*) in either layers III, V, or VI.

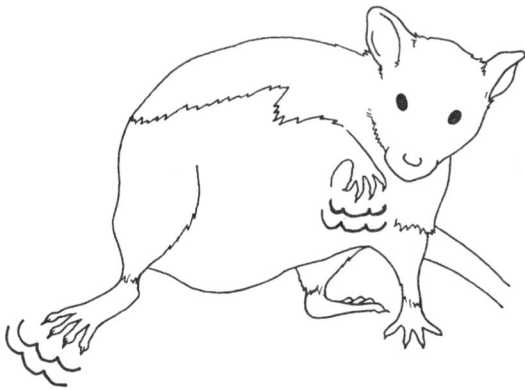

FIGURE 3. Schematic drawing of a typical kindled seizure in a rat triggered from the left amygdala during unilateral spreading depression of the right hemisphere. Note that the unilateral clonic convulsive seizure is sustained only by its right limbs, which is similar to amygdala-kindled seizures in split-brain rats. The drawing was made from a videotaped seizure.

discharge was unilateral and nearly identical to that observed in our "split-brain" preparation (FIG. 3).[22] By contrast, when CSD was induced *ipsilateral* to the kindled amygdala, the triggered convulsive behavior was entirely blocked and, in most cases, the associated amygdala afterdischarge was substantially reduced.[21] The latter results suggested that the frontal cortex might be part of the neural circuit that elaborates amygdala discharges and, if suppressed with CSD, permits only brief amygdala discharges with no convulsive expression. In addition, the contralateral CSD findings suggest that if the ipsilateral cortex is not suppressed, seizure discharge in the kindled amygdala will be normal and will recruit a typical convulsive response (in duration), albeit hemiconvulsive in nature. We suspect, based on split-brain studies,[22] that the hemiconvulsions occur in the contralateral CSD group, because normal bilateralization of convulsive responses is realized through recruitment of the contralateral frontal cortex via its homotopic callosal projections from the kindled hemisphere.[21] Thus, when the contralateral cortex is rendered inoperative because of CSD, hemiconvulsions occur. By contrast, Ferland *et al.*[23] believe that the bilaterality of amygdala-kindled convulsions is based on recruitment of perirhinal projections in the kindled hemisphere to the contralateral perirhinal area and from there to the ipsilateral frontal cortex. Indeed, this could be the case, if the critical *interhemispheric* projection from one perirhinal cortex to the other is realized through the corpus callosum, where callosal bisection lateralizes the convulsion. Independent of this conjecture, our CSD experiment supports the importance of the neocortex for convulsive expression of amygdala-kindled seizures and begs the question as to how necessary the perirhinal/piriform cortex is in the recruitment process leading to convulsive seizure expression.

A

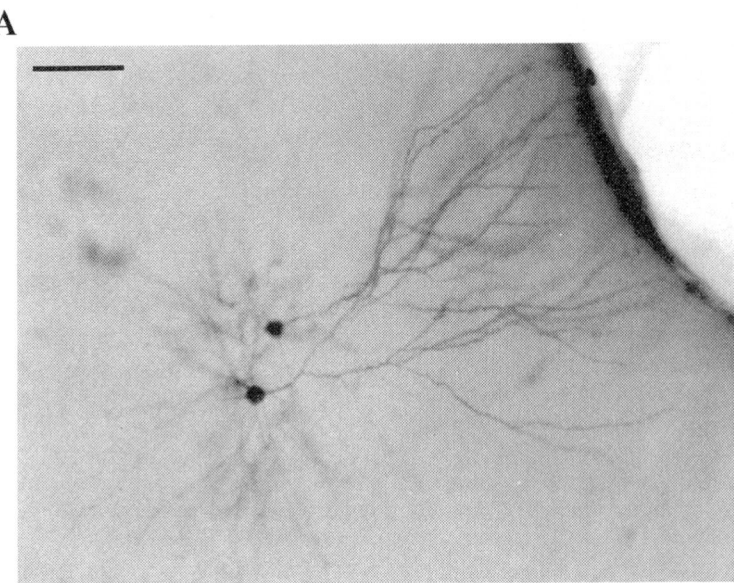

B

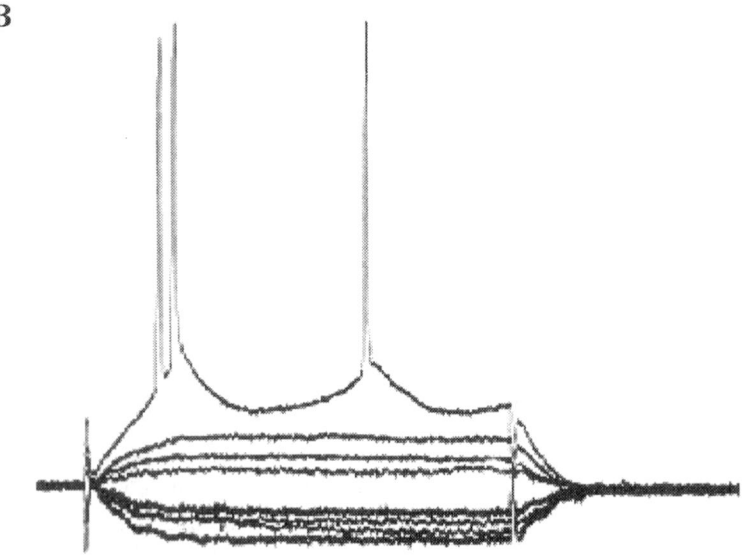

FIGURE 4. The morphology (**A**) and intrinsic electrophysiological responses to both depolarizing and hyperpolarizing current injections (**B**) into a typical layer III perirhinal cortex neuron. Note the dye coupling between two adjacent cells, a phenomenon that was frequent in layer III. Scale bar in **A** is 40 μm.

A

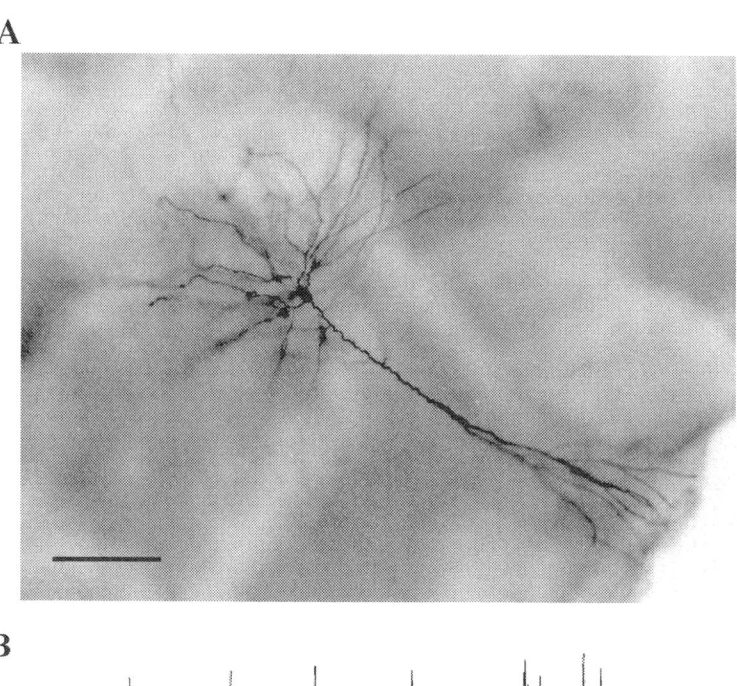

B

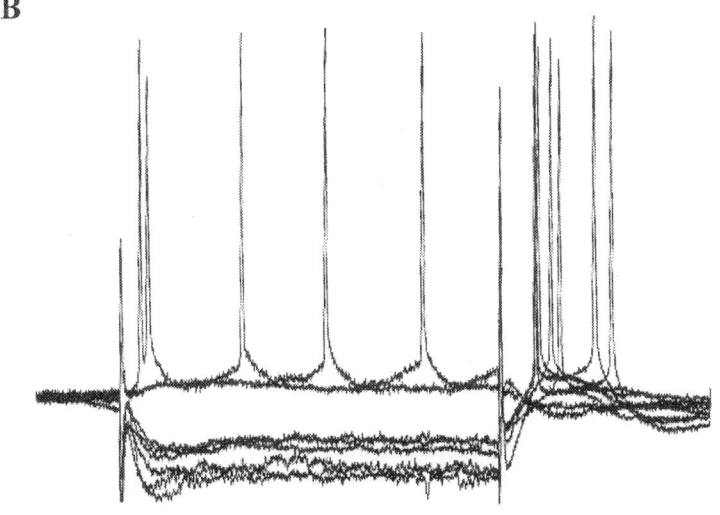

FIGURE 5. The morphology (**A**) and intrinsic electrophysiological responses to both depolarizing and hyperpolaring current injections (**B**) into a typical layer V perirhinal cortex neuron. Note the low threshold for a spike response during the depolarizing injections and the inward rectification during the hyperpolarizing injections. Scale bar in **A** is 80 μm, which is notably different from that of FIGURE 4.

PERIRHINAL CORTEX SEIZURE THRESHOLDS

In approaching this question, we first assessed the intrinsic properties of the perirhinal neurons in layers III and V. In this assessment, clear laminar differences between cells were observed in both their morphology and intrinsic electrophysiological properties. For example, in the lateral two thirds of layer III, most cells were relatively small in size with ovoid-to-pyramidal shaped cell bodies and thin, diffusely arborized dendritic fields, extending broadly to the rhinal fissure (FIG. 4A). All such cells were regular spiking with relatively high spike thresholds, which rapidly accommodated during depolarizing current injections (FIG. 4B). By contrast, at the medial border of layer III and the lateral half of layer V (as there is no layer IV in the agranular perirhinal cortex), much larger pyramidal cells were observed. These cells supported broad apical dendrites that extended to the rhinal fissure (FIG. 5A), the branches of which were covered with spiny terminals. During depolarizing pulses, these cells exhibited relatively low spike thresholds and usually emitted doublet and triplets of spikes that were often followed by several single spikes. Also, they showed inward rectification and anodal break responses to hyperpolarizing current injections (FIG. 5B).[7] Because the main axon of these cells entered the external capsule in a rostral direction, we anticipate that they represent some of the cells in layer V that project directly to the frontal cortex, as noted in our anatomical studies.[19] Many of the characteristics observed in these layer V perirhinal cells were reported recently by others[24,25] and are shared by layer V cells in other cortical areas (e.g., Ref. 26).

Based on the different response profiles evident between perirhinal neurons in layers III versus layer V, we compared the kindling profiles of the perirhinal cortex (3 anteroposterior levels) to the postrhinal cortex,[27] using kindling electrodes that were located either superficially (layers I–III) or deep (layers V–VI) in the cortex. In this kindling study, several important observations were made. First, the afterdischarge thresholds before kindling were significantly higher in superficial cortical layers than in deep layers. This was true for all three perirhinal groups as well as for the postrhinal group. Second, the afterdischarge thresholds during kindling in all four groups dramatically decreased, by approximately an order of magnitude. Importantly, this magnitude of change never occurs locally in a kindled amygdala or kindled hippocampus. Regarding these latter structures, one can observe a focal threshold decrease of 10–50% in the amygdala following kindling, whereas an increase is often seen in the hippocampus, particularly in the dentate gyrus (e.g., Ref. 28). Third, before kindling, the afterdischarge threshold of the anterior perirhinal cortex was significantly less than that of more posterior sites, particularly the postrhinal cortex (~350 μA vs ~1100 μA, respectively). Fourth, the kindling rates of the anterior perirhinal site were significantly faster than those of the posterior sites and, in most groups, the deep sites were significantly faster kindling than were the superficial sites. Finally, the latencies to forelimb clonus also were much shorter from the anterior perirhinal sites than the posterior sites and, in most groups, were significantly shorter for deep versus superfical placements.[29] These results are consistent with results from both the electrophysiological studies, reporting a greater intrinsic excitability of cells in the deeper perirhinal layers (layers V–VI) compared to the superficial layers (layers I–III), and the anatomical analysis, demonstrating a greater concentration of neurons projecting to the frontal motor cortex from (a) deep versus superficial layers and (b) anterior versus posterior sites. One can readily abstract from these results the notion that if recruitment of the perirhinal networks is important for the convulsive expression of kindled seizures, then a kindling-based decrease in afterdischarge threshold in the perirhinal/postrhinal area might be important to recruitment of the convulsive response.

If expression of the convulsive response is based on changes in seizure threshold in certain critical neural networks, as just described for perirhinal and postrhinal cortex kindling, then such a threshold change might also occur in these same structures during kindling from other limbic sites, such as the hippocampus or the amygdala. This possibility is particularly important, because (as indicated herein) the afterdischarge thresholds observed in the kindled amygdala or hippocampus *per se* normally change relatively little by comparison to the changes indicated during direct perirhinal and postrhinal cortex kindling. To answer this question, we kindled the amygdala or dorsal hippocampus and measured changes in the afterdischarge threshold in both the directly kindled structure (amygdala or hippocampus) and the laterally adjacent unkindled perirhinal and postrhinal cortices. Importantly, the large afterdischarge threshold decreases reported during *direct* kindling of the perirhinal and postrhinal cortices[29] also occurred during kindling of either the amygdala or the dorsal hippocampus. On the other hand, the afterdischarge threshold in the kindled structure itself (amygdala or hippocampus) was much less altered (Bureau and McIntyre, in progress). Thus, a decrease of seizure threshold in several important parahippocampal structures (such as the piriform and perirhinal cortices) might be critically important for the recruitment, propagation, and generalization of focal seizures initiated or kindled from a variety of different limbic sites or structures.

CONVULSIVE SEIZURES FOLLOWING STATUS EPILEPTICUS

In recent years, we[30] and others[31] have attempted to directly assess the involvement of the piriform and perirhinal cortices in the expression of kindled motor seizures by lesioning these areas prior to the beginning of kindling. If these parahippocampal structures are important for the development and manifestation of kindled convulsive seizures, destruction of the piriform/perirhinal area should prevent the recruitment necessary to secondarily generalize the focal seizure into its convulsive form.

Racine and colleagues[31] were the first to attempt an examination of this issue. Before kindling the septum, they created *bilateral* lesions in the amygdala-piriform area using electrolytic or radiofrequency techniques. Although the lesions delayed septal kindling, they did not prevent it. However, equally important, the lesions also were incomplete. Unfortunately, these researchers found that creating more complete lesions with these techniques was lethal for their subjects.

In our assessment of the problem, we chose a different vehicle for selectively and completely destroying the piriform/perirhinal area, a technique that involved the induction of status epilepticus (SE). There are many ways experimentally to induce SE, for example, using chemical agents such as kainic acid or pilocarpine. For reasons discussed elsewhere,[32] however, we chose continuous, low-intensity electrical stimulation of a kindled amygdala as the means of SE induction. This technique results in continuous, self-sustained limbic seizures that terminate spontaneously after 10–20 hours and results (in many rats) in complete loss of the piriform cortex, with varying additional damage to the perirhinal cortex.[8] Because this pathology is unilateral in many rats (although bilateral in others), we decided to restrict the experiment to one hemisphere by administering a forebrain commissurotomy before kindling and SE induction. Thus, 3 weeks prior to amygdala kindling, all experimental rats underwent forebrain bisection that included most of the corpus callosum and hippocampal commissure as well as several other midline structures.[30] Subsequently, the rats were amygdala kindled until they experienced a total of six stage-5 convulsive seizures (note that if the anterior half of the corpus callosum is bisected, seizures are hemiconvulsive, involving the contralateral limbs). Three weeks later, SE induction was attempted by stimulating the kindled site continuously for 1 hour. Two weeks after the SE experience, kindling of the dorsal hippocampus was begun. It was predicted that if rats experienced extensive brain damage during SE, which injured the critical neural substrate underwriting convulsive behavior, then subsequent kindling of the dorsal hippocampus to levels of convulsive expression would not occur. The results of the study indicated that near-complete loss of the piriform cortex did not change the rate of hippocampal kindling or the form of convulsive expression compared to that of the appropriate controls, that is, rats that had minimal or no piriform damage. It was only the few rats with extensive piriform damage *plus* extensive perirhinal damage that indicated an inability to manifest a kindled convulsive seizure via the damaged hemisphere.[30] Thus, piriform cortex damage alone did not prevent the development or expression of hippocampal kindled convulsions, but additional damage to the perirhinal cortex, particularly its posterior aspects, blocked the convulsive expression.

Currently, we are testing further the importance of the perirhinal area in the development of hippocampal or amygdala kindling by creating bilateral aspiration lesions restricted singly to either the perirhinal or the postrhinal cortices before the kindling procedure. In this way, we will learn if it is the combined lesions of the piriform and perirhinal cortices that interfere with convulsive expression during kindling or simply the perirhinal cortex lesions alone (Bureau and McIntyre, study in progress).

Studies using the pilocarpine model of TLE give further evidence that the perirhinal area may be important to the development and/or expression of convulsive seizures. Systemic administration of pilocarpine (350–380 mg/kg) results in the development of strong SE, which typically is arrested after 1 hour with diazepam to prevent death of the subject. Despite SE arrest, considerable brain damage to temporal lobe structures follows from this treatment. Over the course of the next few weeks, the majority of these pilocarpine-treated rats begin to show signs of discrete, spontaneous convulsive seizures. The etiology of this behavior was described previously by others (e.g., Refs. 33 and 34).

Mello *et al.*[35] have questioned the neural substrate that is activated during the genesis of these delayed, spontaneous seizures following pilocarpine SE. To do so, rats were perfused approximately 1 hour after a discrete spontaneous seizure, and their brains were examined histologically for evidence of activation of the immediate early gene, *c-fos*. The results showed surprisingly little evidence of *c-fos* expression, but the expression that was evident showed greatest activity in the piriform/perirhinal cortex. These observations are very similar to the results of Ferland *et al.*[23] using the amygdala kindling model.

We also examined rats after exposure to pilocarpine SE and observed that most rats develop spontaneous convulsive seizures within 2 weeks of the SE experience.

However, we have seen two populations of rats that did not develop spontaneous convulsive seizures. On histological examination, those two populations include (a) rats that had little or no brain damage, and (b) rats that had substantial brain damage involving all of the piriform cortex and most of the perirhinal cortex. However, if only the piriform cortex was lost, spontaneous convulsive seizures invariably occurred (McLeod, Kelly, and McIntyre, work in progress). Clearly, if there was little or no brain damage following SE, one might not expect the spontaneous convulsions to occur like those observed with piriform cortex damage alone. Thus, presumably, it was the additional perirhinal cortex damage coupled with the piriform damage that blocked the development of spontaneous convulsive seizures in those few rats exhibiting substantial damage but no convulsive behavior.

In summary, considerable evidence suggests that the perirhinal cortex has, among other things, an important role in the convulsive generalization of limbic triggered seizures. Whether the perirhinal cortex is critically and preemptively important in that regard remains to be determined. Very possibly it plays a powerful role in controlling convulsive behavior, but perhaps only when combined with changes in other parahippocampal structures such as the piriform cortex and/or the entorhinal cortex.[36] Future experiments, however, will be necessary to test these various possibilities.

REFERENCES

1. HAUSER, W.A. 1997. Incidence and prevalence. *In* Epilepsy: A Comprehensive Textbook. J. Engel & T. A. Pedley, Eds.: 47–57. Lippincott-Raven. Philadelphia.
2. HAUSER, W.A. & L.T. KURLAND. 1975. The epidemiology of epilepsy in Rochester, Minnesota, 1935 through 1967. Epilepsia **16:** 1–66.
3. DUCHOWNY, M.S., A.S. HARVEY, M.R. SPERLING & P.D. WILLIAMSON. 1997. Indications and criteria for surgical intervention. *In* Epilepsy: A Comprehensive Textbook. J. Engel & T. A. Pedley, Eds.: 1677–1685. Lippincott-Raven. Philadelphia.
4. FALCONER, M.A., D. HILL, A. MEYER, W. MITCHELL & D.A. POND. 1955. Treatment of temporal-lobe epilepsy by temporal lobectomy. Lancet **:** 827–835.
5. SATO, M., R.J. RACINE & D.C. MCINTYRE. 1990. Kindling: basic mechanisms and clinical validity. Electroenceph. Clin. Neurophysiol. **76:** 459–472.
6. GODDARD, G.V., D.C. MCINTYRE & C.K. LEECH. 1969. A permanent change in brain function resulting from daily electrical stimulation. Exp. Neurol. **25:** 295–330.
7. BATTYE, R.A. & D.C. MCINTYRE. 1995. Intrinsic responses and morphological features of neurons in the rat perirhinal cortex. Soc. Neurosci. Abstr. **21:** 1971.
8. MCINTYRE, D.C., D. NATHANSON & N. EDSON. 1982. A new model of partial status epilepticus based on kindling. Brain Res. **250:** 53–63.
9. KAIRISS, E.W., R.J. RACINE & G.K. SMITH. 1984. The development of the interictal spike during kindling in the rat. Brain Res. **322:** 101–110.
10. PIREDDA, S. & K. GALE. 1985. A crucial epileptogenic site in the deep prepiriform cortex. Nature **317:** 623–625.
11. MCINTYRE, D.C. & R.J. RACINE. 1986. Kindling mechanisms: current progress on an experimental epilepsy model. Prog. Neurobiol. **27:** 1–12.
12. MCINTYRE, D.C. & R.K. WONG. 1985. Modification of local neuronal interactions by amygdala kindling examined *in vitro*. Exp. Neurol. **88:** 529–537.
13. MCINTYRE, D.C. & R.K. WONG. 1986. Cellular and synaptic properties of amygdala-kindled pyriform cortex in vitro. J. Neurophysiol. **55:** 1295–1307.
14. MCINTYRE, D.C. & J.R. PLANT. 1993. Long-lasting changes in the origin of spontaneous discharges from amygdala-kindled rats: piriform vs. perirhinal cortex *in vitro*. Brain. Res. **624:** 268–276.

15. WALTHER, H., J.D.C. LAMBERT, R.S.G. JONES, U. HEINEMANN & B. HAMON. 1986. Epileptiform activity in combined slices of hippocampus, subiculum and entorhinal cortex during perfusion with low magnesium medium. Neurosci. Lett. **69:** 156–161.

16. WILSON, W.A., H.S. SWARTZWELDER, W.. ANDERSON & D.V. LEWIS. 1988. Seizure activity *in vitro*: a dual focus model. Epilepsy Res. **2:** 289–293.

17. McINTYRE, D.C., M.E. KELLY & J.N. ARMSTRONG. 1993. Kindling in the perirhinal cortex. Brain Res. **615:** 1–6.

18. CORCORAN, M.E., H. URSTAD, J. McCAUGHRAN & J.A. WADA. 1976. Frontal lobe and kindling in the rat. *In* Kindling. J. A. Wada, Ed.: 215–228. Raven Press. New York.

19. McINTYRE, D.C., M.E. KELLY & W.A. STAINES. 1996. Efferent projections of the anterior perirhinal cortex in the rat [published erratum appears in J. Comp. Neurol. 1996. **370:** 563–564]. J. Comp. Neurol. **369:** 302–318.

20. TESKEY, G.C. & R.J. RACINE. 1993. Increased spontaneous unit discharge rates following electrical kindling in the rat. Brain Res. **624:** 11–18.

21. KELLY, M.E., R.A. BATTYE & D.C. McINTYRE. 1999. Cortical spreading depression reversibly disrupts convulsive motor seizure expression in amygdala-kindled rats. Neuroscience **91:** 305–313.

22. McINTYRE, D.C. 1975. Split-brain rat: transfer and interference of amygdala kindled convulsions. Can. J. Neurol. Sci. **2:** 419–426.

23. FERLAND, R.J., J. NIERENBERG & C.D. APPLEGATE. 1998. A role for the bilateral involvement of perirhinal cortex in generalized kindled seizure expression. Exp. Neurol. **151:** 124–137.

24. BEGGS, J.M. & E.W. KAIRISS. 1994. Electrophysiology and morphology of neurons in rat perirhinal cortex. Brain Res. **665:** 18–32.

25. FAULKNER, B. & T.H. BROWN. 1999. Morphology and physiology of neurons in the rat perirhinal-lateral amygdala area. J. Comp. Neurol. **411:** 613–642.

26. CHAGNAC-AMITAI, Y., H.J. LUHMANN & D.A. PRINCE. 1990. Burst generating and regular spiking layer 5 pyramidal neurons of rat neocortex have different morphological features. J. Comp. Neurol. **296:** 598–613.

27. BURWELL, R.D., M.P. WITTER & D.G. AMARAL. 1995. Perirhinal and postrhinal cortices of the rat: a review of the neuroanatomical literature and comparison with findings from the monkey brain [published erratum appears in Hippocampus 1996;6(3):340]. Hippocampus **5:** 390–408.

28. McINTYRE, D.C., M.E. KELLY & C. DUFRESNE. 1999. FAST and SLOW amygdala kindling rat strains: comparison of amygdala, hippocampal, piriform and perirhinal cortex kindling. Epilepsy Res. **35:** 197–209.

29. FELSTEAD, L.L., M.E. KELLY & D.C. McINTYRE. 1995. Laminar and topographical analysis of perirhinal cortex kindling in the rat. Soc. Neurosci. Abstr. **21:** 1971.

30. KELLY, M.E. & D.C. McINTYRE. 1996. Perirhinal cortex involvement in limbic kindled seizures. Epilepsy Res. **26:** 233–243.

31. RACINE, R.J., G. PAXINOS, J.M. MOSHER & E.W. KAIRISS. 1988. The effects of various lesions and knife-cuts on septal and amygdala kindling in the rat. Brain Res. **454:** 264–274.

32. KELLY, M.E. & D.C. McINTYRE. 1994. Hippocampal kindling protects several structures from the neuronal damage resulting from kainic acid-induced status epilepticus. Brain Res. **634:** 245–256.

33. OLNEY, J.W., T. DE GUBAREFF & J. LABRUYERE. 1983. Seizure-related brain damage induced by cholinergic agents. Nature **301:** 520–522.

34. TURSKI, W.A., E.A. CAVALHEIRO, S.J. SCHWARZ, Z. CZUCZWAR, S.J. KLEINROK & L. TURSKI. 1983. Limbic seizures produced by pilocarpine in rats: behavioural, electroencephalographic and neuropathological study. Behav. Brain Res. **9:** 315–335.

35. MELLO, L.E.A., C.M. KOHMAN, M.T. AIKO, E.A. CAVALHEIRO & D.M. FINCH. 1996. Lack of Fos-like immunoreactivirty after spontaneous seizures or reinduction of status epilepticus by pilocarpine in rats. Neurosci. Lett. **208:** 133–137.

36. BURCHFIEL, J.L., C.D. APPLEGATE, G.M. SAMORISKI & J. NIERENBERG. 1998. The role of rhinencephalic networks in early stage kindling. *In* Kindling 5. M.E. Corcoran & S. L. Moshé, Eds.: 133–149. Plenum Press. New York.

Memory Deficits Characterized by Patterns of Lesions to the Hippocampus and Parahippocampal Cortex

VÉRONIQUE D. BOHBOT,[a,d] JOHN J.B. ALLEN,[b] AND LYNN NADEL[b,c]

[a]McConnell Brain Imaging Centre, Montreal Neurological Institute, McGill University, Montreal, Quebec, Canada, H3A 2B4

[b]Psychology Department, University of Arizona, Tucson, Arizona 85721, USA

[c]ARL Division of Neural Systems, Memory and Aging, University of Arizona, Tucson, Arizona 85724, USA

ABSTRACT: Spatial and nonspatial memory tests were given to patients with small thermal lesions administered to the medial temporal lobes in an attempt at alleviating pharmacologically resistant epilepsy. In all three spatial memory experiments presented in this paper, patients with lesions that included the right parahippocampal cortex were seriously impaired. Their impairment, together with the performance of patients with lesions to the right hippocampus (sparing the right parahippocampal cortex), provides the different patterns of deficits that lead to different interpretations of the function of the parahippocampal cortex. The distinction between the effects of functional damage in hippocampus and the effects of a lesion to the hippocampus or to regions surrounding the hippocampus, such as the parahippocampal cortex, is emphasized. We conclude that the right parahippocampal cortex participates in spatial memory beyond serving as a gateway to the hippocampus.

INTRODUCTION

Important contributions to our understanding of human memory come from the study of brain-damaged patients whose etiologies differ widely, including cerebrovascular damage (infarct), progressive diseases (such as Alzheimer's and Parkinson's), infectious diseases (herpes encephalitis), closed or open head injuries, surgical removal of tumors or cysts, resections of epileptogenic tissue, and hypoxia. Much of the past and current research on human memory focused on patients with extensive brain damage resulting from one of the above-mentioned etiologies.[1–9] There are, however, reports of memory deficits after lesions restricted to small areas.[10–12] Important contributing factors to these kinds of studies are the recent advances in neuroimaging techniques allowing high-resolution visualization of the brain (such as magnetic resonance imaging, MRI); visualization of brain damage had traditionally been limited to postmortem analyses.

[d]Address for correspondence: Dr. Véronique Bohbot, McConnell Brain Imaging Centre, Montreal Neurological Institute, McGill University, 3801 University St., Montreal, Quebec, Canada, H3A 2B4. Tel.: (514) 398-4965; fax: (514) 398-8948.
e-mail: vero@bic.mni.mcgill.ca

Studies of brain-damaged patients that have large lesions do not allow for the study of the mnemonic role of single structures (defined by distinct cytoarchitecture). In the medial temporal lobe for example, the hippocampus (proper and dentate gyrus) and amygdala are surrounded by the tail of the caudate nucleus and the parahippocampal gyrus, composed of the peri-amygdaloid cortex, the subiculum, the piriform, entorhinal, perirhinal, and parahippocampal cortices. In addition, structures neighboring the medial temporal lobes include the fusiform cortex, lateral temporal neocortices, and, medially, the lingual gyrus and the posterior tip of the cingulate gyrus.[13] Despite the knowledge that cytoarchitectonic fields other than the hippocampus were compromised in studies with human subjects, for several decades it has been thought that the hippocampus was the medial temporal lobe structure primarily responsible for the memory loss observed in amnesic patients. In addition to the hippocampus, lesion studies of rodents, nonhuman primates, and brain-imaging studies with positron emission tomography (PET) and functional MRI (fMRI) now point to regions surrounding the hippocampus, as also contributing to memory processes.[14–24]

The encoding and recall of verbal material[6] or of the location of objects[25,26] and other spatial memory processes[27–29] has been thought to rely on the hippocampal region (hippocampus, subicular complex, and entorhinal cortex[30]). The patients in these studies had unilateral damage that included other neocortical regions of the medial temporal lobe. Thus, damage to structures surrounding the hippocampal region might have contributed to the memory loss.

Topographical amnesia, on the other hand, has been linked to more posterior regions, including areas around the occipital–parietal–temporal junction.[31–33] Topographical amnesia is the inability to find one's way in the environment, in the context of intact visuo-spatial perception. A study by Habib and Sirigu[32] showed that the area common to their patients who suffered from topographical amnesia was the parahippocampal gyrus. Because a lesion to the parahippocampal gyrus will also largely de-afferent the hippocampus, it is possible that topographical learning requires the contribution of the hippocampus.

Given that the various regions of the medial temporal lobes are interconnected, studies that dissociate regions from one another are necessary in order to establish which region is critical for a task.[34–36] Consider the following two possibilities.

(1) *Functional lesion in hippocampus*: Suppose that the parahippocampal cortex was involved in processing *perceptual* information about scenes, but was not involved in *memory* for scenes, then a lesion to the parahippocampal cortex could deprive target structures such as the perirhinal cortex, entorhinal cortex, and hippocampus of their "scene" input. It would not be surprising then to find *memory* deficits for scenes in patients with lesions of the parahippocampal cortex, even if their hippocampus was intact. One could conclude that the parahippocampal cortex was involved in memory, whereas in reality the deficit was produced by a functional lesion of the hippocampus.

(2) *Memory representation in parahippocampal cortex*: Suppose that patients with lesions to the parahippocampal cortex are impaired at remembering "scenes" after a delay period, and patients with lesions to the hippocampus, sparing the parahippocampal cortex, are not impaired, then the interpretation of a functional lesion in the hippocampus can be eliminated. In this case the parahippocampal cortex itself assumed the memory capacity for scenes.

TABLE 1. Subjects

Group	Sex M	F	Age Mean	Range	Wechsler IQ Mean	Range	Wechsler Memory Scale Mean	Range
Back-pain patient control	5	3	41.4	29–57	119	96–133	126	98–143
Epileptic patient control	5	5	26.5	17–43	99.3	80–129	107.1	99–143
Right hippocampal	5	2	36.9	29–49	103.7	88–131	102.9	84–126
Right parahippocampal	3	2	45	38–59	94	82–105	102	81–129
Left hippocampal	1	3	44.5	37–53	91.8	87–96	94.8	89–103
Left parahippocampal	1	0	34	—	99	—	87	—

In the present paper, we attempted to make the distinction between the effects of functional damage in the hippocampus and effects of a lesion to the hippocampus or to regions surrounding the hippocampus, such as the parahippocampal cortex. The patients studied had small stereotaxic thermal lesions performed in an attempt at alleviating intractable epilepsy. Despite the fact that our patients had small lesions, their lesions invaded several different cytoarchitectonic fields. Our contribution, however, is based on the fact that the small lesions do not invade all the different cytoarchitectonic fields, in the same way, in all patients. Consequently, the patients with lesions to the right or left hippocampus or parahippocampal cortex had either an intact entorhinal or perirhinal cortex, and some patients with lesions to the parahippocampal cortex had intact hippocampi. Importantly, all the patients in the parahippocampal lesion groups had damage to the parahippocampal cortex (FIG. 1), and all the patients in the hippocampal groups had intact parahippocampal cortices (FIG. 2). The three experiments described below provide evidence for three different patterns of deficits (1) a functional hippocampal lesion and critical involvement of the hippocampus, (2) involvement of both the hippocampus and parahippocampal cortex, and (3) critical involvement of the parahippocampal cortex.

METHODS AND RESULTS

Subjects

Two control groups and four brain-operated patient groups were tested in the present experiments (see TABLE 1). These patients have been described elsewhere.[12] One control group consisted of patients with back pain problems, but no epileptic problems, and the other consisted of patients with epilepsy who did not undergo brain surgery. Of the two control groups, the epileptic patient control group resembles more closely the experimental groups and therefore serves as a better control.

Back Pain Control Group

Eight patients with back pain were chosen as controls because, as the experimental groups, they were patients who suffered a disorder; however, the disorder was not localized to the brain.

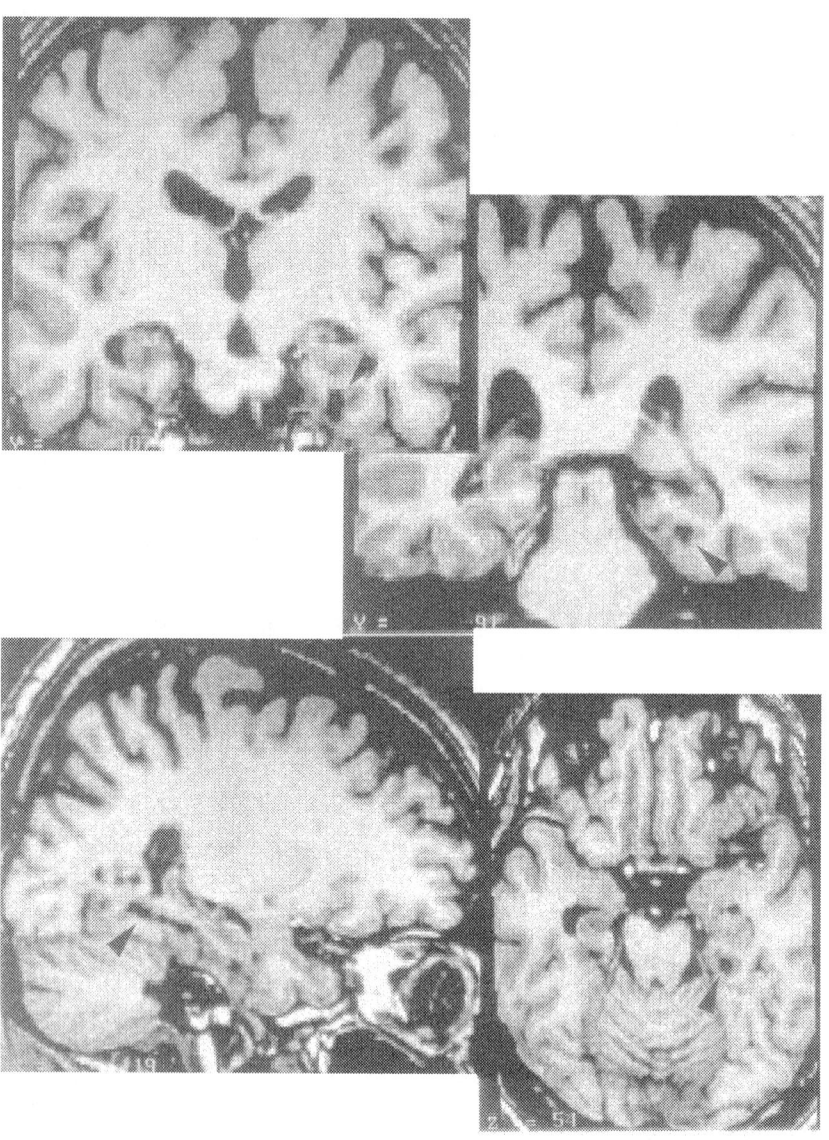

FIGURE 1. Thermal lesion to the right parahippocampal cortex. MRI sections in coronal, horizontal, and sagittal planes of a brain transformed into Talairach[42] standard stereotaxic space. *Arrows* point to the lesion in the right parahippocampal cortex sparing the hippocampus.

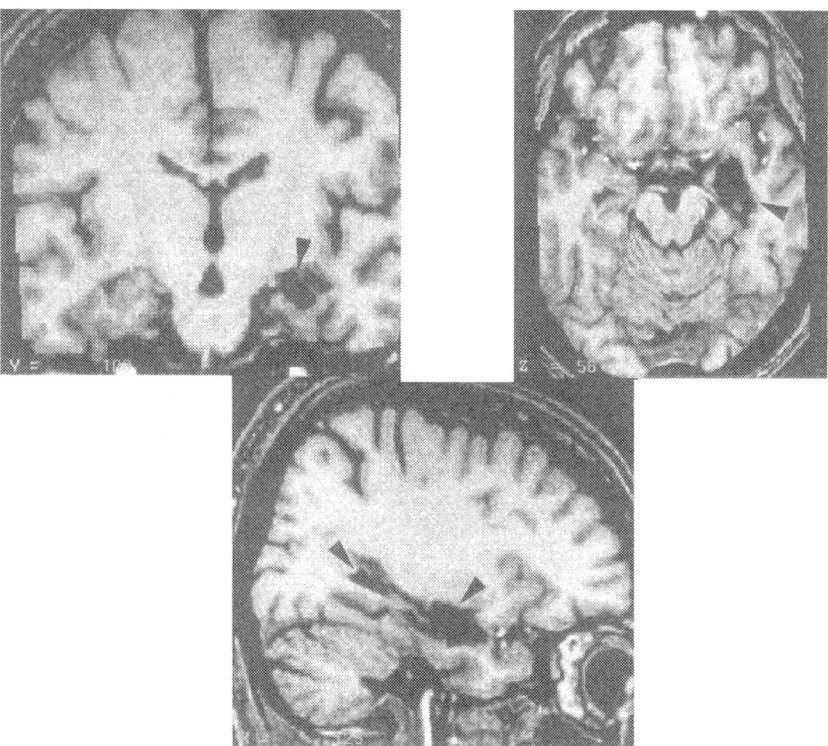

FIGURE 2. Thermal lesion to the right hippocampus. MRI sections in coronal, horizontal, and sagittal planes of a brain transformed into Talairach[42] standard stereotaxic space. *Arrows* point to the lesion in the right hippocampus sparing the parahippocampal cortex.

Epileptic Patient Control Group

Ten epileptic patients without brain resection or thermal lesion were used as controls. They were on nontoxic antiepileptic drug (AED) therapy similar to that received by the operated patients, but their epilepsy was controlled with medication, and they were not surgical candidates. Their epilepsy was of probable temporal origin. This group was considered a good control group because they suffer from the same neurological disorder as the brain-operated patients.

Brain-Operated Groups

Fourteen of 17 patients who underwent selective thermo-coagulation lesions (FIGS. 1 and 2) in an attempt to alleviate pharmacologically intractable epilepsy are reported in each experiment. Patients with Wechsler IQs below 75, psychiatric disorders, or with gross brain atrophy were excluded from the study. All patients were right-handed. The patients were tested 4 to 17 years postoperatively. All patients were on antiepileptic drug therapy at the time of testing. None of the patients had clinical symptoms of overdose, and the patients' performance was not affected by clinical or EEG seizures on the day of testing.

The patients with thermal lesions were divided into four groups: right hippocampus, right parahippocampal cortex, left hippocampus, and left parahippocampal cortex. The anatomical landmarks that were used to identify the patients' lesions have been described elsewhere.[12] In summary, patients with lesions were divided into groups depending on whether or not they had damage to the parahippocampal cortex. Lesions to the hippocampus can include the hippocampus proper, the dentate gyrus, and the subicular complex (FIG. 2). Lesions of the parahippocampal cortex refer to the posterior parahippocampal gyrus (FIG. 1), the neocortical region posterior to the entorhinal cortex and perirhinal cortex. Many but not all patients in these groups had damage to the entorhinal and perirhinal cortices, see Bohbot *et al.*,[12,37] for more details.

Analysis

Because the assumption of a normal distribution cannot be made in groups with small sizes, a nonparametric analysis of variance, the Kruskal-Wallis H test, was used to analyze the data. The single patient with a left parahippocampal lesion was not included in any of the statistical analyses. The five groups included in the analyses were: the back pain control (BPC) and the epilepsy patient control (EPC) groups, as well as the patient groups with lesions to the right hippocampus (RH), right parahippocampal cortex (RPH), and left hippocampus (LH). Further analysis was done with the Wilcoxon rank sum test for comparing two independent samples. First we compared the BPC group to the EPC group, and there were no significant differences on any test. The BPC group and the EPC group were compared with each brain-operated patient group.

Object Location Task

Procedure

This recall task was designed to test memory for several objects and their different spatial locations. The subject was allowed to observe the location of four objects (briefcase, stand, kettle, and flowerpot) in the experimental room, for 10 seconds. Soon afterwards, the subject had to reconstruct the spatial layout of the four objects on an outline of the room presented on a sheet of paper. The coordinates of the object icons on the paper were measured and translated into real space coordinates. The error was defined as the distance between the real location of objects and their estimated location by the subject. To solve this task, the patients must encode spatial relations and the location that each object occupied and their relation to the room.

Results

The mean error for the estimated position of each one of the four objects for the different groups is shown in FIGURE 3. The Kruskal-Wallis analysis of variance indicated that there were significant differences between the groups ($H = 9.65$, $df = 4$, $p < 0.05$). Further analysis with the Wilcoxon Rank Sum Test showed that relative to the epileptic patient controls, both the right hippocampal group ($z = 1.90$, $p < 0.05$) and the right parahippocampal cortex group ($z = 1.77$, $p < 0.05$) were significantly

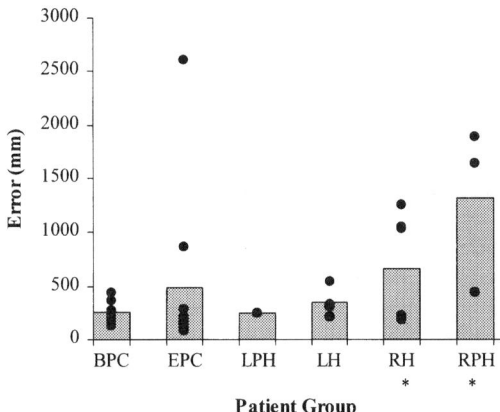

FIGURE 3. Object location task. The error (in millimeters) is the difference between the estimated position of the objects and the real position. Each bar represents the mean of a group. The scores of individual subjects for each group are displayed. BPC: back pain controls; EPC: epileptic patients controls; LPH: left parahippocampal cortex; LH: patients with damage to the left hippocampus; RH: right hippocampus; RPH: right parahippocampal cortex. *Different from EPC, $p < 0.05$.

impaired; in addition, the right parahippocampal cortex group was significantly impaired relative to back-pain controls ($z = 2.14$, $p < 0.05$). The left hippocampal group was unimpaired on this task.

Although there was only one left parahippocampal patient, precluding statistical analysis, descriptively it appeared that the left parahippocampal patient was unimpaired on this task.

Spatial Oddball Task

Procedure

Computerized tasks were developed to assess memory for two types of information about objects: changes in the spatial configuration of objects and changes in the particular objects displayed. These tasks were designed in the oddball fashion for use with evoked potentials.[38] In each task, a standard display depicting five unrelated objects appeared on 80% of the trials (standards), and alterations of this standard display appeared on 20% of the trials. On 10% of the trials, a new object appeared in place of one of the objects on the standard display (object identity change). On another 10% of the trials, two of the objects from the standard display switched locations (spatial configuration change). In each sequence of 10 displays, one spatial configuration change and one object identity change occurred, with a standard display following each of these changes. The standard displays that followed the object identity or the spatial configuration changes were never included in the analyses, as these represented a change back to the standard condition.

In the spatial task, subjects were instructed to respond to spatial configuration changes (targets) and ignore the object identity changes (distractors). They indicated

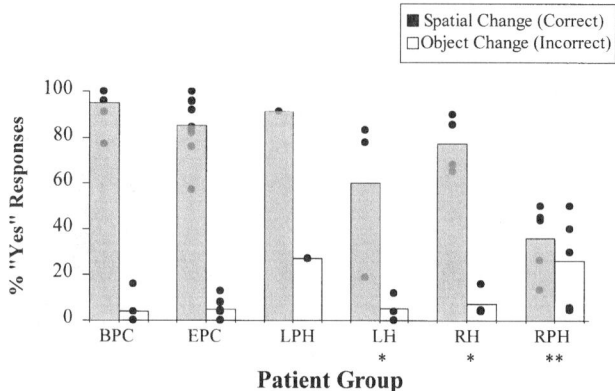

FIGURE 4. Spatial oddball task. Percent scores of correct detection of the spatial configuration change (target), and incorrect detection of the irrelevant object identity change (distractor). Each bar represents the mean of a group. The scores of individual subjects for each group are displayed. Details and labels are described in the legend of FIGURE 3. *Significantly different from the BPC group in responses to spatial changes ($p < 0.05$). **In responses to spatial changes, significantly different from the BPC and EPC groups ($p < 0.005$) and from the RH group ($p < 0.05$); in responses to the object changes, significantly different from the BPC ($p < 0.01$) and EPC ($p < 0.05$) groups.

their response by pressing the left key for standards and distractors ("NO" response), or a right key for the targets ("YES" response). The subject's target detection was "correct" if the right key was pressed for the change in configuration of objects in the spatial task. A response was incorrect if the right key was pressed for either the standards or irrelevant changes. Only the results from the spatial task are presented here. Further details on an object task equivalent to the spatial task are published elsewhere.[37]

Results

The patients with lesions to the right parahippocampal cortex, and to some extent the patients with lesions to the right and left hippocampus showed poor discrimination of the spatial configuration from the object identity changes in the spatial task (FIG. 4). The detection of spatial configuration change ("YES" response) was different across the groups (Kruskal-Wallis rank test, $H = 17.71$, $df = 4$, $p < 0.001$). The Wilcoxon rank sum test for two independent samples showed that the two control groups performed similarly. The right parahippocampal subjects were impaired relative to the EPC subjects ($z = 2.93$, $p < 0.005$), and relative to the BPC subjects ($z = 2.89$, $p < 0.005$). The left and right hippocampal subjects were impaired relative to the BPC subjects (*left*: $z = 1.98$, $p < 0.05$; *right*: $z = 2.33$, $p < 0.05$); however, they were not impaired relative to the EPC subjects (*left*: $z = 1.48$, n.s.; *right*: $z = 0.85$, n.s.). This implies that the left or right hippocampal thermal lesion itself did not significantly change the performance beyond that seen in individuals with epilepsy. The group with lesions to the right parahippocampal cortex was impaired relative to the group with lesions to the right hippocampus ($z = 2.33$, $p < 0.05$), indicating that the impairment resulting from the right parahippocampal cortex lesion could be dissociated from any impairments caused by dysfunction in the right hippocampus.

While subjects were engaged in the spatial task, there were differences (Kruskal-Wallis rank test, $H = 9.76$, $df = 4$, $p < 0.05$) in the number of incorrect "YES" responses to the object identity change (distractors; FIG. 4). The Wilcoxon rank sum test showed that only patients with lesions to the right parahippocampal cortex were impaired relative to the patient control group with epilepsy ($z = 2.15$, $p < 0.05$) and relative to the BPC subjects ($z = 2.59$, $p < 0.01$). None of the other tested comparisons differed. These results show clearly that the only patients who were affected by the presence of distractors in the spatial task were those with lesions to the right parahippocampal cortex.

Invisible Sensor Task

Procedure

A dry version of the Morris water task[39,40] was created for human subjects by hiding a sensor under the carpet of the room. The sensor was placed away from the walls and away from major cues, such as the heater or the sink. The sensor emitted a pleasant sound when stepped on and the subject was asked to locate it as quickly as possible, note its position with respect to the room landmarks, and then to return to the entrance (trial 1). About 30 seconds later, the subject was asked to enter the same room by the other door and to try to go straight to the location of the invisible sensor (trial 2). After a 30-minute delay, trial 3 was administered starting from the same door as in trial 1.

Results

On the first trial, all subjects found the sensor through trial and error by walking around the room. On immediate recall, all groups of patients rapidly found the invisible sensor (FIG. 5); there were no significant differences (Kruskal-Wallis rank test, $H = 1.15$, $df = 4$, n.s.) across all groups. Planned comparisons showed no differences between patients with lesions to the right hippocampus and the epilepsy patient controls in the Wilcoxon rank sum test. Latencies to find the invisible sensor after the 30-minute delay are also shown in FIGURE 5. After this delay, significant differences between the groups on the recall of the location of the invisible sensor were found (Kruskal-Wallis rank test, $H = 11.33$, $df = 4$, $p < 0.05$). The one-tailed Wilcoxon test showed that only the patients with lesions to the right parahippocampal cortex were impaired relative to the BPCs ($z = 2.35$, $p < 0.01$), and relative to the EPCs ($z = 2.45$, $p < 0.01$). Patients with right or left hippocampal lesions were unimpaired on this task.

DISCUSSION

We presented evidence from patients who underwent small stereotaxic thermocoagulation lesions to the medial temporal lobes (FIGS. 1 and 2), done in an attempt to alleviate intractable epilepsy. Patients were tested on various spatial memory tests reported elsewhere.[12,37] Because the lesions were small, we were able to separate the patients into two groups per hemisphere: those with and those without lesions to

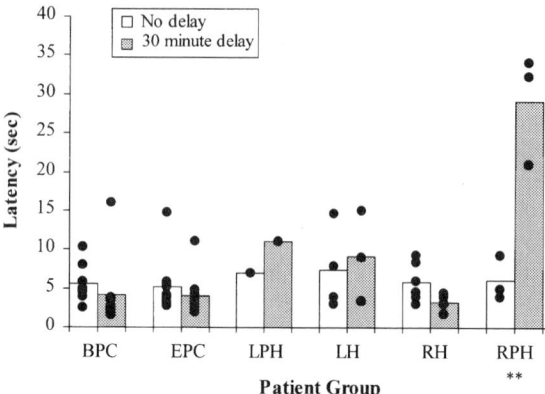

FIGURE 5. Invisible sensor task. Latencies for reaching the invisible sensor (trial 2: no delay and trial 3 at a 30-minute delay). Each bar represents the mean of a group. The scores of individual subjects for each group are displayed. Details and labels are described in the legend of FIGURE 3. **RPH different from BPC and from EPC at the 30-minute delay interval only, $p < 0.01$.

the parahippocampal cortex. Our results showed that patients with lesions to the left hippocampus were unimpaired compared with their epilepsy controls on all spatial memory tasks. Consistent with other reports, only patients with lesions to the right medial temporal lobe were impaired,[26,41] suggesting that the right side is specialized in spatial memory. Within the right medial temporal lobe, three different patterns of deficits were observed.

(1) *Deficit in patients with lesions to the right hippocampus and right parahippocampal cortex.* Patients with lesions to the right hippocampus, sparing the parahippocampal cortex, showed deficits in the object location task (FIG. 3) and the Rey-Osterreith complex figure.[12] Patients with lesions to the right parahippocampal cortex showed similar impairments. Because patients in the right hippocampal group ($n = 6$) had an intact parahippocampal cortex, this suggests that the parahippocampal cortex itself was not capable of sustaining these memory functions. In the group with lesions to the right parahippocampal cortex, one of three patients had an intact hippocampus; this patient's deficit can be attributed to a functional hippocampal lesion. These two tests critically require the involvement of the right hippocampus but do not inform us about the role played by the right parahippocampal cortex: it remains unclear whether it is implicated in memory or in processing perceptual information that it transmits to the hippocampus.

(2) *Mild deficit in patients with lesions to the right hippocampus, severe deficit in patients with lesions to the right parahippocampal cortex.* Patients whose lesions included the right parahippocampal cortex were severely impaired (35% correct) relative to patients with lesions to the right hippocampus, on the spatial oddball task (FIG. 4). Patients with lesions to the right hippocampus sparing the parahippocampal cortex showed no deficit (77% correct) relative to control subjects with epilepsy (85% correct) but had a deficit compared with back pain patient controls (95% cor-

rect). This is best interpreted as evidence that the medial temporal lobes are involved, including the participation of the hippocampus. However, when intact, the right parahippocampal cortex alone can sustain some spatial memory function (up from 35% to 77% correct performance in patients with lesions to the right hippocampus). The deficit in patients with right parahippocampal lesions is therefore not due merely to a functional hippocampal lesion. The right parahippocampal cortex itself is critical for this task, in addition to the right hippocampal involvement.

(3) *No deficit in patients with right hippocampal lesions, severe deficit in patients with lesions to the right parahippocampal cortex.* Patients with lesions to the right parahippocampal cortex were severely impaired after the 30-minute delay of the invisible sensor task and not impaired at all on the immediate recall (FIG. 5). Patients with lesions to the right hippocampus showed no deficit on the invisible sensory task, even when recall was tested after a 30-minute delay. Clearly, the deficit in patients with right parahippocampal lesions was not due to a functional hippocampal lesion, showing that the right parahippocampal cortex itself can sustain long-term memory.

We showed that the pattern of deficits in patients with lesions to the right hippocampus and right parahippocampal cortex differed in the three examples provided. In all three experiments, our patients with lesions that included the right parahippocampal cortex were seriously impaired. Their impairment, together with the performance of patients with lesions to the right hippocampus (sparing the right parahippocampal cortex) provide the different patterns of deficits that lead to different interpretations of parahipocampal function. Specifically, patients with right hippocampal damage were no different from control subjects in the 30-minute delay recall of the invisible sensor task, thus showing that their intact parahippocampal cortex can sustain this memory function. In the spatial oddball task, patients with lesions to the right hippocampus were mildly impaired, showing that the right hippocampus may be involved, but that the intact parahippocampal cortex could sustain some memory for this task. And finally, the object location task showed that both right-sided groups of patients were impaired, indicating that the hippocampus was critical for this task, despite the role of the parahippocampal cortex in some aspects of spatial memory. In a normal brain, both these structures may be recruited if they are intact.

Several hypotheses regarding the different roles of the hippocampus and the parahippocampal cortex can be posed.

(1) The hippocampus is important for allocentric spatial memory, and the parahippocampal cortex for egocentric spatial memory. The data from the invisible sensor task do not support this hypothesis since it is an allocentric task and subjects with right hippocampal damage were not impaired.

(2) The hippocampus is important for the computations involved in navigation and the parahippocampal cortex is important for spatial representations. Results on the object location task and invisible sensor task fail to support this hypothesis, suggesting the opposite if anything.

(3) The hippocampus is important for memory of multiple items, the parahippocampal cortex for single items. Because the difference between the object location task and invisible sensor task lies in the number of items stored in memory, not in the nature of the material to be studied, these data support this hypothesis.

(4) The hippocampus is involved in memory for object locations, and the parahippocampal cortex is involved in memory for scenes. These latter would be crucial in navigation, hence the role of the parahippocampal cortex in the invisible sensor task.

(5) The parahippocampal cortex is involved in memory for two-dimensional static spatial information, such as snapshots, and the hippocampus links these parahippocampal snapshots into three-dimensional representations. This is consistent with the results in the invisible sensor task and the spatial oddball task, since snapshots could subserve performance of the right hippocampal group in these tasks, and results in the object location task, where they could not.

(6) The hippocampus is important for episodes that include memory for single events as well as the context, and the parahippocampal cortex is involved in memory for single events alone (this is a variant of #3).

Our results to date seem to eliminate the first two hypotheses, but the remaining hypotheses are consistent with what has been observed so far. Future studies using subjects with damage limited to small areas in the medial temporal lobe should help distinguish among these various possibilities.

ACKNOWLEDGMENTS

We would like to thank Katerina Stepankova for her comments on an earlier version of this manuscript. This research was supported by the Granting Agency of the Czech Republic (Grant No. 309/95/0730) and by grants from the James S. McDonnell Foundation to Lynn Nadel and Veronique Bohbot (JSMF 92-57, JSMF 97-34). Veronique Bohbot's research is currently funded by the Natural Sciences and Engineering Research Council of Canada.

REFERENCES

1. SCOVILLE, W.B. & B. MILNER. 1957. Loss of recent memory after bilateral hippocampal lesions. J. Neurol. Neurosurg. Psychiatry 20: 11–21.
2. WARRINGTON, E.K. & L. WEISKRANTZ. 1982. Amnesia: a disconnection syndrome? Neuropsychologia 20: 233–248.
3. DAMASIO, A.R., N.R. GRAFF-RADFORD, P.J. ESLINGER, et al. 1985. Amnesia following basal forebrain lesions. Arch. Neurol. 42: 263–271.
4. TUCKER, D.M., D.P. ROELTGEN, R. TULLY, et al. 1988. Memory dysfunction following unilateral transection of the fornix: a hippocampal disconnection syndrome. Cortex 24: 465–472.
5. KOHLER, S. et al. 1998. Memory impairments associated with hippocampal versus parahippocampal- gyrus atrophy: an MR volumetry study in Alzheimer's disease. Neuropsychologia 36: 901–914.
6. DOBBINS, I.G., N.E. KROLL, E. TULVING, et al. 1998. Unilateral medial temporal lobe memory impairment: type deficit, function deficit, or both? Neuropsychologia 36: 115–127.
7. JONES-GOTMAN, M. et al. 1997. Learning and retention of words and designs following excision from medial or lateral temporal-lobe structures. Neuropsychologia 35: 963–973.
8. REMPEL-CLOWER, N.L., S.M. ZOLA, L.R. SQUIRE & D.G. AMARAL. 1996. Three cases of enduring memory impairment after bilateral damage limited to the hippocampal formation. J. Neurosci. 16: 5233–5255.

9. KITCHENER, E.G., J.R. HODGES & R. MCCARTHY. 1998. Acquisition of post-morbid vocabulary and semantic facts in the absence of episodic memory. Brain **121:** 1313–1327.
10. ZOLA-MORGAN, S., L.R. SQUIRE & D.G. AMARAL. 1986. Human amnesia and the medial temporal region: enduring memory impairment following a bilateral lesion limited to field CA1 of the hippocampus. J. Neurosci. **6:** 2950–2967.
11. VARGHA-KHADEM, F. *et al.* 1997. Differential effects of early hippocampal pathology on episodic and semantic memory. Science **277:** 376–380.
12. BOHBOT, V.D. *et al.* 1998. Spatial memory deficits in patients with lesions to the right hippocampus and to the right parahippocampal cortex. Neuropsychologia **36:** 1217–1238.
13. DUVERNOY, H.M. 1988. The Human Hippocampus. J.F. Bergmann Verlag. Munich.
14. BUSSEY, T.J., J.L. MUIR & J.P. AGGLETON. 1999. Functionally dissociating aspects of event memory: the effects of combined perirhinal and postrhinal cortex lesions on object and place memory in the rat. J. Neurosci. **19:** 495–502.
15. MEUNIER, M., J. BACHEVALIER, M. MISHKIN & E.A. MURRAY. 1993. Effects on visual recognition of combined and separate ablations of the entorhinal and perirhinal cortex in rhesus monkeys. J. Neurosci. **13:** 5418–5432.
16. MURRAY, E.A. & M. MISHKIN. 1998. Object recognition and location memory in monkeys with excitotoxic lesions of the amygdala and hippocampus. J. Neurosci. **18:** 6568–6582.
17. MALKOVA, L. & M. MISHKIN. 1997. Memory for the location of objects after separate lesions of the hippocampus and parahippocampal cortex in rhesus monkeys. Soc. Neurosci. Abstr. **23:** 12.
18. AGUIRRE, G.K., J.A. DETRE, D.C. ALSOP & M. D'ESPOSITO. 1996. The parahippocampus subserves topographical learning in man. Cereb. Cortex **6:** 823–829.
19. OWEN, A.M., B. MILNER, M. PETRIDES & A. EVANS. 1996. A specific role for the right parahippocampal gyrus in the retrieval of object-location—a positron emission tomography study. J. Cogn. Neurosci. **8:** 588–602.
20. STERN, C.E. *et al.* 1996. The hippocampal formation participates in novel picture encoding: evidence from functional magnetic resonance imaging. Proc. Natl. Acad. Sci. USA **93:** 8660–8665.
21. WAGNER, A.D. *et al.* 1998. Building memories: remembering and forgetting of verbal experiences as predicted by brain activity. Science **281:** 1188–1191.
22. BREWER, J.B., Z. ZHAO, J.E. DESMOND, *et al.* 1998. Making memories: brain activity that predicts how well visual experience will be remembered. Science **281:** 1185–1187.
23. MAGUIRE, E.A. & L. CIPOLOTTI. 1998. Selective sparing of topographical memory. J. Neurol. Neurosurg. Psychiatry **65:** 903–909.
24. BUFFALO, E.A., P.J. REBER & L.R. SQUIRE. 1998. The human perirhinal cortex and recognition memory. Hippocampus **8:** 330–339.
25. SMITH, M.L. & B. MILNER. 1984. Differential effects of frontal-lobe lesions on cognitive estimation and spatial memory. Neuropsychologia **22:** 697–705.
26. SMITH, M.L. & B. MILNER. 1989. Right hippocampal impairment in the recall of spatial location: encoding deficit or rapid forgetting? Neuropsychologia **27:** 71–81.
27. PIGOTT, S. & B. MILNER. 1993. Memory for different aspects of complex visual scenes after unilateral temporal- or frontal-lobe resection. Neuropsychologia **31:** 1–15.
28. MAGUIRE, E.A., T. BURKE, J. PHILLIPS & H. STAUNTON. 1996. Topographical disorientation following unilateral temporal lobe lesions in humans. Neuropsychologia **34:** 993–1001.
29. MORRIS, R.G., A. PICKERING, S. ABRAHAMS & J.D. FEIGENBAUM. 1996. Space and the hippocampal formation in humans. Brain Res. Bull. **40:** 487–490.
30. AMARAL, D.G. 1993. Emerging principles of intrinsic hippocampal organization. Curr. Opin. Neurobiol. **3:** 225–229.
31. LANDIS, T., J.L. CUMMINGS, D.F. BENSON & E.P. PALMER. 1986. Loss of topographic familiarity. An environmental agnosia. Arch. Neurol. **43:** 132–136.
32. HABIB, M. & A. SIRIGU. 1987. Pure topographical disorientation: a definition and anatomical basis. Cortex **23:** 73–85.

33. HUBLET, C. & G. DEMEURISSE. 1992. Pure topographical disorientation due to a deep-seated lesion with cortical remote effects. Cortex **28:** 123–128.
34. VAN HOESEN, G.W. 1982. The parahippocampal gyrus. Trends Neurosci. **5:** 345–350.
35. SUZUKI, W.A. & D.G. AMARAL. 1994. Perirhinal and parahippocampal cortices of the macaque monkey: cortical afferents. J. Comp. Neurol. **350:** 497–533.
36. SUZUKI, W.A. & D.G. AMARAL. 1990. Cortical inputs to the CA1 field of the monkey hippocampus originate from the perirhinal and parahippocampal cortex but not from area TE. Neurosci. Lett. **115:** 43–48.
37. BOHBOT, V.D., J.J.B. ALLEN, M. KALINA, *et al.* 1999. Severe deficit in memory for the configuration but not the identy of objects in patients with lesions to the right para-hippocampal cortex. Submitted.
38. ALLEN, J.J.B., Z.V. DIKMAN & L. NADEL. 1994. Scalp distribution of P3 in hippocampus-dependent and hippocampus-independent visual tasks: Support for multiple P3 generators. Psychophysiology **31:** S22.
39. MORRIS, R.G.M. 1981. Spatial localization does not require the presence of local cues. Learn. Motiv. **12:** 239–260.
40. MORRIS, R.G.M., P. GARRUD, J.N. RAWLINS & J. O'KEEFE. 1982. Place navigation impaired in rats with hippocampal lesions. Nature **297:** 681–683.
41. MILNER, B. 1965. Visually-guided maze learning in man: effects of bilateral hippocampal, bilateral frontal, and unilateral cerebral lesions. Neuropsychologia **3:** 317–338.
42. TALAIRACH, J. & P. TOURNOUX. 1988. Co-planar stereotaxic atlas of the human brain: 3-dimensional proportional system—an approach to cerebral imaging. Thieme Medical Publishers. New York.

Reciprocal Connections between the Amygdala and the Hippocampal Formation, Perirhinal Cortex, and Postrhinal Cortex in Rat

A Review

ASLA PITKÄNEN,[a,b,d] MARIA PIKKARAINEN,[a] NINA NURMINEN,[c] AND AARNE YLINEN[b,c]

[a]A.I. Virtanen Institute for Molecular Sciences, University of Kuopio, POBox 1627, FIN-70 211 Kuopio, Finland

[b]Department of Neurology, Kuopio University Hospital, POBox 1777, FIN-70 211 Kuopio, Finland

[c]Department of Neurosciences, University of Kuopio, POBox 1627, FIN-70 211 Kuopio, Finland

ABSTRACT: Recent anterograde and retrograde studies in the rat have provided detailed information on the origin and termination of the interconnections between the amygdaloid complex and the hippocampal formation and parahippocampal areas (including areas 35 and 36 of the perirhinal cortex and the postrhinal cortex). The most substantial inputs to the amygdala originate in the rostral half of the entorhinal cortex, the temporal end of the CA1 subfield and subiculum, and areas 35 and 36 of the perirhinal cortex. The amygdaloid nuclei receiving the heaviest inputs are the lateral, basal, accessory basal, and central nuclei as well as the amygdalohippocampal area. The heaviest projections from the amygdala to the hippocampal formation and the parahippocampal areas originate in the lateral, basal, accessory basal, and posterior cortical nuclei. These pathways terminate in the rostral half of the entorhinal cortex, the temporal end of the CA3 and CA1 subfields or the subiculum, the parasubiculum, areas 35 and 36 of the perirhinal cortex, and the postrhinal cortex. The connectional data are summarized and the underlying principles of organization of these projections are discussed.

INTRODUCTION[e]

The amygdala is a multinuclear complex located at the medial edge of the temporal lobe. The various amygdaloid nuclei differ cytoarchitectonically, chemoarchitectonically, and connectionally.[48] Consistent with anatomic data, major outputs to functional systems generating motor, mnemonic, attentional, autonomic, or endo-

[d]Address for correspondence: Dr. Asla Pitkänen, A.I. Virtanen Institute for Molecular Sciences, University of Kuopio, P.O. Box 1627, FIN-70 211 Kuopio, Finland. Tel.: *-358-17-16 3296; fax: *-358-17-16 3025.

e-mail: asla.pitkanen@uku.fi.

[e]A list of abbreviations can be found after the Acknowledgments.

crine responses to emotionally significant stimuli originate largely in different nuclei.[5,17,19,33,47,48]

Interest in the amygdala in both normal and pathologic brains recently increased due largely to new imaging data on humans. These studies demonstrate the role of the amygdala in determining the emotional significance of visual, auditory, and olfactory signals,[1,7,52,62] which is needed for successful coping in the everyday social environment.[2,39] Another major function of the amygdala is the enhancement of memory formation for emotionally arousing events (see Refs. 11 and 21), which becomes compromised in brain diseases with amygdaloid damage, such as Alzheimer's disease.[38] Ikegaya et al.[22–24] demonstrated that electrical stimulation of the amygdala in rats enhances the formation of long-term potentiation (LTP) in the dentate gyrus, whereas amygdaloid lesions impair LTP, which suggests a role for amygdalohippocampal interconnections in memory modulation. Temporal lobe epilepsy is another condition in which the amygdalohippocampal interconnections have a critical role; these pathways provide routes for epileptogenesis and the spread of seizure activity.[20]

Extensive data indicate that the amygdaloid complex is reciprocally connected with the hippocampus and the surrounding cortex. Until recently, however, many details of these connections were better understood in primates than in rodents (for reviews, see Refs. 5 and 48). Small tracer injections into nuclei or nuclear divisions of the amygdaloid complex or different parts of the hippocampus and surrounding cortex have provided new data regarding the organization of these interconnections in the rat, which will be briefly reviewed.

NOMENCLATURE

Amygdala. The amygdaloid complex is partitioned into various nuclei and cortical areas based on the nomenclature described by Price et al.[48] with modifications.[26,45] Briefly, the *deep nuclei* include the lateral nucleus, basal nucleus, and accessory basal nucleus. The *superficial nuclei* include the anterior cortical nucleus, bed nucleus of the accessory olfactory tract, medial nucleus, nucleus of the lateral olfactory tract, periamygdaloid cortex, and posterior cortical nucleus. The *remaining nuclei* include the anterior amygdaloid area, central nucleus, amygdalohippocampal area, and the intercalated nuclei. The location of the different amygdaloid regions is shown in FIGURE 1.

Hippocampal formation. The hippocampal formation includes the entorhinal cortex, dentate gyrus, hippocampus, subiculum, presubiculum, and parasubiculum.[4] The entorhinal cortex was divided into six subfields according to the nomenclature of Insausti et al.[25]: caudal entorhinal subfield (CE), medial entorhinal subfield (ME), ventral intermediate entorhinal subfield (VIE), amygdaloentorhinal transitional subfield (AE), dorsal intermediate entorhinal subfield (DIE), and dorsal lateral entorhinal subfield (DLE). The other regions of the hippocampal formation were defined according to Amaral and Witter.[4] Schematic presentation of various components of the hippocampal formation is shown in FIGURES 2 through 6.

Perirhinal and postrhinal cortex. The cortex located around the rhinal sulcus is partitioned into the perirhinal and postrhinal cortices according to guidelines of Burwell and colleagues[9,10] (FIG. 6). According to this nomenclature, the perirhinal cor-

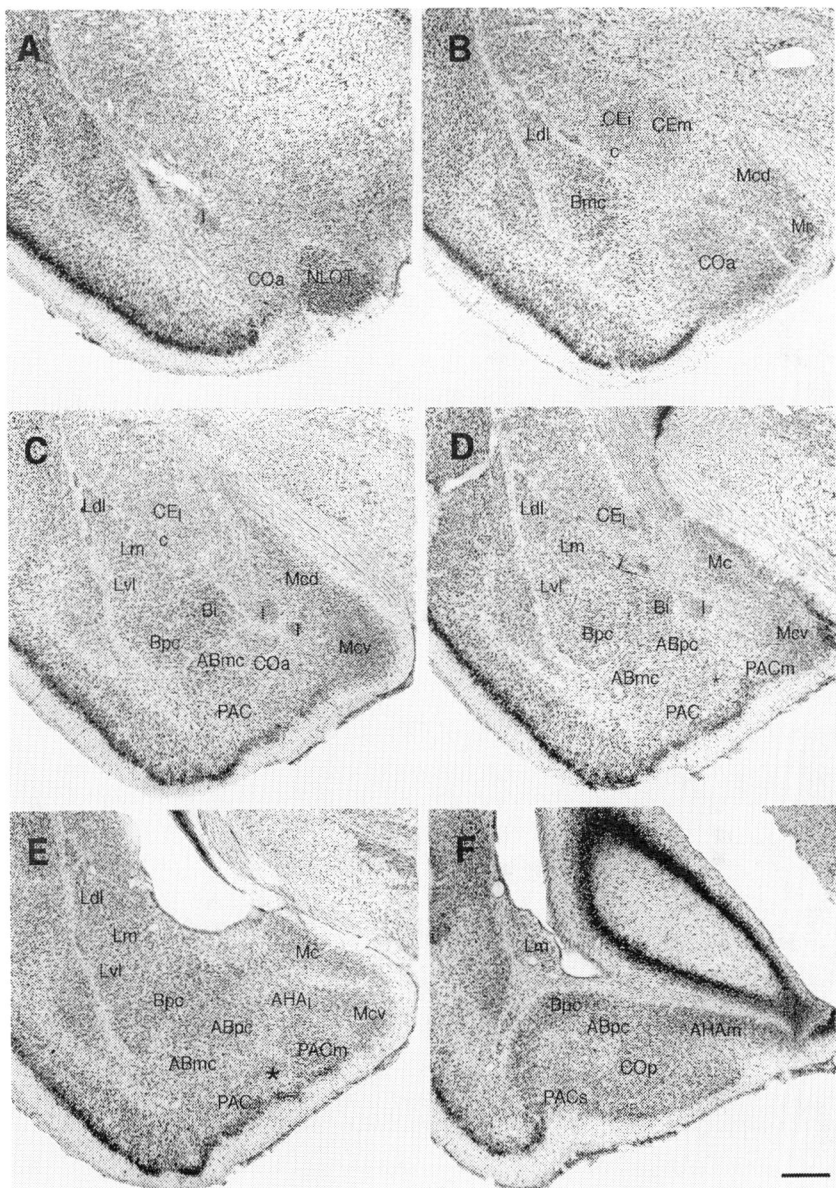

FIGURE 1. Brightfield photomicrographs from thionin-stained coronal sections of the rat amygdaloid complex showing the location of various amygdaloid nuclei and nuclear divisions. Six rostrocaudal levels are presented (panel **A** is the most rostral and panel **F** the most caudal). *Asterisks* in panels **D** and **E** indicate the location of the small-celled group of neurons described by Canteras *et al.*[13] as a portion of the stria terminalis. Scale bar equals 0.5 mm.

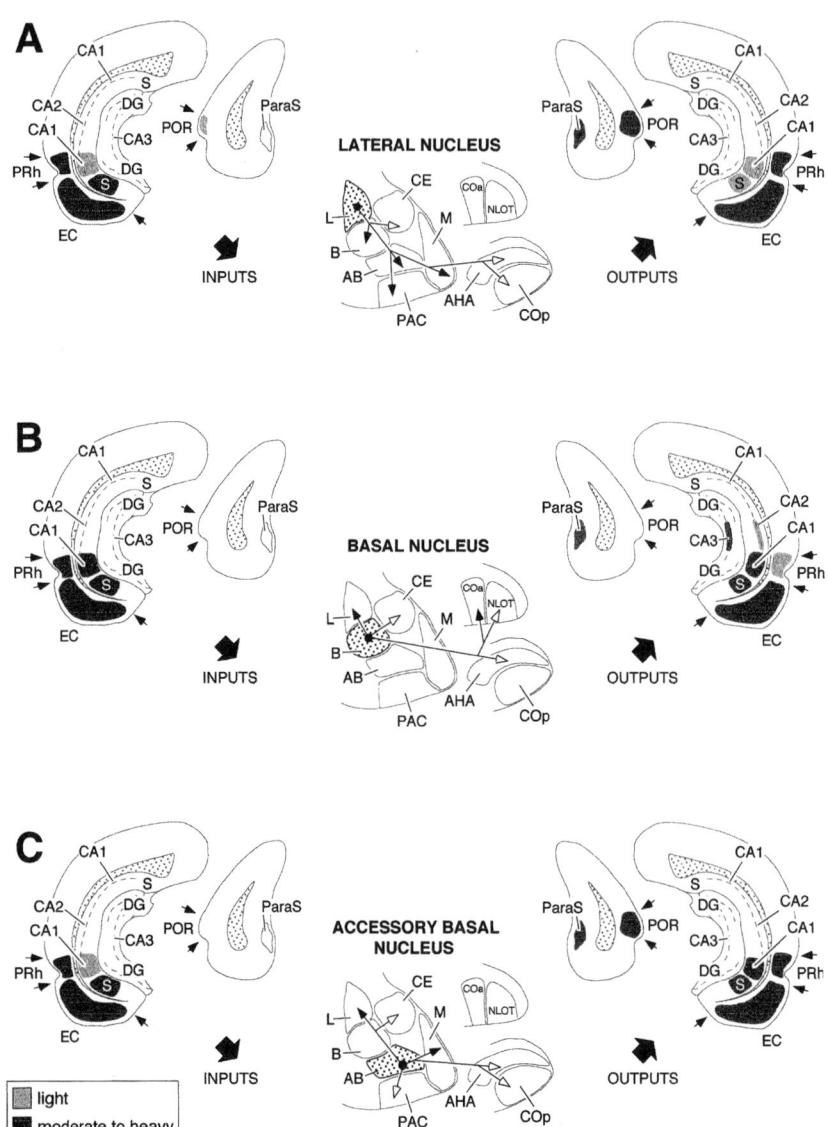

FIGURE 2. Schematic illustrations summarizing the afferent and efferent connections of the amygdaloid complex with the hippocampal formation and the perirhinal and postrhinal cortices. See text for details of topography. (**A**) Interconnections with the lateral nucleus; (**B**) interconnections with the basal nucleus; and (**C**) interconnections with the accessory basal nucleus. The inputs and outputs are labeled with *gray shading*. Darkness of shading (light or moderate to heavy) is based on the description of projections in the original articles (see text for references). *Arrows* within the amygdaloid complex indicate the intra-amygda-

tex begins at the caudal limit of the claustrum (−2.50 caudal to bregma, according to the atlas of Paxinos and Watson[41]). It can be divided into areas 35 and 36. Area 35 primarily occupies the ventral bank and the fundus of the rhinal sulcus. Area 36 is located dorsal to area 35 and includes much of the dorsal bank of the rhinal sulcus as well as a portion of the dorsally adjacent cortex. The postrhinal cortex is located caudal to the perirhinal cortex and begins approximately −7.80 mm caudal to bregma.[9] Recent connectional studies by McDonald[37] and Shi and Cassell[54] provide a somewhat different view of the anatomic boundaries of the perirhinal cortex, particularly rostrally and dorsally. These observations are taken into account in the present analysis, and therefore, the data presented includes cortical projections that originate or terminate −3.5 mm or more caudally relative to bregma. Schematic presentation of the location of area 35, area 36, and the postrhinal cortex is shown in FIGURE 6.

CONNECTIONS BETWEEN THE AMYGDALA AND THE HIPPOCAMPAL FORMATION

Entorhinal Cortex

Projections from the amygdala to the entorhinal cortex. Anterograde[13,14,28,30–32,34,42,44] and retrograde[6] tracer studies demonstrate substantial topographically organized projections from the amygdaloid complex to various subfields of the entorhinal cortex (FIGS. 2–6). The heaviest projections originate in the lateral, basal, accessory basal, medial, and posterior cortical nuclei and terminate in layers 3 or 5 of the entorhinal cortex (FIG. 6).

The medial division of the *lateral nucleus* sends moderate to heavy projections to layers 3 and 5 of the VIE and layer 3 of the DIE subfields. The parvicellular division of the *basal nucleus* provides projections to layers 3 through 6 of the AE and layers 3 and 5 of the VIE and DIE subfields. Also, upper layer 3 of the ME subfield receives a moderate projection. In addition, the magnocellular division of the basal nucleus gives origin to moderate projections to layer 3 of the AE and DLE subfields. The magnocellular division of the *accessory basal nucleus* sends a moderate projection to layer 3 of the DIE subfield, whereas the parvicellular division moderately innervates layer 5 of the VIE subfield.[44] The dorsal part of the central division of the *medial nucleus* projects moderately to the part of the entorhinal cortex that corresponds to the AE and DIE subfields. Most of the labeled terminals in the AE appear in layers 1 through 3 and in the DIE in layers 3 through 6 (see FIG. 4 in Canteras *et al.*[14]). The ventral part of the central division of the medial nucleus projects to the AE (layers 1–3) and VIE (layers 3–6) subfields (see FIG. 5 in Canteras *et al.*[14]). The *posterior cortical nucleus* gives origin to a moderate projection to layers 2 through 5 of the DIE and layer 2 of the VIE subfields (see FIG. 8 in Canteras *et al.*;[13] Kemppainen

---

loid connections of the nucleus. A *closed arrowhead* refers to a reciprocal connection and an *open arrowhead* refers to a unidirectional connection. Only the known moderate-to-heavy intra-amygdaloid projections are indicated (for review see Ref. 47). Abbreviations: AB, accessory basal nucleus; AHA, amygdalohippocampal area; B, basal nucleus; CE, central nucleus; EC, entorhinal cortex; L, lateral nucleus; M, medial nucleus. Other abbreviations are listed in the list of abbreviations.

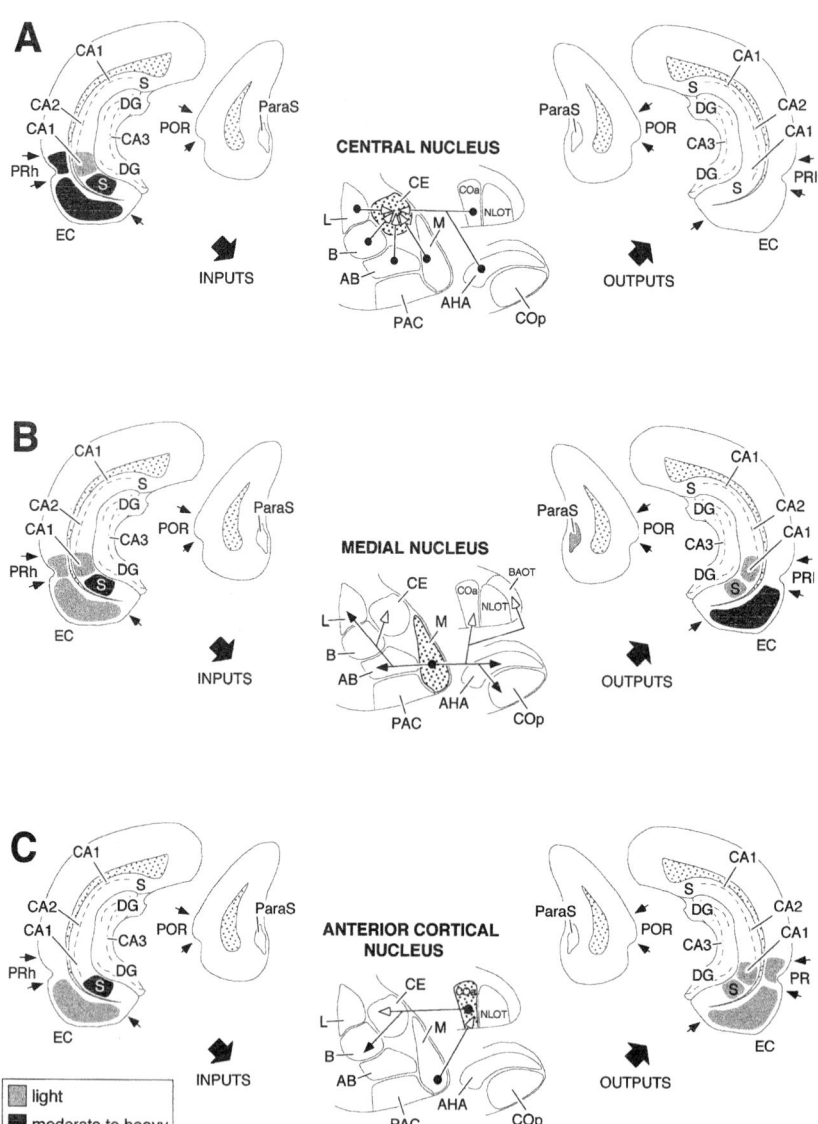

FIGURE 3. See legend to FIGURE 2. (**A**) Interconnections with the central nucleus; (**B**) interconnections with the medial nucleus; and (**C**) interconnections with the anterior cortical nucleus.

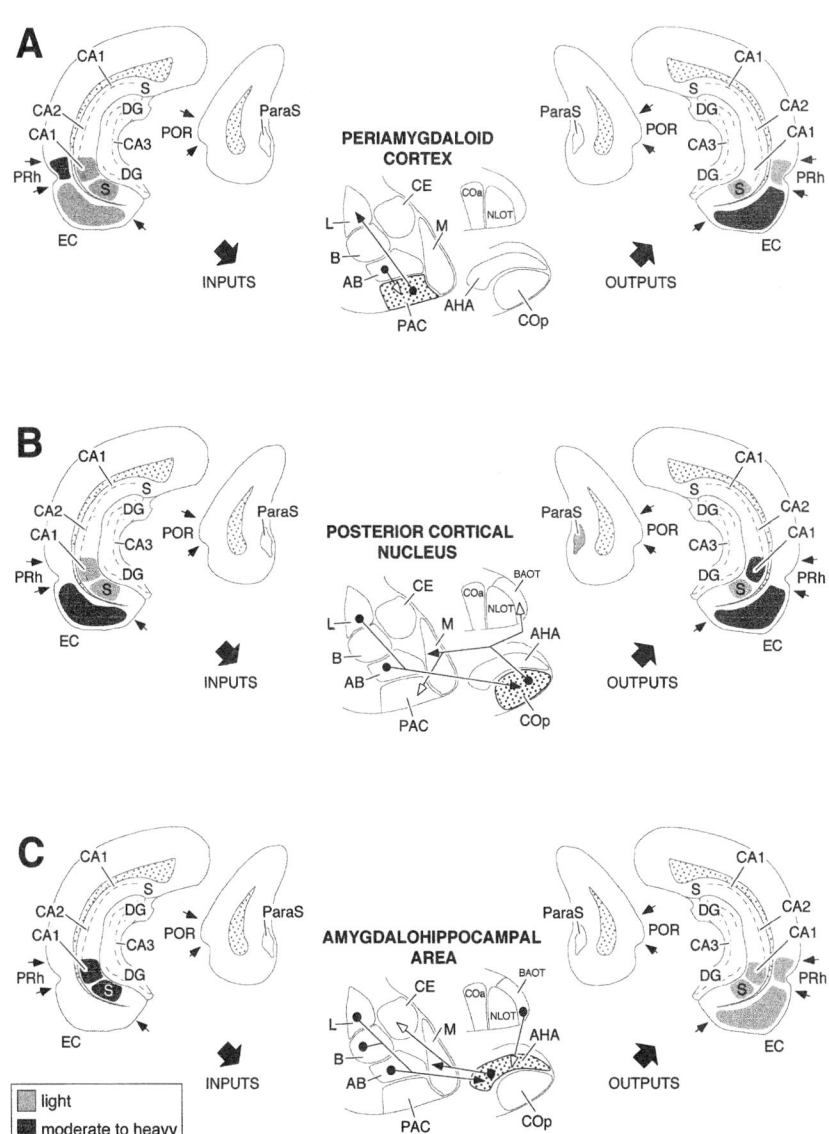

FIGURE 4. See legend to FIGURE 2. (**A**) Interconnections with the periamygdaloid cortex; (**B**) interconnections with the posterior cortical nucleus; and (**C**) interconnections with the amygdalohippocampal area.

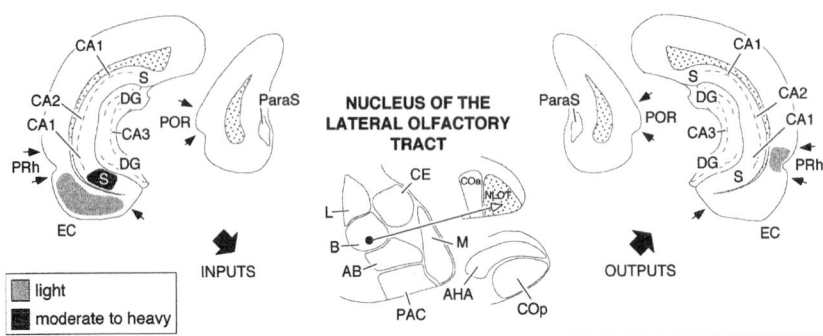

FIGURE 5. See legend to FIGURE 2. Interconnections with the nucleus of the lateral olfactory tract.

and Pitkänen[28]). Injection of radioactive amino acids into the *periamygdaloid cortex* results in anterograde labeling in the entorhinal cortex that corresponds roughly to the VIE and DIE subfields (see FIG. 19 in Krettek and Price[32]).

Lighter projections from the amygdala to the entorhinal cortex are observed from the lateral division of the amygdalohippocampal area (called the deep portion of the lateral zone of the posterior part of the cortical nucleus in FIG. 7 by Canteras *et al.*[13]) and the anterior cortical nucleus.[6,32,34,42] These projections appear to terminate in the AE and DIE subfields.

Projections from the entorhinal cortex to the amygdala. Both anterograde[34,36,55,61] and retrograde[15,40,54,59] studies indicate that various subfields of the entorhinal cortex project to selective amygdaloid nuclei or nuclear subdivisions (FIGS. 2–5).

Anterograde tracer injections located in the *DIE/DLE subfields* label projections that terminate most heavily in the lateral aspects of the magnocellular and parvicellular divisions of the basal nucleus. Moderate projections are observed in the medial and ventrolateral divisions of the lateral nucleus, parvicellular division of the accessory basal nucleus, capsular division of the central nucleus, anterior cortical nucleus, layer 1 of the nucleus of the lateral olfactory tract, and the posterior cortical nucleus.[36] Injections located in the *VIE subfield* result in moderate-to-heavy labeling in the medial division of the lateral nucleus, medial aspect of the parvicellular division of the basal nucleus, parvicellular division of the accessory basal nucleus, capsular division of the central nucleus, and the posterior cortical nucleus.[36] Injections of PHA-L into the cortex corresponding to the *AE subfield* result in robust labeling in the capsular and lateral divisions of the central nucleus, the parvicellular division of the basal nucleus, and layers 1 and 2 of the nucleus of the lateral olfactory tract.[27,36]

Consistent with anterograde tracer studies, injections of retrograde tracers into the lateral nucleus result in retrograde labeling of cells in the VIE and DIE subfields, and injections into the basal nucleus result in labeling in the DLE, DIE, and VIE subfields of the entorhinal cortex.[54] Most of the retrogradely labeled neurons are located in layers 5 and 6.[54]

To summarize, most of the amygdala-entorhinal interconnections occur between the lateral, basal, and accessory basal nuclei of the amygdaloid complex and the AE,

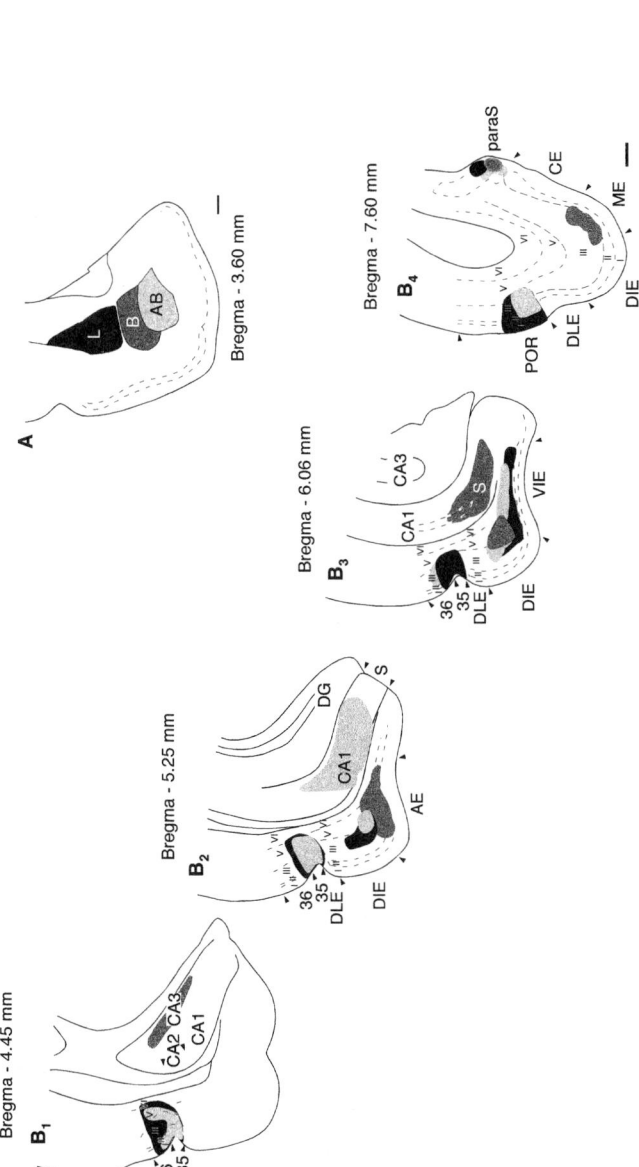

FIGURE 6. Schematic drawing summarizing the projections from the lateral, basal, and accessory basal nuclei of the amygdala to the hippocampal formation and the perirhinal and postrhinal cortices. Only the moderate-to-heavy projections are illustrated. Note the topographic and largely nonoverlapping organization of projections originating in the different amygdaloid nuclei. (Data were taken from Refs. 44 and 51; Pikkarainen and Pitkänen, unpublished data.)

DLE, DIE, and VIE subfields of the entorhinal cortex. Many of these connections appear reciprocal. Perhaps the clearest exception is the central nucleus, which receives inputs from the entorhinal cortex but does not project back to the entorhinal cortex.

Dentate Gyrus

According to the available data, there are no monosynaptic interconnections between the amygdaloid complex and the dentate gyrus.

CA3 Subfield

Projections from the amygdala to the CA3 subfield. The caudomedial parvicellular division of the basal nucleus provides a substantial projection to the *stratum oriens* and *stratum radiatum* of the temporal end of the CA3 subfield[44] (FIGS. 2–5).

Projections from the CA3 subfield to the amygdala. There are no data showing that the CA3 subfield projects to the amygdaloid complex.

CA2 Subfield

Projections from the amygdala to the CA2 subfield. The magnocellular division of the basal nucleus projects lightly to the *stratum oriens* and *stratum radiatum* of the CA2 subfield[44] (FIGS. 2–5).

Projections from the CA2 subfield to the amygdala. There are no data indicating that the CA2 subfield projects to the amygdaloid complex.

CA1 Subfield

Projections from the amygdala to the CA1 subfield. Anterograde tracer studies[13,14,28,42,44] indicate that the basal, accessory basal, and posterior cortical nuclei are the major sources of projections from the amygdala to the CA1 subfield (FIGS. 2–5).

The caudomedial portion of the parvicellular division of the *basal nucleus* projects moderately throughout the temporal half of the CA1 subfield. Most of the labeled terminals are located in the *stratum oriens* and *stratum radiatum*. In distal CA1 (the portion of CA1 that is located closer to the subiculum), the pyramidal cell layer also contains varicose fibers that are closely apposed to pyramidal cell somata. Projections from the lateral portion of the parvicellular division are substantially lighter. Unlike the other amygdaloid areas, the magnocellular division of the basal nucleus gives origin to a light projection that terminates in the *stratum oriens* and *stratum pyramidale* of the most septal end of the CA1/subiculum border.[44] The magnocellular division of the *accessory basal nucleus* also sends a moderate projection to the CA1 subfield, which extends throughout its temporal two thirds. Most of the labeled terminals are located in the *stratum lacunosum moleculare*. At the most temporal and distal portion of the CA1 subfield, labeled terminals are also observed in the pyramidal cell layer. The moderate projection from the parvicellular division of the accessory basal nucleus to the CA1 subfield extends only to the temporal one third of the *stratum lacunosum moleculare* of CA1 and to the most temporal region of the CA1/subiculum border.[42,44] The *posterior cortical nucleus* also provides a heavy projection to the temporal end of CA1. Labeled terminals are located primarily in the *stratum lacunosum moleculare* and *stratum radiatum*.[13,28]

Lighter projections originate in the ventrolateral and medial divisions of the lateral nucleus,[44] the central and caudal divisions of the medial nucleus,[14] the anterior cortical nucleus (area called the anterior basomedial nucleus[42]), and the medial division of the amygdalohippocampal area.[13]

Projections from the CA1 subfield to the amygdala. According to anterograde[37,43,58] and retrograde[13,15,40] tracer studies, only the temporal end of the CA1 subfield projects to the amygdala (FIGS. 2–5).

Projections that are moderate to heavy in density terminate in the region of the basal nucleus that appears to correspond to the medial aspect of the parvicellular division and/or intermediate division of the basal nucleus (see FIG. 34 in McDonald[37]). The lateral and medial divisions of the amygdalohippocampal area also receive a projection.[13,15,37] Lighter projections terminate in the lateral,[40,43,58] accessory basal,[37,43] central,[40] medial,[15] and posterior cortical[40] nuclei as well as in the periamygdaloid cortex.[15,40]

To summarize, the dentate gyrus does not have interconnections with the amygdala. The CA3 and CA2 subfields of the hippocampus proper receive light-to-moderate projections from the basal nucleus but do not project back to the amygdala. The temporal end of the CA1 subfield is the only hippocampal region that has substantial reciprocal connections with the amygdala. Within the amygdaloid complex, the basal nucleus has the most extensive interconnections with the hippocampus. Overall, it appears that the amygdaloid complex provides more projections to the hippocampus than *vice versa*.

Subiculum

Projections from the amygdala to the subiculum. As the anterograde[13,14,30,32,42,44] studies reveal, the subiculum receives substantial projections from the basal and accessory basal nuclei of the amygdala (FIGS. 2–5).

Projections from the caudomedial portion of the parvicellular division of the *basal nucleus* terminate most heavily in the temporal half of the subiculum, where PHA-L-labeled terminals are distributed throughout the entire transverse axis of the subiculum. These terminals are mostly located in the superficial portion of the cellular layer. The projection from the lateral portion of the parvicellular division, as well as from the magnocellular and intermediate divisions of the basal nucleus, is lighter and is directed primarily to the proximal portion (i.e., closer to the CA1 subfield) of the subiculum.[44] The magnocellular division of the *accessory basal nucleus* projects more heavily to the proximal portion of the subiculum, whereas the parvicellular division projects throughout the mediolateral extent of the subiculum with the projection slightly heavier distally (i.e., closer to the presubiculum). The projection is mostly directed to the deep portion of the molecular layer, although varicose terminals are also observed in the superficial portion of the pyramidal cell layer. All projections from the accessory basal nucleus terminate in the temporal one third of the subiculum.[44]

Lighter projections from the amygdala to the temporal end of the subiculum also originate in the medial and ventrolateral divisions of the lateral nucleus,[44] the central and caudal divisions of the medial nucleus,[14] the anterior cortical nucleus,[42] the posterior cortical nucleus,[13] the amygdalohippocampal area,[13] and the periamygdaloid cortex.[30,32]

Projections from the subiculum to the amygdala. As the anterograde[12,16,37,43] and retrograde[40,59] studies reveal, the temporal end of the subiculum provides substantial projections to a large number of amygdaloid nuclei (FIGS. 2–5). The proximal and distal portions of the subiculum have somewhat different target areas in the amygdaloid complex.

The proximal part of the temporal subiculum projects to the medial division of the lateral nucleus, parvicellular division of the basal nucleus, accessory basal nucleus, medial division of the central nucleus, layers 2 and 3 of the anterior cortical nucleus, medial division of the amygdalohippocampal area, the nucleus of the lateral olfactory tract, and the posterior cortical nucleus.[16,37] Most of these projections are moderate to heavy in density (see FIG. 33 in McDonald[37]).

The major targets for projections originating in the distal part of the temporal subiculum include the magnocellular and parvicellular divisions of the accessory basal nucleus, caudal part of the parvicellular division of the basal nucleus, medial division of the amygdalohippocampal area, and the posterior cortical nucleus. Lighter projections also terminate in the capsular and lateral divisions of the central nucleus, central division of the medial nucleus (both dorsal and ventral parts), periamygdaloid cortex, nucleus of the lateral olfactory tract, and intercalated nuclei.[12]

To summarize, the temporal end of the subiculum gives origin to substantial projections to a large number of amygdaloid nuclei (e.g., compared to the CA1 subfield). The basal and accessory basal amygdaloid nuclei provide moderate-to-heavy projections back to the subiculum.

Presubiculum

To date, there have not been any reports of monosynaptic connections between the amygdaloid complex and the presubiculum.

Parasubiculum

Projections from the amygdala to the parasubiculum. Studies with anterograde tracers[13,14,32,42,44,57] indicate that the parasubiculum receives substantial projections from the lateral, basal, and accessory basal nuclei of the amygdala (FIGS. 2–6).

Within the *lateral nucleus*, the heaviest projections originate in the caudal portion of the medial division. The highest density of labeled terminals is found in layer 1 and in the superficial portion of layers 2 and 3 in the ventral aspect of the parasubiculum, which abuts the caudal entorhinal subfield of the entorhinal cortex.[44] All divisions of the *basal nucleus* originate a light-to-heavy projection to the parasubiculum. The projection is heaviest from the caudomedial portion of the parvicellular division. Most of the labeled fibers are observed in the deep portion of layer 1 and superficially in layers 2 and 3 of the ventral aspect of the parasubiculum.[44] Both the magnocellular and parvicellular divisions of the *accessory basal nucleus* provide a light-to-moderate projection to the parasubiculum. The magnocellular division projects primarily to the larger dorsally located portion of the parasubiculum, whereas most of the terminals originating in the parvicellular division terminate in layer 1 and superficial layers 2 and 3 of the ventral aspect of the parasubiculum.[42,44] Also, the dorsal and ventral parts of the central division of the medial nucleus[14] and the posterior cortical nucleus[13] project lightly to the parasubiculum.

Projections from the parasubiculum to the amygdala. There are no data available demonstrating monosynaptic projections from the parasubiculum to the amygdaloid complex (Dr. T. van Groen, personal communication).

To summarize, interconnections between the amygdala and the parasubiculum are unidirectional, that is, from the amygdala to the parasubiculum.

CONNECTIONS BETWEEN THE AMYGDALA AND THE PERIRHINAL CORTEX

Projections from the amygdala to the perirhinal cortex. Both anterograde[31,32,34, 37,42,49,50,51,54] and retrograde[18,35] studies reveal that the amygdala gives origin to heavy topographically organized projections to the perirhinal cortex (FIGS. 2–6).

Area 35: The heaviest projections from the amygdala to the perirhinal cortex originate in the lateral and accessory basal nuclei and terminate in area 35. The medial division of the lateral nucleus heavily innervates layers 1 through 5, and the dorsolateral division heavily innervates layers 1 through 3 of area 35. The parvicellular division of the accessory basal nucleus projects moderately to layers 2–3 and heavily to layer 5.

Area 36: Overall, projections from the lateral, basal, and accessory basal nuclei to area 36 are light compared to projections to area 35. According to recent observations, however, the dorsolateral division of the lateral nucleus and the magnocellular division of the accessory basal nuclei provide dense projections to layer 1 of area 36 (Pikkarainen and Pitkänen, unpublished data).

Studies with retrograde and anterograde tracers also reveal light projections to the perirhinal cortex from the basal nucleus,[31,32,35,49,51], anterior cortical nucleus,[31,35,42,49] periamygdaloid cortex,[18,34,35] amygdalohippocampal area,[35] and nucleus of the lateral olfactory tract.[18,35]

Projections from the perirhinal cortex to the amygdala. Both anterograde[37,50,54] and retrograde[40,54] studies demonstrate that the perirhinal cortex provides substantial projections to the amygdala (FIGS. 2–5).

Area 35: The ventral bank and the fundus of the perirhinal cortex (corresponding to area 35) project to the amygdala. Projections terminate most heavily in the basal nucleus, particularly in the magnocellular division.[37,54] This projection originates in layer 2 and also in the deep layers.[54] Injections of anterograde tracers into area 35 involving the fundus also result in labeling in the lateral and accessory basal nuclei.

Area 36: Recent anterograde tracer studies with biocytin,[54] biotinylated dextran amine,[54] and PHA-L[37] reveal that the dorsal bank of the perirhinal cortex corresponding to area 36 projects heavily to the lateral nucleus (see also FIG. 11 in Burwell and Amaral[10]). The projection is heaviest in the caudal two thirds of the nucleus and terminates in all three divisions of the lateral nucleus. Retrograde tracer studies demonstrate that the projection to the lateral nucleus originates in all cellular layers 2 through 6.[40,54] Moderate projections terminate in the accessory basal nucleus and layer 3 of the periamygdaloid cortex. Light projections are observed in the magnocellular division of the basal nucleus and a few fibers in the dorsal part of the central division of the medial nucleus and in the capsular division of the central nucleus.[37,54] It is still under dispute, however, whether the perirhinal cortex provides any inputs to the central nucleus. This partly relates to the definition of the cytoarchitectonic borders of the central nucleus. According to Shi and Cassell, the perirhinal cortex does not project to the central nucleus. McDonald,[37] however, reports a moderate projection from area 36 ("dorsal portion of the perirhinal cortex") to the capsular division of the central nucleus. A lighter projection originates from the "ventral portion of the perirhinal cortex" (area 35). In his camera lucida drawings, labeled terminals extend down to the ventral aspects of the capsular division, which also appears to be innervated in the illustrations of Shi and Cassell.[54] See FIGURES 29A and 30A in McDonald[37] and compare them with FIGURES 6A-B and 12A-B in Shi and Cassell.[54] This region has also been included into the capsular division in the recent chemoarchitectonic and connectional study by Jolkkonen and Pitkänen.[26]

To summarize, lateral and accessory basal nuclei provide the most substantial projections from the amygdala to the perirhinal cortex, which terminate most heavily in area 35. The heaviest projections from the perirhinal cortex to the amygdala terminate in the lateral nucleus.

CONNECTIONS BETWEEN THE AMYGDALA AND THE POSTRHINAL CORTEX

Projections from the amygdala to the postrhinal cortex. Most of the connectional studies have not specifically addressed the projections from the amygdala to the postrhinal cortex. Our recent data indicate that the medial division of the lateral nucleus projects to layers 1 through 3 and the dorsolateral division projects to layer 1 of the postrhinal cortex. Projections from the accessory basal nucleus terminate in a narrow strip of the postrhinal cortex adjacent to the border of the entorhinal cortex (Pikkarainen and Pitkänen, unpublished data; FIGS. 2–6).

Projections from the postrhinal cortex to the amygdala. Relatively few data are available on the projections from the postrhinal cortex to the amygdala (FIGS. 2–5). A classical work of Ottersen,[40] in which HRP injections were placed into the lateral nucleus, resulted in retrograde labeling in the superficial layers of the cortical area that corresponds to the postrhinal cortex (see FIG. 2 in Ottersen[40]). No labeled cells were observed, however, in cases where the HRP injection was located in the parvicellular division of the basal nucleus (see FIG. 5 in Ottersen[40]). Recently, Shi and Cassell[54] injected retrograde tracers into the lateral and basal nuclei. They demonstrate that the superficial layers of the cortical region corresponding to the postrhinal cortex (levels −7.6 and −8.0 in their FIGS. 18-19) project to the lateral nucleus. The density of retrogradely labeled cells was, however, substantially lower than that in the perirhinal cortex.

To summarize, the postrhinal cortex projects to the lateral nucleus. Amygdalopostrhinal projections originate in the lateral and accessory basal nuclei.

DISCUSSION

Projections from the Hippocampal and Parahippocampal Areas to the Amygdaloid Complex

Analysis of the connectional data suggests several principles in the organization of projections from the hippocampal/parahippocampal areas to the amygdaloid complex (FIG. 7). First, the major inputs to the amygdala originate in the deep layers of the rostral half of the entorhinal cortex, temporal end of the CA1 subfield and the subiculum, and areas 35 and 36 of the perirhinal cortex. Therefore, different regions of the hippocampal and parahippocampal areas project to the amygdaloid complex in parallel. Second, each one of these regions provides parallel inputs to several amygdaloid nuclei. For example, the subiculum provides substantial projections to the lateral, basal, accessory basal, central, medial, and anterior cortical nuclei as well as to the amygdalohippocampal area and the nucleus of the lateral olfactory tract. Whether the parallel inputs represent axon collaterals of the same neuron or whether they originate in different populations of subicular neurons remains to be studied. Finally, it is the distal end of the hippocampal trisynaptic circuitry in the temporal end of the hippocampus that projects to the amygdaloid complex. Also, the entorhinal subfields innervating the amygdala are those that are more heavily interconnected with the temporal rather than the septal hippocampus.

Amygdaloid Nuclei Receiving Inputs from the Hippocampal and Parahippocampal Areas

The major targets for inputs to the amygdala are the lateral, basal, accessory basal, and central nuclei, and the amygdalohippocampal area, all of which receive inputs from at least two levels of the hippocampal/parahippocampal system. As mentioned earlier, however, the innervation of the central nucleus by the entorhinal and perirhinal cortices is still somewhat controversial. The entorhinal and perirhinal inputs terminate largely in the capsular division of the central nucleus according to McDonald and Mascagni[36] and McDonald.[37] Terminals located in this region were considered to belong to the projection terminating in the amygdalostriatal area by Shi and Cassell,[54] who state that the perirhinal cortex does not project to the central nucleus. Otherwise, the rostral part of the entorhinal cortex, which is partly included into the AE subfield of the entorhinal cortex by Insausti *et al.*,[25] is often considered to be the amygdalopiriform transition area.[41,56] This area provides a robust projection to the lateral division of the central nucleus.[27,36] According to our recent observation, this area does not project to the dentate gyrus (Jolkkonen and Pitkänen, unpublished data), which is considered a hallmark for the connectivity of the entorhinal cortex, and therefore favors the idea that the heavy input to the lateral division of the central nucleus does not originate in the entorhinal cortex.

Projections terminating in the amygdala might (a) converge in the same amygdaloid nucleus or (b) remain segregated by innervating different amygdaloid nuclei. As an example of convergence, areas 35 and 36, the entorhinal cortex, and the subiculum all project to the medial division of the lateral nucleus. Whether all these areas innervate the same neurons or the same population of neurons is unclear. It is more difficult to find examples in which the projections from the two components of the

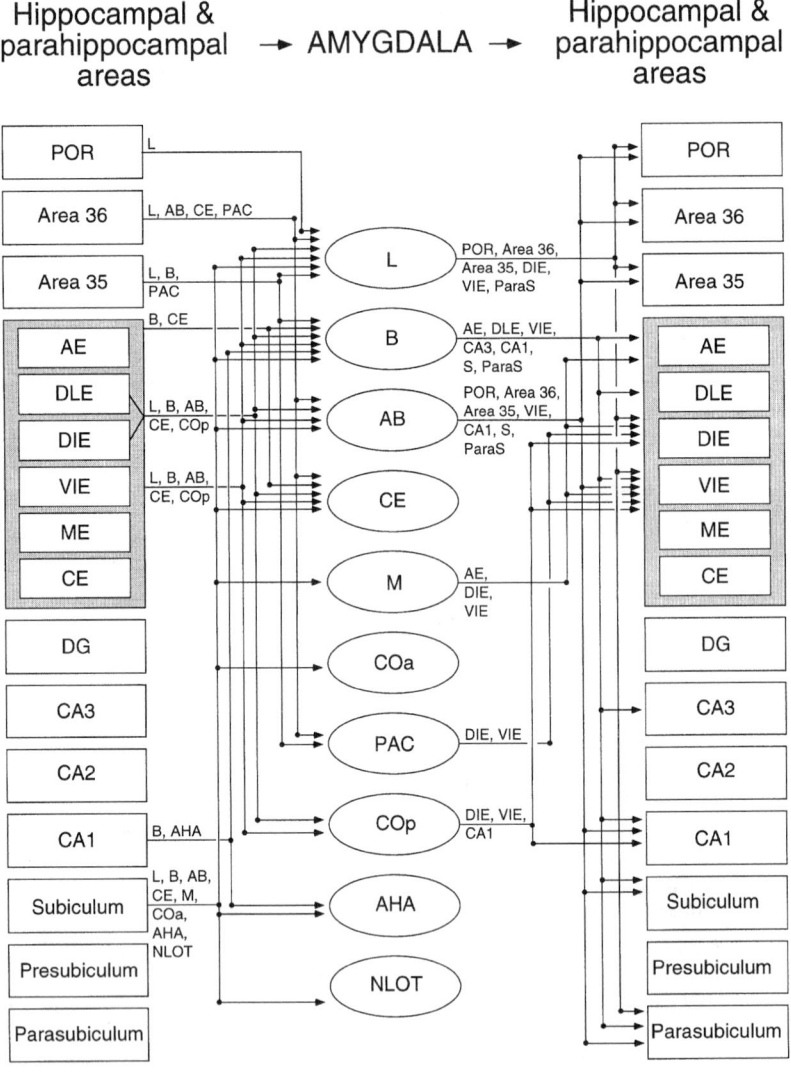

FIGURE 7. Summary of parallel inputs and outputs of the amygdaloid complex with the hippocampal formation and the perirhinal and postrhinal cortices. Only the projections that are moderate to heavy in density are included in the drawing. See text for references.

hippocampal/parahippocampal system remain segregated and terminate in non-overlapping amygdaloid regions. The projections from the postrhinal area terminate in the lateral nucleus, however, whereas the projection from the CA1 subfield innervates the basal nucleus and the amygdalohippocampal area. In these cases, dense intra-amygdaloid connections provide pathways for association of information within the amygdaloid circuitries.

Amygdaloid Projections to the Hippocampal and Parahippocampal Areas

The largest number of amygdaloid outputs originate in the lateral, basal, accessory basal, and posterior cortical nuclei, all of which innervate at least two components of the hippocampal/parahippocampal system. Therefore, the hippocampal and parahippocampal regions receive monosynaptic inputs from those amygdaloid nuclei that are interconnected with the sensory-related cortical and thalamic areas, the prefrontal cortex, olfactory system, and striatal motor system. Otherwise, amygdaloid nuclei that are most heavily interconnected with the autonomic and endocrine centers in the brainstem and hypothalamus (central and medial nuclei, respectively) do not provide substantial monosynaptic inputs to the hippocampal and parahippocampal areas (except the projection from the medial nucleus to the entorhinal cortex).

One amygdaloid nucleus or nuclear division might innervate different hippocampal and parahippocampal areas in parallel, that is, one nuclear division might influence the information processing at different levels of the hippocampal circuitries. Whether the parallel projections from one amygdaloid subnucleus represent axon collaterals of the same neuron or whether they originate in different neuronal populations remains unknown. We recently started to explore this question with single cell labeling studies. Preliminary data shown in FIGURE 8 demonstrate that the axonal tree of the neuron located in the lateral nucleus innervates both the entorhinal cortex and the postrhinal area, in addition to the other amygdaloid nuclei and the amygdalostriatal area (Nurminen, Ylinen, and Pitkänen, unpublished data).

The different amygdaloid nuclei provide parallel outputs to the hippocampus and surrounding cortex, which might (a) converge in the same subregion or (b) remain segregated. Even though the projections from the lateral, basal, and accessory basal nuclei all innervate the entorhinal cortex, however, projections originating in different amygdaloid nuclei terminate largely in the different entorhinal subfields or different layers of the same subfield. Therefore, these projections presumably innervate different target cells or different portions of the target cell within the entorhinal cortex. Similar point-to-point organization of innervation is found in the amygdaloid projections to the CA1 subfield and the subiculum (see Pikkarainen et al.[44] for details). Perhaps the best examples of regional segregation in the amygdalohippocampal projections are the projections to the CA2 and CA3 subfields, which appear to originate exclusively in the basal nucleus of the amygdala.

Hippocampal and Parahippocampal Areas Receiving Inputs from the Amygdaloid Complex

Regions receiving inputs from at least two amygdaloid nuclei include the rostral aspects of the entorhinal cortex, temporal aspects of the CA1 subfield and subiculum, and the parasubiculum as well as the perirhinal and postrhinal cortices.

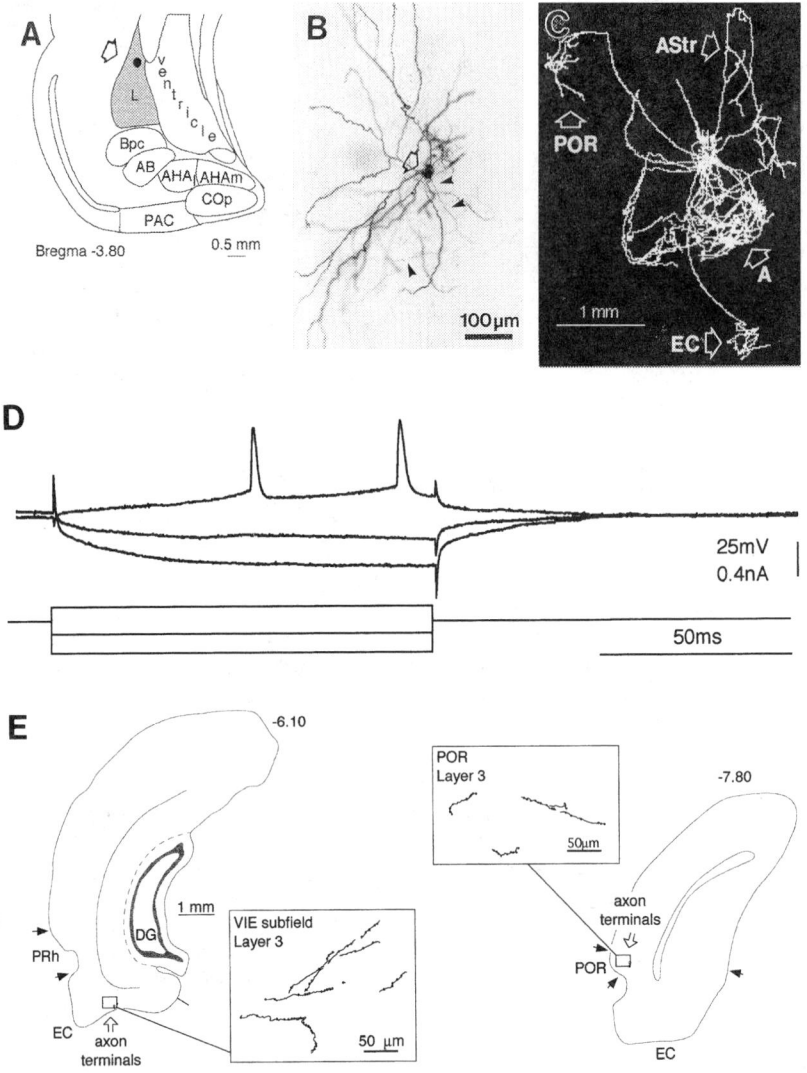

FIGURE 8. One neuron might innervate several regions in the hippocampal formation and parahippocampal areas. As an example we show the axonal tree of a densely spiny pyramidal neuron that was characterized electrophysiologically and, thereafter, filled intracellularly with biocytin in a urethane-anesthetized rat. The soma is located caudally in the lateral nucleus. The entire axonal tree was reconstructed three-dimensionally using Neurolucida software (Microbrightfield, Colchester, VT). **(A)** Schematic drawing showing the location of the filled neuron (a dot pointed by an *open arrow*) in the lateral nucleus. **(B)** A brightfield photomicrograph of the filled neuron (*open arrow*) and dendritic tree. The axon is indicated with *small arrowheads*. **(C)** Coronal wireframe of the reconstructed axonal tree of the filled neuron. The densest clusters of axon terminals are located within the amygdala (A), amygdalostriatal

Typically, each of these regions receives inputs from at least two amygdaloid nuclei except the CA3 subfield, which is innervated by only the basal nucleus. Amygdaloid projections to the hippocampal/parahippocampal areas innervate most heavily (a) the distal aspect of the trisynaptic hippocampal circuitry, (b) the temporal half of the septotemporal axis of the hippocampus, and (c) regions of the entorhinal cortex that project to the mid- and temporal third of the hippocampus. Projections to area 35 and the postrhinal cortex might provide a route *via* which the amygdala modulates the ongoing activity in the septal end of the hippocampus. In particular, the magnocellular division of the basal nucleus projects to the septal CA1/subiculum border as well as to the DLE subfield of the entorhinal cortex, which is interconnected with the septal hippocampus.[44] Therefore, the magnocellular division of the basal nucleus might also serve as a link between the amygdala and the septal hippocampus, even though these projections are very light compared to those directed to the temporal end.

To summarize, the major aspect in the topography of the amygdala-hippocampal/parahippocampal interconnections is that the projections are heaviest between the amygdala and the temporal end of the hippocampus. The lateral nucleus is heavily interconnected with cortical areas and the parasubiculum, whereas the basal nucleus is also interconnected with the hippocampus proper. Many of the connections between the amygdala and the hippocampal and parahippocampal areas are reciprocal. Perhaps the most conspicuous exception is the central nucleus, which receives substantial projections but does not project back to the hippocampal and parahippocampal areas. Another exception is the parasubiculum, which receives heavy projections from the amygdaloid complex but does not project back to the amygdala.

Functional Considerations

All areas of the hippocampal/parahippocampal system that project to the amygdala innervate the lateral nucleus, except for the CA1 subfield, which innervates the basal nucleus and the amygdalohippocampal area. Because the lateral nucleus provides the most extensive intra-amygdaloid projections,[45] the information coming from the medial temporal lobe memory system will have multiple representations in various amygdaloid locations either monosynaptically or by intra-amygdaloid pathways. Via these projections, mnemonic information might become associated with other kinds of information processed in various amygdaloid nuclei (e.g., projections from the prefrontal cortex to the lateral, basal, medial, and central nuclei; from the hypothalamic endocrine centers to the medial and central nuclei; and from the striatal motor system to the basal nucleus). Or, multiple representations of mnemonic information in various amygdaloid locations might "fine tune," in parallel, the different components of the behavioral response that the amygdala generates

---

area (AStr), the entorhinal cortex (EC), and the postrhinal area (POR). (**D**) Response of the neuron to depolarizing and hyperpolarizing current steps. The resting membrane potential was approximately −60 mV and the cell fired spontaneously at a rate of 6–7 Hz. (**E**) Camera lucida drawing of labeled varicose terminals in layer 3 of the VIE subfield of the entorhinal cortex. (**F**) Camera lucida drawing of labeled varicose terminals in layer 3 of the postrhinal cortex. In panels **E** and **F** the terminals were drawn from one 100-μm section.

in response to emotionally significant stimuli via its multiple output connections originating in different amygdaloid nuclei.

The central nucleus is often considered an output station of the amygdala, because it converges inputs from most of the other amygdaloid nuclei but has only meager projections back to the other amygdaloid nuclei.[27,45] The projections of the central nucleus terminate in the midbrain, pons, and medulla as well as in the bed nucleus of the stria terminalis, hypothalamus, and the cholinergic and aminergic systems of the brain (for review see Ref. 47). Therefore, the perirhinal and entorhinal projections to the capsular division of the central nucleus as well as the subicular projections to the medial division might provide pathways by which the mnemonic experiences modulate autonomic, endocrine, and attentive responses even at the latest steps of the intra-amygdaloid information processing. The central nucleus, however, does not provide any projections back to the hippocampal/parahippocampal system.

The interconnections between the amygdaloid complex and the hippocampal and parahippocampal regions are highly topographically organized. This finding suggests that a "knock-out" of amygdaloid regions by a disease process, such as the medial division of the lateral nucleus and the parvicellular division of the basal nucleus in temporal lobe epilepsy,[46] the central nucleus and periamygdaloid cortex in Parkinson's disease,[8] the lateral, basal, and accessory basal nuclei in depression,[53] or the basal and accessory basal nuclei in Alzheimer's disease,[60] might compromise the information flow in a specific set of amygdala-hippocampal/parahippocampal networks and consequently impair the functions that they mediate. Supporting this idea are some experimental data already available in both rat[29] and monkey.[3] The large amount of parallel information flow between the amygdaloid complex and hippocampal and parahippocampal regions might, however, compensate for a defect caused by a circumscribed lesion. One of the critical questions to be explored is, how much damage is needed and where, to induce functional impairments associated with these circuitries, such as the modulation of memory formation by emotional experiences.

ACKNOWLEDGMENTS

This study was supported by the Academy of Finland, the Vaajasalo Foundation, and the Sigrid Juselius Foundation.

ABBREVIATIONS

AB_{mc}, accessory basal nucleus, magnocellular division; AB_{pc}, accessory basal nucleus, parvicellular division; AE, entorhinal cortex, amygdalo-entorhinal transitional subfield; AHA_l, amygdalohippocampal area, lateral division; AHA_m, amygdalohippocampal area, medial division; BAOT, bed nucleus of the accessory olfactory tract; B_i, basal nucleus, intermediate division; B_{mc}, basal nucleus, magnocellular division; B_{pc}, basal nucleus, parvicellular division; c, central nucleus, capsular division; CA1, CA1 field of the hippocampus; CA2, CA2 field of the hippocampus; CA3, CA3 field of the hippocampus; CE, entorhinal cortex, caudal entorhinal subfield; CE_l, central nucleus, lateral division; CE_m, central nucleus, medial division; CO_a, anterior cortical nucleus; CO_p, posterior cortical nucleus; DG, dentate gyrus; DIE, entorhinal cortex, dorsal intermediate entorhinal subfield; DLE, entorhinal cortex, dorsal lateral entorhinal subfield; I, intercalated nucleus; L_{dl}, lateral nucleus, dorsolateral division; L_m, lateral nucleus, medial division; L_{vl}, lateral nucleus, ventrolateral division; M_c, medial nucleus, caudal division; M_{cd}, medial nucleus, dorsal portion of the central division; M_{cv}, medial nucleus, ventral portion of the central division; ME, entorhinal cortex, medial entorhinal subfield; M_r, medial nucleus, rostral division; NLOT, nucleus of the lateral olfactory tract; PAC, periamygdaloid cortex; PAC_m, periamygdaloid cortex, medial division; paraS, parasubiculum; POR, postrhinal cortex; PRh, perirhinal cortex; S, subiculum; VIE, entorhinal cortex, ventral intermediate entorhinal subfield; 35, perirhinal cortex, area 35; 36, perirhinal cortex, area 36.

REFERENCES

1. ADOLPHS, R., D. TRANEL, H. DAMASIO & A. DAMASIO. 1994. Impaired recognition of emotion in facial expressions following bilateral damage to the human amygdala. Nature **372:** 669–672.
2. ADOLPHS, R., D. TRANEL & A.R. DAMASIO. 1998. The human amygdala in social judgement. Nature **393:** 470–474.
3. AGGLETON, J.P. & R.E. PASSINGHAM. 1981. Syndrome produced by lesions of the amygdala in monkeys (*Macaca mulatta*). J. Comp. Physiol. Psychol. **99:** 961–977.
4. AMARAL, D.G. & M.P. WITTER. 1989. The three-dimensional organization of the hippocampal formation: a review of anatomical data. Neuroscience **31:** 571–591.
5. AMARAL, D.G., J.L. PRICE, A. PITKÄNEN & S.T. CARMICHAEL. 1992. Anatomical organization of the primate amygdaloid complex. *In* The Amygdala. J.P. Aggleton, Ed.: 1–66. Wiley-Liss Publishers. New York.
6. BECKSTEAD, R.M. 1978. Afferent connections of the entorhinal area in the rat as demonstrated by retrograde cell-labeling with horseradish peroxidase. Brain Res. **152:** 249–264.
7. BONDA, E., M. PETRIDES, D. OSTRY & A. EVANS. 1996. Specific involvement of human parietal systems and the amygdala in the perception of biological motion. J. Neurosci. **16:** 3737–3744.
8. BRAAK, H., E. BRAAK, D. YILMAZER *et al.* 1994. Amygdala pathology in Parkinson's disease. Acta Neuropathol. **88:** 493–500.
9. BURWELL, R.D., M.P. WITTER & D.G. AMARAL. 1995. Perirhinal and postrhinal cortices of the rat: a review of the neuroanatomical literature and comparison with findings from the monkey brain. Hippocampus **5:** 390–408.
10. BURWELL, R.D. & D.G. AMARAL. 1998. Perirhinal and postrhinal cortices of the rat: interconnectivity and connections with the entorhinal cortex. J. Comp. Neurol. **391:** 293–321.
11. CAHILL, L. & J.L. MCGAUGH. 1998. Mechanisms of emotional arousal and lasting declarative memory. Trends Neurosci. **21:** 294–299.
12. CANTERAS, N.S. & L.W. SWANSON. 1992. Projections of the ventral subiculum to the amygdala, septum, and hypothalamus: a PHA-L anterograde track-tracing study in the rat. J. Comp. Neurol. **324:** 180–194.
13. CANTERAS, N.S., R.B. SIMERLY & L.W. SWANSON. 1992. Connections of the posterior nucleus of the amygdala. J. Comp. Neurol. **324:** 143–179.
14. CANTERAS, N.S., R.B. SIMERLY & L.W. SWANSON. 1995. Organization of projections from the medial nucleus of the amygdala: a PHA-L study in the rat. J. Comp. Neurol. **360:** 213–245.
15. CHRISTENSEN, M.-K. & C.J. FREDERICKSON. 1998. Zinc-containing afferent projections to the rat corticomedial amygdaloid complex: a retrograde tracing study. J. Comp. Neurol. **400:** 375–390.

16. CULLINAN, W.E., J.P. HERMAN & J.S. WATSON. 1993. Ventral subicular interaction with the hypothalamic paraventricular nucleus: evidence for a relay in the bed nucleus of the stria terminalis. J. Comp. Neurol. 332: 1–20.
17. DAVIS, M. 1992. The role of the amygdala in conditioned fear. In The Amygdala. J.P. Aggleton, Ed.: 255–306. Wiley-Liss Publishers. New York.
18. DEACON, T.W., H. EICHENBAUM, P. ROSENBERG et al. 1983. Afferent connections of the perirhinal cortex in the rat. J. Comp. Neurol. 220: 168–190.
19. GALLAGHER, M. & P.C. HOLLAND. 1994. The amygdala complex: multiple roles in associative learning and attention. Proc. Natl. Acad. Sci. USA 91: 11771–11776.
20. GLOOR, P. 1992. Role of amygdala in temporal lobe epilepsy. In The Amygdala: Neurobiological Aspects of Emotion, Memory, and Mental Dysfunction. J.P. Aggleton, Ed.: 505–538. Wiley-Liss. New York.
21. HAMANN, S.B., T.D. ELY, S.T. GRAFTON & C.D. KILTS. 1999. Amygdala activity related to enhanced memory for pleasant and aversive stimuli. Nature Neurosci. 3: 289–293.
22. IKEGAYA, Y., H. SAITO & K. ABE. 1994. Attenuated hippocampal long-term potentiation in basolateral amygdala-lesioned rats. Brain Res. 656: 157–164.
23. IKEGAYA, Y., H. SAITO & K. ABE. 1995. High-frequency stimulation of the basolateral amygdala facilitates the induction of long-term potentiation in the dentate gyrus in vivo. Neurosci. Res. 22: 203–207.
24. IKEGAYA, Y., H. SAITO & K. ABE. 1996. Dentate gyrus field potentials evoked by stimulation of the basolateral amygdaloid nucleus in anesthetized rats. Brain Res. 718: 53–60.
25. INSAUSTI, R., M.T. HERRERO & M.P. WITTER. 1997. Entorhinal cortex of the rat: cytoarchitectonic subdivisions and the origin and distribution of cortical efferents. Hippocampus 7: 146–183.
26. JOLKKONEN, E. & A. PITKÄNEN. 1998. Intrinsic connections of the rat amygdaloid complex: projections originating in the central nucleus. J. Comp. Neuorol. 395: 53–72.
27. JOLKKONEN, E. & A. PITKÄNEN. 1998. Projections from the amygdala piriform transition area to the central nucleus of the amygdala: a PHA-L study in the rat. Soc. Neurosci. Abstr. 24: 675.
28. KEMPPAINEN, S. & A. PITKÄNEN. 1998. Projections from the posterior cortical nucleus of the amygdala to other temporal lobe areas in rat. Soc. Neurosci. Abstr. 24: 676.
29. KILLCROSS, S., T.W. ROBBINS & B.J. EVERITT. 1997. Different types of fear-conditioned behaviour mediated by separate nuclei within amygdala. Nature 388: 377–380.
30. KRETTEK, J.E. & J.L. PRICE. 1974. Projections from the amygdala to the perirhinal and entorhinal cortices and the subiculum. Brain Res. 71: 150–154.
31. KRETTEK, J.E. & J.L. PRICE. 1977. Projections from the amygdaloid complex to the cerebral cortex and thalamus in the rat and cat. J. Comp. Neurol. 172: 687–722.
32. KRETTEK, J.E. & J.L. PRICE. 1977. Projections from the amygdaloid complex and adjacent olfactory structures to the entorhinal cortex and to the subiculum in the rat and cat. J. Comp. Neurol. 172: 723–752.
33. LEDOUX, J.E. 1992. Emotion and the amygdala. In The Amygdala. J.P. Aggleton, Ed.: 339–352. Wiley-Liss Publishers. New York.
34. LUSKIN, M.B. & J.L. PRICE. 1983. The topographic organization of associational fibres of the olfactory system in the rat, including centrifugal fibres to the olfactory bulb. J. Comp. Neurol. 216: 264–291.
35. MCDONALD, A.J. & T.R. JACKSON. 1987. Amygdaloid connections with posterior insular and temporal cortical areas in the rat. J. Comp. Neurol. 262: 59–77.
36. MCDONALD, A.J. & F. MASCANGNI. 1997. Projections of the lateral entorhinal cortex to the amygdala: A Phaseolus vulgaris leucoagglutinin study in the rat. Neuroscience 445–460.
37. MCDONALD, A.J. 1998. Cortical pathways to the mammalian amygdala. Progr. Neurobiol. 55: 257–332.
38. MORI, E., M. IKEDA, N. HIRONO et al. 1999. Amygdalar volume and emotional memory in Alzheimer's disease. Am. J. Psychiatry 156: 216–222.
39. MORRIS, J.S., A. ÖHMAN & R.J. DOLAN. 1998. Conscious and unconscious emotial learning in the human amygdala. Nature 393: 467–470.

40. OTTERSEN, O.P. 1982. Connections of the amygdala of the rat. Corticoamygdaloid and intraamygdaloid connections as studied with axonal transport of horseradish peroxidase. J. Comp. Neurol. **205:** 30–48.
41. PAXINOS, G. & C. WATSON. 1986. The Rat Brain in Stereotaxic Coordinates. Academic Press. New York.
42. PETROVICH, G.D., P.Y. RISOLD & L.W. SWANSON. 1996. Organization of projections from the basomedial nucleus of the amygdala: a PHAL study in the rat. J. Comp. Neurol. **374:** 387–420.
43. PHILLIPS, R.G. & J.E. LEDOUX. 1992. Overlapping and divergent projections of CA1 and ventral subiculum to the amygdala. Soc. Neurosci. Abstr. **18:** 518.
44. PIKKARAINEN, M., S. RÖNKKÖ, V. SAVANDER *et al.* 1999. Projections from the lateral, basal, and accessory basal nuclei of the amygdala to the hippocampal formation in rat. J. Comp. Neurol. **403:** 229–260.
45. PITKÄNEN, A., V. SAVANDER & J.E. LEDOUX. 1997. Organization of intra-amygdaloid circuitries in the rat: an emerging framework for understanding functions of the amygdala. Trends Neurosci. **20:** 517–523.
46. PITKÄNEN, A., J. TUUNANEN, R. KÄLVIÄINEN *et al.* 1998. Amygdala damage in experimental and human epilepsy. Epilepsy Res. **328:** 233–253.
47. PITKÄNEN, A. 2000. Connectivity of the rat amygdaloid complex. *In* The Functional Analysis of the Amygdala. J. Aggleton, Ed. Wiley-Liss Publishers.
48. PRICE, J.L., F.T. RUSSCHEN & D.G. AMARAL. 1987. The Limbic Region. **II.** The amygdaloid complex. *In* Handbook of Chemical Neuroanatomy, vol. 5. Integrated systems of the CNS, Part I. A. Björklund, T. Hökfelt & L.W. Swanson, Ed.: 279–388. Elsevier. Amsterdam.
49. RAY, J.P. & J.L. PRICE. 1992. The organization of the thalamocortical connections of the mediodorsal thalamic nucleus in the rat, related to the ventral forebrain-prefrontal cortex topography. J. Comp. Neurol. **323:** 167–197.
50. ROMANSKI, L.M. & J.E. LEDOUX. 1993. Information cascade from primary auditory cortex to the amygdala: corticocortical and corticoamygdaloid projections of temporal cortex in the rat. Cerebr. Cortex **3:** 515–532.
51. SAVANDER, V., M. MIETTINEN, S. RÖNKKÖ *et al.* 1997. Projections from the lateral, basal and accessory basal nuclei of the amygdala to the perirhinal and postrhinal cortices: a Phaseolus vulgaris leucoagglutinin study in rat. Soc. Neurosci. Abstr. **23:** 2101.
52. SCOTT, S.K., A.W YOUNG, A.J. CALDER *et al.* 1997. Impaired auditory recognition of fear and anger following bilateral amygdala lesions. Nature **385:** 254–257.
53. SHELINE, Y.I., M.H. GADO & J.L. PRICE. 1998. Amygdala core nuclei volumes are decreased in recurrent major depression. NeuroReport **9:** 2023–2028.
54. SHI, C.-J. & M.D. CASSELL. 1999. Perirhinal cortex projections to the amygdaloid complex and hippocampal formation in the rat. J. Comp. Neurol. **406:** 299–328.
55. SWANSON, L.W. & C. KOHLER. 1986. Anatomical evidence for direct projections from the entorhinal area to the entire cortical mantle in the rat. J. Neurosci. **6:** 3010–3023.
56. SWANSON, L.W. 1992. Brain Maps: Structure of the Rat Brain. Elsevier. Amsterdam.
57. VAN GROEN, T. & J.M. WYSS. 1990. The connections of presubiculum and parasubiculum in the rat. Brain Res. **518:** 227–243.
58. VAN GROEN, T. & M.J. WYSS. 1990. Extrinsic projections from area CA1 of the rat hippocampus: olfactory, cortical, subcortical, and bilateral hippocampal formation projections. J. Comp. Neurol. **302:** 515–528.
59. VEENING, J.G. 1978. Cortical afferents of the amygdaloid complex in the rat: an HRP study. Neurosci. Lett. **8:** 191–195.
60. VEREECKEN, T.H.L.G, O.J.M. VOGELS & R. NIEUWENHUYS. 1994. Neuron loss and shrinkage in the amygdala in Alzheimer's disease. Neurobiol. Aging **15:** 45–54.
61. WYSS, J.M. 1981. An autoradiographic study of the efferent connections of the entorhinal cortex in the rat. J. Comp. Neurol. **199:** 495–512.
62. ZALD, D.H. & J.V. PARDO. 1997. Emotion, olfaction, and the human amygdala: amygdala activation during aversive olfactory stimulation. Neurobiology **94:** 4119–4124.

Networks of the Hippocampal Memory System of the Rat

The Pivotal Role of the Subiculum[a]

PIETERKE A. NABER,[b,c,d] MENNO P. WITTER,[d] AND
FERNANDO H. LOPES DA SILVA[c]

Graduate School Neurosciences Amsterdam

[c]*Institute of Neurobiology, University of Amsterdam*

[d]*Institute of Neurosciences, Department of Anatomy, Free University,
Amsterdam, the Netherlands*

ABSTRACT: The hippocampal system, consisting of the hippocampus, subiculum, and adjacent parahippocampal region, is known to play an important role in learning and memory processes. It is also known that the originally proposed trisynaptic circuit is a simplified representation of the organization of this system. In this paper, we present evidence, both anatomically and electrophysiologically, for the existence of direct and indirect parallel pathways through the hippocampal memory system arising from the perirhinal and postrhinal cortex. These pathways form nested loops. The subiculum occupies a central position within these loops. In the subiculum, both "raw" and highly processed information will converge. Therefore, we propose that the subiculum occupies a pivotal position in the hippocampal memory system, both as recipient and comparator of signals and as a distributor of processed information.

THE HIPPOCAMPAL MEMORY SYSTEM: THE CLASSICAL REPRESENTATION

A contribution to a better understanding of the mechanisms by which the hippocampal system mediates memory functions depends on detailed information regarding the flow of sensory information into, through, and out of the various fields that comprise this system. The classical representation of the organization within the hippocampal memory system is referred to as the "trisynaptic circuit." The first link of this circuit arises in the entorhinal cortex (EC) and terminates in the dentate gyrus (DG) [FIG. 1, dark gray line for the lateral (LEC) and light gray line for the medial (MEC) entorhinal cortex]. The second link originates in the granule cells of the DG and terminates onto CA3-pyramidal cells (not shown in FIG. 1). The third link is between CA3-pyramidal cells and CA1-pyramidal cells (FIG. 1, medium gray lines). It is generally accepted that this is a simplified scheme of what is currently known

[a]This research was supported by Grant No. 903-47-008 of The Netherlands Organization for Scientific Research (NWO) and the Human Frontier Science Program.

[b]Current address: Netherlands Institute for Brain Research, Meibergdreef 33, 1105 AZ Amsterdam, the Netherlands. Tel.: +31 20 5665495; fax: +31 20 6961006.

e-mail: R.Naber@nih.knaw.nl

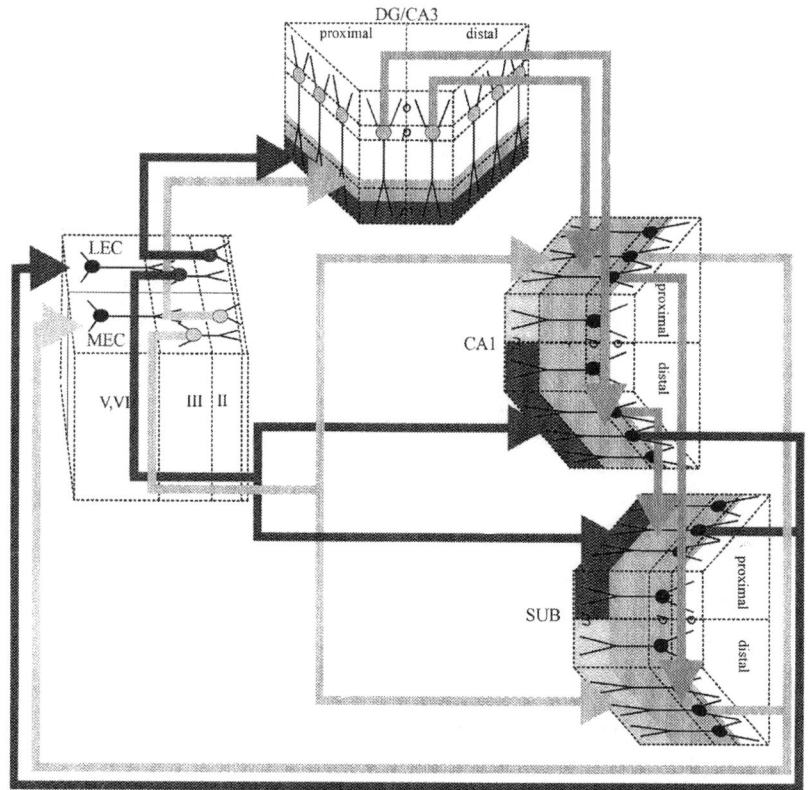

FIGURE 1. Scheme of the organization of the hippocampal memory system in the rat: cells in layer II of LEC project to the outer one-third of the DG molecular layer and the outer portion of the CA3 stratum lacunosum-moleculare, whereas cells in layer II of MEC project to the middle one-thirds of the respective layers of DG and CA3. Note that DG and CA3 are indicated here as one part. This is done to simplify the scheme since we want to put the emphasis of this scheme on area CA1 and SUB. In contrast to the laminar and radial pattern of EC to DG and CA3 projections, EC projections arising from layers III, distributing to area CA1 and SUB, terminate throughout the depth of the molecular layer and exhibit a transverse topographic pattern. This transverse organization is such that fibers from MEC terminate in the portion of CA1 that is located closer to CA3 and in the portion of SUB that is closer to the presubiculum. Fibers from LEC terminate closer to the border of CA1 with SUB. Area CA1 and SUB, in turn, reciprocate the LEC and MEC projections to the same area from which the EC projections originated.

about hippocampal connectivity. To the classical trisynaptic pathway, several additional connections should be added. One is that there are actually two distinct projections from the EC, both referred to as the perforant path, which project to all hippocampal fields and to the subiculum (SUB) (FIG. 1, dark gray lines for LEC and light gray lines for MEC; see also chapter by Witter *et al.* in this volume). Neurons in layer II of the EC project to DG and CA3, in contrast to layer III cells, which

Dorsal-distal subiculum

retrosplenial cortex
presubiculum (dorsal)
medial mammillary nucleus (CM)
medial entorhinal cortex (CL)

Dorsal-proximal subiculum

perirhinal cortex
prelimbic cortex
nucleus accumbens (RL)
lateral septum (dorsal)
medial mammillary nucleus (RL)
lateral entorhinal cortex (L)

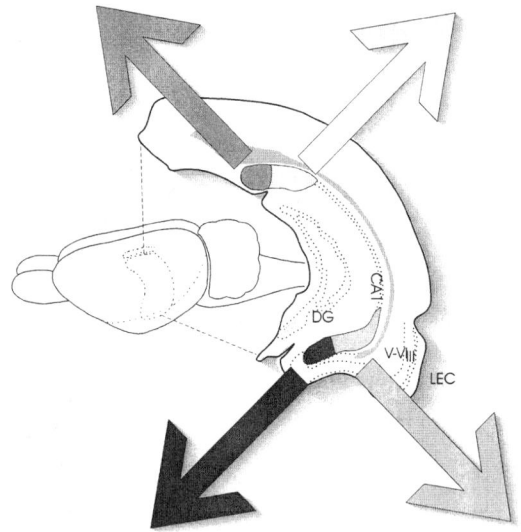

Ventral-distal subiculum

presubiculum (ventral)
ventromedial hypothalamic nucleus (shell)
medial mammillary nucleus (CM)
medial entorhinal cortex (RM)

Ventral-proximal subiculum

infralimbic cortex
nucleus accumbens (CM)
lateral septum (ventral)
ventromedial hypothalamic nucleus (core)
amygdala
medial mammillary nucleus (RL)
lateral entorhinal cortex (RM)

FIGURE 2. Schematic drawing of a coronal brain slice with the four different regions of the SUB, that is, dorsal-distal, dorsal-proximal, ventral-distal, and ventral-proximal, indicated with different shadings. The connected boxes show the specific sets of target structures for each area that characterize the different areas of the subiculum. Abbreviations: DG, dentate gyrus; LEC, lateral entorhinal cortex; V–VI, deep cortical layers; III, superficial cortical layer; CM, caudomedial; CL, caudolateral; RL, rostrolateral; RM, rostromedial; L, lateral. (Reproduced from ref. 11, with permission from Wiley–Liss, New York.)

project to CA1 and SUB. Also, the important projection from CA1 to SUB, which can be seen as the "fourth link," was not included in the classical representation.

From this description, it is clear that the organization of the hippocampal memory system exhibits two main features: (1) parallel pathways exist throughout the hippocampus and SUB, within which (2) several nested circuits are present (FIG. 1). As regards the former, we refer to the two components of the perforant path originating in LEC or MEC, respectively. It has been suggested that these two pathways, that is, the lateral and medial perforant pathway, transmit functionally different types of information.[1–5] These two parallel perforant paths have the same type of divergent distribution along the longitudinal axis of the hippocampus, but have a more selective distribution along the transverse and radial axes.[6–9] Whereas layer II cells of LEC send fibers to the outer one-third of DG/CA3, the projections from layer II cells of MEC terminate in the respective middle one-thirds of these layers. This means that these two pathways can influence the same cells; that is, there is convergence of the pathways. In contrast, at the level of CA1/SUB, these two parallel input routes stay separate from each other. It is therefore most likely that the functional relevance of DG/CA3 is different from that of CA1/SUB. With respect to the projections to CA1 and SUB, the existence of nested circuits must be stressed. One possible route to reach CA1 and SUB is via a long, polysynaptic route through the whole hippocampus (EC $\Rightarrow$ DG $\Rightarrow$ CA3 $\Rightarrow$ CA1 $\Rightarrow$ SUB). The other route represents a short, monosynaptic pathway that consists of the entorhinal fibers that terminate directly in CA1/SUB (EC $\Rightarrow$ SUB), bypassing the long route. It is most likely that both long and short circuits may eventually influence the same neurons in CA1/SUB. The projections from CA1/SUB back to EC close the circuit. Both the long and the short loop may function independently, but one can also modulate the other. Since SUB is the last station within the hippocampus and gives rise to the most widespread output connections to the septal area, nucleus accumbens, and hypothalamus among other areas[10,11] (see FIG. 2), it may be proposed that SUB occupies a pivotal position in the hippocampal memory system.

In addition to the role of the hippocampal formation in memory functions, there is evidence that the perirhinal cortex (PER) and the postrhinal cortex (POR), which serve as the major input sources of LEC and MEC, respectively, have important functions in learning tasks.[12–22] Moreover, some anatomical data indicate that PER may have a direct input to SUB[23,24] and can thus also directly influence this pivotal output structure. In order to assess the functions of these various structures, it is important to know more precisely how the system is organized. The research presented in this article therefore focuses on the subiculum and its complex parallel and nested connections with the parahippocampal region, in particular with PER and POR.

PERI- AND POSTRHINAL CORTEX PROJECTIONS TO THE SUBICULUM

Electrical stimulation of PER evoked a field potential with two components with different latencies in the hippocampus.[25] CSD analysis revealed that the early component most likely was caused by a synaptic input to the molecular layer of area CA1/SUB (FIG. 3). This conclusion was supported by additional recordings of unit activity at approximately the same latency as the early component. From these electrophysiological results, combined with the anatomical observations of ourselves[25] and those of other authors,[23,24] showing the presence of a direct projection from PER to an area around the border of CA1 and SUB, we conclude that the hippocampal area CA1 and SUB can be directly activated from PER. This implies that cortical information entering PER can monosynaptically be transferred to CA1/SUB. In

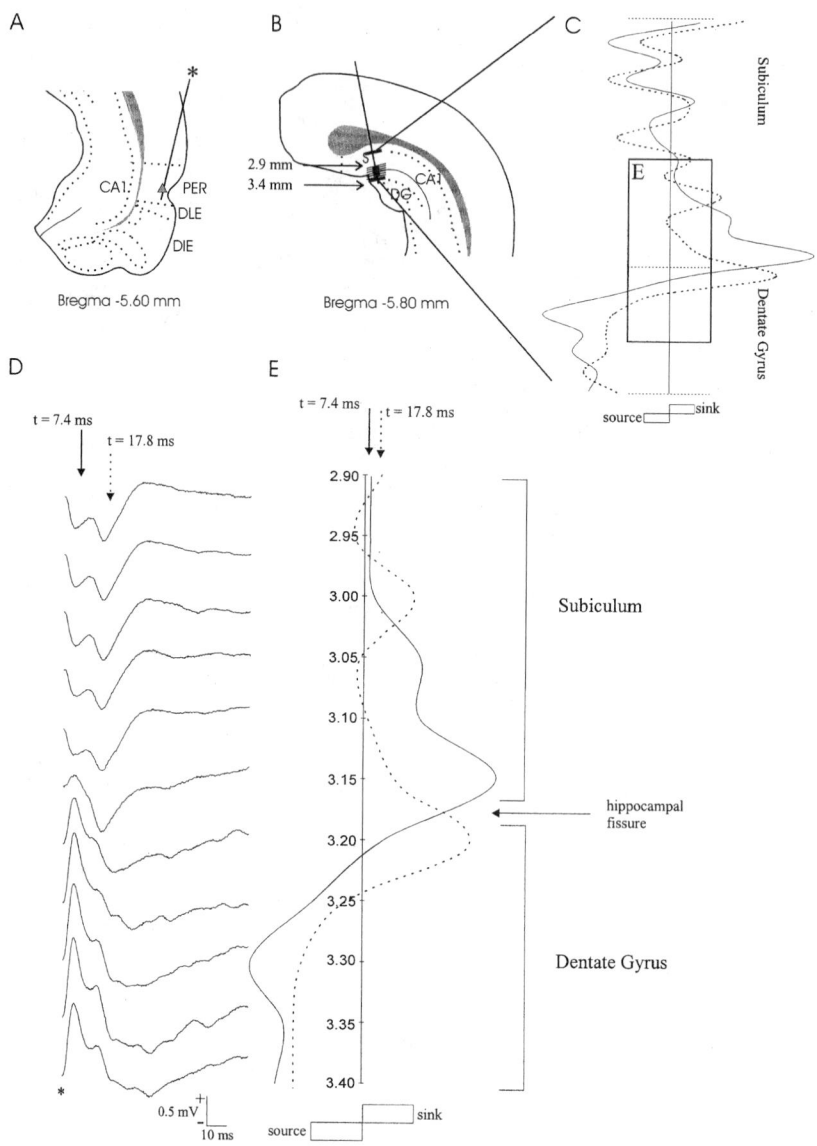

FIGURE 3. Example of a current source density (CSD) analysis of a representative experiment in which the perirhinal cortex (PER) was stimulated. **A** and **B** are schematic drawings of parts of two coronal sections, indicating the stimulation site in PER (**A**) and the recording track through the subiculum (SUB) (**B**), at the level around 5.6 mm and 5.8 mm behind bregma, respectively. In **C**, the result of a CSD analysis of the complete recording track is indicated. In **D** and **E**, the depth profile of the recorded field potentials recorded in SUB around the hippocampal fissure after PER stimulation and the corresponding detailed

addition, CSD analysis revealed that the second, longer latency, component of the field potential was due to synaptic input to the outer molecular layer of DG. When the synaptic transmission in LEC was partly interrupted by a local injection of CNQX to reversibly block synaptic transmission in LEC, the second component was largely diminished, leaving the first component intact. This suggests that, in addition to the direct pathway, PER can activate DG via activation of a synaptic relay in LEC.[25,26] Using a similar experimental strategy, we found also evidence for a direct projection from POR to SUB. An indirect route from POR, reaching DG via MEC, was also found.[27] This suggests that, like PER, POR also reaches SUB via both a direct and an indirect route.

CONVERGENT AND SEGREGATED PROJECTIONS TO CA1/SUB

There is evidence that PER and POR project along distinct pathways to LEC and MEC, respectively.[25,27–29] A question of interest is whether these two parallel pathways are kept segregated at the level of CA1/SUB. As illustrated in the chapter by Witter *et al.* (in this volume), the anatomical findings clearly show that the terminal distribution in SUB of the projection from PER is clearly distinct from that of the projection arising from POR. In area CA1, the terminal density of the projection is weaker compared to that in SUB, but even here the projections originating from PER and POR are separated. This is also the case for the projection from LEC and MEC to SUB and CA1.[6,30] The organization is such that the projections of LEC and of PER to the SUB overlap with each other, and those arising from MEC and POR also do. The termination areas of PER or POR projections, however, are more restricted than those of the projections arising from layer III of LEC or MEC, respectively. The projections from PER/LEC, as much as those arising from POR/MEC, thus do not directly influence the same neuronal populations in SUB. This is different from the situation with respect to the projections from PER and POR to DG and area CA3 by way of the perforant path originating in LEC and MEC. Since LEC and MEC terminate in DG and CA3 on the same granular or pyramidal neurons, respectively, the signals originally arising from PER and POR can converge on the same neurons. Thus, in contrast to area CA1/SUB, where information relayed from PER and POR is kept segregated, in DG/CA3 these different types of information are most likely integrated. Via the intrinsic hippocampal connections, area CA1 and SUB may be reached by these integrated signals from DG/CA3. At the end of the trisynaptic path-

---

cross-section CSD, respectively, are shown. The depths indicated hold for both **D** and **E** and correspond to the track indicated in **B**. The field potentials in **D** constitute two distinct negative-going components when recorded in SUB. At the level of the hippocampal fissure, the potentials reverse. The solid lines in **C** and **E** represent the computed CSD from the field potential of the first, short latency, component, while the dotted lines represent the CSD from the field potential of the second, longer latency, component. The CSD of the first component has a maximal sink just above the hippocampal fissure in SUB, which contrasts to the sink of the second component, which is situated underneath the hippocampal fissure, in the outer molecular layer of the dentate gyrus. Abbreviations: CA, cornu Ammonis; DG, dentate gyrus; S, subiculum. (Reproduced from ref. 25, with permission of Oxford University Press, London/New York.)

way, these signals may reach the same neurons in CA1 and SUB that also receive separate inputs either from PER and LEC or from POR and MEC. This hypothesis was tested experimentally by stimulating electrically either PER or POR and both jointly, while recording at different sites along the transverse and longitudinal axes of SUB. Despite the specific topographic relations between stimulating and recording sites, we were able to record at some sites responses either to PER or POR. In FIGURE 4, the results of such an experiment are illustrated. The point was to determine whether the responses to stimulation of the two pathways would summate linearly (as it should be expected in the case that they were independent) or not. Thus, the responses obtained separately to either PER or POR were summed in the com-

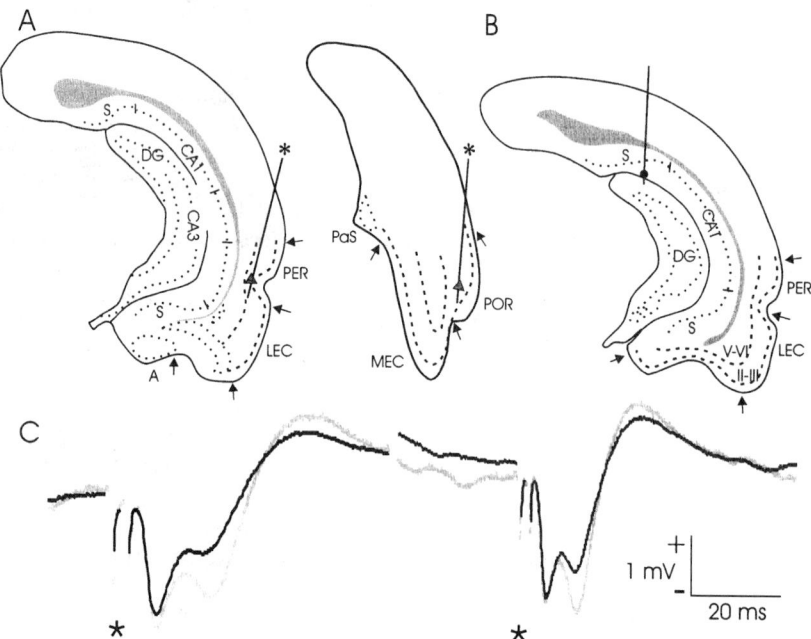

FIGURE 4. Example of evoked field potentials (EFPs; averages of 16 sweeps) recorded in the SUB after combined stimuli of PER and POR. **(A)** The stimulation sites in PER (left) and POR (right). **(B)** The recording site in the SUB. **(C)** A characteristic EFP recorded in the molecular layer of the SUB after PER and POR stimulation is indicated with the black line. The gray line indicates the theoretical EFP when single PER and POR stimuli were manually added, thus assuming that the two stimuli do not influence each other. A slight difference between the black and gray line is only observed in the second component of the response. This suggests that direct inputs to the SUB, which is most likely represented by the first component, originating from PER or POR do not terminate on the same neuronal population. Asterisks in **C** indicate the moments of stimuli. Abbreviations: A, amygdala; CA, cornu Ammonis; DG, dentate gyrus; LEC, lateral entorhinal cortex; MEC, medial entorhinal cortex; PaS, parasubiculum; PER, perirhinal cortex; POR, postrhinal cortex; S, subiculum; mV, millivolts; ms, milliseconds; II–III, superficial cortical layers; V–VI, deep cortical layers.

puter and we compared this theoretical "joint response" to that obtained by real joint stimulation of PER and POR, compensating for the difference in latencies. FIGURE 4 shows that the first component was almost equal for the theoretical and experimental responses, but this was not the case for the second component. This means that the direct pathways give rise to segregated responses that add linearly, while the indirect pathway shows interference; that is, the pathways converge and share, at least partly, the same neuronal elements. It is likely that this convergence takes place in the trisynaptic hippocampal circuit.

INPUTS FROM VISUAL AND BARREL CORTEX TO THE PERI- AND POSTRHINAL CORTEX

In order to understand the functional relevance of PER and POR, it is necessary to know the nature of the inputs they receive from other cortical structures. In a parallel study, we demonstrated that stimulation of the visual and somatosensory cortices indeed can activate neurons in both cortices.[31] Therefore, we may conclude that it is likely that visual and somatosensory (namely, barrel cortex that receives information from the whiskers) signals reach PER and POR. In view of the available anatomical evidence[32] (however, see ref. 33), the effects of stimulation of the barrel cortex might be mediated through other cortical areas, such as adjacent temporal or insular cortex. The effects measured following stimulation of the visual cortex are likely to be both mono- as well as polysynaptic.[29] Electrical stimulation of the barrel cortex resulted in responses distributed almost equally along the longitudinal extent of PER and POR. Stimulation of the visual cortex also resulted in activation of PER and POR; however, in contrast to barrel cortex stimulation, no responses were observed in the rostral part of PER, while in its caudal part and in POR strong responses were almost always observed. These results provide physiological evidence for a topological distribution of cortical inputs to PER and POR and are thus in line with previously published anatomical reports[32,34–36] (see also chapter by Burwell in this volume). In view of the unequal distribution of information originating from the barrel cortex and from the visual cortex in PER and POR, it is of interest that anatomical evidence supports the notion that strong reciprocal connections exist between PER and POR.[28,29] Moreover, activation studies in the rat and in the guinea pig with the use of voltage-dependent dye imaging have indicated that spread of activity along the rostro-caudal axis of PER and POR is likely to occur (Iijima and de-Curtis, personal communication; and our unpublished results).

THE PIVOTAL ROLE OF THE SUBICULUM

Our experimental results demonstrate that SUB receives inputs from specific sensory areas (e.g., somatosensory barrel cortex and visual cortex), relayed via PER and POR and mediated by direct and indirect pathways. Regarding the latter, we should distinguish two pathways that reach the CA1/SUB area: one has only one synaptic relay in EC (LEC and MEC, respectively), while the other, after this relay in EC, follows the perforant path and the trisynaptic hippocampal circuit. These pathways are

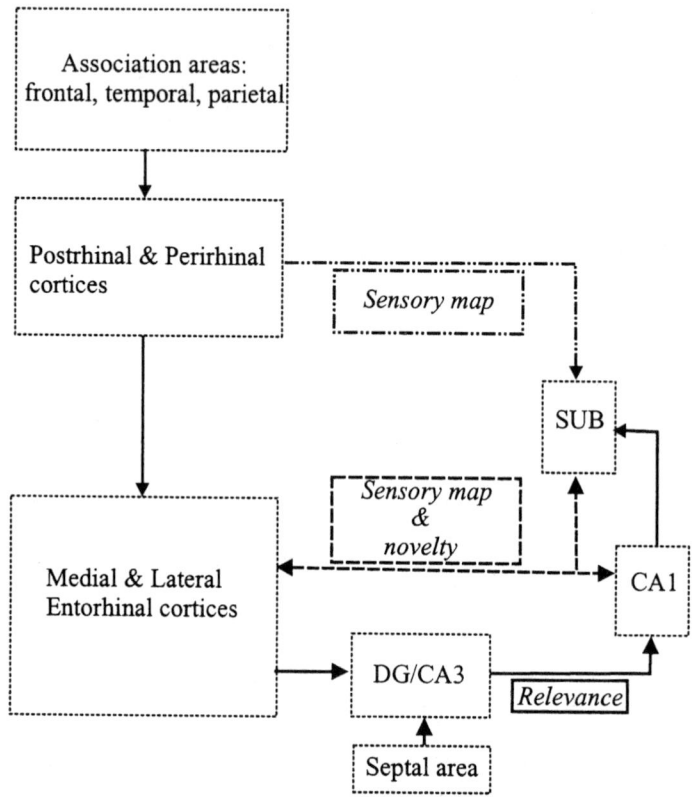

FIGURE 5. Diagram of the anatomical organization of the parahippocampal-hippocampal system with emphasis on the pivotal role of the subiculum, receiving three, differently processed copies of the same sensory information that originates in the association areas: (1) A direct projection from PER and POR to SUB, which transfers a sensory map to the SUB, bypassing the EC and hippocampal structures. This same map is transferred to the EC as well. (2) The interaction, by way of the reciprocal connections between the EC and CA1/SUB, may allow the system to decide whether the current sensory map is different from that previously stored; that is, a novelty flag is added to the sensory map, which may subsequently enter the SUB by way of the layer III projection. (3) The classic trisynaptic loop, starting with the projection of entorhinal layer II cells to the dentate gyrus (DG) (indicated with solid lines), allows the system to add information about relevance (septal input) to the sensory map present in the SUB.

nested within each other. This functional organization implies that SUB is in a position to receive at least three different versions of the same kind of sensory information according to the following scheme (as illustrated in FIG. 5):

(i) First, a raw associative sensory map of the input relayed directly from PER and POR.

(ii) Second, a modified version of the same sensory map, but now processed by the superficial layers of the EC. What kind of processing might this be? This is not yet clear, but we should take into account that there exists a closed loop connecting layer III of EC to CA1/SUB and from the latter to deep layers of EC,[8,9] which in turn project back to the superficial EC. In this circuit, layer III neurons may be reactivated by information reentering in such a way that the circuit may function as a system to hold information for a short time.[37] Thus, we may advance the hypothesis that, in this circuit, a continuous comparison between new inputs and temporarily stored information takes place. In this way, the quality of novelty of any new input could be estimated. Hence, the sensory map would get a "novelty flag" or not, depending on previous experience.

(iii) Third, another modified version of the same sensory map, but now after being processed in the long entorhinal-hippocampal trisynaptic circuit. Two main features of this circuit may help us to understand what type of processing may take place here. In contrast with the other projections discussed above, in this case there is considerable convergence of different inputs, particularly in DG/ CA3, whereas these neuronal networks receive important modulating signals relayed from the septal area. These signals mediate information about the state of the basic functions of the organism through the parallel neurochemical systems of the brain stem and hypothalamus. These modulating signals would provide a "flag of the relevance" to the sensory map, namely, its emotional connotation in relation to the context of the situation where the organism was stimulated. Although this proposal for a role of the layer II projection is different from that proposed by Buzsáki (in this volume), both hypotheses share the same notion that the layer II signal becomes integrated with that of the parallel layer III input, in this way contributing to the final hippocampal output signal. According to this scheme (FIG. 5), the nested circuits that assure the transfer and processing of sensory maps from PER and POR to SUB would enable the latter structure to perform a comparison between sensory maps processed in different ways. Based on such a comparison that takes into account the novelty and relevance of a particular sensory map, in SUB a decision could be made to transfer the information to other brain systems. From SUB, a distributed set of projections arise, namely, to the entorhinal, perirhinal, and postrhinal cortices; to the retrosplenial, infralimbic, and prelimbic cortices; and to the septal nuclei, the ventral striatum, the amygdala, and several thalamic and hypothalamic nuclei[10,11] (see FIG. 2). Thus, SUB occupies a pivotal position in the hippocampal memory system, both as recipient and comparator of sensory associative signals and as a distributor of the processed information.

REFERENCES

1. MCNAUGHTON, B.L. 1980. Evidence for two physiologically distinct perforant pathways to the fascia dentate. Brain Res. **199:** 1–19.
2. TIELEN, A.M., F.H. LOPES DA SILVA, W.J. MOLLEVANGER & F.H. DE JONGE. 1981. Differential effects of enkephalin within hippocampal areas. Exp. Brain Res. **44:** 343–346.
3. ABRAHAM, W.C. & N. MCNAUGHTON. 1984. Differences in synaptic transmission between medial and lateral components of the perforant path. Brain Res. **303:** 251–260.
4. DAHL, D., E.C. BURGARD & J.M. SARVEY. 1990. NMDA receptor antagonists reduce medial, but not lateral, perforant path–evoked EPSPs in dentate gyrus of rat hippocampal slice. Exp. Brain Res. **83:** 172–177.

5. COLINO, A. & R.C. MALENKA. 1993. Mechanisms underlying induction of long-term potentiation in rat medial and lateral perforant paths *in vitro*. J. Neurophysiol. **69:** 1150–1159.
6. WITTER, M.P. 1993. Organization of the entorhinal-hippocampal system: a review of current anatomical data. Hippocampus **3:** 33–44.
7. AMARAL, D.G. 1993. Emerging principles of intrinsic hippocampal organization. Curr. Opin. Neurobiol. **3:** 225–229.
8. TAMAMAKI, N. & Y. NOJYO. 1995. Preservation of topography in the connections between the subiculum, field CA1, and the entorhinal cortex in rats. J. Comp. Neurol. **353:** 379–390.
9. NABER, P.A., F.H. LOPES DA SILVA & M.P. WITTER. 2000. Reciprocal connections between the entorhinal cortex and hippocampal fields CA1 and the subiculum are in register with the projections from CA1 to the subiculum. Hippocampus. In press.
10. WITTER, M.P. & H.J. GROENEWEGEN. 1990. The subiculum: cytoarchitectonically a simple structure, but hodologically complex. *In* Understanding the Brain through the Hippocampus: The Hippocampal Region as a Model for Studying Structure and Function. Vol. 83, pp. 47–58. Elsevier. Amsterdam/New York.
11. NABER, P.A. & M.P. WITTER. 1998. Subicular efferents are organized mostly as parallel projections: a double-labeling, retrograde-tracing study in the rat. J. Comp. Neurol. **393:** 284–297.
12. ZOLA-MORGAN, S., L.R. SQUIRE, D.G. AMARAL & W.A. SUZUKI. 1989. Lesions of perirhinal and parahippocampal cortex that spare the amygdala and hippocampal formation produce severe memory impairment. J. Neurosci. **9:** 4355–4370.
13. ZOLA-MORGAN, S., L.R. SQUIRE, R.P. CLOWER & N.L. REMPEL. 1993. Damage to the perirhinal cortex exacerbates memory impairments following lesions to the hippocampal formation. J. Neurosci. **13:** 251–265.
14. ROSEN, J.B., J.M. HITCHCOCK, M.J.D. MISERENDINO, W.A. FALLS, S. CAMPEAU & M. DAVIS. 1992. Lesions of the perirhinal cortex, but not of the frontal, medial prefrontal, visual, or insular cortex block fear-potentiated startle using a visual conditioned stimulus. J. Neurosci. **12:** 4624–4633.
15. MEUNIER, M., J. BACHEVALIER, M. MISHKIN & E.A. MURRAY. 1993. Effects on visual recognition of combined and separate ablations of the entorhinal and perirhinal cortex in rhesus monkeys. J. Neurosci. **13:** 5418–5432.
16. MEUNIER, M., W. HADFIELD, J. BACHEVALIER & E.A. MURRAY. 1996. Effects of rhinal cortex lesions combined with hippocampectomy on visual recognition memory in rhesus monkeys. J. Neurophysiol. **75:** 1190–1205.
17. MURRAY, E.A. & D. GAFFAN. 1993. Effects of lesions of rhinal cortex, hippocampus, or parahippocampal gyrus in rhesus monkeys on object and spatial reversals. Soc. Neurosci. Abstr. **19:** 438.
18. SUZUKI, W.A., S. ZOLA-MORGAN, L.R. SQUIRE & D.G. AMARAL. 1993. Lesions of the perirhinal and parahippocampal cortices in the monkey produce long-lasting impairment in the visual and tactual modalities. J. Neurosci. **13:** 2430–2451.
19. RAMUS, S.J., S. ZOLA-MORGAN & L.R. SQUIRE. 1994. Effects of lesions of perirhinal cortex or parahippocampal cortex on memory in monkeys. Soc. Neurosci. Abstr. **20:** 1074.
20. HERZOG, C. & T. OTTO. 1997. Odor-guided fear conditioning in rats: 2. Lesions in the anterior perirhinal cortex disrupt fear conditioning to the explicit conditioned stimulus, but not to the training context. J. Neurosci. **111:** 1265–1272.
21. TENG, E., L.R. SQUIRE & S. ZOLA. 1997. Different memory roles for the parahippocampal and perirhinal cortices in spatial reversal. Soc. Neurosci. Abstr. **23:** 12.
22. BUSSEY, T.J., J.L. MUIR & J.P. AGGLETON. 1999. Functionally dissociating aspects of event memory: the effects of combined perirhinal and postrhinal cortex lesions on object and place memory in the rat. J. Neurosci. **19:** 495–502.
23. KOSEL, K.C., G.W. VAN HOESEN & D.L. ROSENE. 1983. A direct projection from the perirhinal cortex area 35 to the subiculum in the rat. Brain Res. **269:** 347–351.
24. MCINTYRE, D.C., M.E. KELLY & W.A. STAINES. 1996. Efferent projections of the anterior perirhinal cortex in the rat. J. Comp. Neurol. **369:** 302–318.
25. NABER, P.A., M.P. WITTER & F.H. LOPES DA SILVA. 1999. Perirhinal cortex input to the hippocampal formation in the rat: evidence for parallel pathways, both direct and

indirect—a combined physiological and anatomical study. Eur. J. Neurosci. **11:** 4119–4133.

26. CANNING, K.J. & L.S. LEUNG. 1997. Lateral-entorhinal, perirhinal, and amygdala-entorhinal transition projections to hippocampal CA1 and dentate gyrus in the rat: a current source density study. Hippocampus **7:** 643–655.

27. NABER, P.A., M.P. WITTER & F.H. LOPES DA SILVA. 2000. Evidence for a direct projection from postrhinal cortex to subiculum in the rat. Hippocampus. In press.

28. BURWELL, R.D. & D.G. AMARAL. 1998. Perirhinal and postrhinal cortices of the rat: interconnectivity and connections with the entorhinal cortex. J. Comp. Neurol. **391:** 293–321.

29. NABER, P.A., M. CABALLERO-BLEDA, B. JORRITSMA-BYHAM & M.P. WITTER. 1997. Parallel input to the hippocampal memory system through peri- and postrhinal cortices. Neuroreport **8:** 2617–2621.

30. WITTER, M.P. & D.G. AMARAL. 1991. Entorhinal cortex of the monkey: V. Projections to the dentate gyrus, hippocampus, and subicular complex. J. Comp. Neurol. **307:** 437–459.

31. NABER, P.A., M.P. WITTER & F.H. LOPES DA SILVA. 2000. Differential distribution of barrel or visual cortex–evoked responses along the rostro-caudal axis of the peri- and postrhinal cortices. Brain Res. In press.

32. BURWELL, R.D. & D.G. AMARAL. 1998. Cortical afferents of the perirhinal, postrhinal, and entorhinal cortices of the rat. J. Comp. Neurol. **398:** 179–205.

33. HOOGLAND, P.V., E. WELKER & H. VAN DER LOOS. 1987. Organization of the projections from barrel cortex to thalamus in mice studied with *Phaseolus vulgaris*–leucoagglutinin and HRP. Exp. Brain Res. **68:** 73–87.

34. ROOM, P. & H.J. GROENEWEGEN. 1986. Connections of the parahippocampal cortex. I. Cortical afferents. J. Comp. Neurol. **251:** 415–450.

35. SUZUKI, W.A. & D.G. AMARAL. 1994. The perirhinal and parahippocampal cortices of the macaque monkey: cortical afferents. J. Comp. Neurol. **350:** 497–533.

36. SUZUKI, W.A. & D.G. AMARAL. 1994. Topographic organization of the reciprocal connections between the monkey entorhinal and the perirhinal and parahippocampal cortices. J. Neurosci. **14:** 1856–1877.

37. IIJIMA, T., M.P. WITTER, M. ICHIKAWA, T. TOMINAGA, R. KAJIWARA & G. MATSUMOTO. 1996. Entorhinal-hippocampal interactions revealed by real-time imaging. Science **272:** 1176–1179.

Imaging Epileptiform Discharges in Slices of Piriform Cortex with Voltage-sensitive Fluorescent Dyes

REZAN DEMIR, LEWIS B. HABERLY, AND MEYER B. JACKSON[a]

Departments of Physiology and Anatomy, University of Wisconsin Medical School, Madison, Wisconsin 53706, USA

ABSTRACT: Voltage imaging techniques were used to investigate epileptiform discharges in brain slices containing piriform cortex (PC). These experiments pinpointed the site of discharge onset in the endopiriform nucleus (En). Under some conditions, discharge onset also occurred simultaneously in adjoining neocortex. With slightly suprathreshold electrical stimulation, discharge generation was a two-stage process in which onset was preceded by a sustained spatially localized depolarization denoted as plateau activity. Plateau activity was seen away from the onset site, in a border region between En and layer III of PC. A similar two-stage sequence was seen for slices taken from a variety of planes, using two different interictal models as well as an ictal model. Plateau activity was found to be necessary for the generation of both kinds of discharge. Synaptic transmission at the site of onset was found to be required for the generation of interictal-like discharges, but ictal-like discharges were different in that they could still be generated when synaptic transmission at this site was impaired. These studies identify specialized regions with potentially important roles in epileptogenesis and help to elucidate the neuronal circuitry that can produce epileptiform activity.

During seizure discharges, large numbers of neurons fire synchronously as abnormal activity is initiated and subsequently spreads within the brain. This activity arises from the complex interactions of a very large number of individual neurons. When an intracellular recording is made from a single cell during an epileptiform discharge, the information obtained is necessarily a very small part of a much larger picture. To overcome this general limitation, techniques have been developed to image voltage in intact neural systems.[1–3] One of the most popular variations of this technique is based on the use of fluorescent dyes that stain neuronal tissue by insertion into the plasma membrane. These dyes orient within the lipid bilayer such that the transmembrane potential influences the electronic transitions of the chromophore. As a result, when the membrane potential changes, the spectral properties of the dye change. This sensitivity to voltage can be exploited to provide a voltage-dependent fluorescent signal. When tissue stained with such a dye is imaged, the fluorescent light provides a readout of membrane potential and allows the imaging of electrical activity.

[a]Corresponding author: Department of Physiology, SMI 127, University of Wisconsin Medical School, 1300 University Ave., Madison, WI 53706.
e-mail: MJackson@Physiology.Wisc.Edu

Voltage imaging has been used to study epileptiform activity in a number of laboratories.[4–7] These studies described the onset of epileptiform discharges, primarily in brain slices, and showed how electrical activity spreads under various conditions used to make neural tissue hyperexcitable. Our laboratory has studied epileptiform activity in slices of piriform cortex (PC). The PC has an unusually high seizure susceptibility,[8–10] and slices of PC can easily be induced to generate epileptiform discharges.[11,12] What makes the PC especially interesting in the study of epilepsy is that it contains specific foci with special roles in discharge generation.[13–16] Voltage imaging of epileptiform discharges with interictal and ictal character in slices of PC has helped pinpoint these sites with high resolution and has indicated the roles played by these sites in the generation of paroxysmal neuronal activity.

METHODS

Voltage Imaging

The technique of voltage imaging has been described in detail by Wu and Cohen;[3] a similar system is used in this laboratory.[15,17] FIGURE 1 shows this instrumentation

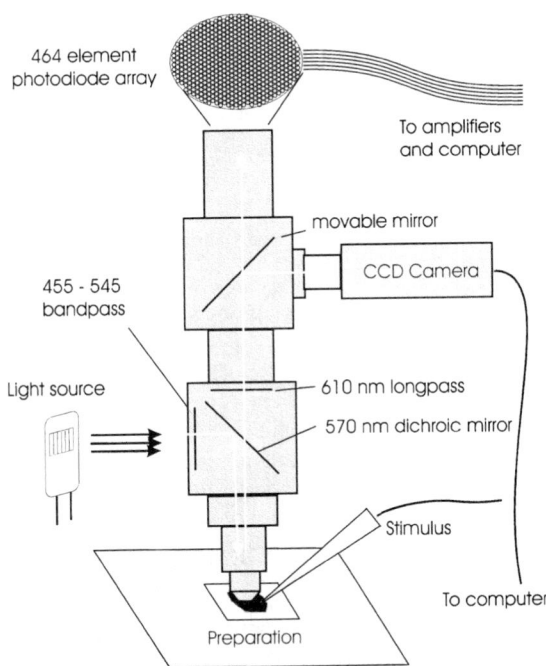

FIGURE 1. Instrumental setup for imaging voltage. Light from a 100-W halogen bulb passes through an excitation filter and is reflected off of a dichroic mirror onto the preparation. Fluorescent light passes through the dichroic mirror and through an emission filter, and is then focused onto the 464-element photodiode–fiber optic camera for recording dye fluorescence in real time. Light can also be directed to a CCD camera by inserting a movable mirror to take video pictures of the preparation.

schematically. A conventional upright fluorescent microscope is used to view a brain slice stained with the voltage-sensitive dye RH414 (200 μM) for 30–45 min (Molecular Probes, Eugene, OR). The preparation is illuminated with an intense light source and, because the fluorescence changes associated with electrical activity are quite small, it is important that the light source be driven by a very stable power supply. An excitation filter transmits light with a wavelength between 475 and 565 nm to illuminate within the absorbance band of the dye. A 570-nm dichroic mirror reflects the light onto the preparation, and an emission filter selects fluorescent light with a wavelength longer than 610 nm to be focused on a detector. The imaging device used to record fluorescence is an array of 464 photodiodes arranged in a hexagonal pattern. Photodiodes are not widely used for imaging studies, but in voltage imaging they have the advantage of being able to detect the small fractional changes in fluorescence produced by voltage-sensitive dyes. Each photodiode has its own amplifier circuit, and the 464 signals are amplified and read sequentially into a computer. The data acquisition system reads an entire image into the computer in less than 1 ms. The computer is then used to display and analyze the traces and associate each trace with a corresponding location in the slice from which the recording was made.

Piriform Cortex Slices

Slices were prepared from the PC as described previously.[11,15] A block of brain containing PC is removed from a rat and mounted in a vibratome. Slices, 350 μm thick, are cut approximately perpendicular to the cortical surface. For cutting, storage, and recording, slices are kept in artificial cerebrospinal fluid (aCSF) consisting of 124 mM NaCl, 5 mM KCl, 26 mM NaHCO$_3$, 1.2 mM KH$_2$PO$_4$, 2.4 mM CaCl$_2$, 1.3 mM MgCl$_2$, and 10 mM glucose, bubbled with 95% O$_2$/5% CO$_2$.

Epileptiform Activity

Slices of PC can generate discharges that are either interictal-like or ictal-like, depending on the choice of experimental conditions. For inducing ictal-like discharges, slices are bathed in a low-Cl$^-$ version of aCSF in which 93% of the Cl$^-$ is replaced by isethionate. The low Cl$^-$ shifts the Nernst potential so that GABA-gated Cl$^-$ channels conduct an inward, depolarizing current. Slices bathing in this solution at 34°C for 30 to 90 min are thought to burst spontaneously. Evoked paroxysmal discharges under these conditions are seizure-like, providing a model for ictal epileptiform behavior. An episode of bursting in low Cl$^-$ produces a lasting change in the excitability of a slice of PC so that, if it is subsequently returned to normal aCSF, it continues to exhibit epileptiform behavior. Slices returned to control saline no longer produce spontaneous seizure-like bursts, but very weak electrical stimulation evokes a discharge strongly resembling an interictal spike. Slices treated in this way are said to be "induced" and provide an excellent model for interictal epileptiform activity. In addition to this induction model, we have employed the "disinhibition" model, entailing addition of the GABA$_A$ receptor antagonist bicuculline (5–10 μM) while recording from the slice. These disinhibited slices behave similarly to induced slices, generating interictal-like spikes in response to relatively weak electrical stimulation.

Electrical stimulation in the form of current pulses was applied from a stimulus isolator through a saline-filled glass micropipette with a tip diameter of ~50 μm.

A. Control   B. Disinhibited

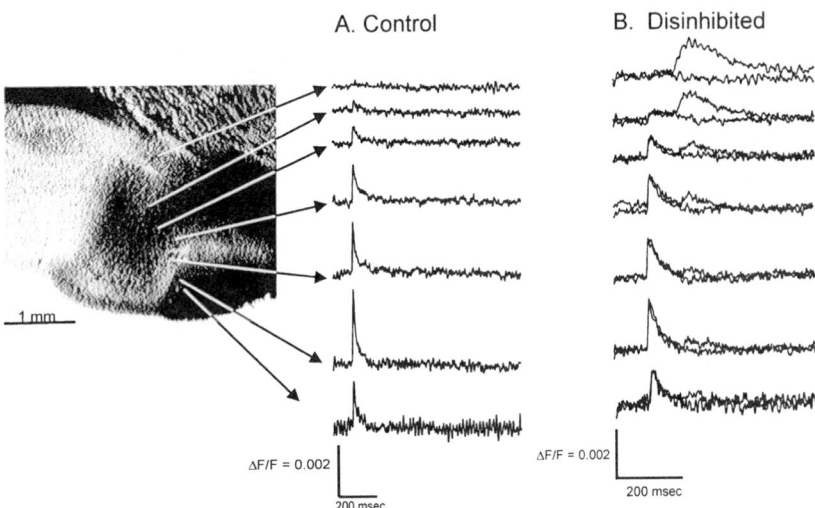

FIGURE 2. Stimulus-evoked changes in dye fluorescence are shown from selected locations of an anterior slice under control and disinhibited conditions. The video image on the left shows the slice from which the recordings were made, indicating the locations where fluorescence traces were taken. The site of electrical stimulation was in layer Ib (indicated by the white double-zigzag symbol). **(A)** Fluorescence traces show responses in the indicated regions. The sites shown are (from top to bottom) En, deep layer III, superficial layer III, layer II, layer Ib, layer Ia, and lateral olfactory tract. The stimulus was a 200-μA, 200-μs current pulse applied at 100 ms. **(B)** Recordings from the same slice after disinhibition with 5 μM bicuculline methiodide. Stimulus-evoked fluorescence changes were recorded from the same locations. Sub- and suprathreshold responses from each site are superimposed. Both were evoked by a threshold stimulus current (80 μA). (Adapted from ref. 15.)

Drugs were applied to the bath or locally by pressure ejection from a micropipette with a 3–4-μm-tip diameter.[16]

RESULTS

Fluorescence traces recorded in slices of PC stained with voltage-sensitive fluorescent dye show local graded responses to electrical stimulation in a control slice (FIG. 2A). Following disinhibition, weak electrical stimulation evokes epileptiform discharges characterized by an abnormal discharge that occurs with a discrete threshold (FIG. 2B). Electrical stimulation can be varied to find the threshold for discharge generation; FIGURE 2B shows subthreshold and suprathreshold responses superimposed. When a slightly suprathreshold stimulus is applied, the discharge is evoked with a latency of up to 150 ms. This depolarization then sweeps through the entire slice, generally with a velocity below the conduction velocity for action potentials in intrinsic excitatory fiber systems.[14,15] It has been pointed out that the slower conduction velocity rules out action potential propagation as the sole mechanism of discharge spread.[18] In general, there is a dramatic decrement in the inten-

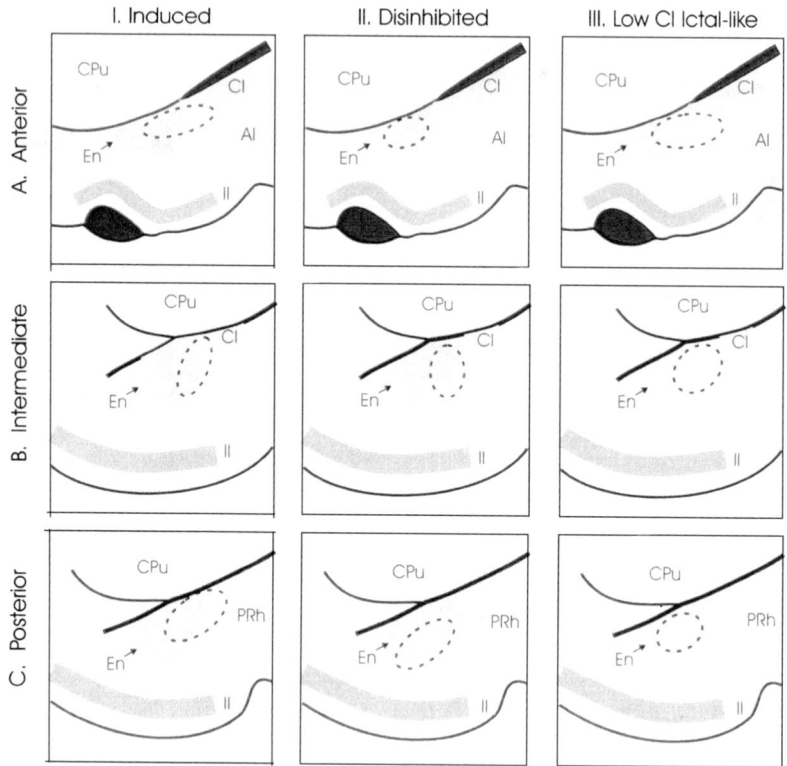

FIGURE 3. Summary of sites of onset. Anterior, intermediate, and posterior slices of PC are as defined in Demir et al.[15] Interictal-like discharges were elicited in either induced slices (prepared by a transient period of bursting in low-Cl⁻ aCSF) or disinhibited slices (recorded in 5–10 μM bicuculline). Ictal-like discharges were elicited in low-Cl⁻ aCSF. Contours indicate the general locations estimated from examination of four or more individual experiments, but there was some variation between slices.[15,20] Labels: En, endopiriform nucleus; Cl, claustrum; II, layer II of piriform cortex; AI, agranular insula; PRh, anterior perirhinal cortex; CPu, caudate-putamen.

sity of the discharge as it propagates from the site of onset in the deepest regions of the slice toward more superficial cortical layers; this is clearly seen in FIGURE 2B.

Site of Onset

Previous studies had identified the endopiriform nucleus (En) as a site of especially high excitability in slices of PC.[13] Microelectrodes showed that interictal-like discharges were seen with the shortest latency in the En, indicating that it is the site of discharge onset.[14,19] Voltage imaging revealed the site of onset as the first region to depolarize during a discharge. To display the site of onset, we drew contours around the first detectors to reach 50–70% of their maximal fluorescence intensity (FIG. 3). Imaging experiments with both interictal-like and ictal-like discharges revealed onset in a similar location, but the higher resolution and distributed recording capability of the imaging technique revealed a number of new features, including differences in spatial pattern under different generating conditions, sublocalization of different phases of burst development, and involvement of neighboring structures in addition to the En. Different spatiotemporal patterns of burst development were also seen, depending on the plane along the anterior-posterior axis from which slices were taken.[15,20] In all cases, the site of onset included the En. However, for interictal-like activity in induced slices, the site of onset included a neighboring portion of layer VI of the adjoining neocortex. For slices taken from an anterior level, discharges appeared in the agranular insula with the same latency as in the En (FIG. 3). For slices taken from a posterior level, discharges appeared in the anterior perirhinal cortex with the same latency as in the En. It should be noted that these sites of onset were independent of the site of stimulation within the PC. Regardless of whether the stimulus electrode was positioned in layer I, II, or III of the overlying PC, onset was always seen in the En and adjoining layer VI of neocortex. Furthermore, increasing the stimulus intensity above threshold did not alter the site of onset, although it did shorten the latency to discharge and increase the size of the site of onset.

There were some variations to the general trend of onset in En and adjoining neocortex. In slices from a rostro-caudal level where the adjoining neocortex was intermediate in cytoarchitecture between agranular insula and perirhinal cortex, the site of onset was contained entirely within the En. Furthermore, when interictal-like discharges were generated with the disinhibition model (using bicuculline), the site of onset was contained entirely in the En regardless of the location of the slice along the anterior-posterior axis.[15] The general trend of involvement of the En underscores the importance of this region in seizure generation,[13,14,19] but the participation of layer VI of the adjoining neocortex under some conditions indicates that there are important regional variations in neuronal properties and circuitry.

Ictal-like discharges were initiated in the En, but the site of onset was somewhat larger than that for interictal-like discharges.[20] The adjoining neocortex participated as well, provided that the slice was taken from a more anterior plane and included agranular insula. In posterior slices containing anterior perirhinal cortex, the site of onset was confined to the En. These results further underscore the importance of the En as a site with unique neuronal properties and circuitry that predispose this region to generate seizures.

Plateau Activity

The results just presented show that epileptiform discharges evoked by electrical stimulation originate at a highly characteristic site. However, prior to the onset of a discharge, microelectrode recordings had suggested that a slice is relatively quiescent.[21] The events leading up to a discharge were poorly understood. In particular, it was considered paradoxical that a slice could be largely quiescent during the latent period and subsequently generate a paroxysmal discharge. Imaging voltage in slices during the latent period has shed some light on this problem.

When discharges were evoked by slightly suprathreshold electrical stimuli, the latent period was about 100 ms in duration. During this time period, imaging revealed a low level of sustained depolarization that began a few milliseconds after the

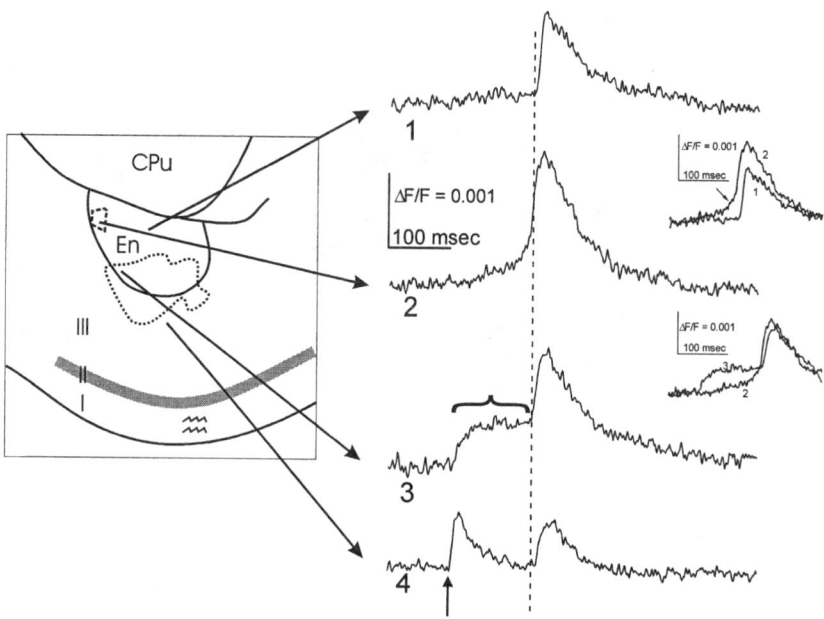

FIGURE 4. Voltage-sensitive dye fluorescence at selected locations during an epilepti-form discharge. The locations are indicated in the sketch on the left, with labels as in FIGURE 3. Epileptiform discharges were evoked by a 132-μA, 200-μs stimulus in layer Ib (site indicat-ed by the double-zigzag symbol). Trace 1 was from a central part of the En, outside the sites of onset and plateau activity, where activity started abruptly after onset activity and plateau activity at other sites. Trace 2 was from the site of onset (indicated by the dashed contour) in dorsalmost En and shows ramplike onset activity, building to an epileptiform discharge. Com-parison of latencies at the different sites with the aid of the dashed vertical line shows that the discharge appeared at this location first. Trace 3 shows plateau activity (indicated by the brack-et). The site of plateau activity is indicated by a dotted contour. Trace 4 from a site in layer III outside the plateau activity region shows that the local response decayed before the discharge began. The arrow indicates the time of stimulus. The upper inset superimposes traces 1 and 2, and the lower inset superimposes traces 2 and 3. These superpositions highlight the different time courses of latent period activity. (Adapted from ref. 16.)

stimulus pulse and continued until the discharge started (FIG. 4, trace 3). As the re-sponses near the stimulus electrode died out, the depolarization in one small region continued at a nearly constant level. Because of its distinct time course, this depo-larization was named plateau activity. A surprising feature of plateau activity was its location. It was observed at a site that was near to, but clearly distinct from, the site of discharge onset. At the onset site, activity displayed a slowly accelerating buildup that began ~50 ms after the abrupt onset of plateau activity (FIG. 4, trace 2). This ramplike depolarization was referred to as onset activity because of the site where it was seen and because it leads directly to the earliest phase of the discharge. The site of plateau activity generally showed little, if any, overlap with the site where the dis-charge actually began. The upper inset of FIGURE 4 superimposes a trace from the site of onset with a trace from another nearby site to emphasize the distinct time

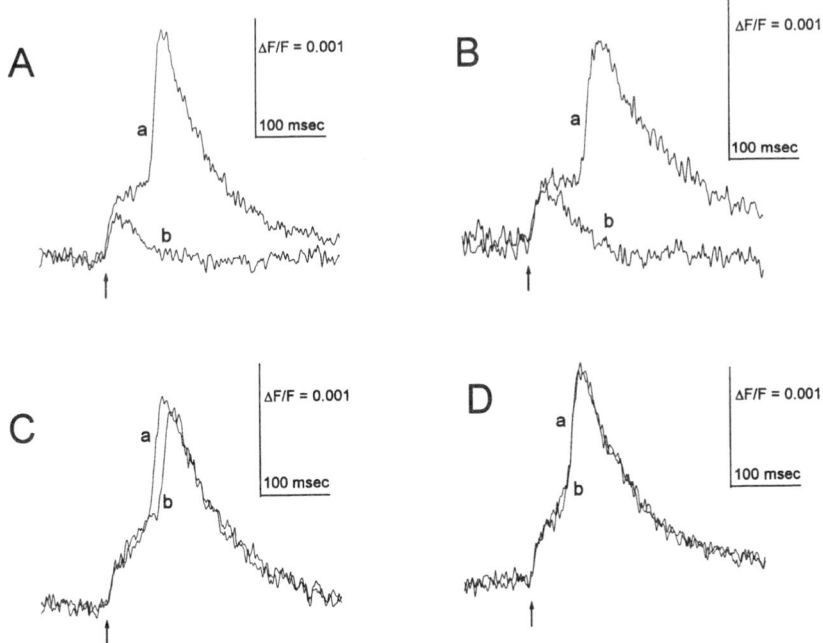

FIGURE 5. Blockade of discharges by application of CoCl₂ to selected sites. Fluorescence traces were taken from the site of plateau activity **(A)**, the site of onset **(B)**, elsewhere in En **(C)**, and in nearby neocortex **(D)** [**(a)** before CoCl₂ application; **(b)** immediately after]. CoCl₂ at the onset and plateau sites blocked discharges, whereas CoCl₂ elsewhere did not. (Adapted from ref. 16.)

course of onset activity. Likewise, the lower inset contrasts the distinct temporal characters of onset and plateau activity.

The finding of plateau activity during the latent period preceding discharge onset suggested that plateau activity plays a role in discharge generation. To test this hypothesis, blockers of electrical activity were applied locally to specific sites within slices of PC. Application of blockers to the site of plateau activity immediately prior to electrical stimulation blocked the discharge. Blockade was seen with 10 mM CoCl₂ (FIG. 5), a nonspecific blocker of Ca^{2+} channels, or 5 mM kynurenic acid, a nonspecific blocker of glutamate receptors. FIGURE 5B makes the important point that blockade of activity at the site of onset changes the time course of activity at the plateau site; the depolarization there is no longer sustained, but instead decays smoothly back to baseline. Thus, feedback from the site of onset is necessary for the flat time course of plateau activity.

Ictal-like discharges also depend on plateau activity (FIG. 6A). These results indicate that plateau activity plays an essential role in the generation of epileptiform discharges by weak, slightly suprathreshold stimulation. Plateau activity is thus a precursor for both ictal- or interictal-like discharges.

Ictal Discharges and Synaptic Transmission

Ictal-like discharges could be evoked in PC slices maintained in low-Cl^- aCSF. These discharges were similar to those evoked in low Mg^{2+}.[11] In low Cl^-, electrical stimulation evokes a discharge that lasts much longer than an interictal-like discharge and often shows repeated bursts indicative of distinct temporal phases.[20] When the electrical stimulus is only slightly suprathreshold, plateau activity can be seen at essentially the same site as for interictal-like discharges (FIG. 6A, traces 1 and 3). As noted above for interictal-like discharges, blocker application to the site of plateau activity prevented the generation of ictal-like discharges. However, when blockers were applied to the site of discharge onset, an interesting difference was found between interictal- and ictal-like activity. The local application of an inhibitor to the site of onset blocked interictal-like discharges (FIG. 5B), but not ictal-like discharges (FIG. 6B). Either $CoCl_2$ or kynurenic acid applied to the plateau site blocked ictal-like discharges, but neither of these two inhibitors blocked ictal-like discharges when they were applied to the site of onset. Twofold higher concentrations of kynurenic acid were tested with the same result. Mixtures of blockers were also tested. Furthermore, because $GABA_A$ receptor activation is depolarizing under the conditions used to generate ictal-like activity (low-Cl^- aCSF), bicuculline was also tested and found to be equally ineffective in blocking discharges.[20] These results suggest that the mechanisms of generation of ictal-like discharges differ from those of interictal-like discharges. The high resistance to blockade of synaptic transmission suggests more spatially distributed generator circuitry or, perhaps, the involvement of nonsynaptic mechanisms.

DISCUSSION

Voltage imaging has provided a direct view of the spatiotemporal pattern of electrical activity during epileptiform discharges in PC slices. This allowed us to monitor the generation and propagation of discharges under a variety of experimental conditions. This technique has localized the site of onset with high precision and revealed previously unidentified foci of activity. One of the new sites found by these studies is layer VI of the neocortex adjoining the En. In anterior slices, the agranular insula participated in discharge onset; and in posterior slices, the anterior perirhinal cortex participated in discharge onset.[15] These results focus attention on the cellular properties and circuitry of these regions. In conjunction with ongoing studies of the spatial localization of molecular markers associated with different types of neurons, imaging studies will help identify cellular and molecular processes with possible pathophysiological roles in epilepsy. Voltage imaging has also revealed subtle differences in the site of onset between different models of epilepsy, and it will be interesting to see if these sites can be correlated with different cellular or molecular mechanisms. Comparisons between these models may help us to understand how different conditions influence the choice between different pathways to paroxysmal activity.

Voltage imaging has also identified a form of electrical activity with a special role in the generation of epileptiform discharges. This weak sustained depolarization, termed plateau activity, was seen during the latent period that precedes epileptiform

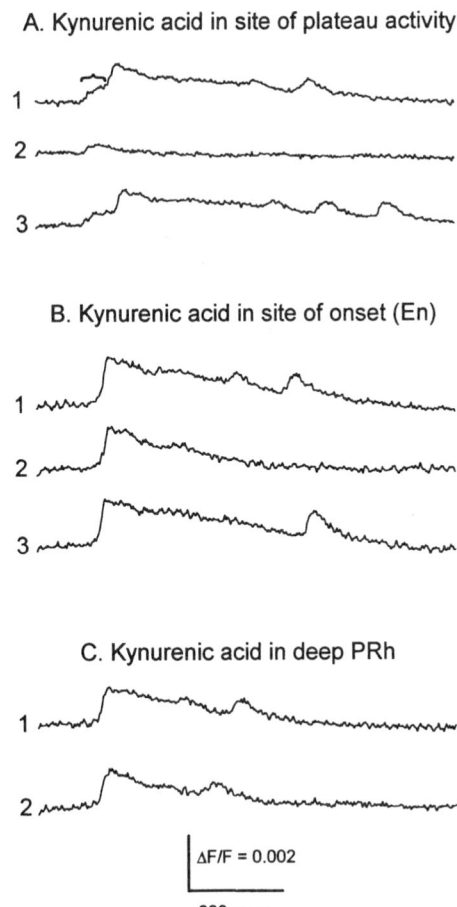

FIGURE 6. Ictal-like activity and blockade by local application of kynurenic acid. Kynurenic acid (5 mM) was locally applied at various sites to determine the role of excitatory synaptic transmission in the generation of ictal-like discharges. **(A)** Responses from the site of plateau activity in an intermediate PC slice prior to (1), immediately after (2), and a few minutes after (3) kynurenic acid application. The bracket over part of trace 1 indicates plateau activity. The ictal-like discharge was blocked and recovered completely after washout. **(B)** Kynurenic acid application at the site of onset did not block the discharge, although the response was usually attenuated locally (2). The amplitude recovered fully after a few minutes (3). **(C)** Kynurenic acid application at a site in deep anterior perirhinal cortex did not block the ictal-like discharge. Discharges were evoked by 200-μs current pulses of (A) 140 μA, (B) 110 μA, and (C) 95 μA, applied in layer Ib. (Adapted from ref. 20.)

discharges evoked by slightly suprathreshold electrical stimulation.[16] Plateau activity was generally seen in a more superficial part of the En, as well as in an adjoining part of deep layer III of the PC. Further, depending on the choice of conditions, plateau activity also occurred in an adjoining part of layer V of neocortex.[22] These are sites clearly distinct from the site of discharge onset and thus represent important additional regions with crucial roles in discharge generation.

The importance of plateau activity is that it is a precursor to epileptiform discharges. A great deal of attention has been devoted to understanding the activity that precedes a discharge in the hope of clarifying the mechanisms by which discharges are generated. Computer models based on the hippocampus suggest that discharges are generated by a gradual buildup of electrical activity through reciprocal excitatory synaptic interactions.[18,23] These modeling studies suggest that, in the hippocampus, the activity that leads up to a discharge is widely distributed over a large area and increases continually throughout the latent period prior to discharge onset. The situation in the PC differs in both respects. Electrical activity during the latent period is localized to two key sites—the site of onset and the site of plateau activity. Further, while an acceleration reminiscent of the hippocampal buildup occurs at the site of onset in PC slices,[14] plateau activity is fairly constant during the latent period.[16] In fact, the buildup of activity in slices of PC appears to result from the interplay between these two distinct regions. Activity at the site of onset is necessary to keep plateau activity from decaying. Application of blockers at the site of onset alters the response at the site of plateau activity so that it decays smoothly back to baseline (FIG. 5B).[16]

Based on these results, we envision the generation of an interictal-like epileptiform discharge as an emergent process dependent on interactions between two distinct regions. This process is depicted with the circuit diagram shown in FIGURE 7. The electrical stimulus activates fibers with excitatory synapses within the site of plateau activity. Activating these synapses evokes a depolarization, which first sustains itself through reciprocal excitatory synaptic interactions within this site. Excitatory projections from the site of plateau activity to the site of onset initiate onset activity at that site. This depolarization is initially very weak, but grows as the latent period continues. Excitatory projections back to the site of plateau activity provide reciprocal excitation. These projections play a key role in maintaining the constant level of activity at the plateau site. Presumably, a balance between these synaptic pathways allows plateau activity to continue without decrement, while onset activity gradually increases. Onset activity builds with an accelerating trajectory until it exceeds a threshold for the regenerative positive feedback that gives rise to discharges. At that point, the discharge can propagate from the site of onset to other regions in the slice.

The generation of ictal-like discharges starts on a similar pathway as that taken in the generation of interictal-like discharges. Once again, plateau activity plays an essential role and synaptic transmission within the plateau site is required (FIG. 6A). However, synaptic transmission at the site of onset appears to be less critical.[20] Discharges still appear when synaptic transmission at the site of onset is blocked (FIG. 6B). These results bring to mind a number of studies in hippocampal slices showing that ictal-like discharges can be generated without functional chemical synapses.[24,25] However, one of the key differences between slices of hippocampus and PC as models of epilepsy appears to be the degree to which specific aspects of epileptiform activity can be spatially localized. Therefore, in the PC, functional chemical synapses are still required for the generation of an ictal-like discharge, but this requirement is restricted to the site of plateau activity. At the site of onset, syn-

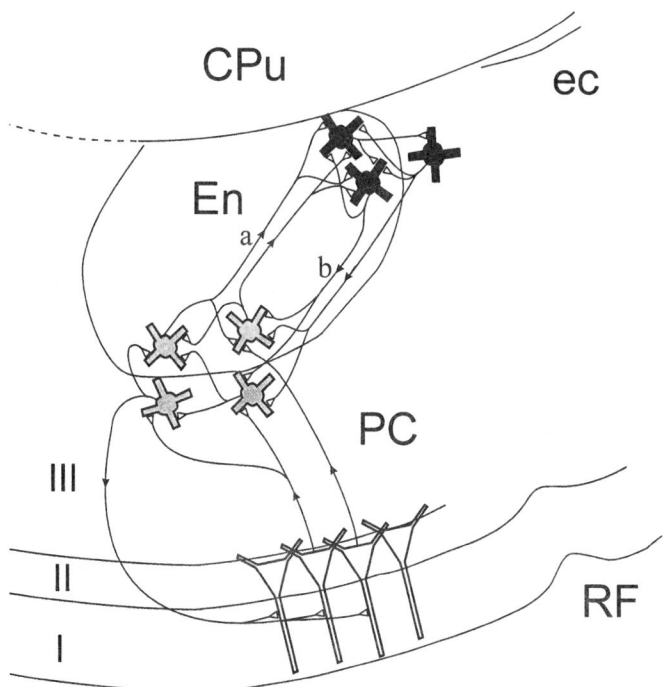

FIGURE 7. A circuit diagram illustrates the key elements that generate discharges in PC slices. The structures and labels are as in FIGURE 3; RF, rhinal fissure; ec, external capsule. Deep multipolar cells (windmills) concentrated in the En are reciprocally connected with each other and with layer II pyramidal cells (triangles). A suprathreshold stimulus anywhere in the PC or En activates a cluster of multipolar cells at the border of the En with deep layer III (light gray). These multipolar cells sustain plateau activity with the aid of reciprocal excitation within this population and project to other multipolar cells (*a*) at the site of discharge onset (dark gray). Excitatory feedback from the site of onset to the site of plateau activity (*b*) may contribute to sustaining plateau activity. As plateau activity continues, onset activity accelerates. The excitatory drive from the site of plateau activity to the site of onset may also be amplified by local reciprocal excitation (between the dark gray cells) to produce ramplike onset activity, culminating in an epileptiform discharge.

aptic transmission may be less critical for ictal-like discharges. Thus, the ictal- and interictal-like discharges start along a common pathway and then diverge. How these two forms of epileptiform activity bifurcate along different trajectories following plateau activity remains an open question, but further investigation will be aided by the precise knowledge of the locations where the initial events are seen.

The PC is important in the study of epilepsy because of its extraordinarily high seizure susceptibility, along with the high excitability of the En and deep layers of adjoining neocortex. Another reason for focusing attention on the PC is its anatomical relation to other regions to which seizures are known to spread. The dense projections from the PC to neocortical regions involved in temporal lobe seizures closely parallel projections from the En.[26] These pathways provide a means for discharges generated by the mechanisms investigated here to spread over a substantial portion of the cerebral cortex.

REFERENCES

1. GRINVALD, A., A. MANKER & M. SEGAL. 1982. Visualization of the spread of electrical activity in rat hippocampal slices by voltage-sensitive optical probes. J. Physiol. **333:** 269–291.
2. GRINVALD, A., R.D. FROSTIG, E. LIEKE & R. HILDESHEIM. 1988. Optical imaging of neuronal activity. Physiol. Rev. **68:** 1285–1366.
3. WU, J.Y. & L.B. COHEN. 1993. Fast multisite optical measurements of membrane potential. *In* Fluorescent and Luminescent Probes for Biological Activity, pp. 389–404. Academic Press. New York/London.
4. ALBOWITZ, B., U. KUHNT & L. EHRENREICH. 1990. Optical recording of epileptiform voltage changes in the neocortical slice. Exp. Brain Res. **81:** 241–256.
5. COLOM, L.V. & P. SAGGAU. 1994. Spontaneous interictal-like activity originates in multiple areas of the CA2–CA3 region of hippocampal slices. J. Neurophysiol. **71:** 1574–1585.
6. LONDON, J.A., L.B. COHEN & J.Y. WU. 1989. Optical recordings of the cortical response to whisker stimulation before and after the addition of an epileptogenic agent. J. Neurosci. **9:** 2182–2190.
7. SUTOR, R., J.J. HABLITZ, R. RUCKER & G. TEN BRUGGENCATE. 1994. Spread of epileptiform activity in the immature rat neocortex studied with voltage sensitive dyes and laser scanning microscopy. J. Neurophysiol. **72:** 1756–1768.
8. LOSCHER, W. & U. EBERT. 1996. The role of the piriform cortex in kindling. Prog. Neurobiol. **50:** 427–481.
9. PIREDDA, S. & K. GALE. 1985. A crucial epileptogenic site in the deep prepiriform cortex. Nature **317:** 623–625.
10. RACINE, R.J., M. MOSHER & E.W. KAIRISS. 1988. The role of the pyriform cortex in the generation of interictal spikes in the kindled preparation. Brain Res. **454:** 251–263.
11. HOFFMAN, W.H. & L.B. HABERLY. 1989. Bursting induces persistent all-or-none EPSPs by an NMDA-dependent process in piriform cortex. J. Neurosci. **9:** 206–215.
12. McINTYRE, D.C. & R.K.S. WONG. 1986. Cellular and synaptic properties of amygdala-kindled pyriform cortex *in vitro*. J. Neurophysiol. **55:** 1295–1307.
13. HOFFMAN, W.H. & L.B. HABERLY. 1991. Bursting-induced epileptiform EPSPs in slices of piriform cortex are generated by deep cells. J. Neurosci. **11:** 2021–2031.
14. HOFFMAN, W.H. & L.B. HABERLY. 1993. Role of synaptic excitation in the generation of bursting-induced epileptiform potentials in the endopiriform nucleus and piriform cortex. J. Neurophysiol. **70:** 2550–2561.
15. DEMIR, R., L.B. HABERLY & M.B. JACKSON. 1998. Voltage imaging of epileptiform activity in slices from rat piriform cortex: onset and propagation. J. Neurophysiol. **80:** 2727–2742.
16. DEMIR, R., L.B. HABERLY & M.B. JACKSON. 1999. Sustained and accelerating activity at two discrete sites generates epileptiform discharges in slices of piriform cortex. J. Neurosci. **19:** 1294–1306.
17. JACKSON, M.B. & H.E. SCHARFMAN. 1996. Positive feedback from hilar mossy cells to granule cells in the dentate gyrus revealed by voltage-sensitive dye and microelectrode recording. J. Neurophysiol. **76:** 601–616.
18. MILES, R., R.D. TRAUB & R.K.S. WONG. 1988. Spread of synchronous firing in longitudinal slices from the CA3 region of the hippocampus. J. Neurophysiol. **60:** 1481–1496.
19. HOFFMAN, W.H. & L.B. HABERLY. 1996. Kindling-induced epileptiform potentials in piriform cortex slices originate in the underlying endopiriform nucleus. J. Neurophysiol. **76:** 1430–1438.

20. DEMIR, R., L.B. HABERLY & M.B. JACKSON. 1999. Sustained plateau activity precedes and can generate ictal-like discharges in slices from rat piriform cortex. J. Neurosci. **19:** 10738–10746.
21. TRAUB, R.D. & R. MILES. 1991. Neuronal Networks of the Hippocampus. Cambridge University Press. London/New York.
22. DEMIR, R., L.B. HABERLY & M.B. JACKSON. 2000. Characteristics of plateau activity during the latent period prior to epileptiform discharges from rat piriform cortex. J. Neurophysiol. **83:** 1088–1098.
23. TRAUB, R.D., R. MILES & R.K.S. WONG. 1989. Model of the origin of rhythmic population oscillations in the hippocampal slice. Science **243:** 1319–1325.
24. KONNERTH, A., U. HEINEMANN & Y. YAARI. 1986. Nonsynaptic epileptogenesis in the mammalian hippocampus *in vitro*. I. Development of seizure-like activity in low extracellular calcium. J. Neurophysiol. **56:** 409–423.
25. TAYLOR, C.P. & F.E. DUDEK. 1982. Synchronous neural discharges in rat hippocampal slices without active chemical synapses. Science **218:** 810–812.
26. BEHAN, M. & L.B. HABERLY. 1999. Intrinsic and efferent connections of the endopiriform nucleus in rat. J. Comp. Neurol. **408:** 532–548.

Computational Modeling of Entorhinal Cortex

MICHAEL E. HASSELMO,[a,d] ERIK FRANSEN,[b,e] CLAYTON DICKSON,[c,f]
AND ANGEL A. ALONSO[c,f]

[a]*Department of Psychology, Boston University, Boston, Massachusetts 02215, USA*

[b]*Department of Numerical Analysis and Computing Science,
Royal Institute of Technology, Stockholm, Sweden*

[c]*Montreal Neurological Institute, McGill University, Montreal, Quebec, Canada*

ABSTRACT: Computational modeling provides a means for linking the physiological and anatomical characteristics of entorhinal cortex at a cellular level to the functional role of this region in behavior. We have developed detailed simulations of entorhinal cortical neurons and networks, with an emphasis on the role of acetylcholine in entorhinal cortical function. Computational modeling suggests that when acetylcholine levels are high, this sets appropriate dynamics for the storage of stimuli during performance of delayed matching tasks. In particular, acetylcholine activates a calcium-sensitive nonspecific cation current which provides an intrinsic cellular mechanism which could maintain neuronal activity across a delay period. Simulations demonstrate how this phenomena could underlie entorhinal cortex delay activity as described in previous unit recordings.[191,164] Acetylcholine also induces theta rhythm oscillations which may be appropriate for timing of afferent input to be encoded in hippocampus and for extraction of individual stored sequences from multiple stored sequences. Lower levels of acetylcholine may allow sharp wave dynamics which can reactivate associations encoded in hippocampus and drive the formation of additional traces in hippocampus and entorhinal cortex during consolidation.

INTRODUCTION

Experimental data about the parahippocampal region is available on a number of different levels, including detailed anatomical descriptions,[23,24,127] physiological characterization of intrinsic properties using entorhinal slice preparations,[96–98,39] correlations between unit spiking activity and behavior,[191,164] and lesion effects in rats and primates.[117,126] Computational modeling provides a means for bridging across these different levels of experimental analysis, for linking data at a physiological and anatomical level to the possible functional role of the parahippocampal region.

We have been developing detailed compartmental simulations of entorhinal cortical neurons based on data obtained from the Alonso laboratory. Initially, we have

[d]Address for correspondence: Dr. Michael E. Hasselmo, Dept. of Psychology, Boston University, 64 Cummington St., Boston, MA 02215. Tel.: (617) 353-1397; fax: (617) 353-1424.

e-mail: hasselmo@berg.bu.edu

[e]e-mail: erikf@sans.kth.se

[f]e-mail: mdao@music.mcgill.ca

focused on specific features of the intrinsic properties of layer II neurons, and their potential functional role in network dynamics. Here we will focus on three major topics: (1) Simulations of layer II pyramidal neurons demonstrate the potential role of muscarinic cholinergic activation of a calcium-sensitive nonspecific cation current for allowing neurons to maintain self-sustained spiking activity during performance of delay tasks. This research will be described in the first portion of this paper. (2) Cholinergic modulation induces theta rhythm oscillations in both parahippocampal structures and the hippocampus. We will briefly describe simulations of layer II stellate neurons used to analyze the membrane currents underlying subthreshold oscillations, which may be important for generation and synchronization of network oscillatory dynamics in the theta range.[41,53,54] In addition, we will describe how theta oscillations might interact with a comparison function in region CA1 and subiculum, for enhancing encoding and retrieval of individual stored associations from among multiple stored associations. (3) Lower levels of acetylcholine may set appropriate dynamics for consolidation, allowing sharp wave activity generated in hippocampus or layer V of entorhinal cortex to reactivate memories for encoding of additional representations in the hippocampus and parahippocampal regions. Models demonstrate how changes in network dynamics associated with lowering of acetylcholine levels may be appropriate for setting dynamics for sharp wave generation.

CHOLINERGIC MODULATION AND MEMORY BUFFERING IN ENTORHINAL CORTEX

The entorhinal cortex and perirhinal cortex appear to play an important role in the formation of episodic memories. Lesions of the hippocampus alone cause anterograde amnesia, as tested with tasks such as free recall and paired associate memory.[62,193,194,162] But these effects on episodic memory tasks appear to be stronger in cases where portions of the entorhinal and perirhinal cortex have also been affected.[155,149] Blockade of cholinergic effects by systemic injections of the muscarinic cholinergic antagonist scopolamine also appears to impair the encoding of new episodic memories in humans. Scopolamine strongly impairs encoding of new words into memory for subsequent free recall, without affecting recall of words learned before injections of scopolamine.[36,60,142] Scopolamine does not impair simple measures of short-term memory such as digit span[20] and the recency component of a serial position curve,[36] but does impair performance on the Brown-Peterson task—a short-term memory task with a distractor during the delay.[12] Similarly, damage to the hippocampus does not impair digit span[34] or the recency component of a serial position curve,[10] but does impair performance in tasks requiring longer retention of stimuli, such as a delayed nonmatch to sample task.[161] The important role of entorhinal cortex in encoding of information can be seen in fMRI studies which demonstrate that level of activity in entorhinal cortex during encoding of sets of five words correlates with subsequent retrieval performance for those individual five word sets.[49] This suggests that slow changes in modulatory state in entorhinal cortex may determine the efficacy of encoding within this system.

The delayed nonmatch to sample task (DNMS) has been used extensively as a test of memory function in studies of lesion effects in monkeys.[57,192,196,195,8,101,117,22] In this task, monkeys see an individual object from a large set of stimuli during the sample phase. After a delay, the monkey is presented with two objects, one of which was seen previously. The monkey must respond to the object which they did not previously see in order to get a reward. Hippocampal lesions cause impairments in this task,[192] but the impairment is much more severe if lesions include damage to surrounding cortical areas.[195,117] In fact, adding hippocampal and parahippocampal lesions to perirhinal lesions may actually reduce the deficit.[117] Lesions of parahippocampal and perirhinal cortex alone cause a severe impairment,[196] whereas lesions of entorhinal cortex alone cause a less severe memory impairment which decreases over time, potentially due to collateral growth of perirhinal input to region CA1.[101] Entorhinal and perirhinal cortex ablations also impair performance in delayed match to sample tasks.[58] All these impairments appear at longer delays (e.g., 1 minute, 10 minutes) but not short delays (0.5, 1, or 3 seconds).[58,8] This is consistent with the notion that entorhinal cortex and perirhinal cortex are important for maintaining memory across many seconds. See the paper by Murray for more extensive discussion of this work on lesion effects.

A variant of the task has been developed for research on rats in the Eichenbaum laboratory.[136,191] This task has been described more extensively in the paper by Eichenbaum, and is called the continuous delayed nonmatch to sample task (cDNMS). In this task, rats are presented with a series of single odors. For each odor, they must respond on the basis of the comparison with the odor presented on the previous trial. If the odor on the previous trial was different than the odor on the current trial, then they can respond with a nose poke to receive a water reward. If the odor on the previous trial was the same as the odor on the current trial, then they must withhold their nose poke response. Lesions of the entorhinal cortex and perirhinal cortex cause impairments of performance in the cDNMS task in rats at long delays (30 seconds and 60 seconds), but not at shorter delays.[136]

Entorhinal neurons show responses which could mediate memory function in these tasks. Some entorhinal neurons show decreased responses to familiar stimuli[21,48] similar to the suppression of response to repeated (match) stimuli observed in inferotemporal cortex.[121,118] This match suppression may be an automatic process for any repeated stimulus, whereas match enhancement may be an active process occurring only for a match with the stimulus seen as sample.[118] Recent studies have shown both enhancement and suppression of responses to matching stimuli as well as sustained activity during the delay period of the DNMS task in rats.[191] In rats, sustained activity during the delay was found primarily in 15% of entorhinal cortex neurons, but less than 3% of neurons in perirhinal cortex or subiculum. These delay responses sometimes showed selectivity for individual odors, and could therefore underlie the storage of individual odors.[191] Changes in neuronal response during matching have also been observed in hippocampal region CA1 of rats,[137] and hippocampal neurons have been shown to demonstrate sustained activity during task delays.[66] These results are generally consistent with recordings from neurons of the entorhinal cortex of monkeys, which have been performed in a delayed match to sample task in which different numbers of visual stimuli are presented as distractors between the initial sample stimulus and its subsequent reappearance as a match stimulus[164] That study also demonstrated neurons which showed stimulus-selective activity persisting during the delay period, as well as some neurons showing either match enhancement or match suppression. See the paper by Suzuki for more extensive description of this research.

Cholinergic modulation in the entorhinal cortex may be particularly important for performance in delayed nonmatch and delayed match to sample tasks. Systemic injections of the muscarinic cholinergic antagonists has been shown to impair performance on recognition memory tasks at longer delays in monkeys, while sparing performance at zero second delay—this occurs with both the antagonists scopolamine[11] and atropine.[140] Injections of scopolamine appear to impair the encoding of new stimuli for recognition but not retrieval of stimuli learned before scopolamine injection.[2,167] Systemic injections of scopolamine also impair arm choice behavior in an 8-arm radial maze in rats when there is a delay between the individual choices.[16] The locus of cholinergic effect has been tested with localized injection of cholinergic antagonists in monkeys. Tang, Mishkin, and Aigner[167] demonstrated that infusion of scopolamine into perirhinal cortex before encoding impairs performance on a recognition memory task, whereas infusion into adjacent structures did not cause impaired performance. The location of the perirhinal infusion cannula in this experiment was probably close enough to entorhinal cortex to affect that structure as well.[167] Microdialysis shows a 41% increase in acetylcholine levels in perirhinal cortex during performance of this visual recognition task.[166]

These data suggest that acetylcholine plays an important role in regulating neuronal activity patterns during memory task performance. Cholinergic modulation causes changes in the intrinsic properties of entorhinal neurons which may set a dynamical state appropriate for buffering of activity.[96,97,39] This could be important both for maintaining memories during the delay of a DNMS task and for maintaining memories while they are encoded in the hippocampus. Cholinergic effects could enhance sustained activity during a delay period, or underlie match enhancement.[191,164] Consistent with this hypothesis are the data showing that ACh effects in other cortical structures might enhance the encoding of sensory input, and may alter or enhance the subsequent response to these sensory stimuli.[170,45,116,115,156]

Cholinergic Modulation of Plateau Potentials in Nonstellate Cells

In collaboration with Dr. Alonso's laboratory, we have used the GENESIS simulation package[17] to model intrinsic properties of neurons in layer II of entorhinal cortex. We have developed biophysical compartmental models of layer II nonstellate (pyramidal-like) neurons, focusing on how acetylcholine causes sustained plateau potentials and rhythmic bursting in these cells. These phenomena might underlie sustained activity and match enhancement during performance of delayed nonmatch to sample tasks.[191,164] The model used Hodgkin-Huxley representations of a range of intrinsic currents which underlie generation of action potentials, and additional phenomena such as spike frequency adaptation, as shown in FIGURE 1.

In physiological recordings from nonstellate cells in brain slice preparations,[96,97] application of the cholinergic agonist carbachol causes long-term depolarizations, which have been termed plateau potentials. Modeling demonstrates that plateau potentials could arise from cholinergic activation of calcium-dependent nonspecific

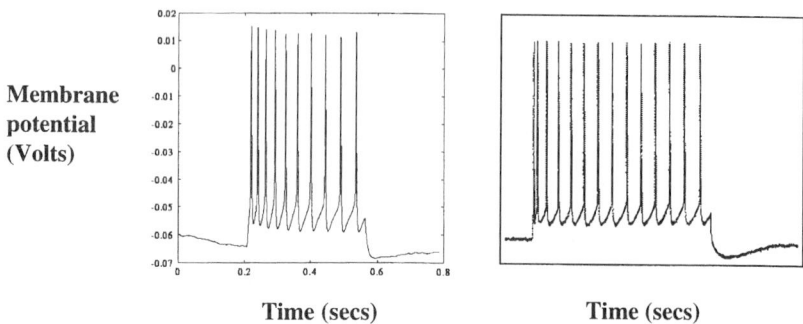

Membrane potential (Volts)

Time (secs)   Time (secs)

FIGURE 1. *Right*: Spike frequency adaptation in response to a sustained current injection to a layer II nonstellate cell. *Left*: Simulated layer II nonstellate cell. This cell contains a full range of voltage and calcium-dependent currents, including the fast sodium and delayed rectifier potassium currents underlying spiking activity, and the calcium-dependent potassium current which underlies spike frequency adaptation and the slow afterhyperpolarization.

cation currents (ICAN). The intracellular calcium which activates these channels could come from two sources: (1) release of calcium from intracellular stores via muscarinic activation of the IP3 pathway; and/or (2) calcium influx via voltage gated channels. Cholinergic activation of the ICAN current causes the membrane potential to depolarize in response to any intracellular calcium. When the cell is further depolarized with a current injection in the presence of cholinergic modulation, then the cell can go into a state of sustained activation characterized by repeated periods of spike generation with intermittent periods of less depolarization. The self-sustained generation of spiking activity results from the following cycle: (1) each action potential causes influx of calcium through voltage-sensitive calcium channels, (2) the increase in intracellular calcium causes further activation of the ICAN current, (3) the activation of the ICAN current depolarizes the cell sufficiently to cause generation of another action potential. Physiological traces and computational modeling of the phases of rhythmic spike generation during plateau potentials is shown in FIGURE 2. This provides a mechanism which would be ideal for performance in the delayed nonmatch to sample task. In the presence of cholinergic modulation, neurons depolarized by afferent input will respond in a sustained manner suitable for maintaining that representation. In contrast, neurons will not fire in a sustained manner if they receive insufficient depolarization from afferent input, or if cholinergic modulation is not present. While this example shows experimental data and simulation of pyramidal cell activity, the stellate cells in layer II have also been shown to generate self-sustained spiking activity in response to cholinergic activation combined with depolarizing current injection.

The properties of the ICAN current underlying plateau potential generation provide an intrinsic mechanism ideal for maintaining memory-related activity in the entorhinal cortex during short delay periods. Thus, the activation of ICAN by cholinergic modulation may be important for the entorhinal cortex unit activity observed during the delay period of delayed match or delayed nonmatch to sample tasks.[191,164]

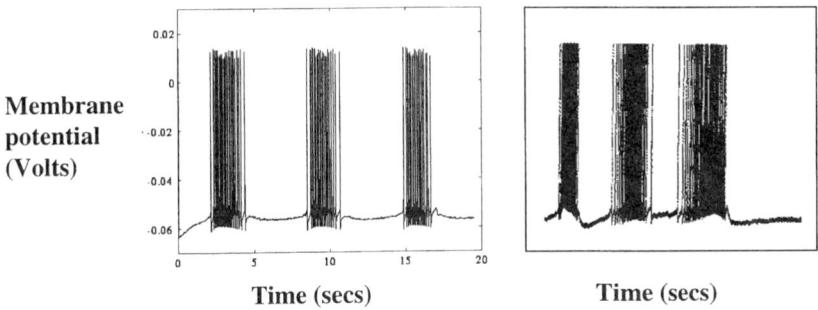

Membrane
potential
(Volts)

Time (secs)   Time (secs)

FIGURE 2. *Right*: Physiological recording showing a sustained plateau potential in an entorhonal cortex layer II nonstellate cell.[97] *Left*: Sustained spiking activity in a simulated entorhinal nonstellate cell, with Hodgkin-Huxley currents mediating spiking activity. The simulation includes muscarinic receptor activation of the calcium sensitive nonspecific cation currrent (ICAN), which causes depolarization. The sustained spiking activity depends upon additional extrinsic activation of the neuron by current injection, which brings the cell over threshold and induces sustained oscillatory depolarization. The activity is sustained because each spike causes calcium influx through voltage-sensitive calcium channels which causes activation of the ICAN current which depolarizes the cell sufficiently to generate subsequent spiking, allowing the cycle to repeat. This effectively simulates oscillatory bursting activity induced in entorhinal cells by cholinergic activation combined with intracellular current injection.

Simulation of Entorhinal Cortex Unit Activity
during Delayed Nonmatch to Sample Tasks

The simulations of single cells and slice dynamics described above provide a framework for simulation of neural activity during performance of a delayed non-matching to sample task. Cholinergic effects on the intrinsic properties of neurons could alter network dynamics in a manner which allows the network to mediate performance of delayed matching tasks. In particular, the induction of plateau potentials might allow individual neurons to hold information about the particular odor viewed in a previous sample trial. In the presence of acetylcholine, neurons respond to depolarization with strong plateau potentials. If there is an increase in acetylcholine levels when a particular stimulus is viewed, this will cause neurons activated by that stimulus to hold their activity levels during the delay period, allowing a matching function at the end of the delay. Thus, cholinergic modulation would be well suited to account for data from the Eichenbaum laboratory[191] showing that a percentage of neurons show activity during the delay period in the cDNMS task. These cells were seen most frequently in the lateral entorhinal cortex. In some cases, these neurons would show enhanced stimulus selective activity during the end of the sample period which would be maintained throughout a three second delay period until the next stimulus was presented.

Even without persistent spiking activity, cholinergic modulation of ICAN could mediate memory type function in the form of match enhancement. In a number of studies, some neurons have been demonstrated to show enhancement of response to a stimulus which matches the preceding sample stimulus, as compared to the same

High ACh   Low ACh

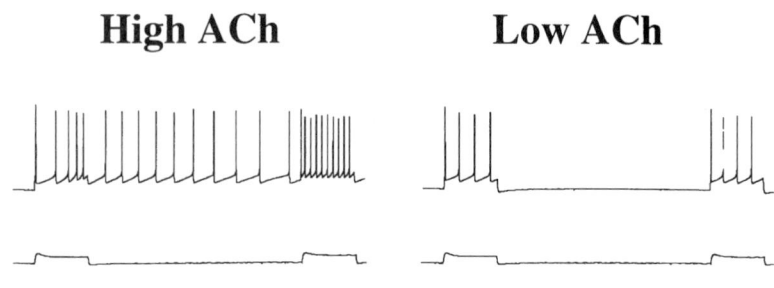

500 msec

FIGURE 3. Simulation of delay activity and match enhancement during cDNMS task due to cholinergic enhancement of ICAN current. *Top traces* show responses to two 600-msec suprathreshold current injections with a 2400-msec delay between injections. *Bottom traces* show responses to subthreshold current injection. *Left*: Cholinergic enhancement of ICAN current allows sustained delay activity and match enhancement. Suprathreshold depolarizing input causes spiking in the neuron. This causes influx of calcium through voltage-sensitive calcium channels, which causes further activation of ICAN. This causes depolarization of the neuron sufficient to cause action potential generation even after the end of the period of current injection. This new spike causes further calcium influx which causes further ICAN activation. Thus, a cycle of self-sustained spiking activity is maintained during the delay period. Afferent input to the same neuron after the delay period is over will now evoke a larger response than during the initial stimulus period, corresponding to match enhancement. *Right*: Without cholinergic enhancement of ICAN, the neuron responds to suprathreshold depolarization with the same number of spikes before and after the delay. Lack of regenerative ICAN activation prevents match enhancement from occurring.

stimulus when it does not match the preceding sample stimulus.[118,164,191] This could provide another neurobiological mechanism for performing matching which does not depend upon maintaining activity during the delay.

Simulation of the ICAN current provides an intrinsic mechanism for both sustained delay activity and match enhancement, as shown in FIGURE 3. In this figure, the cDNMS task is simulated with a 600-msec current injection representing afferent input to the entorhinal cortex during sniffing of one odor during the stimulus period of the task, followed by a 2400-msec delay period with no current injection, followed by a 600-msec current injection representing afferent input to the entorhinal cortex during sniffing of the same odor during the next stimulus period (corresponding to a match condition). The traces on the left show how a neuron responds after simulated cholinergic activation of the ICAN current. A subthreshold input (bottom) does not cause spiking in the cell, and therefore does not cause any sustained activity during the delay period, but a suprathreshold input (top) causes spiking. This spiking during the stimulus period causes calcium influx through voltage-sensitive calcium channels, this calcium influx causes further activation of the ICAN current, which depolarizes the membrane sufficient to cause another action potential even after the end of the depolarizing current injection. Each subsequent spike causes sufficient depolarization to induce another spike, allowing self-sustained spiking activity throughout the delay period until the next stimulus is given. When the second presentation of the same stimulus occurs, the cell is already depolarized by ICAN activation, such that it responds to the "match" stimulus with considerably greater spiking than the initial response to that same stimulus. A comparison of this "match" period with the preceding stimulus period would correspond to the match enhancement observed in experimental work.[191] Thus, ICAN provides mechanisms appropriate for both the sustained delay activity and the match enhancement phenomenon. This mechanism is similar to the afterdepolarization mechanism proposed for short-term memory on different gamma cycles of the theta rhythm.[201]

In contrast, the traces on the right side of the figure show the response of the neuron without cholinergic enhancement of ICAN. The subthreshold response is the same, but the suprathreshold response shows how the neuron will spike during the initial stimulus period, but the absence of ICAN activation prevents the neuron from showing sustained depolarization and spike generation during the delay period. In addition, the absence of a self-sustained depolarization during the delay prevents the neuron from generating increased spiking activity during the match stimulus. Thus, it fires the same number of spikes in response to the match stimulus that it did in response to the previous input. Thus, in this framework, cholinergic modulation is important to the intrinsic mechanisms for sustained activity.

If cholinergic activation of ICAN is important to provide intrinsic mechanisms for self-sustained spiking activity, then blockade of this cholinergic activation should prevent sustained spiking activity during the delay period and match enhancement. This effect of muscarinic antagonists could underlie the behavioral impairments in delayed matching tasks seen with systemic injections of muscarinic antagonists.[11,140] In addition to this role in short-term memory function, sustained activity in entorhinal cortex could also be very important for effective encoding of long-term representations through synaptic modification in the hippocampal formation. The blockade of sustained entorhinal activity by muscarinic antagonists could also underlie the impairments of encoding for subsequent recognition or recall observed with local infusion of the antagonist scopolamine into perirhinal cortex in monkeys[167] or with systemic injections of scopolamine in human subjects.[36,60,142]

In addition to the match enhancement described above, many researchers have described suppression of the response to the second viewing of a particular stimulus in entorhinal cortex[48,164] and inferotemporal cortex.[118,119] Match suppression could reflect lateral inhibition from neurons undergoing match enhancement—usually both types of responses are reported. It is also possible that during the initial viewing of a stimulus, cholinergic modulation is at high levels, whereas subsequent viewing of a matching stimulus might cause feedback suppression of cholinergic modulation which decreases the neuronal activity in response to the stimulus.[158] This type of match suppression should be sensitive to cholinergic blockade. In contrast, match suppression might also arise from the spike frequency accomodation properties of individual neurons, or the self-organization of feedforward connections with a combination of synaptic enhancement and synaptic depression.[158] These mechanisms might be less sensitive to cholinergic blockade, and this is supported by the absence of change in match suppression with local infusion of cholinergic antagonists during recording in inferotemporal cortex.[119] In these cases, match suppression may be more sensitive to increases in cholinergic influences due to local infusion of the acetylcholinesterase blocker physostigmine. Some studies describe an active reset mechanism such that consecutive presentation of a stimulus as a sample does not induce match suppression, even if the intervening match presentations show suppression.[120,121] This phenomena could arise if spike frequency accomodation mediates match suppression and higher levels of acetylcholine during the sample phase suppresses this accomodation. In this case, scopolamine should block the active reset mechanism.

In previous network simulations from this laboratory, neuronal activity during matching of stimuli has been analyzed extensively. In contrast to the intrinsic properties presented above, these simulations used changes in synaptic connectivity to mediate matching function. In a simulation of piriform cortex, it was shown that enhancement of synaptic connectivity during the sample period allows the network to respond more strongly to a subsequent stimulus matching the sample stimulus.[102] This enhancement of activity associated with matching has also been analyzed in network simulations of hippocampal region CA1[74] and region CA3.[75] In these simulations, cholinergic enhancement of synaptic modification is specifically important for allowing subsequent enhancement of response to matching stimuli, in contrast to nonmatching stimuli. Thus, as with the intrinsic properties described above, this match enhancement should be decreased by blockade of muscarinic cholinergic receptors by the antagonist scopolamine.

THETA RHYTHM GENERATION AND COMPARISON
FUNCTION IN HIPPOCAMPUS

Acetylcholine may also enhance memory storage by enhancing the theta rhythm, a 3–10 Hz oscillation observed in the EEG of hippocampus and entorhinal cortex when a rat actively explores its environment.[63,31,110] Theta rhythm has also been reported in medial temporal areas in monkeys[163] and humans.[199] Theta rhythm oscillations are strongest in the superficial layers of entorhinal cortex,[3,4,31] and the entorhinal cortex and hippocampus show strong interactions during theta rhythm oscillations. Current source density analysis demonstrates that entorhinal input to the hippocampus is a major driving force for theta rhythm oscillations.[29] Thus, the mechanisms for generation and synchronization of theta rhythm oscillations are vital to understanding the interaction of entorhinal cortex with hippocampus. Input from the medial septum and vertical limb of the diagonal band provides a prominent driving force for the theta rhythm in the hippocampus.[168] The entorhinal cortex also receives strong anatomical input from these structures.[6] This innervation consists of both cholinergic and GABAergic fibers.[99] The GABAergic input appears to selectively target inhibitory interneurons, and may drive theta oscillations through rhythmic disinhibition within hippocampus and entorhinal cortex.[168] However, the cellular effects of the cholinergic input also strongly contribute to the theta rhythm, as lesions of the medial septum eliminate theta rhythm in the entorhinal cortex,[123] and the AChE blocker physostigmine enhances theta here.[4,37] Intracellular recording from slice preparations of the entorhinal cortex have demonstrated cholinergic induction of subthreshold oscillations and rhythmic spike firing which could contribute to the theta rhythm oscillations observed on a systems level.[7,95,96]

Subthreshold Membrane Potential Oscillations in Stellate Cells

We have developed models of subthreshold oscillations in layer II stellate cells. These subthreshold oscillations may enhance theta oscillations in entorhinal cortex which could synchronize input for optimal encoding in the hippocampus. Most previous work on subthreshold oscillations in neurons has focused on a potential interaction between a persistent sodium channel and a slow potassium conductance, as in models of subthreshold oscillations in somatosensory cortex,[177] frontal cortex,[64] and amygdala.[138] Previous simulations of entorhinal cortex stellate cells have used models with this mechanism in a bifurcation analysis of oscillations[178] and simulations analyzing the role of channel noise.[179] However, recent data (Dickson *et al.*, in press) suggest that interactions between the persistent sodium current and the hyperpolarization-activated inward current (IH) are necessary and sufficient for the generation of membrane potential oscillations in entorhinal stellate cells.

The biophysical simulations shown here were developed using recent voltage clamp data on the slowly inactivating "persistent type" Na-current,[203] along with voltage-clamp data on the hyperpolarization activated H-current (Dickson *et al.*, in press). The model was utilized to simulate current clamp phenomena recorded in entorhinal cortex stellate cells[98] (see also Dickson *et al.*, in press), including the "sag" in membrane potential during hyperpolarizing current steps and the subthreshold membrane potential oscillations.

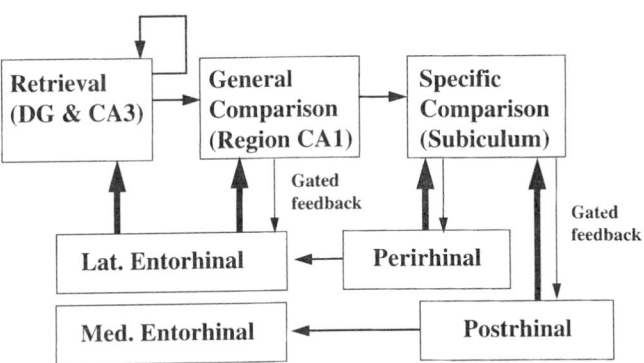

FIGURE 4. Schematic representation of comparison function at different stages of feedback from hippocampal region CA3 to parahippocampal cortices. In this framework, input from parahippocampal regions activates representations in the dentate gyrus and region CA3 that mediate retrieval based on previously encoded representations. The activity caused by this retrieval then spreads to region CA1, where it can be compared with direct afferent input from entorhinal cortex. If the afferent input is familiar, it will evoke familiar representations in region CA3 which should then match the afferent input from entorhinal cortex. If the afferent input is novel, the initial retrieval from CA3 may be based on related memories, and might not accurately match the entorhinal input. This stage of comparison may be more coarse, as region CA1 sends more distributed collaterals which could be representative of general context. If the inputs match, activity can flow on to the subiculum, where a more specific comparison process may evaluate the detailed features of the retrieval before this activity can spread along the more localized connections from subiculum back to perirhinal and postrhinal cortices.

The simulations show that an interplay between IH and INaP is sufficient to account for the generation of membrane potential oscillations in layer II stellate cells, the persistent sodium current increases during the depolarizing phase of oscillations, followed by a decrease in IH during the hyperpolarizing phase of oscillations. Simulation of the blockade of IH by ZD7288 effectively prevented generation of the subthreshold membrane potential oscillations in the model. We have also modeled subthreshold membrane potential oscillations in a more detailed simulation containing a full range of additional membrane currents, including the Na^+ and K^+ currents responsible for fast action potentials, a high-threshold Ca^{2+} current, a calcium-dependent K^+ current, a fast calcium- and voltage-dependent K^+ current, a slowly inactivating Ca-independent K^+ current, and a nonspecific Ca^{2+}-dependent cationic current. These additional currents allow testing of the parameters influencing spike clustering.

Functional Role of Theta Oscillations and Comparison for Disambiguating Stored Sequences

Considerable work has focused on the mechanisms of generation of theta rhythm oscillations, but few models have addressed the functional role of these oscillations. Network simulations of theta oscillatory dynamics have demonstrated that these oscillations could assist in the effective encoding and retrieval of overlapping pattern sequences in sparsely connected networks. Recent modeling has focused on encoding of sequences of activity in region CA3.[175,176,73,200,204–206] This sequence storage is easier to implement in fully connected networks than in networks where connectivity approaches the biologically observed percentages. For low connection probabilities, sequence encoding and retrieval is more effective when additional neurons not directly activated by afferent input are active and become associated with segments of the encoded sequence. These additional neurons are referred to as "local context units."[175,176,200] Without theta rhythm oscillations, it can be difficult to gradually recruit these additional neurons, as their background activation then depends only on variation in synaptic connectivity and intrinsic parameters. Too many units tend to be recruited initially, and if these undergo adaptation subsequently too few units are available. In contrast, with theta rhythm oscillations of the full network, individual subpopulations of units can be progressively recruited in a more gradual manner. As the theta oscillation progresses, changes in the average level of inhibition and depolarization across the network allow a small subset of units to fire. These prevent firing of other units through fast $GABA_A$ inhibition. Then on the next cycle, the units which previously fired are prevented from firing by the afterhyperpolarization due to the calcium-dependent potassium current. Without theta rhythm oscillations, this might cause difficulties in recruiting new neurons, but with theta rhythm oscillations a broader range of inhibition and depolarization levels are sampled. Thus, slightly later in the cycle a different set of neurons can now be activated, which then inhibit other neurons. In this manner, progressive cycles of theta more effectively pick out different subgroups of neurons to participate as local context units. This type of function appears to have been obtained in the Levy models through normalization of network activity. But that normalization property is difficult to obtain in more realistic simulations, and may be more effectively obtained via theta oscillations. In previous simulations, systematic changes in $GABA_B$ receptor activation were shown to be important for encoding of new sequences in the network.[175,176, 205] Analytical work and recent simulation suggest that theta oscillations may be important for sampling across a wide range of values for multiple different parameters, including strength of feedback inhibition, strength of feedback excitation, and depolarization of pyramidal cells.

Theta might play the same sort of role during retrieval dynamics. Analytical work and computational models of region CA3[204,205] demonstrate that when multiple sequence associations are stored in the network, theta rhythm changes in dynamics can assist in disambiguation of stored sequences. In these studies, a fixed strength of excitatory intrinsic connections makes it difficult to retrieve one sequence without activating other overlapping sequences. In contrast, a modeled change in strength of excitatory intrinsic connections allows a sequence picked out with stronger afferent bias to become sufficiently active that it dominates the attractor state before other sequences are activated.

This previous work focused on retrieval dynamics within region CA3, but the same type of principles may be important for setting the learning dynamics of hippocampus or gating of feedback to parahippocampal regions. A number of researchers have suggested that the direct afferent input to region CA1 from entorhinal cortex would allow a comparison of the retrieval from region CA3 with the direct afferent input.[74,30,69,78,197] This comparison function has been used to determine whether an input is novel or familiar, because novel patterns will have a mismatch between the output of region CA3 and the input from entorhinal cortex.[74] Familiar patterns would have a match between region CA3 output and entorhinal cortex input, resulting in stronger activity (match enhancement). Match enhancement does occur in some region CA1 neurons.[136,137,67] This match enhancement could reduce modulatory input from the medial septum to put the network into more of a "retrieval" state when there is a consistent match between retrieval and afferent input.[74,69] Physiological data does support the possibility that activity of region CA1 could inhibit modulatory input from the septum.[114,43]

In addition to setting modulatory dynamics in the hippocampus, the comparison process in region CA1 could also gate the feedback to entorhinal cortex and other parahippocampal structures, as summarized in FIGURE 4. This is relevant for both the reciprocal connections between entorhinal cortex and region CA1[165] and the more recently described reciprocal connections between the subiculum and the perirhinal and postrhinal cortices.[127] This gating could occur through the same comparison process used for the matching function in Hasselmo and Schnell.[74] In that paper, entorhinal input to region CA1 alone was subthreshold, but when this input matched the output pattern from region CA3, the neurons could fire. A functional network of this sort would only allow propagation of activity back to parahippocampal regions when the retrieval proved sufficiently accurate relative to the direct afferent input—in a sense, this would provide a sort of test of the validity of hippocampal retrieval. The transition from more collateralized connectivity arising from region CA1 to more specific projections from subiculum[127] could reflect different stages of testing of the validity of retrieval—with perhaps a looser criterion of validity at the region CA1 level as compared to the subicular level. The interaction of synaptic input from entorhinal cortex with hippocampal input to the subiculum could contribute to this comparison function in the subiculum.[13]

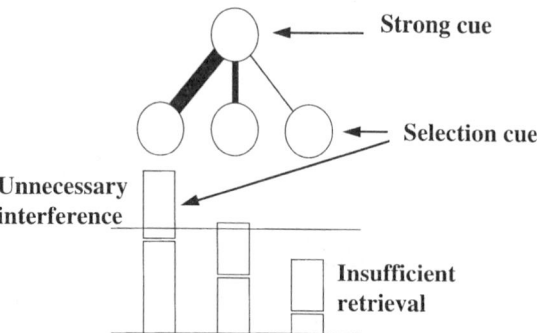

FIGURE 5. Memory retrieval must account for the fact that memories might have many different strengths dependent upon the strength of associations (as illustrated by width of connecting lines) or the number of units representing features of the memory. The retrieval cue does not have access to the strength of the individual memories. Thus, a selection cue may be sufficient to bring an intermediate size memory over threshold (*center*), but if there are other stronger memories present it may erroneously evoke related strong memories, or it may be insufficient to retrieve a weak memory. In this representation, the size of the histograms represents differences in retrieval activity due to different strengths of associations and number of features. The histograms represent three different memories which could be evoked by different appropriate selection cues. A selection cue has appropriately evoked a memory if it brings it over the threshold line.

As shown in FIGURES 5 and 6, the theta rhythm could play an important role for this comparison function, both in terms of timing the afferent input from region CA3 and entorhinal cortex to arrive with the appropriate synchrony in region CA1 and subiculum, and in terms of sampling across multiple parameter values. Memory retrieval suffers from the fact that the strength and size of a memory representation is not known when trying to cue that memory. Thus, a very strong memory might require only a very weak cue to be elicited and for comparison. A stronger cue might elicit multiple associations which would also pass through the gating process because the cue input to region CA1 and subiculum would be strong and would allow multiple neurons to cross threshold. In contrast, a weak memory would require a much stronger cue to elicit retrieval in CA3 and to pass through the gating process. The theta rhythm provides a means of allowing a cue of a single size to sample across multiple memory strengths—searching first for memories with the best match with current input, even if they are very weak, and in failing to find an optimal match, then allowing retrieval of stronger memories with a poorer match with current input. Finally, if no match is determined, then the incoming information could induce the formation of a new representation. This process would be enhanced by progressive changes in strength of excitatory transmission during different phases of the theta rhythm. Progressive changes in strength of excitatory evoked potentials have been demonstrated at different phases of theta in recordings from region CA1,[188,189] and previous studies showed progressive changes in ease of eliciting population spikes.[153,26] An effective transition through these different matching states would require resetting of theta rhythm in response to stimulus input to the phase of weak retrieval matching, to prevent a familiar stimulus from being encoded as new before

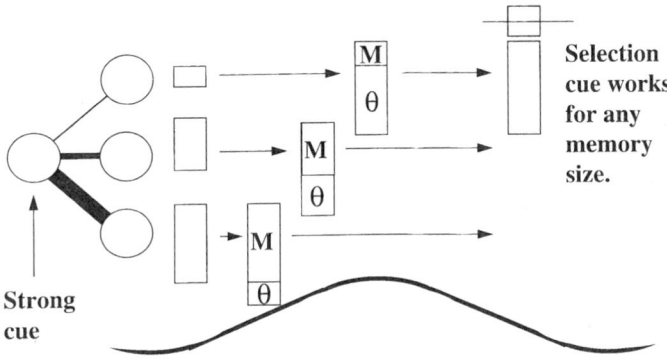

FIGURE 6. Theta rhythm oscillations provide a means for sampling across different memory strengths. Theta oscillations are associated with phasic changes in strength of synaptic transmission and depolarization of pyramidal cells. This will result in phasic changes of the magnitude of network activity, which could be seen as adding some activity level (marked with θ) to the activity evoked by a specific memory (M). This means that a selection cue of the same size can pick out memories of different strengths, as the theta oscillation will change the magnitude of activity. Once a specific memory crosses threshold due to the selection cue, feedback inhibition could prevent other stronger memory activation from interfering with this initial retrieval.

the retrieval process had been exhausted. In fact, resetting of theta rhythm phase has been observed in working memory tasks.[61]

Even without the use of a comparison process, the changes in physiological properties within each cycle of the theta rhythm could allow phasic switching between encoding and retrieval dynamics. In particular, the phase of strongest synaptic input from the entorhinal cortex differs from the phase of strongest synaptic input to stratum radiatum of region CA1 from region CA3,[29,19,18] an effect which would be enhanced by the inhibition in stratum radiatum induced by entorhinal layer III input to region CA1.[47] The phase of strong entorhinal input and weaker region stratum radiatum input could allow accurate encoding of afferent input, as long as the magnitude of long-term potentiation is strongest at that phase. In fact, physiological experiments suggest that long-term potentiation in stratum radiatum can be most effectively induced at the phase of local theta when synaptic input in stratum radiatum is weakest, though these experiments have only been performed *in vitro*[85] and in urethane anesthetized animals.[82]

LOW ACETYLCHOLINE MAY SET DYNAMICS FOR CONSOLIDATION

Lesions restricted to subregions of the hippocampal formation cause moderate anterograde memory impairments with very short retrograde memory impairments.[194,149] In contrast, lesions including entorhinal cortex and subiculum cause much more extensive gradients of retrograde amnesia.[149,129] This suggests that after initial encoding, episodic memories may be consolidated in a manner which depends upon formation of additional traces in the entorhinal cortex. In this section, we will explore the proposal that lower levels of acetylcholine may enhance consolidation of memory traces in the entorhinal cortex.

When measured by microdialysis techniques, acetylcholine shows higher levels during active waking (exploration of the environment) than during quiet waking (immobility, or behaviors such as grooming and eating).[110] ACh levels are higher during acquisition of a new behavioral task than during performance of a previously learned task.[134] In sleep, ACh levels drop to less than one third of waking levels during slow-wave sleep, then rebound dramatically during REM sleep.[92,110] Changes in ACh levels may be vital for setting dynamics of encoding versus consolidation. Theories of memory function propose initial storage in hippocampus during active waking, followed by transfer from the hippocampus to the neocortex during quiet waking or slow-wave sleep.[28,185] Cholinergic suppression of feedback from hippocampus to neocortex during waking could enhance encoding by preventing interference from previously stored memories,[199] whereas removal of this suppression during slow-wave sleep should aid consolidation by enhancing the driving influence of the hippocampus on the neocortex.[77] In support of this, evoked synaptic potentials in stratum radiatum of hippocampal region CA1 have been shown to increase during slow-wave sleep.[186,187] During the theta rhythm oscillations associated with sensory stimulation, field EPSPs are decreased by cholinergic modulation in hippocampal region CA1.[80,81] During quiet waking and slow-wave sleep, when acetylcholine levels are low, phenomena termed sharp waves spread back from hippocampus to entorhinal cortex.[27,31] These sharp waves could drive the formation of multiple memory traces.

These dynamical changes are relevant to several different clinical syndromes. Blockade of muscarinic receptors causes impairments in the encoding of new information (see Ref. 69 for review), and loss of cholinergic innervation may contribute to amnesia in Alzheimer's disease.[100] Blockade of cholinergic suppression during waking will allow a dominant influence of feedback excitation in the cortex. This might underlie the hallucinations induced by muscarinic cholinergic antagonists,[35] and associated with Lewy Body dementia—which involves a selective loss of cholinergic but not monoaminergic innervation.[141] Continuous spike and wave seizures during slow-wave sleep would be expected to distort normal consolidation mechanisms. This phenomena in children has been associated with a disintegration of cognitive capabilities such as language function.[108] Finally, depression has been associated with early onset and increased amount of REM sleep during the night, and most antidepressants very effectively suppress the acetylcholine increases necessary for REM sleep.[203] These data suggest the importance of understanding the changes in dynamics induced by acetylcholine during different stages of waking and sleep.

Network Dynamics in Entorhinal Slice Preparations

As an initial step toward understanding the function of large scale circuits, it is useful to model the network properties observed in slice preparations. In particular, cholinergic modulation has been shown to induce synchronized population activity in slice preparations of the entorhinal cortex. Simulation of these data provides a useful initial step in characterizing network dynamics. Single compartment simulations of stellate cells were incorporated in biophysical network simulations containing 1000 stellate neurons and 200 inhibitory interneurons. (The exact numbers and proportion of neurons were not crucial to the dynamical properties of the network, as the synaptic weights needed to be scaled up to compensate for the small size of the population.) This allowed simulation of field potentials induced by synchronous activity in a large number of simulated neurons. Application of carbachol to the slice preparation was modeled by altering intrinsic neuron properties to reflect the membrane changes induced by muscarinic activation. These changes in intrinsic properties caused field events similar to those observed experimentally in the slice preparation.[39] The field events started with a long period of synchronous population activity (termed a long-duration ictiform event in the paper) followed by periodic occurrence at regular long intervals of shorter bursts of synchronous population activity (termed short-duration ictiform events in the paper).

Simulations were used to explore the cellular basis of some of the properties of this synchronous population activity. In the model, induction of synchronous population activity could be obtained through activation of the calcium-sensitive nonspecific cation current (ICAN). Simulations then addressed other properties of the population activity. In particular, the long-duration ictiform event starts with an initial high frequency oscillation (about 15 Hz) which gradually decreases to lower frequencies (about 3 Hz).[39] In the simulation, this change in frequency appeared due to increased concentrations of GABA causing activation of presynaptic GABA-B receptors on the presynaptic terminals of inhibitory interneurons. Activation of presynaptic GABA-B receptors has been shown to decrease release of GABA and thereby to decrease inhibitory potentials.[135] This causes a progressive change in the relative size of GABA-A and GABA-B currents in the model which causes a progressive decrease in frequency of oscillations. Future experiments will investigate whether application of GABA-B receptor antagonists prevents this progressive change in frequency during the long-duration ictiform events. In the simulations, the short-duration ictiform events required a mechanism for rapidly shutting down activity after a brief period of oscillations. This was obtained in the model with activation of presynaptic metabotropic glutamate receptors, causing decreases in excitatory glutamatergic transmission and thereby shutting off the recurrent drive which maintained the network oscillation. Future experiments will investigate whether blockade of metabotropic glutamate receptors will increase the length of short-duration ictiform events.

Changes in Acetylcholine Levels and Sharp Wave Dynamics

Theta oscillations appear during active waking, when an animal is actively exploring its environment, and acetylcholine levels are high in hippocampus and neocortex.[92,109] In contrast, during quiet waking and slow-wave sleep, there is much less appearance of hippocampal and entorhinal cortex theta rhythm,[63,173,122] and levels of acetylcholine decrease substantially in hippocampus and neocortex.[92,109] As the amount of theta rhythm decreases in the EEG, recordings show increased appearance of hippocampal sharp waves which appear in region CA1 and entorhinal cortex.[27,31] These sharp waves are correlated with extensive spiking activity in hippocampus and the output layers of entorhinal cortex.

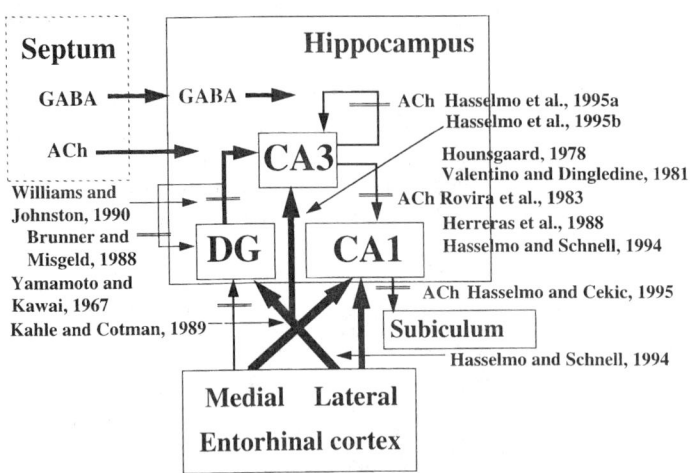

FIGURE 7. Summary of experimental data showing cholinergic suppression of excitatory synaptic connections within the hippocampal formation. Numerous studies have demonstrated this phenomenon at excitatory feedback connections from region CA3 toward cortical structures, but most excitatory feedforward connections appear to show much less cholinergic suppression of excitatory transmission (e.g., lateral entorhinal cortex to outer molecular layer and lateral entorhinal cortex to region CA1).[74] This supports the notion that cholinergic modulation may selectively reduce excitatory feedback to parahippocampal regions, which is consistent with changes in evoked potential size in waking and sleeping animals.[187]

Computational modeling suggests that decreases in cholinergic modulation could set parameters which would enhance the propensity for initiation and propagation of sharp wave activity. Sharp waves have characteristics suggestive of exponential growth in activity which could result from runaway excitatory feedback, yet at the same time they appear when there is less overall background activity. More abstract simulations of interacting populations of excitatory and inhibitory units[184,75,76,79,139] can give some insight into the dynamical underpinnings of sharp waves. In particular, changes in cholinergic modulation may shift the network between theta rhythm and sharp wave generation dependent upon the relative magnitude of the modulation of membrane depolarization (by influences on ICAN) and modulation of recurrent and feedback excitation (by influences on glutamatergic synaptic transmission).

As summarized in FIGURE 7, extensive physiological data suggests strong cholinergic suppression of the recurrent excitatory connections in region CA3,[75] the Schaffer collaterals from region CA3 to region CA1,[84,172,44,80,81,74] and the connections from region CA1 to subiculum.[71] Thus, when acetylcholine levels are high, region CA3 should have less capacity for runaway excitatory feedback and influence on region CA1, whereas when acetylcholine levels fall, this should result in more powerful excitatory feedback, with potential for exponential growth of excitatory activity (FIG. 8). However, as acetylcholine levels reach a very low level, the loss of

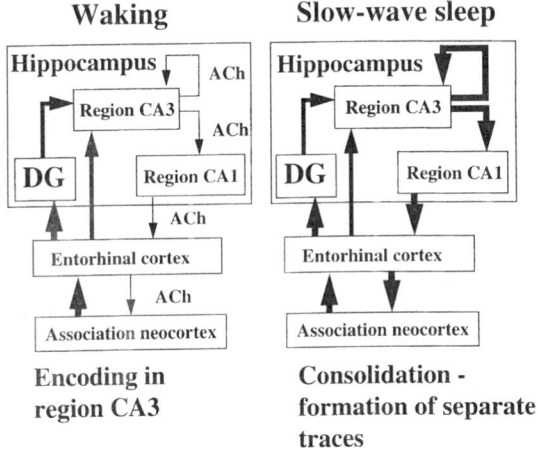

FIGURE 8. Schematic representation of changes in flow of activity during active waking (high acetylcholine) versus slow-wave sleep (low acetylcholine). The decrease in levels of acetylcholine will release the cholinergic suppression of excitatory feedback from region CA3 back to parahippocampal cortices. This should allow associations encoded initially in region CA3 of hippocampus to guide formation of additional associations in hippocampus and parahippocampal regions.

cholinergic depolarization of principal cells should prevent activity from propagating in the network.

Previous research in the Hasselmo laboratory[76,79,139] has analyzed network dynamics using highly simplified network models involving representations of the average firing rate across a large population of excitatory and inhibitory units. These models use continuous variables to represent these different firing rates, analogous to the representation used in other simplified dynamical models of neural circuits.[184] These models show that stable self-sustained activity can be maintained in a population of excitatory and inhibitory neurons if the strength of excitatory feedback connections W is greater than the decay constant η and less than $\eta + HW'/\eta$ (where H is the strength of feedback inhibition, W' is the excitatory input to feedback interneurons, and η is the decay constant). As acetylcholine levels fall, the network should go from stable activity to explosive activity, because lower levels of acetylcholine will reduce the cholinergic suppression of excitatory transmission. Hence, as acetylcholine levels fall, the influence of excitatory connections W will increase to levels until $W > \eta + HW'/\eta$, and the network will go from stable levels of activity to exponential growth of activity during brief explosive periods followed by a strong wave of feedback inhibition. This effect is illustrated in FIGURE 9. The transition from stable sustained activity to brief waves of strong activity is consistent with the appearance of sharp waves during the period immediately following the presence of stable theta oscillations (James Chrobak, personal communication). However, note that the decrease in cholinergic modulation will also result in a decrease in depolarization of excitatory neurons. This will cause a decrease in the likelihood of individual neurons getting over threshold and initiating spiking activity. Thus, decreases in

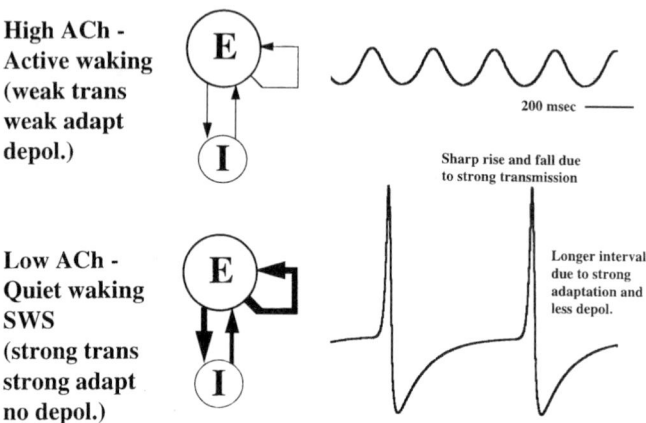

High ACh -
Active waking
(weak trans
weak adapt
depol.)

200 msec ————

Sharp rise and fall due
to strong transmission

Low ACh -
Quiet waking
SWS
(strong trans
strong adapt
no depol.)

Longer intervals
due to strong
adaptation and
less depol.

FIGURE 9. Abstract model representing changes in dynamics as acetylcholine levels drop from high levels during active waking to lower levels during quiet waking or slow-wave sleep. In this model, a population of excitatory neurons is represented by the output of a single unit (E) and a population of inhibitory neurons is represented by the output of a single unit (I). *Top*: When acetylcholine levels are high, excitatory and inhibitory synaptic connectivity is weakened in the model, consistent with experimental data *in vivo* and *in vitro*. In certain parameter ranges, stable oscillatory dynamics can be obtained with weak synaptic connectivity. Theta frequency oscillations can be obtained dependent upon adaptation properties of the excitatory neurons. *Bottom*: When acetylcholine levels drop, the excitatory and inhibitory synaptic connectivity becomes stronger due to a decrease in muscarinic modulation of transmission. This results in a change to parameter ranges where excitatory feedback causes explosive growth of activity, followed by abrupt decreases due to feedback inhibition. This might be analogous to changes underlying sharp wave generation in hippocampus and entorhinal cortex.[31] At the same time, the neurons undergo less depolarization thereby decreasing the frequency of generation of suprathreshold activity.

acetylcholine levels should result in less frequent activity, but when activity gets over threshold it should show explosive increases. Gradually, the loss of depolarization should result in a slowing in the generation of explosive excitatory activity and eventually a state of quiescence.

These types of properties should arise as well in networks of spiking neurons. Phenomena of this sort have already been observed in a network of simulated cortical neurons.[51] In that network, excitatory interactions between neurons would cause explosive growth in activity followed by abrupt cessation of activity due to spike frequency accomodation caused by activation of calcium-dependent potassium currents. The modulatory suppression of calcium-dependent potassium currents would allow the network to instead enter a state of sustained lower levels of spiking activity. Thus, cholinergic modulation of the calcium-dependent potassium current could also contribute to a shift from intermittent periods of strong and brief activation to periods of more temporally distributed and sustained activation.

SUMMARY

In summary, modeling of entorhinal cortical networks provides a technique for linking specific cellular physiological properties of neurons to their functional role in behavior. The research reviewed here demonstrates three theories of this link between physiological properties and function: 1) Cholinergic activation of the ICAN current could provide an intrinsic mechanism for the maintenance of information during performance of a delayed nonmatch to sample task, 2) Theta rhythm generation in the hippocampus and entorhinal cortex could provide a mechanism enhancing encoding of overlapping sequences, and gating the retrieval of these sequences during the flow of information back to entorhinal cortex and parahippocampal cortices during retrieval, and 3) decreases in cholinergic modulation could set dynamics for sharp wave generation to rapidly reactivate encoded representations and guide the modification of additional traces in hippocampus and parahippocampal regions.

REFERENCES

1. AIGNER, T.G., D.L. WALKER & M. MISHKIN. 1991. Comparison of the effects of scopolamine administered before and after acquisition in a test of visual recognition memory in monkeys. Behav. Neural Biol. **55**(1): 61–67.
2. AIGNER, T.G. & M. MISHKIN. 1986. The effects of physostigmine and scopolamine on recognition memory in monkeys. Behav. Neural Biol. **45**(1): 81–87.
3. ALONSO, A. & E. GARCIA-AUSTT. 1987. Neuronal sources of theta rhythm in the entorhinal cortex of the rat. I. Laminar distribution of theta field potentials. Exp. Brain Res. **67**: 493–501.
4. ALONSO, A. & E. GRACIA-AUSTT. 1987. Neuronal sources of theta rhythm in the entorhinal cortex of the rat. II. Phase relations between unit discharges and theta field potentials. Exp. Brain Res. **67**: 502–509.
5. ALONSO, A. & R. KLINK. 1993. Differential electroresponsiveness of stellate and pyramidal-like cells of medial entorhinal cortex layer II. J. Neurophysiol. **70**: 128–143.
6. ALONSO, A. & C. KOHLER. 1984. A study of the reciprocal connections between the septum and the entorhinal area using anterograde and retrograde axonal transport methods in the rat brain. J. Comp. Neurol. **225**: 327–343.
7. ALONSO A. & R.R. LLINAS. 1989. Subthreshold Na$^+$-dependent theta-like rhythmicity in stellate cells of entorhinal cortex layer II. Nature **342**: 175–177.
8. ALVAREZ, P., S. ZOLA-MORGAN & L.R. SQUIRE. 1994. The animal model of human amnesia: long-term memory impaired and short-term memory intact. Proc. Natl. Acad. Sci. USA **91**(12): 5637–5641.
9. ALVAREZ-ROYO, P., S. ZOLA-MORGAN & L.R. SQUIRE. 1992. Impairment of long-term memory and sparing of short-term memory in monkeys with medial temporal lobe lesions: a response to Ringo. Behav. Brain Res. **52**: 1–5.
10. BADDELEY, A.D. & E.K. WARRINGTON. 1970. Amnesia and the distinction between long- and short-term memory. J. Verb. Learn. Verb. Behav. **9**: 176–189.
11. BARTUS, R.T. & H.R. JOHNSON. 1976. Short-term memory in the rhesus monkey: disruption from the anti-cholinergic scopolamine. Pharmacol. Biochem. Behav. **5**(1): 39–46.
12. BEATTY, W.W., N. BUTTERS & D.S. JANOWSKY. 1986. Patterns of memory failure after scopolamine treatment: implications for cholinergic hypotheses of dementia. Behav. Neural Biol. **45**: 196–211.
13. BEHR, J., T. GLOVELI & U. HEINEMANN. 1998. The perforant path projection from the medial entorhinal cortex layer III to the subiculum in the rat combined hippocampal-entorhinal cortex slice. Eur. J. Neurosci. **10**: 1011–1018.
14. BERZHANSKAYA, J., N.N. URBAN & G. BARRIONUEVO. 1998. Electrophysiological and pharmacological characterization of the direct perforant path input to hippocampal area CA3. J. Neurophysiol. **79**: 2111–2118.

15. BLANTON, M.G., J.J. LoTURCO & A.R. KRIEGSTEIN. 1989. Whole cell recordings from neurons in slices of reptilian and mammalian cerebral cortex. J. Neurosci. Methods **30:** 203–210.
16. BOLHUIS, J.J., A.M. STRIJKSTRA & R.J. KRAMERS. 1988. Effects of scopolamine on performance of rats in a delayed-response radial maze task. Physiol. Behav. **43:** 403–409.
17. BOWER, J.M. & D. BEEMAN. 1995. The Book of GENESIS: Exploring Realistic Neural Models with the GEneral NEural SImulation System. Springer-Verlag. New York.
18. BRAGIN, A., G. JANDO, Z. NADASDY, J. HETKE, K. WISE & Y. BUZSAKI. 1995. Gamma (40–100 Hz) oscillation in the hippocampus of the behaving rat. J. Neurosci. **15:** 47–60.
19. BRANKACK, J., M. STEWART & S.E. FOX. 1993. Current source density analysis of the hippocampal theta rhythm: associated sustained potentials and candidate synaptic generators. Brain Res. **615:** 310–327.
20. BROKS, P., G.C. PRESTON, M. TRAUB, P. POPPLETON, C. WARD & S.M. STAHL. 1988. Modelling dementia: effects of scopolamine on memory and attention. Neuropsychologia **26:** 685–700.
21. BROWN, M.W., F.A. WILSON & I.P. RICHES. 1987. Neuronal evidence that inferomedial temporal cortex is more important than hippocampus in certain processes underlying recognition memory. Brain Res **409:** 158–162.
22. BUCKLEY, M.J., D. GAFFAN & E.A. MURRAY. 1997. Functional double dissociation between two inferior temporal cortical areas: perirhinal cortex versus middle temporal gyrus. J. Neurophysiol. **77**(2): 587–598.
23. BURWELL, R.D. & D.G. AMARAL. 1998. Cortical afferents of the perirhinal, postrhinal, and entorhinal cortices of the rat. J. Comp. Neurol. **398**(2): 179–205.
24. BURWELL, R.D. & D.G. AMARAL. 1998. Perirhinal and postrhinal cortices of the rat: interconnectivity and connections with the entorhinal cortex. J. Comp. Neurol. **391**(3): 293–321.
25. BURWELL, R.D., M.P. WITTER & D.G. AMARAL. 1995. Perirhinal and postrhinal cortices of the rat: a review of the neuroanatomical literature and comparison with findings from the monkey brain. Hippocampus **5**(5): 390–408.
26. BUZSAKI, G., E. GRASTYAN, J. CZOPF, L. KELLENYI & O. PROHASKA. 1981. Changes in neuronal transmission in the rat hippocampus during behavior. Brain Res. **225:** 235–247.
27. BUZSAKI, G. 1986. Hippocampal sharp waves: their origin and significance. Brain Res. **398:** 242–252.
28. BUZSAKI, G. 1989. Two-stage model of memory trace formation: a role for "noisy" brain states. Neuroscience **31:** 551–570.
29. BUZSAKI, G., J. CZOPF, I. KONDAKOR & L. KELLENYI. 1986. Laminar distribution of hippocampal rhythmic slow activity (RSA) in the behaving rat: current-source density analysis, effects of urethane and atropine. Brain Res. **365**(1): 125–137.
30. BUZSAKI, G., M. PENTTONEN, A. BRAGIN, Z. NADASDY & J.J. CHROBAK. 1995. Possible physiological role of the perforant path-CA1 projection. Hippocampus **5**(2): 141–146.
31. CHROBAK, J.J. & G. BUZSAKI. 1994. Selective activation of deep layer (V–VI) retrohippocampal cortical neurons during hippocampal sharp waves in the behaving rat. J. Neurosci. **14:** 6160–6170.
32. CHROBAK, J.J. & G. BUZSAKI. 1996. High-frequency oscillations in the output networks of the hippocampal-entorhinal axis of the freely behaving rat. J. Neurosci. **16**(9): 3056–3066.
33. CHROBAK, J.J. & G. BUZSÁKI. 1998. Gamma oscillations in the entorhinal cortex of the freely behaving rat. J. Neurosci. **18:** 388–398.
34. CORKIN, S. 1984. Lasting consequences of bilateral medial temporal lobectomy: clinical course and experimental findings in H.M. Semin. Neurol. **4:** 249–259.
35. CRAWSHAW, J.A. & P.E. MULLEN. 1984. A study of benzhexol abuse. Br. J. Psychiatry **145:** 300–303.
36. CROW, T.J. & I.G. GROVE-WHITE. 1973. An analysis of the learning deficit following hyoscine administration to man. Br. J. Pharmacol. **49:** 322–327.
37. DICKSON, C.T., C. TREPEL & B.H. BLAND. 1994. Extrinsic modulation of theta field activity in the entorhinal cortex of the anesthetized rat. Hippocampus **4:** 37–52.
38. DICKSON, C.T., I.J. KIRK, S.D. ODDIE & B.H. BLAND. 1995. Classification of theta-related cells in the entorhinal cortex: cell discharges are controlled by the ascending

brainstem synchronizing pathway in parallel with hippocampal theta-related cells. Hippocampus **5**(4): 306–319.

39. DICKSON, C.T. & A. ALONSO. 1997. Muscarinic induction of synchronous population activity in the entorhinal cortex. J. Neurosci. **17:** 6729–6744.

40. DICKSON, C.T., A. MENA & A. ALONSO. 1997. Electroresponsiveness of medial entorhinal cortex layer III neurons *in vitro*. Neuroscience **81:** 937–950.

41. DICKSON, C.T., J. MAGISTRETTI, M.H. SHALINSKY, E. FRANSÉN, M.E. HASSELMO & A. ALONSO. 2000. Properties and role of I(h) in the pacing of subthreshold oscillations in entorhinal cortex layer II neurons. J. Neurophysiol. **83:** 2562–2579.

42. DIFRANCESCO, D., M. FERRONI, M. MAZZANTI & C. TROMBA. 1986. Properties of the hyperpolarizing-activated current (If) in cells isolated from the rabbit sino-atrial node. J. Physiol. (Lond.) **377:** 61–88.

43. DRAGOI, G., D. CARPI, M. RECCE, J. CSICSVARI & G. BUZSAKI. 1999. Interactions between hippocampus and medial septum during sharp waves and theta oscillation in the behaving rat. J Neurosci. **19**(14): 6191–6199.

44. DUTAR, P. & R.A. NICOLL. 1988. Classification of muscarinic responses in hippocampus in terms of receptor subtypes and second-messenger systems: electrophysiological studies *in vitro*. J. Neurosci. **8**(11): 4214–4224.

45. DYKES, R.W. 1997. Mechanisms controlling neuronal plasticity in somatosensory cortex. Can. J. Physiol. Pharmacol. **75**(5): 535–545.

46. EICHENBAUM, H., T. OTTO & N.J. COHEN. 1994. Two functional components of the hippocampal memory system. Behav. Brain Sci. **17:** 449–472.

47. EMPSON, R.M. & U. HEINEMANN. 1995. The perforant path projection to hippocampal area CA1 in the rat hippocampal-entorhinal cortex combined slice. J. Physiol. (Lond.) **484:** 707–720.

48. FAHY, F.L., I.P. RICHES & M.W. BROWN. 1993. Neuronal activity related to visual recognition memory: long term memory and the encoding of recency and familiarity information in the primate anterior and medial inferior temporal and rhinal cortex. Exp. Brain Res. **96:** 457–472.

49. FERNANDEZ, G., J.B. BREWER, Z. ZHAO, G.H. GLOVER & J.D. GABRIELI. 1999. Level of sustained entorhinal activity at study correlates with subsequent cued-recall performance: a functional magnetic resonance imaging study with high acquisition rate. Hippocampus **9**(1): 35–44.

50. FOX, S.E., S. WOLFSON & J.B.J. RANCK. 1986.. Hippocampal theta rhythm and the firing of neurons in walking and urethane anesthetized rats. Exp. Brain Res. **62:** 495–508.

51. FRANSÉN, E. & A. LANSNER. 1995. Low spiking rates in a population of mutually exciting pyramidal cells. Network **6:** 271–288.

52. FRANSEN, E., C.T. DICKSON, J. MAGISTRETTI, A.A. ALONSO & M.E. HASSELMO. 1998. Modeling the generation of subthreshold membrane potential oscillations of entorhinal cortex layer II stellate cells. Soc. Neurosci. Abstr. **24:** 814.5.

53. FRANSEN, E., G.V. WALLENSTEIN, A. ALONSO, C.T. DICKSON & M.E. HASSELMO. 1999. A biophysical simulation of intrinsic and network properties of entorhinal cortex. Neurocomputing. In press.

54. FRANSEN, E., A. ALONSO & M.E. HASSELMO. 1999. Intrinsic properties of rat entorhinal cells relevant to working memory. Soc. Neurosci. Abstr. In press.

55. FREEMAN, J.A. & C. NICHOLSON. 1975. Experimental optimization of current source-density technique for anuran cerebellum. J. Neurophysiol. **38**(2): 369–382.

56. FRIEL, D.D. 1995. [Ca^{2+}]$_i$ oscillations in sympathetic neurons: an experimental test of a theoretical model. Biophys. J. **68:** 1752.

57. GAFFAN, D. 1974. Recognition impaired and association intact in the memory of monkeys after transection of the fornix. J. Comp. Physiol. Psychol. **86:** 1100–1109.

58. GAFFAN, D. & E.A. MURRAY. 1992. Monkeys (*Macaca fascicularis*) with rhinal cortex ablations succeed in object discrimination learning despite 24-hr intervals and fail at matching to sample despite double sample presentations. Behav. Neurosci. **106:** 30–38.

59. GALLYAS, F., F.H. GULDNER, G. ZOLTAY & J.R. WOLFF. 1990. Golgi-like demonstration of "dark" neurons with an argyrophil III method for experimental neuropathology. Acta Neuropathol. (Berl.) **79:** 620–628.

60. GHONHEIM, M.M. & S.P. MEWALDT. 1975. Effects of diazepam and scopolamine on storage, retrieval and organization processes in memory. Psychopharmacologia **44:** 257–262.

61. GIVENS, B. 1996. Stimulus-evoked resetting of the dentate theta rhythm: relation to working memory. Neuroreport **8:** 159–163.
62. GRAF, P.A., L.R. SQUIRE & G. MANDLER. 1984. The information that amnesic patients do not forget. J. Exp. Psychol. Hum. Learn. Mem. **10:** 164–178.
63. GREEN, J.D. & A.A. ARDUINI. 1954. Hippocampal electrical activity and arousal. J. Neurophysiol. **17:** 533–557.
64. GUTFREUND, Y., Y. YAROM & I. SEGEV. 1995. Subthreshold oscillations and resonant frequency in guinea-pig cortical neurons: physdiology and modelling. J. Physiol. **483**(3): 621–640.
65. HAMAM, B.N., C.T. DICKSON & A. ALONSO. 1997. Electrophysiological characterization and cholinergic modulation of entorhinal cortex (EC) layer V neurons in rat brain slices. Soc. Neurosci. Abstr. **23:** 488.
66. HAMPSON, R.E. & S.A. DEADWYLER. 1989. Effects of delta-9-tetrahydrocannabinol on sensory evoked hippocampal activity in the rat: principal components analysis and sequential dependency. J. Pharmacol. Exp. Ther. **251**(3): 870–877.
67. HAMPSON, R.E., C.J. HEYSER & S.A. DEADWYLER. 1993. Hippocampal cell firing correlates of delayed-match-to-sample performance in the rat. Behav. Neurosci. **107**(5): 715–739.
68. HAMPSON, R.E., L.E. JARRARD & S.A. DEADWYLER. 1999. Effects of ibotenate hippocampal and extrahippocampal destruction on delayed-match and -nonmatch-to-sample behavior in rats. J. Neurosci. **19**(4): 1492–1507.
69. HASSELMO, M.E. 1995. Neuromodulation and cortical function: modeling the physiological basis of behavior. Behav. Brain Res. **67:** 1–27.
70. HASSELMO, M.E. & J.M. BOWER. 1992. Cholinergic suppression specific to intrinsic not afferent fiber synapses in rat piriform cortex. J. Neurophysiol. **67:** 1222–1229.
71. HASSELMO, M.E. & M. CEKIC. 1995. A simulation of episodic memory function in the hippocampal formation. Soc. Neurosci. Abstr. **21:** 376.1.
72. HASSELMO, M.E. & M. CEKIC. 1996. Suppression of synaptic transmission may allow combination of associative feedback and self-organizing feedforward connections in the neocortex. Behav. Brain Res. **79:** 153–161.
73. HASSELMO, M.E. & A. KAPUR. 2000. Modeling of large networks. *In* Computational Neuroscience: Realistic Modeling for Experimentalists. E. DeSchutter, Ed. CRC Press. New York.
74. HASSELMO, M.E. & E. SCHNELL. 1994. Laminar selectivity of the cholinergic suppression of synaptic transmission in rat hippocampal region CA1: computational modeling and brain slice physiology. J. Neurosci. **14:** 3898–3914.
75. HASSELMO, M.E., E. SCHNELL & E. BARKAI. 1995. Dynamics of learning and recall at excitatory recurrent synapses and cholinergic modulation in hippocampal region CA3. J. Neurosci. **15:** 5249–5262.
76. HASSELMO, M.E., E. SCHNELL, J. BERKE & E. BARKAI. 1995. A model of the hippocampus combining self-organization and associative memory function. *In* Advances in Neural Information Processing Systems. G. Tesauro, D. Touretzky & T. Leen, Eds. Vol. 7: 77–84. MIT Press. Cambridge, MA.
77. HASSELMO, M.E., B.P. WYBLE & G.V. WALLENSTEIN. 1996. Encoding and retrieval of episodic memories: role of cholinergic and GABAergic modulation in the hippocampus. Hippocampus **6**(6): 693–708.
78. HASSELMO, M.E. & B.P. WYBLE. 1997. Simulation of the effects of scopolamine on free recall and recognition in a network model of the hippocampus. Behav. Brain Res. **89:** 1–34.
79. HASSELMO, M.E., C. LINSTER, M. PATIL, D. MA & M. CEKIC. 1997. Noradrenergic suppression of synaptic transmission may influence cortical signal-to-noise ratio. J. Neurophysiol., **77:** 3326–3339.
80. HERRERAS, O., J.M. SOLIS, M.D. MUNOZ, R. MARTIN DEL RIO & J. LERMA. 1988. Sensory modulation of hippocampal transmission. I. Opposite effects on CA1 and dentate gyrus synapsis. Brain Res. **461:** 290–302.
81. HERRERAS, O., J.M. SOLIS, A.S. HERRANZ, R. MARTIN DEL RIO & J. LERMA. 1988. Sensory modulation of hippocampal transmission. II. Evidence for a cholinergic locus of inhibition in the Schaffer-CA1 synapse. Brain Res. **461:** 303–313.

82. HOLSCHER, C., R. ANWYL & M.J. ROWAN. 1997. Stimulation on the positive phase of hippocampal theta rhythm induces long-term potentiation that can be depotentiated by stimulation on the negative phase in area CA1 *in vivo*. J. Neurosci. **17:** 6470–6477.

83. HOLSHEIMER, J., C.J. STOK & F.H. LOPES DA SILVA. 1983. Theta rhythm related hippo-campal cell discharges in the urethan anaesthetized rat: evidence for a predominant entorhinal input. Electroencephalogr. Clin. Neurophysiol. **55:** 464–467.

84. HOUNSGAARD, J. 1978. Presynaptic inhibitory action of acetylcholine in area CA1 of the hippocampus. Exp. Neurol. **62:** 787–797.

85. HUERTA, P.T. & J.E. LISMAN. 1996. Synaptic plasticity during the cholinergic theta-frequency oscillation *in vitro*. Hippocampus **6:** 58–61.

86. HUGUENARD, J.R, O.P. HAMILL & D.A. PRINCE. 1988. Developmental changes in Na^+ conductances in rat neocortical neurons: appearance of a slowly inactivating component. J. Neurophysiol. **59**(3)**:** 778–795.

87. HUGUENARD, J.R. & D.A. MCCORMICK. 1992. Simulation of the currents involved in rhythmic oscillations in thalamic relay neurons. J. Neurophysiol. **68:** 1373–1383.

88. HUTCHEON, B., R.M. MIURA & E. PUIL. 1996. Subthreshold membrane resonance in neocortical neurons. J. Neurophysiol. **76:** 683–697.

89. HUTCHEON, B., R.M. MIURA & E. PUIL. 1996. Models of subthreshold membrane res-onance in neocortical neurons. J. Neurophysiol. **76:** 698–714.

90. ITOH, A., A. NITTA, Y. KATONO, M. USUI, K. NARUHASHI, R. IIDA, T. HASEGAWA & T. NABESHIMA. 1997. Effects of metrifonate on memory impairment and cholinergic dysfunction in rats. Eur. J. Pharmacol. **322**(1)**:** 11–19.

91. JONES, R.S. & U. HEINEMANN. 1988. Synaptic and intrinsic responses of medical entorhinal cortical cells in normal and magnesium-free medium *in vitro*. J. Neurophysiol. **59**(5)**:** 1476–1496.

92. KAMETANI, H. & H. KAWAMURA. 1990. Alterations in acetylcholine release in the rat hippocampus during sleep-wakefulness detected by intracerebral dialysis. Life Sci. **47:** 421–426.

93. KAPUR, A., M.F. YECKEL, R. GRAY & D. JOHNSTON. 1998. L-type calcium channels are required for one form of hippocampal mossy fiber LTP. J. Neurophysiol. **79:** 2181–2190.

94. KAPUR, A., R.A. PEARCE, W.W. LYTTON & L.B. HABERLY. 1997. $GABA_A$-mediated IPSCs in piriform cortx have fast and slow components with different properties and locations on pyramidal cells. J. Neurophysiol. **78:** 2531–2545.

95. KLINK, R. & A. ALONSO. 1993. Ionic mechanisms for the subthreshold oscillations and differential electroresponsiveness of medial entorhinal cortex layer II neurons. J. Neurophysiol. **70:** 144–157.

96. KLINK, R. & A. ALONSO. 1997. Muscarinic modulation of the oscillatory and repeti-tive firing properties of entorhinal cortex layer II neurons. J. Neurophysiol. **77:** 1813–1828.

97. KLINK, R. & A. ALONSO. 1997. Ionic mechanisms of muscarinic depolarization in entorhinal cortex layer II neurons. J. Neurophysiol. **77:** 1829–1843.

98. KLINK, R. & A. ALONSO. 1997. Morphological characteristics of layer II projection neurons in the rat medial entorhinal cortex. Hippocampus **7:** 571–583.

99. KOHLER, C., V. CHAN-PALAY & J.Y. WU. 1984. Septal neurons containing glutamic acid decarboxylase immunoreactivity project to the hippocampal region in the rat brain. Anat. Embryol. (Berl.) **169**(1)**:** 41–44.

100. KOPELMAN, M.D. 1986. The cholinergic neurotransmitter system in human memory and dementia: a review. Quart. J. Exp. Psychol. **38:** 535–573.

101. LEONARD, B.W., D.G. AMARAL, L.R. SQUIRE & S. ZOLA-MORGAN. 1995. Transient memory impairment in monkeys with bilateral lesions of the entorhinal cortex. J. Neurosci. **15**(8)**:** 5637–5659.

102. LINSTER, C. & M.E. HASSELMO. 1997. Short-term memory function in a model of the olfactory system. *In* Computational Neuroscience, Trends in Research, 1997. J.M. Bower, Ed. Plenum Press. New York.

103. LUDVIG, N., P.E. POTTER & S.E. FOX. 1994. Simultaneous single-cell recording and microdialysis within the same brain site in freely behaving rats: a novel neurobiolog-ical method. J. Neurosci. Methods **55**(1)**:** 31–40.

104. MACEK, T.A., D.G. WINDER, R.W. GEREAU IV, C.O. LADD & P.J. CONN. 1996. Differential involvement of group II and group III mGluRs as autoreceptors at lateral and medial perforant path synapses. J. Neurophysiol. **76**(6): 3798–3806.
105. MAGISTRETTI, J. & A. ALONSO. 1999. Slow voltage-dependent inactivation of a sustained sodium current in stellate cells of rat entorhinal cortex layer II. *In* Molecular and Functional Diversity of Ion Channels and Receptors. Ann. N.Y. Acad. Sci. **868**: 84–88.
106. MAGISTRETTI, J., D. RAGSDALE & A. ALONSO. 1999. High conductance sustained single channel activity responsible for the low threshold persistent Na$^+$ current in entorhinal cortex neurons. J. Neurosci. **19**: 7334-7341.
107. MANNS, I.D., A. ALONSO & B.E. JONES. 1998. Characterization of juxtacellularly recorded and labelled basal forebrain units in relation to cortical EEG activity. Soc. Neurosci. Abstr. **24**: 1694.
108. MAQUET, P., E. HIRSCH, M.N. METZ-LUTZ, J. MOTTE, D. DIVE, C. MARESCAUX & G. FRANCK. 1995. Regional cerebral glucose metabolism in children with deterioration of one or more cognitive functions and continuous spike-and-wave discharges during sleep. Brain **118**: 1497–1520.
109. MARROSU, F., A. COZZOLINO, M. PULIGHEDDU, M. GIAGHEDDU & G. DI CHIARA. 1997. Hippocampal theta activity after systemic administration of a non-peptide delta-opioid agonist in freely-moving rats: relationship to D1 dopamine receptors. Brain Res. **776**(1–2): 24–29.
110. MARROSU, F., C. PORTAS, M.S. MASCIA, M.A. CASU, M. FA, M. GIAGHEDDU, A. IMPERATOR & G.L. GESSA. 1995. Microdialysis measurement of cortical and hippocampal acetylcholine release during sleep-wake cycle in freely moving cats. Brain Res. **671**: 329–332.
111. MATSUOKA, N. & T.G. AIGNER. 1996. Cholinergic-glutamatergic interactions in visual recognition memory in rhesus monkeys. Neuroreport **7**: 565–568.
112. MCCORMICK, D.A. & J.R. HUGUENARD. 1992. A model of the electrophysiological properties of thalamocortical relay neurons. J. Neurophysiol. **68**: 1384–1400.
113. MCCORMICK, D.A. & H.C. PAPE. 1990. Properties of a hyperpolarization-activated cation current and its role in rhythmic oscillations in thalamic relay neurons. J. Physiol. **431**: 291–318.
114. MCLENNAN, H. & J.J. MILLER. 1974. The hippocampal control of neuronal discharges in the septum of the rat. J. Physiol. **237**: 607–624.
115. METHERATE, R. & N.M. WEINBERGER. 1989. Acetylcholine produces stimulus-specific receptive field alterations in cat auditory cortex. Brain Res. **480**(1–2): 372–377.
116. METHERATE, R., J.H. ASHE & N.M. WEINBERGER. 1990. Acetylcholine modifies neuronal acoustic rate-level functions in guinea pig auditory cortex by an action at muscarinic receptors. Synapse **6**(4): 364–368.
117. MEUNIER, M., W. HADFIELD, J. BACHEVALIER & E.A. MURRAY. 1996. Effects of rhinal cortex lesions combined with hippocampectomy on visual recognition memory in rhesus monkeys. J. Neurophysiol. **75**(3): 1190–1205.
118. MILLER, E.K. & R. DESIMONE. 1994. Parallel neuronal mechanisms for short-term memory. Science **263**: 520–522.
119. MILLER, E.K. & R. DESIMONE. 1993. Scopolamine affects short-term memory but not inferior temporal neurons. Neuroreport **4**(1): 81–84.
120. MILLER, E.K., L. LIN & R. DESIMONE. 1991. A neural mechanism for working and recognition memory in inferior temporal cortex. Science **254**: 1377–1379.
121. MILLER, E.K., L. LIN & R. DESIMONE. 1993. Activity of neurons in anterior inferior temporal cortex during a short-term memory task. J. Neurosci. **13**: 1460–1478.
122. MITCHELL, S.J. & J.B. RANCK, JR. 1980. Generation of theta rhythm in medial entorhinal cortex of freely moving rats. Brain Res. **178**: 49–66.
123. MITCHELL, S.J., J.N. RAWLINS, O. STEWARD & D.S. OLTON. 1982. Medial septal area lesions disrupt theta rhythm and cholinergic staining in medial entorhinal cortex and produce impaired radial arm maze behavior in rats. J. Neurosci. **2**: 292–302.
124. MIZUMORI, S.J.Y., C.A. BARNES & B.L. MCNAUGHTON. 1989. Reversible inactivation of the medial septum: selective effects on the spontaneous unit activity of different hippocampal cell types. Brain Res. **500**: 99–106.

125. MUMBY, D.G. & J.P.J. PINEL. 1994. Rhinal cortex lesions and object recognition in rats. Behav Neurosci **108:** 11–18.
126. MURRAY, E.A., M.G. BAXTER & D. GAFFAN. 1998. Monkeys with rhinal cortex damage or neurotoxic hippocampal lesions are impaired on spatial scene learning and object reversals. Behav. Neurosci. **112**(6): 1291–1303.
127. NABER, P.A. & M.P. WITTER. 1998. Subicular efferents are organized mostly as parallel projections: a double-labeling, retrograde-tracing study in the rat. J. Comp. Neurol. **393**(3): 284–297.
128. NABER, P.A., M. CABALLERO-BLEDA, B. JORRITSMA-BYHAM & M.P. WITTER. 1997. Parallel input to the hippocampal memory system through peri- and postrhinal cortices. Neuroreport **8**(11): 2617–2621.
129. NADEL, L. & M. MOSCOVITCH. 1997. Memory consolidation, retrograde amnesia and the hippocampal complex. Curr. Opin. Neurobiol. **7**(2): 217–227.
130. NAGAO, T., A. ALONSO & M. AVOLI. 1996. Epileptiform activity induced by pilocarpine in the rat hippocampal-entorhinal slice preparation. Neuroscience **72**(2): 399–408.
131. OH, M.M., J.M. POWER, L.T. THOMPSON, P.L. MORIEARTY & J.F. DISTERHOFT. 1999. Metrifonate increases neuronal excitability in CA1 pyramidal neurons from both young and aging rabbit hippocampus. J. Neurosci. **19**(5): 1814–1823.
132. OHISHI, H., R. SHIGEMOTO, S. NAKANISHI & N. MIZUNO. 1993. Distribution of the messenger RNA for a metabotropic glutamate receptor, mGluR2, in the central nervous system of the rat. Neuroscience **53**(4): 1009–1018.
133. OLPE, H.-R., G. KARLSSON, M.F. POZZA, F. BRUGGER, M. STEINMANN, H. VAN RIEZEN, G. FAGG, R.G. HALL, W. FROESTL & H. BITTIGER. 1990. CGP 35348: a centrally active blocker of GABA-B receptors. Eur. J. Pharmacol. **187:** 27–38.
134. ORSETTI, M., F. CASAMENTI & G. PEPEU. 1996. Enhanced acetylcholine release in the hippocampus and cortex during acquisition of an operant behavior. Brain Res. **724:** 89–96.
135. OTIS, T.S., Y. DEKONINCK & I. MODY. 1993. Characterization of synaptically elicited GABA(B) responses using patch-clamp recordings in rat hippocampal slices. J. Physiol. **463:** 391–407.
136. OTTO, T. & H. EICHENBAUM. 1992. Complementary roles of orbital prefrontal cortex and the perirhinal-entorhinal cortices in an odor-guided delayed non-matching to sample task. Behav. Neurosci. **106:** 763–776.
137. OTTO, T. & H. EICHENBAUM. 1992. Neuronal activity in the hippocampus during delayed non-match to sample performance in rats: evidence for hippocampal processing in recognition memory. Hippocampus **2:** 323–334.
138. PAPE, H.C. & R.B. DRIESANG. 1998. Ionic mechanisms of intrinsic oscillations in neurons of the basolateral amygdaloid complex. J. Neurophysiol. **79**(1): 217–226.
139. PATIL, M.M. & M.E. HASSELMO. 1999. Modulation of inhibitory synaptic potentials in the piriform cortex. J. Neurophysiol. **81**(5): 2103–2118.
140. PENETAR, D.M. & J.H. MCDONOUGH, JR. 1983. Effects of cholinergic drugs on delayed match-to-sample performance of rhesus monkeys. Pharmacol. Biochem. Behav. **19**(6): 963–967.
141. PERRY, E.K. & R.H. PERRY. 1995. Acetylcholine and hallucinations: disease-related compared to drug-induced alterations inn consciousness. Brain Cognit. **28:** 2402–2458.
142. PETERSON, R.C. 1977. Scopolamine induced learning failures in man. Psychopharmacology **52:** 283–289.
143. PINAULT, D. 1996. A novel single-cell staining procedure performed *in vivo* under electrophysiological control: morpho-functional features of juxtacellularly labeled thalamic cells and other central neurons with biocytin or Neurobiotin. J. Neurosci. Methods **65**(2): 113–336.
144. PITLER, T.A. & B.E. ALGER. 1992. Cholinergic excitation of GABAergic interneurons in the rat hippocampal slice. J. Physiol. **450:** 127–142.
145. PITLER, T.A. & B.E. ALGER. 1994. Depolarization-induced suppression of GABAergic inhibition in rat hippocampal pyramidal cells: G protein involvement in a presynaptic mechanism. Neuron **13**(6): 1447–1455.
146. PROTOPAPAS, A.D., M. VANIER & J.M. BOWER. 1999. Simulating large networks of neurons. *In* Methods in Neuronal Modeling: From Ions to Networks. C. Koch & I. Segev, Eds.: 461–498. MIT Press. Cambridge, MA.

147. PUIL, E., B. GIMBARZEVSKY & R.M. MIURA. 1986. Quantification of membrane properties of trigeminal root ganglion neurons in guinea pigs. J. Neurophysiol. **55**(5): 995–1016.
148. RAFIQ, A., R.J. DELORENZO & D.A. COULTER. 1993. Generation and propagation of epileptiform discharges in a combined entorhinal cortex/hippocampal slice. J. Neurophysiol. **70**(5): 1962–1974.
149. REMPEL-CLOWER, N.L., S.M. ZOLA, L.R. SQUIRE & D.G. AMARAL. 1996. Three cases of enduring memory impairment after bilateral damage limited to the hippocampal-formation. J. Neurosci. **16**: 5233–5255.
150. RICHES, I.P., F.A.W. WILSON & M.W. BROWN. 1991. The effects of visual stimulation and memory on neurons of the hippocampal formation and the neighboring parahippocampal gyrus and inferior temporal cortex of the primate. J. Neurosci. **11**: 1763–1779.
151. RIEKKINEN, M., B. SCHMIDT, J. KUITUNEN & P. RIEKKINEN, JR. 1997. Effects of combined chronic nimodipine and acute metrifonate treatment on spatial and avoidance behavior. Eur. J. Pharmacol. **322**(1): 1–9.
152. ROVIRA, C., Y. BEN-ARI, E. CHERUBINI, K. KRNJEVIC & N. ROPERT. 1983. Pharmacology of the dendritic action of acetylcholine and further observations on the somatic disinhibition in the rat hippocampus *in situ*. Neuroscience **8**: 97–106.
153. RUDELL, A.P., S.E. FOX & J.B.J. RANCK. 1980. Hippocampal excitability phase-locked to the theta rhythm in walking rats. Exp. Neurol. **68**: 87–96.
154. SANTORO, B., S.G.N. GRANT, D. BARTSCH & E.R. KANDEL. 1997. Interactive cloning with the SH3 domain of N-src identifiers: a new brain specific ion channel protein, with homology to Eag and cyclic nucleotide-gated channels. PNAS **94**: 14815–14820.
155. SCOVILLE, W.B. & B. MILNER. 1957. Loss of recent memory after bilateral hippocampal lesions. J. Neurol. Neurosurg. Psychiatry **20**: 11–21.
156. SILLITO, A.M. & J.A. KEMP. 1983. Cholinergic modulation of the functional organization of the cat visual cortex. Brain Res. **289**(1–2): 143–155.
157. SKAGGS, W.E. & B.L. MCNAUGHTON. 1996. Replay of neuronal firing sequences in rat hippocampus during sleep following spatial experience. Science **271**: 1870–1873.
158. SOHAL, V. & M.E. HASSELMO. 2000. A model for experience-dependent changes in the responses of inferotemporal neurons. Network: Comp. Neural Syst. In press.
159. SPAIN, W.J., P.C. SCHWINDT & W.E. CRILL. 1987. Anomalous rectification in neurons from cat sensorimotor cortex *in vitro*. J. Neurophysiol. **57**: 1555–1576.
160. SPRUSTON, N., D.B. JAFFE, S.H. WILLIAMS & D. JOHNSTON. 1993. Voltage- and space-clamp errors associated with the measurement of electrotonically remote synaptic events. J. Neurophysiol. **70**: 781–802.
161. SQUIRE, L.R., S. ZOLA-MORGAN & K.S. CHEN. 1988. Human amnesia and animal models of amnesia: performance of amnesic patients on tests designed for the monkey. Behav. Neurosci. **102**: 210–221.
162. SQUIRE, L.R., D.G. AMARAL & G.A. PRESS. 1990. Magnetic resonance imaging of the hippocampal formation and mammillary nuclei distinguish medial temporal lobe and diencephalic amnesia. J. Neurosci. **10**: 3106–3117.
163. STEWART, M. & S.E. FOX. 1991. Hippocampal theta activity in monkeys. Brain Res. **538**: 59–63.
164. SUZUKI, W.A., E.K. MILLER & R. DESIMONE. 1997. Object and place memory in the macaque entorhinal cortex. J. Neurophysiol. **78**: 1062–1081.
165. TAMAMAKI, N. & Y. NOJYO. 1995. Preservation of topography in the connections between the subiculum, field CA1, and the entorhinal cortex in rats. J. Comp. Neurol. **353**(3): 379–390.
166. TANG, Y. & T.G. AIGNER. 1996. Release of cerebral acetylcholine increases during visually mediated behavior in monkeys. Neuroreport **7**: 2231–2235.
167. TANG, Y., M. MISHKIN & T.G. AIGNER. 1997. Effects of muscarinic blockade in perirhinal cortex during visual recognition. Proc. Natl. Acad. Sci. USA **94**: 12667–12669.
168. TOTH, K., T.F. FREUND & R. MILES. 1997. Disinhibition of rat hippocampal pyramidal cells by GABAergic afferent from the septum. J. Physiol. **500**: 463–474.
169. TRAUB, R.D., R.K.S. WONG, R. MILES & H. MICHELSON. 1991. A model of a CA3 pyramidal neuron incorporating voltage-clamp data on intrinsic conductances. J. Neurophysiol. **66**: 635–650.

170. TREMBLAY, N., R.A. WARREN & R.W. DYKES. 1990. Electrophysiological studies of acetylcholine and the role of the basal forebrain in the somatosensory cortex of the cat. II. Cortical neurons excited by somatic stimuli. J. Neurophysiol. **64**(4): 1212–1222.

171. URBAN, N.N., D.A. HENZE & G. BARRIONUEVO. 1998. Amplification of perforant-path EPSPs in CA3 pyramidal cells by LVA calcium and sodium channels. J. Neurophysiol. **80**: 1558–1561.

172. VALENTINO, R.J. & R. DINGLEDINE. 1981. Presynaptic inhibitory effect of acetylcholine in the hippocampus. J. Neurosci. **1**: 784–792.

173. VANDERWOLF, C.H., R. KRAMIS & T.E. ROBINSON. 1977. Hippocampal electrical activity during waking behaviour and sleep: analyses using centrally acting drugs. Ciba Found. Symp. **58**: 199–226.

174. WALLENSTEIN, G.V., H. EICHENBAUM & M.E. HASSELMO. 1998. The hippocampus as an associator of discontiguous events. Trends Neurosci. **21**(8): 317–323.

175. WALLENSTEIN, G.V. & M.E. HASSELMO. 1997. GABAergic modulation of hippocampal population activity: sequence learning, place field development and the phase precession effect. J. Neurophysiol. **78**(1): 393–408.

176. WALLENSTEIN, G.V. & M.E. HASSELMO. 1997. Functional transitions between epileptiform-like activity and associative memory in hippocampal region CA3. Brain Res. Bull. **43**(5): 485–493.

177. WANG, X.J. 1993. Ionic basis for intrinsic 40 Hz neuronal oscillations. Neuroreport **5**(3): 221–224.

178. WHITE, J.A., T. BUDDE & A.R. KAY. 1995. A bifurcation analysis of neuronal subthreshold oscillations. Biophys. J. **69**: 1203–1217.

179. WHITE, J.A., R. KLINK, A. ALONSO & A.R. KAY. 1998. Noise from voltage-gated ion channels may influence neuronal dynamics in the entorhinal cortex. J. Neurophysiol. In press.

180. WIIG, K.A. & R.D. BURWELL. 1998. Memory impairment on a delayed non-matching-to-position task after lesions of the perirhinal cortex in the rat. Behav. Neurosci. **112**(4): 827–838.

181. WILLIAMS, S. & D. JOHNSTON. 1990. Muscarinic depression of synaptic transmission at the hippocampal mossy fiber synapse. J. Neurophysiol. **64**(4): 1089–1097.

182. WILLIAMS, S.H. & L. JOHNSTON. 1991. Kinetic properties of two anatomically distinct excitatory synapses in hippocampal CA3 pyramidal neurons. J. Neurophysiol. **66**: 1010–1020.

183. WILLIAMS, S.R., J.P. TURNER, S.W. HUGHES & V. CRUNELLI. 1997. On the nature of anomalous rectification in thalamocortical neurones of the cat ventrobasal thalamus *in vitro*. J. Physiol. (Lond.) **505**: 727–747.

184. WILSON, H.R. & J.D. COWAN. 1972. Excitatory and inhibitory interactions in localized populations of model neurons. Biophys. J. **12**: 1–24.

185. WILSON, M.A. & B.L. MCNAUGHTON. 1994. Reactivation of hippocampal ensemble memories during sleep. Science **265**: 676–679.

186. WINSON, J. & C. ABZUG. 1977. Gating of neuronal transmission in the hippocampus: efficacy of transmission varies with behavioral state. Science **196**: 1223–1225.

187. WINSON, J. & C. ABZUG. 1978. Dependence upon behavior of neuronal transmission from perforant pathway through entorhinal cortex. Brain Res. **147**: 422–427.

188. WYBLE, B.P., C. LINSTER & M.E. HASSELMO. 1997. Evoked synaptic potential size depends on phase of theta rhythm in rat hippocampus. Soc. Neurosci. Abstr. **23**: 197.7.

189. WYBLE, B.P., C. LINSTER & M.E. HASSELMO. 2000. Size of CA1 evoked synaptic potentials is related to theta rhythm phase in rat hippocampus. J. Neurophysiol. In press.

190. YLINEN, A., A. BRAGIN, Z. NADASDY, G. JANDO, I. SZABO, A. SIK & G. BUZSAKI. 1995. Sharp wave-associated high-frequency oscillation (200 Hz) in the intact hippocampus: network and intracellular mechanisms. J. Neurosci. **15**: 30–46.

191. YOUNG, B.J., T. OTTO, G.D. FOX & H. EICHENBAUM. 1997. Memory representation within the parahippocampal region. J. Neurosci. **17**: 5183–5195.

192. ZOLA-MORGAN, S. & L.R. SQUIRE. 1985. Medial temporal lesions in monkeys impair memory on a variety of tasks sensitive to human amnesia. Behav. Neurosci. **99**(1): 22–34.

193. ZOLA-MORGAN, S. & L.R. SQUIRE. 1986. Memory impairment in monkeys following lesions limited to the hippocampus. Behav. Neurosci. **100**(2): 155–160.

194. ZOLA-MORGAN, S., L.R. SQUIRE & D.G. AMARAL. 1986. Human amnesia and the medial temporal region: enduring memory impairment following a bilateral lesion limited to field CA1 of the hippocampus. J. Neurosci. **6**: 2950–2967.
195. ZOLA-MORGAN, S., L.R. SQUIRE, R.P. CLOWER & N.L. REMPEL. 1993. Damage to the perirhinal cortex exacerbates memory impairment following lesions to the hippocampal formation. J. Neurosci. **13**(1): 251–265.
196. ZOLA-MORGAN, S., L.R. SQUIRE, D.G. AMARAL & W.A. SUZUKI. 1989. Lesions of perirhinal and parahippocampal cortex that spare the amygdala and hippocampal formation produce severe memory impairment. J. Neurosci. **9**(12): 4355–4370.
197. EICHENBAUM, H. & J. BUCKINGHAM. 1990. Studies on hippocampal processing: experiment, theory and model. *In* Learning and Computational Neuroscience: Foundations of Adaptive Networks. M. Gabriel & J. Moore, Eds.: 171–231. MIT Press. Cambridge, MA.
198. HASSELMO, M.E. & J.M. BOWER. 1993. Acetylcholine and memory. Trends Neurosci. **16(6)**: 218–222.
199. KAHANA, M.J., R. SEKULER, J.B. CAPLAN, M. KIRSCHEN & J.R. MADSEN. 1999. Human theta oscillations exhibit task dependence during virtual maze navigation. Nature **399**: 781–784.
200. LEVY, W.B. 1996. A sequence predicting CA3 is a flexible associator that learns and uses context to solve hippocampal-like tasks. Hippocampus **6**: 579–590.
201. LISMAN, J.E. & M.A. IDIART. 1995. Storage of 7 +/− 2 short-term memories in oscillatory subcycles. Science **267(5203)**: 1512–1515.
202. MAGISTRETTI, J. & A. ALONSO. 1999. Biophysical properties and slow-voltage-dependent inactivation of a sustained sodium current in entorhinal cortex layer-II principal neurons: a whole-cell and single-channel study. J. Gen. Physiol. **114**: 491–509.
203. MCCARLEY, R.W. 1982. REM sleep and depression: common neurobiological control mechanisms. Am. J. Psychiatry **139**: 565–570.
204. SOHAL, V.S. & M.E. HASSELMO. 1998. Changes in GABA$_B$ modulation during a theta cycle may be analogous to the fall of temperature during annealing. Neural Comp. **10**: 889–902.
205. SOHAL, V.S. & M.E. HASSELMO. 1998. GABA$_B$ modulation improves sequence disambiguation in computational models of hippocampal region CA3. Hippocampus **8**: 171–193.
206. TSODYKS, M.V., W.E. SKAGGS, T.J. SEJNOWSKI & B.L. MCNAUGHTON. 1996. Population dynamics and theta rhythm phase precession of hippocampal place cell firing: a spiking neuron model. Hippocampus **6**: 271–280.

Disruption of the Ventral Visual Stream in a Case of Reduplicative Paramnesia

ANDREW E. BUDSON,[a,b,c,d] HEIDI L. ROTH,[e] DORENE M. RENTZ,[b,c,f] AND MICHAEL RONTHAL[c,f]

[b]Division of Cognitive and Behavioral Neurology, Brigham and Women's Hospital, Boston, Massachusetts, USA

[c]Harvard Medical School, Boston, Massachusetts, USA

[d]Department of Psychology, Harvard University, Cambridge, Massachusetts, USA

[e]Department of Neurology, University of Florida, Gainesville, Florida, USA

[f]Department of Neurology, Beth Israel Deaconess Medical Center, Boston, Massachusetts, USA

INTRODUCTION

Reduplicative paramnesia (RP), a syndrome named by Pick in 1903 to describe a specific and limited disturbance of memory, is characterized by a subjective certainty that a familiar place or person has been duplicated.[1] Most often seen in post-traumatic brain injuries, this syndrome has been described in a variety of neurologic conditions, including strokes, intracerebral hemorrhages, tumors, dementias, encephalopathies, and various psychiatric conditions.[2] The classic and most commonly described neuroanatomical localization is the combination of bilateral frontal lobe and right hemisphere lesions.[3,4] Although many theories have been advanced to explain how these lesions could produce this syndrome, the specific pathophysiology is unknown. We report a patient who provides anatomical and neuropsychological support for the theory that RP is a syndrome that may develop in a vulnerable brain by a lesion in the ventral visual stream, disrupting communication between the visual cortex and both visual processing areas in the inferior temporal lobe and visual memory in the nondominant parahippocampal region.

CASE REPORT

The patient, OB, was a 45-year-old left-handed man with a history of alcoholism, diabetes, and hypertension, who had been admitted to the hospital for a minor operation. Two weeks prior to admission, he stopped drinking. Ten days into his hospital stay, the nursing staff reported that OB was "confused," not knowing where his room was. The neurology service was consulted. Most of the bedside mental status examination, carried out in his hospital room, was normal, including being oriented to

[a]Address for correspondence: Andrew E. Budson, Division of Cognitive and Behavioral Neurology, Brigham and Women's Hospital, 221 Longwood Avenue, Boston, MA 02115. Tel.: (617) 732-8060; fax: (617) 738-9122.

e-mail: abudson@yahoo.com

"Boston, Beth Israel Hospital, 7th floor." However, when OB was asked to put on his glasses for the visual exam, he pointed to his roommate's bed and said that the glasses were in his "other room," explaining that we were presently in his "room in the hallway." When pressed about why he should have a room in the hallway and why he should have two rooms, he acknowledged that he was unable to resolve these contradictions. Over the next few days, when questioned as to where he was (when in his hospital room), he again sometimes reported that he was in his room in the hallway and at other times that he was in his room at his house. At all times, he believed that he had "another room" that was located in the correct place in the hospital, although he never reported being in this "other room."

He was not concerned about his orientation difficulties. He was able to provide a coherent history of his hospitalization. His neurological examination was significant for mild clumsiness and autotopagnosia (incorrect somatotopic localization) of the right hand. Neuropsychological testing was obtained, revealing decreased performance of complex attention and response inhibition tasks, mild right-sided neglect, and moderately impaired visuospatial integration and visual memory (see TABLE 1 for these and other results). An electroencephalogram and lumbar puncture were obtained. Brain MRI revealed a small, linear, nonenhancing lesion in the white matter of the left temporo-parieto-occipital junction, which was hyperintense on T2 and proton density images and isointense on T1, consistent with a subacute stroke (see FIG. 1). The duplication of his hospital room persisted throughout the remainder of his hospitalization. In follow-up visits to the neurology clinic, although his paramnesia and autotopagnosia had resolved, he now complained of memory problems.

DISCUSSION

Explanations as to the etiology of RP began with Pick, who hypothesized that his patient produced the duplication due to a "convulsive attack" interrupting conscious memory.[1] Weinstein and Kahn postulated a psychodynamic theory based upon a patient's denial of illness.[5] Benson, Gardner, and Meadows studied three patients with traumatic brain injury, all of whom had both right hemisphere and bifrontal damage.[3] They suggested that the right hemisphere injury rendered patients unable to correctly update their orientation due to impaired visuospatial perception and visual memory, while their frontal lobe dysfunction left them unable to resolve the conflict that inevitably arose when the assumptions of their orientation were challenged. Other authors have also found disruption of visual perception, including facial recognition, in patients with Capgras syndrome (CS), a subset of RP in which close acquaintances are regarded as imposters.[4,6–8] Because CS can be thought of as the "mirror image" of proposagnosia, Ellis and Young hypothesized that it was likely due to a lesion that disrupts the dorsal visual stream.[6] In their discussion of a case of a patient with CS in the visual (but not the auditory) modality, Hirstein and Ramachandran argued that it was more likely that this syndrome would be caused by disruption of the ventral visual stream, producing in their patient a failure of communication between the temporal lobe and the limbic complex.[9] Imaging studies of this patient, however, did not show the specific lesion that they postulated.

Our patient developed a reduplicative paramnesic disturbance specific to the location of his room following a small left hemisphere stroke. Although one might ar-

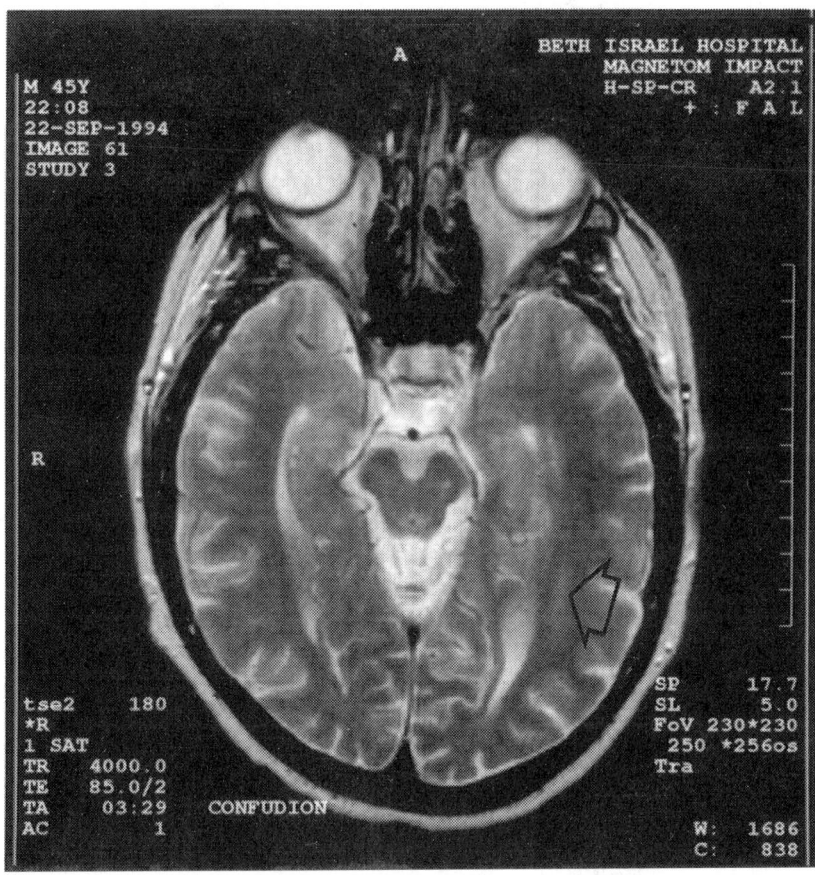

FIGURE 1. T2-weighted axial MRI image demonstrating a small, linear area of hyper-intensity consistent with a subacute stroke (arrow) in the white matter adjacent to Brodmann areas 19 and 37, a localization consistent with the occipitotemporal projection system, the fiber pathway of the ventral visual stream.[10] Location of the stroke was confirmed by lesion analysis as described by Damasio and Damasio.[13]

gue that his paramnesia may have been part of a more general confusional state, this is unlikely given that he showed no evidence of confusion other than for the location of his room, he had no difficulty in providing a coherent history of recent events, and he performed well on tests of simple attention such as Digit Span (7 forward, 7 back-ward). The stroke damaged the white matter adjacent to Brodmann areas 19 and 37 and most likely disrupted the occipitotemporal projection system, the fiber pathway of the ventral visual stream.[10] This disruption, interfering with the communication between the visual cortex and both visual processing areas in the inferior temporal lobe and visual memory of the nondominant parahippocampal region, can explain OB's difficulty with tests of visuospatial perception and visual memory. Our left-handed patient may also have reversed dominance for visual memory, which would

TABLE 1. Results and interpretation of tests and examinations

Tests and examinations	Results	Interpretation
Bedside mental status testing		
Months backward	Intact	Normal
Calculations	Intact	Normal
Confrontational naming	Intact	Normal
Comprehension of complex commands	Intact	Normal
Writing a sentence	Intact	Normal
Repetition	Intact	Normal
Right/left confusion	Absent	Normal
Finger agnosia	Absent	Normal
Recent memory: current events	Intact	Normal
Remote memory: personal history	Intact	Normal
Copy 3-dimensional figure	Normal	Normal
Clock drawing	Intact	Normal
Neurological examination		
Cranial nerves including vision	Intact	Normal
Strength	Normal	Normal
Reflexes	Loss of ankle reflexes	Abnormal
Sensation—General	Mild peripheral neuropathy	Abnormal
Two-point discrimination	Intact	Normal
Autotopagnosia (somatotopic localization)	Mild disruption on right hand	Abnormal
Stereognosis & graphesthesia	Intact	Normal
Coordination	Mild right-sided clumsiness	Abnormal
Plantar reflexes	Flexor	Normal
Asterixis	Absent	Normal
Neuropsychological tests[12]		
General Intelligence		
American National Adult Reading Test	Est. IQ = 118	High average
Simple and complex attention		
Digit Span	7F, 7B	High average
Trails A	58 s, 10th percentile	Mild to moderate impairment
Trails B	115 s, 15th percentile	Mild to moderate impairment
Response inhibition		
Short Stroop	67 s, 2 errors	Mild to moderate impairment
Verbal fluency		
Word generation: F words	20 words	High average
Word generation: animals	18 words	High average
Language		
Boston Naming Test	55/60	Average
Verbal memory		
Wechsler: Logical Memory I—immediate	32nd percentile	Average
Wechsler: Logical Memory II—delayed	62nd percentile	Average
Visual memory		
Wechsler: Visual Memory I—immediate	32nd percentile	Average

— continued

TABLE 1. Results and interpretation of tests and examinations

Tests and examinations	Results	Interpretation
Wechsler: Visual Memory II—delayed	12th percentile	Mild to moderate impairment
Visuospatial ability		
Hooper Visual Organization Test	15/25	Moderate impairment
Ravens Colored Matrices	5th percentile, est. visual IQ = 75	Moderate to severe impairment
Visuospatial attention		
Letter cancellation test	Mild right-sided omissions	Mild impairment
Lumbar puncture	Unremarkable	Normal
Electroencephalogram	Transient bi-temporal and independent left mid-temporal theta activity with hyperventilation	Abnormal
Brain MRI (see FIG. 1)	Left posterior stroke	Abnormal

explain why the disturbance of left parahippocampal pathways could more likely produce the syndrome in his case. (Support for the possibility of reversed dominance comes from the fact that, with a left-sided lesion, our patient's verbal memory was above average and his visual memory—a "nondominant" hemisphere function—was impaired.) In addition, OB had evidence of frontal lobe dysfunction, as can be seen in his poor performance on tests of complex attention and response inhibition. Alcoholism has been shown to be a cause of selective bifrontal dysfunction[11] and is most likely the cause of his difficulty with those tests. Our patient thus provides radiologic evidence to support the theory that the critical pathology in RP is the combination of disruption of the ventral visual stream of the nondominant hemisphere, leading to inaccurate orientation, and bifrontal dysfunction that allows this inaccurate and confused orientation to be tolerated.

ACKNOWLEDGMENTS

We thank Daniel Z. Press, Jeremey D. Schmahmann, and Kirk R. Daffner for their thoughtful discussions.

REFERENCES

1. PICK, A. 1903. Clinical studies: III. On reduplicative paramnesia. Brain **26:** 260–267.
2. FORSTL, H., O.P. ALMEIDA, A.M. OWEN, A. BURNS & R. HOWARD. 1991. Psychiatric, neurological, and medical aspects of misidentification syndromes: a review of 260 cases. Psychiatr. Med. **21:** 905–910.
3. BENSON, D.F., H. GARDNER & J.C. MEADOWS. 1976. Reduplicative paramnesia. Neurology **26:** 147–151.
4. ALEXANDER, M.P., D.T. STUSS & D.F. BENSON. 1979. Capgras syndrome: a reduplicative phenomenon. Neurology **29:** 334–339.

5. WEINSTEIN, E.A. & R.L. KAHN. 1955. Denial of Illness: Symbolic and Physiological
    Aspects. Thomas. Springfield, IL.
6. ELLIS, H.D. & A.W. YOUNG. 1990. Accounting for delusional misidentifications. Br. J.
    Psychiatry 157: 239–248.
7. ELLIS, H.D. 1994. The role of the right hemisphere in the Capgras delusion. Psycho-
    pathology 27: 177–185.
8. SILVA, J.A. & G.B. LEONG. 1995. Visual-perceptual abnormalities in delusional mis-
    identification. Can. J. Psychiatry 40: 6–8.
9. HIRSTEIN, W. & V.S. RAMACHANDRAN. 1997. Capgras syndrome: a novel probe for
    understanding the neural representation of the identity and familiarity of persons.
    Proc. R. Soc. Lond. 264: 437–444.
10. TUSA, R.T. & L.G. UNGERLEIDER. 1985. The inferior longitudinal fasciculus: a reexam-
    ination in humans and monkeys. Ann. Neurol. 18: 583–591.
11. HAKIM, H., N.P. VERMA & M.F. GREIFFENSTEIN. 1988. Pathogenesis of reduplicative
    paramnesia. J. Neurol. Neurosurg. Psychiatry 51: 839–841.
12. LEZAK, M.D. 1995. Neuropsychological Assessment. Oxford Univ. Press. London/
    New York.
13. DAMASIO, H. & A.R. DAMASIO. 1989. Lesion Localization in Neuropsychology. Oxford
    Univ. Press. London/New York.

Predator Exposure Produces Retrograde Amnesia and Blocks Synaptic Plasticity

Progress toward Understanding How the Hippocampus Is Affected by Stress

DAVID M. DIAMOND[a] AND COLLIN R. PARK

Department of Psychology and Neuroscience Program, University of South Florida, Tampa, Florida 33620, USA

Medical Research Service, Veterans Affairs Medical Center, Tampa, Florida 33612, USA

A vast amount of research has been devoted to understanding the role of the hippocampus in learning and memory. Damage to the hippocampus results in severe cognitive impairments in a broad range of species, including humans and rats.[1] Complementary work has shown that chronic stress, which can result in hippocampal cell death, impairs hippocampal-specific learning and memory.[2] For example, spatial learning, which is impaired in animals with lesions of the hippocampus, is impaired in chronically stressed animals.[2] Moreover, acute stress also impairs hippocampal-dependent learning and memory.[3,4] This chapter reviews our studies on the effects of acute stress on hippocampal-dependent memory and synaptic plasticity. Our recent findings indicate that exposing rats to a predator, which is an intense stressor, impairs cognitive and electrophysiological measures of hippocampal functioning.

In electrophysiological studies, we have shown that stress blocks the induction of primed burst potentiation (PBP), a physiological model of memory, in behaving rats.[5,6] PBP is a low-threshold form of plasticity that can be induced by only five physiologically patterned electrical pulses.[7] Because our earlier work studied stress–PBP interactions *in vivo*, it could not be determined whether the blockade of PBP was caused by extrahippocampal influences (such as elevated corticosterone or inhibitory afferent activity) or by stress-induced changes in the intrinsic circuitry of the hippocampus. We addressed this issue by recording PBP in hippocampal slices obtained from rats exposed to a cat for a relatively brief period of time (75 minutes). We found that cat exposure completely blocked PB potentiation *in vitro* (FIG. 1).[8] Thus, stress produces an inhibitory influence on plasticity that can be localized to the intrinsic circuitry of the hippocampus.

Does the stress-induced suppression of PBP indicate that stress completely blocks all forms of electrophysiological plasticity? We evaluated this question by delivering LTP stimulation to slices obtained from rats exposed to a cat. The LTP stim-

[a]Address for correspondence: David M. Diamond, Ph.D., Dept. of Psychology (BEH 339), University of South Florida, 4202 E. Fowler Ave., Tampa, FL 33620. Tel.: (813) 974-0480; fax: (813) 974-4617.
e-mail: ddiamond@chuma1.cas.usf.edu

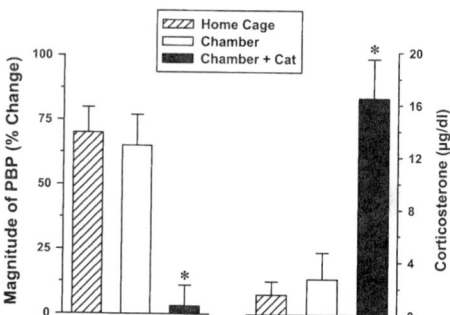

FIGURE 1. *Right side*: Corticosterone levels were elevated 75 minutes after rats were placed in a chamber with the cat. Rats not exposed to the cat (home cage and chamber without cat) had basal corticosterone levels. *Left side*: PBP developed in the two control groups, but did not occur in the cat-exposed group. * = $p < 0.05$, ANOVA, Bonferroni corrected *t*-tests versus the control groups.

ulation was composed of a train of 100 pulses, which is 20 times as many pulses as were used to try to induce PBP. Unlike PBP, the magnitude of LTP was unaffected by the predator stress experience.[8] Taken together, the PB and LTP work indicated that stress inhibits, but does not completely block, the capacity of the hippocampus to develop plasticity.

Because stress impairs the development of hippocampal plasticity, one would expect that stress should impair cognitive measures of hippocampal function. We tested the possibility that exposing rats to a predator would impair hippocampal-dependent memory. Rats were trained in a radial arm water maze (RAWM), which is a tank of water that contains swim paths (arms) radiating out of an open central area, with a hidden platform located at the end of one of the arms. The platform was located in the same arm on each trial within a day, and was in a different arm on different days. Each day rats learned the location of the platform during acquisition trials, after which the rats were removed from the maze for a 30-minute delay period. During the delay period, the rats were placed either in their home cage (nonstress condition) or near a cat (stress condition). At the end of the delay period, the rats were tested in a retention trial, which probed their ability to remember which arm contained the platform on that day.[9] Cat exposure resulted in impaired performance on the retention trial (FIG. 2). Thus, the stress-induced impairment in spatial memory is consistent with the idea that stress interferes with hippocampal functioning. It is important to note, however, that the stress effect on memory was evident only when rats were trained on a spatially complex maze (a six-arm RAWM). When another group of rats was trained on an easier maze (a four-arm RAWM), predator exposure had no effect on spatial memory (FIG. 2).[9]

This series of cognitive and electrophysiological studies reveals much about how stress affects hippocampal functioning. The findings provide strong support for the hypothesis that stress exerts an inhibitory influence on hippocampal processing. Acute stress does not, however, produce the equivalent of complete hippocampal inactivation. Stress appears to reduce the efficiency of hippocampal processing, which

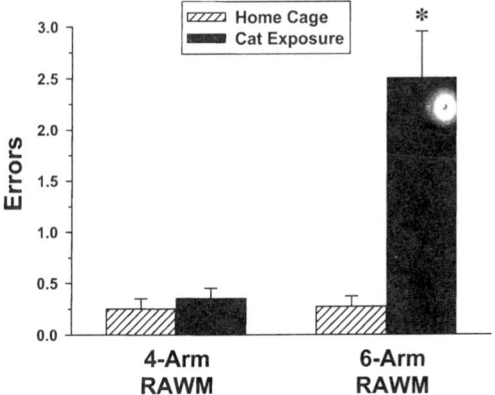

FIGURE 2. Cat exposure impaired spatial memory in rats trained on the six-arm RAWM, but not in rats trained on the four-arm RAWM. Rats placed in their home cage during a 30-minute period between the learning (acquisition) phase and memory (retention) test made approximately 0.25 errors/day. Rats that were trained on the six-arm maze committed significantly more errors after spending the 30-minute delay period with the cat, whereas rats that were trained on the four-arm maze were unimpaired by cat exposure (see Diamond et al.[9] for additional details).

was evident when threshold (PBP), but not suprathreshold (LTP), stimulation was used to induce synaptic plasticity and when subjects were trained in a more complex spatial memory task.

REFERENCES

1. SQUIRE, L.R. & S.M. ZOLA. 1997. Amnesia, memory and brain systems. Philos. Trans. R. Soc. London [Biol.] **352:** 1663–1673.
2. McEWEN, B.S. & A.M. MAGARINOS. 1997. Stress effects on morphology and function of the hippocampus. Ann. N.Y. Acad. Sci. **821:** 271–284.
3. DIAMOND, D.M., M. FLESHNER, N. INGERSOLL & G.M. ROSE. 1996. Psychological stress impairs spatial working memory: relevance to electrophysiological studies of hippocampal function. Behav. Neurosci. **110:** 661–672.
4. KIRSCHBAUM, C., O.T. WOLF, M. MAY, et al. 1996. Stress- and treatment-induced elevations of cortisol levels associated with impaired declarative memory in healthy adults. Life Sci. **58:** 1475–1483.
5. DIAMOND, D.M., M. FLESHNER & G.M. ROSE. 1994. Psychological stress repeatedly blocks hippocampal primed burst potentiation in behaving rats. Behav. Brain Res. **62:** 1–9.
6. BENNETT, M.C., D.M. DIAMOND, M. FLESHNER & G.M. ROSE. 1991. Serum corticosterone level predicts the magnitude of hippocampal primed burst potentiation and depression in urethane-anesthetized rats. Psychobiology **19:** 301–307.
7. DIAMOND, D.M., T.V. DUNWIDDIE & G.M. ROSE. 1988. Characteristics of hippocampal primed burst potentiation in vitro and in the awake rat. J. Neurosci. **8:** 4079–4088.
8. MESCHES, M.H., M. FLESHNER, K.L. HEMAN, et al. 1999. Exposing rats to a predator blocks primed burst potentiation in the hippocampus in vitro. J. Neurosci. **19 (RC18):** 1–5.
9. DIAMOND, D.M., C.R. PARK, K.L. HEMAN & G.M. ROSE. 2000. Exposing rats to a predator impairs spatial working memory in the radial arm water maze. Hippocampus **9:** 542–552.

Higher Cortisol Values Facilitate Spatial Memory in Toddlers

Brief Report

KATHY STANSBURY,[a] DAVID HALEY, AND ANGIE KOENEKER

Department of Psychology, University of New Mexico, Albuquerque, New Mexico 87131, USA

Although it is clear that large increases in glucocorticoids (B) disrupt learning and memory in both humans and animals,[1,2] more recent studies indicate that moderate increases in B have the opposite effect, facilitating learning and memory.[3–5] Indeed, normal binding of B in the hippocampus appears to be necessary for any learning and consolidation of stress-relevant spatial information.[6–8] This effect has also been seen for passive avoidance in birds.[9] The goal of the current study was to demonstrate this B facilitation effect in children in a hippocampal-dependent task.[10] For this purpose, a dry analogue of the Morris water maze was developed.[11]

Participants were 27 parent/child pairs including 15 boys and 12 girls. Children ranged in age from 24 to 36 months (M = 28.22, SD = 3.57). Saliva was collected to assess basal cortisol levels when the participants arrived at the laboratory. A dry analogue of the Morris water maze was used to test cortisol facilitation of learning and memory. The maze consisted of one continuous hallway on the ground floor of a square, approximately symmetrical building. The building had four lobbies, one each at the north, south, east, and west sides, and 30 identical brown doors on the outside perimeter of the hallway. Learning trials began immediately after collection of the saliva sample. For all trials, parents hid behind a prespecified door halfway between the north and east lobby and were signaled to open the door and step out into the hallway as the child approached the door. At the beginning of each trial, the child was encouraged to explore the maze and find his or her parent. After each trial, the child was carried out of the building via one of the four lobby doors and began the next trial in a different lobby, in a preset, randomly determined pattern. Children completed an average of five exposure trials. After approximately 40 minutes of free play in another room with toys, parent, and busy experimenter, children completed a probe trial in which they started in the south lobby and were told that mother was hiding the same place as before. They began their search but the correct door did not open automatically on the probe trial. Search time in each quadrant during the probe trial was recorded for a maximum of 5 minutes. Time spent in the correct (NE) quadrant of the maze was recorded.

[a]Address for correspondence: Kathy Stansbury, Department of Psychology, University of New Mexico, Albuquerque, NM 87131. Tel.: (505) 277-4805; fax (505) 277-1394.
e-mail: kes@unm.edu

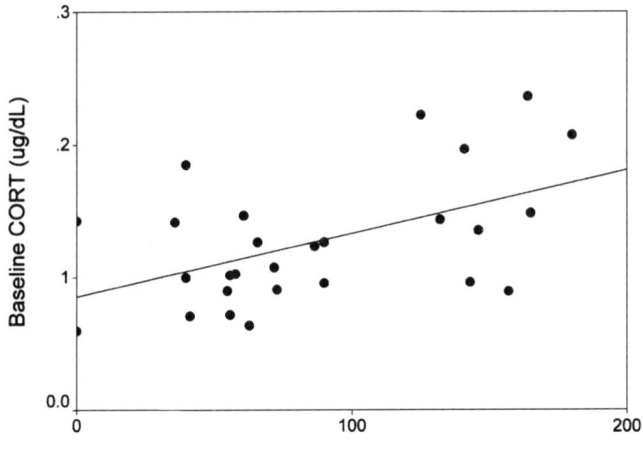

Time in Correct Quadrant (seconds)

FIGURE 1. Positive correlation between toddlers' baseline cortisol [B] levels and time spent in the correct quadrant during the probe trial.

Results indicated that children with higher basal B levels during the learning trials spent more time in the correct quadrant during the probe trial ($r(25) = 0.51$; $p = 0.006$; FIG. 1). In order to control for possible motivational differences, we assessed children's peak levels of distress during the 40-minute waiting period before the probe trial, speculating that higher distress levels would mark greater motivation to find mother in the probe trial. A significant partial correlation between B and time spent in the correct quadrant in the probe, controlling for peak distress in the waiting period, would rule out the influence of motivation. This partial correlation was significant ($r(25) = 0.54$; $p = 0.005$. B, measured as saliva cortisol levels, appeared to facilitate memory for spatial location in toddlers.

REFERENCES

1. DIAMOND, D.M. 2000. Predator exposure produces retrograde amnesia and blocks synaptic plasticity: progress toward understanding how the hippocampus is affected by stress. Ann. N.Y. Acad. Sci. This volume.
2. SAPOLSKY, R.M. 1996. Why stress is bad for your brain. Science **273:** 749–750.
3. MARTINEZ, C.J., M. VILLEGAS & B.S. McEWEN. 1993. Moderate stress enhances acquisition of a spatial memory task in rats. Presented at the meeting of the Society for Neuroscience, Washington, D.C., 1993.
4. McEWEN, B.S. & R.M. SAPOLSKY. 1995. Stress and cognitive function. Curr. Opin. Neurobiol. **5:** 205–216.
5. STANSBURY, K., C. DUGLE BRAINERD & C. GOODSON. 1998. Facilitative effects of stress and cortisol on memory for spatial location in children. Presented at the meeting of the Cognitive Neuroscience Society, San Francisco, CA, April, 1998.
6. MITCHELL, J.B. & M.J. MEANEY. 1991. Effects of corticosterone on response consolidation and retrieval in the forced swim test. Behav. Neurosci. **105:** 798–803.
7. OITZL, M.S. & E.R. DE KLOET. 1992. Selective corticosteroid antagonists modulate specific aspects of spatial orientation learning. Behav. Neurosci. **106:** 62–71.

8. ROUSSE, I.S. BEAULIEU, W. ROWE, *et al.* 1997. Spatial memory in transgenic mice with impaired glucocorticoid receptor function. Neuroreport **8:** 841–845.
9. SANDI, C. & S.P.R. ROSE. 1994. Corticosteroid receptor antagonists are amnestic for passive avoidance learning in day-old chicks. Eur. J. Neurosci. **6:** 1292–1297.
10. SUTHERLAND, R.J., B. KOLB & I.Q. WHISHAW. 1984. Spatial mapping: definitive disruption by hippocampal or frontal cortical damage in the rat. Neurosci. Lett. **31:** 271–276.
11. MORRIS, R.G.M. 1981. Spatial localization does require the presence of local cues. Learn. Motiv. **12:** 239–260.

Functional Characterization of Hippocampal Output to the Entorhinal Cortex in the Rat

FABIAN KLOOSTERMAN,[a,b] THEO VAN HAEFTEN,[b,c] AND
FERNANDO H. LOPES DA SILVA[b]

[b]Institute of Neurobiology, University of Amsterdam, 1098 SM Amsterdam,
The Netherlands

[c]Department of Anatomy, Vrije Universiteit Amsterdam, 1081 BT Amsterdam,
The Netherlands

The entorhinal–hippocampal network plays a central role in memory formation. Synaptic plasticity and reverberatory activity in this network are mechanisms suggested to underlie memory formation.[1] Information from the neocortex is transferred to the hippocampus mainly through superficial layers of the entorhinal cortex (EC). Classically, superficial layers (I–III) of the EC were regarded as "input layers" receiving cortical inputs and relaying this input to all subfields of the hippocampus via the perforant path. In turn, hippocampal area CA1 and subiculum return the processed information to the deep layers (V–VI) of the EC, which project back to the neocortex. Accordingly, the deep layers were regarded as "output layers." In view of recent anatomical data, however, this functional distinction between deep and superficial layers can no longer be held. Indeed, hippocampal outputs also make synaptic contacts with neurons of the superficial layers, whereas deep-layer neurons, the dendrites of which can extend to layers I–III, may receive inputs similar to neurons of the superficial layers. Furthermore, deep-layer neurons give rise to a significant projection to the superficial layers.[2,3] Until recently, anatomical and physiological studies have focused on the entorhinal input to the hippocampus. In contrast, relatively little is known about the physiological characteristics of the hippocampal output to the EC. In this study, we therefore aimed at characterizing the hippocampo-entorhinal pathways by means of field potential recordings.

Female Wistar rats weighing 180 to 240 grams were anesthetized with an intraperitoneal injection of ketamine and xylazine (4:3, 10% solution of Ketaset Aesco, Boxtel, The Netherlands, and 2% solution Rompun, Bayer, Brussels, Belgium; total dose, 1 ml/kg). Rats were mounted in a stereotaxic apparatus and kept at 37°C with the use of a blanket connected to a circulating water bath. The skull was exposed, and a window was drilled above the sagittal sinus, which served as a medio-lateral reference point. Small windows were drilled to enter the right medial EC, the right dorsal subiculum, and the right dorsal CA1 area. The locations of stimulation and recording electrodes were verified by histology.

[a]Address for correspondence: F. Kloosterman, Institute of Neurobiology, University of Amsterdam, Kruislaan 320, 1098 SM Amsterdam, The Netherlands. Tel.: +31 (0)20 525 7622; fax: +31 (0)20 525 7709.

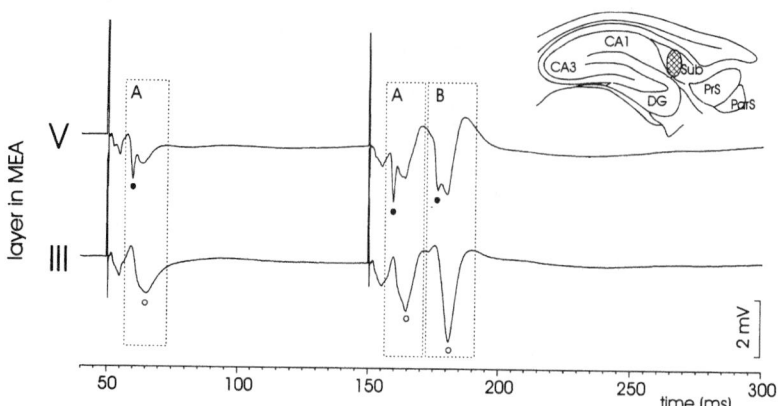

FIGURE 1. Averaged field potentials in layers V and III of the medial entorhinal cortex evoked by subiculum stimulation. Stimuli were given at 50 msec and 150 msec. Short latency **(A)** and long latency **(B)** responses both show a spike component (*closed circle*) in layer V and a slower negative potential with maximum amplitude in layer III (*open circle*). The location of the stimulation electrode in the subiculum (6.1 mm posterior to bregma, 3.2 mm lateral to sagittal sinus) is shown in a schematic sagittal section. DG, dentate gyrus; Sub, subiculum; PrS, presubiculum; ParS, parasubiculum.

Evoked field potentials were recorded in the medial part of the EC (MEA) during subiculum or CA1 stimulation. Using a six-channel probe, which was lowered into MEA parallel to the cortical layers, field potentials in both superficial and deep layers were recorded simultaneously. The evoked field potentials were more prominent in the dorsal part of the MEA than in the ventral part of the MEA. These results are consistent with anatomical data showing a dense terminal field in dorsal parts of the MEA after tracer injection in the dorsal subiculum at the same stereotaxic coordinates used for stimulation.[4] Both short and long latency responses were identified (FIG. 1). To study these responses in more detail, laminar profiles were constructed using glass micropipettes. The latter were placed perpendicular to the EC layers, and recordings were carried out throughout all layers of the EC at 50- or 100-μm intervals. The short latency response usually consists of two components: a spike-like negative potential in deep layers of the MEA and a slower broad negative potential involving both deep layers and superficial layers, having its maximal amplitude in the superficial layers. The peak of the spike-like component occurred 5–7 msec before the peak of the second component. When a paired pulse protocol was used (inter-pulse interval of 100 msec), both components of this early latency response were typically augmented after the test pulse (see FIG. 1).

The long latency response appeared after the test pulse and was only rarely seen after the conditioning pulse. This response was not only evoked by subiculum stimulation, but could also be evoked by stimulation of CA1. The threshold for evoking the long latency response was higher than the threshold for the early latency response. The long latency response had an appearance similar to the early latency response, consisting of a spike-like negative potential in deep layers, which preceded a slower and broader negative potential in more superficial layers.

It can be concluded that the spike-like component of the short latency response is due to orthodromic activation of deep layers of the MEA by subiculum stimulation. In addition, the direct activation of deep layers may concurrently activate superficial layers as demonstrated by the second component of the short latency response. The long latency response may be the result of reverberation of activity, involving activation of the hippocampus via the perforant path. Another possible contribution to the long latency response could be a rebound activity of locally activated neurons in the EC. Further studies will be needed to address the respective roles of (1) intrinsic local circuits in the EC, (2) rebound activation of neurons of the EC, and (3) reverberatory activity in the entorhinal–hippocampal–subiculum–entorhinal pathways.

REFERENCES

1. LOPES DA SILVA, F.H., M.P. WITTER, P.H. BOEIJINGA & A.H. LOHMAN. 1990. Anatomic organization and physiology of the limbic cortex. Physiol. Rev. **70:** 453–511.
2. KÖHLER, C. 1986. Intrinsic connections of the retrohippocampal region in the rat brain. II. The medial entorhinal area. J. Comp. Neurol. **246:** 149–169.
3. DOLORFO, C.L. & D.G. AMARAL. 1998. Entorhinal cortex of the rat: organization of intrinsic connections. J. Comp. Neurol. **398:** 49–82.
4. VAN HAEFTEN, T. & M.P. WITTER. 1997. Topographical organization of subiculum projection to the rhinal cortex in the rat [abstract]. Soc. Neurosci. Abstr. **23:** 2103.

Dopamine, Serotonin, and Noradrenaline Strongly Inhibit the Direct Perforant Path-CA1 Synaptic Input, but Have Little Effect on the Schaffer Collateral Input

NONNA A. OTMAKHOVA AND JOHN E. LISMAN

Department of Biology and Volen Center for Complex Systems, Brandeis University, Waltham, Massachusetts 02454, USA

The CA1 region receives cortical information by two distinct pathways. One pathway reaches CA1 directly through the perforant path (pp) and probably conserves the specificity of the informational context. Another pathway connects via the dentate gyrus (DG) with the CA3 field and reaches the CA1 region by the Schaffer collaterals (sc) (indirect input). The pp input has a topographic organization and terminates on distal apical dendrites of CA1 cells, in the stratum lacunosum-moleculare. The sc input is highly divergent and terminates in the stratum radiatum. The CA1 region is richly innervated by different neuromodulatory systems. Some of them selectively target one or the other stratum. In particular, stratum lacunosum-moleculare appears to have a higher density of nicotinic, D1 and D2 dopamine, and α noradrenaline receptors.[1] The meaning of such selectively was unclear. We have recently demonstrated that dopamine acting through D1 and D2 receptors strongly inhibits the field EPSP (fEPSP) to pp stimulation, but not the response to sc stimulation.[2] Here we compare the pp and the sc input sensitivities to dopamine, serotonin, and noradrenalin on the same hippocampal slices.

We analyzed the two inputs using fEPSP recordings from rat hippocampal slices *in vitro* after the interruption of the trisynaptic pathway (dentate→CA3→CA1). We found that the pp fEPSP had a higher ratio of NMDA/AMPA currents than the sc. In control ACSF, NMDA antagonists did not affect sc fEPSP but decreased the peak amplitude of the pp response by 18%. Under the conditions maximizing the NMDA response (low Mg^{2+} and picrotoxin in ACSF), the peak amplitude of the sc fEPSP was significantly decreased by the antagonist ($\sim$20%) but still to a lesser degree than the pp amplitude ($\sim$40%).[2]

We found that the pp input is strongly affected by three monoamine neuromodulators (FIG. 1). At 20 μM, dopamine (FIG. 1A) and serotonin (FIG. 1B) inhibited the pp fEPSP by 30–40%, but did not affect the sc response. Noradrenaline (FIG. 1C) suppressed the pp responses even more ($\sim$50%), but also inhibited the sc fEPSP ($\sim$15%).

The fact that three neuromodulatory systems selectively control the pp suggests that this input is very important for hippocampal function and may be a site relevant

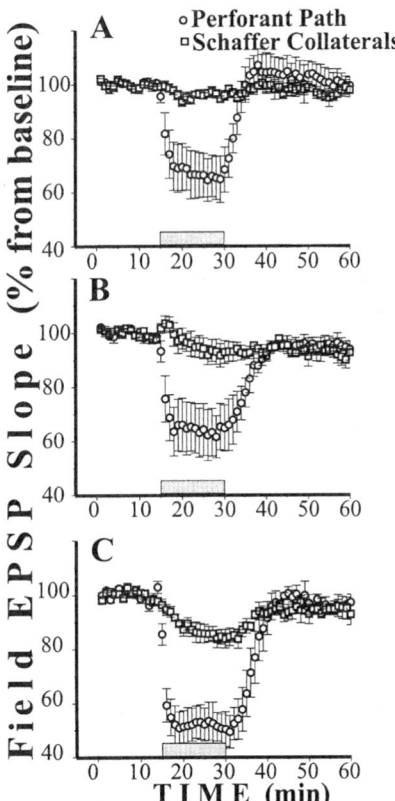

FIGURE 1. Dopamine, serotonin and noradrenaline strongly and selectively inhibit the pp fEPSP. (**A**) Dopamine suppressed the pp fEPSP ($p < 0.001$; $n = 5$). The response fully recovered in 5 minutes of washout. The sc input was not affected. (**B**) Serotonin suppressed the pp fEPSP slope ($p < 0.001$; $n = 5$) to the same degree as dopamine ($F = 3.22$; $p > 0.08$) and had no significant effect on the sc input. The recovery of the pp response was longer (about 10 minutes). (**C**) Noradrenaline suppressed the pp responses ($p < 0.001$; $n = 5$) more strongly than dopamine ($F = 24.35$; $p < 0.001$) and serotonin ($F = 8.37$; $p < 0.006$). Noradrenaline also weakly suppressed the sc fEPSP ($p < 0.001$). Both inputs recovered during 10 minutes of washout. All three monoamines were applied at 20 mM to each slice (regular ACSF). Time of application is marked by rectangles.

to cognitive abnormalities in schizophrenia, depression, and drug addiction. Interestingly, the atypical neuroleptic clozapine completely blocked the effect of dopamine on the pp fEPSP (100% inhibition, $F = 113.2$; $p < 0.0001$; $n = 4$). Clozapine also significantly but relatively weakly inhibited the effect of serotonin (by 25–30%, $F = 14.86$; $p < 0.001$; $n = 5$) and noradrenaline (by 35–40%; $F = 18.51$; $p < 0.001$; $n = 4$).

According to some data,[3,4] the direct pp is the main source of specific sensory information to the CA1 field. Our current understanding of hippocampal circuitry suggests how pathological hyperactivity of monoaminergic sytems and/or hypofunction of NMDA receptors might isolate CA1 from the specific sensory feedback and cause abnormalities in information processing.[2,5]

ACKNOWLEDGMENTS

Supported by 2R01 NS27337/09 and RG3-96-015 Alzheimer Association Grants to J.L.; 1F32 MH11720-01 NIMH INRSA, NARSAD Young Investigator Award, and the Supreme Council 33° Scottish Rite Schizophrenia Research Program, N.M.J., U.S.A., grants to N.O.

REFERENCES

1. SWANSON L, C. KÖHLER & A. BJÖRKLUND. 1987. The limbic region. I: The septohippocampal system. In Integrated Systems of the CNS. A. Björklund, T. Hökfelt & L. Swanson, Eds.: 125–269. Elsevier. New York.
2. OTMAKHOVA, N.A. & J.E. LISMAN. 1999. Dopamine selectively inhibits the direct cortical pathway to the ca1 hippocampal region. J. Neurosci. 19: 1437–1445.
3. VINOGRADOVA, O. 1984. Functional organization of the limbic system in the process of registration of information: facts and hypotheses. In The Hippocampus. R.L. Isaacson & K.H. Pribram, Eds.: 1–69. Plenum. New York.
4. MCNAUGHTON, B.L., C.A. BARNES, J. MELTZER & R.J. SUTHERLAND. 1989. Hippocampal granule cells are necessary for normal spatial learning but not for spatially-selective pyramidal cell discharge. Exp. Brain Res. 76: 485–965.
5. LISMAN, J.E. 1999. Relating hippocampal circuitry to function: recall of memory sequences by reciprocal dentate–CA3 interactions. Neuron 22: 233–242.

Age-related Deficits in Episodic Memory May Result from Decreased Responsiveness of Hippocampal Place Cells to Changes in Context

JONATHAN A. OLER[a] AND ETAN J. MARKUS

Behavioral Neuroscience Division, Department of Psychology, University of Connecticut, Storrs, Connecticut 06269, USA

The hippocampal formation (HF) is a vital processing stage for episodic memory[1] and for the performance of spatial memory tasks.[2,3] Aging has been shown to impair episodic memory in humans,[4] as well as behavioral performance on spatial tasks in rats.[5,6] These behavioral findings, taken together with anatomical and physiological changes, indicate impaired hippocampal function during aging. The principal cells of the rodent HF display location-dependent activity,[7–9] and these "place cells" may form a cognitive map of the animal's environment.[10] Furthermore, the fact that the HF can change its representation of the environment in response to behavioral manipulations may form the basis for episodic memory processing.[11] The present study was designed to examine the effects of altering *behavioral demands* on hippocampal place cell activity in middle-aged and old rats, while the testing environment remained relatively stable, and the animals were not removed from the apparatus. The results suggest that age-related memory deficits associated with a loss of normal hippocampal function result from decreased sensitivity of the hippocampal network to respond to meaningful changes in the environment.

METHODS

Five middle-aged (12–16 months) and six old (24–28 months) F-344 male rats were trained to run in both directions on a "figure-8" track in order to receive a food reward (see FIG. 1A). The track consisted of four arms forming a symmetrical "✚", with two removable arcs connecting the top and bottom of the figure-8. A few chocolate sprinkles were placed in small food cups at the four corners of the track, and the rats were consistently rewarded each time they reached a corner (task A). With the connecting arcs removed, the track was transformed into a traditional four-arm plus maze with identical, symmetrical arms, each with a food cup at the end (task B, see FIG. 1B). This permitted recording cells as the animal sampled the same locations under two different behavioral conditions. During task B, the baiting procedure was also changed to create a working memory task. The experiment was designed so there would be sufficient sampling of the track arms, in both directions, between task

[a]Address for correspondence: Jonathan A. Oler, M.A., Behavioral Neuroscience Division, Department of Psychology, University of Connecticut, 406 Babbidge Rd., Box U-20, Storrs, CT 06269. Tel.: (860) 486-3671; fax: (860) 486-2760.
e-mail: jonathan.oler@uconn.edu

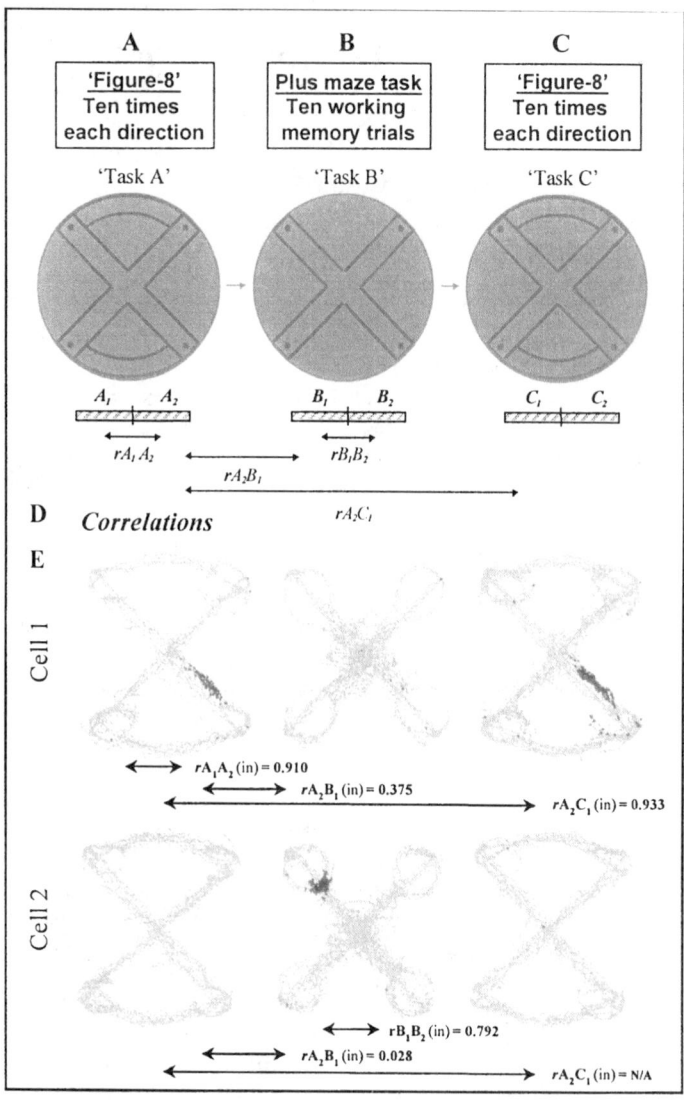

FIGURE 1. Training/recording procedure. **(A)** Configuration of the behavioral apparatus during task A. The rats were trained to run five laps in one direction, 10 laps in the reverse direction, and five additional laps in the original direction ($5 \times 10 \times 5$ procedure). The animals were consistently rewarded with a few chocolate sprinkles at each corner. **(B)** At the end of task A, the top and bottom arcs of the track were removed. With the apparatus in this configuration, the corners were rebaited only after the rat ate from all four arms. This "working memory" procedure was repeated for 10 trials. **(B)** Following the 10th working memory trial, the arcs were returned and the food cups rebaited. The animals again performed the $5 \times 10 \times 5$ procedure, receiving a food reward each time a corner was reached. **(C)** Correlation analysis. The correlation of firing-rate maps between the two halves of a behavioral task

A and task B. At the end of task B, the experimenter replaced the connecting arcs and rebaited the food cups, and the animal again ran the figure-8 task (task C; see FIG. 1C).

The animals were surgically implanted with microelectrodes for single-unit recording from the dorsal hippocampus. The recording environment was divided up into a 64×64 bin array and smoothed firing-rate maps were constructed for each cell.[12] Place fields were defined as an area of at least 15 bins sharing adjacent edges, with a firing rate per bin greater than two standard deviations above the mean firing rate of the cell. To compare changes in place fields between tasks, rate map correlations within and between the different tasks were calculated (see FIG. 1D). To statistically analyze changes in place fields between behavioral tasks, several relative scores were calculated for each place cell. The following formula was used to calculate the relative score:

$$R = \frac{(r \text{ within task})}{(r \text{ within task}) + (r \text{ between tasks})}$$

Where "r within task" is the correlation between the first and second half of a given task, and "r between tasks" is the correlation between the second half of one task and the first half of the other task. Thus, a relative score of 0.5 indicates no change in place fields across the two tasks because the within-task correlation is equal to the between-tasks correlation. A relative score closer to 1.0 indicates a change in spatial firing across tasks because the between-tasks correlation is smaller than the within-task correlation (see Oler and Markus[17]).

RESULTS

A total of 187 complex spike cells were recorded as the animals performed the full sequence of tasks ($A \rightarrow B \rightarrow C$). An analysis of variance, by animal, of the middle-aged and old rats showed no effect of age on the basic spatial firing properties of the cells (all, $p > 0.1$). Place fields were unchanged between tasks A and C, with the average R_{AC} score for both age groups almost exactly 0.5 (FIG. 2A). This indicates a high degree of consistency in the representation of the environment under similar behavioral circumstances. However, a substantial proportion of place fields from both middle-aged and old animals displayed "re-mapping" in response to changing the task. As can be seen in the examples in FIGURE 1E, some place fields were strongly affected. The average R_{AB} scores were significantly different from 0.5 for both the middle-aged and old rats (FIG. 2B). These relative scores denote smaller between-task correlations (rA_2B_1) than within-task correlations (rA_1A_2), indicating dissimilar

---

("within-task" correlations; rA_1A_2, rB_1B_2) were compared to the correlation of firing-rate maps between the second half of task A and the first half of the tasks B and C ("between-tasks" correlations; rA_2B_1, rA_2C_1, respectively). (E) Hippocampal place cell responses to a change in task. Two examples of the spatial firing of single hippocampal neurons, recorded from different animals, during the entire sequence of the change in behavioral task, and rate map correlations. Grey depicts the position of the animal and black a spike from the neuron. Cell 1, A place field on the southeast arm only during the figure-8 track (task A and task C). Cell 2, Place field that appeared only during task B.

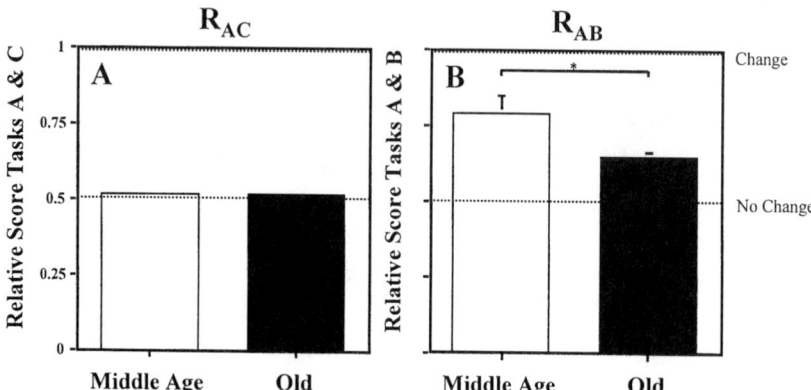

FIGURE 2. Relative scores. *A*, Task A ↔ Task C. The relative score (R_{AC}) was calculated as the ratio of within-task correlation (rA_1A_2) over the sum of the within-task correlation and the between-tasks correlation ($rA_1A_2 + rA_2C_1$). Therefore, a score of 0.5 indicates that the within-task correlation is equal to the between-tasks correlation, whereas a score closer to 1.0 denotes a change in spatial firing across tasks. Note that for both age groups the mean R_{AC} was almost exactly 0.5, indicating that place fields represented tasks A and C in a highly similar fashion. Additionally, these relative scores are evidence for electrode stability during recording sessions. **(B)** Task A ↔ Task B. The relative score (R_{AB}) was calculated as the ratio of within task correlation (rA_1A_2) over the sum of the within task correlation and the between tasks correlation ($rA_1A_2 + rA_2B_1$). Note that the mean R_{AB} for both age groups (middle aged: 0.773 ± 0.04; old: 0.648 ± 0.03, mean and SEM, respectively) was significantly greater than 0.5 (*t*-tests, $p < 0.01$), indicating that place fields represented tasks A and B differently. Additionally, the change in representation across behavioral tasks was greater for the middle-aged than for old animals (*$p < 0.05$).

hippocampal representations of the environment between tasks A and B. It was found that this change in representation was greater for middle-aged than for old animals.

DISCUSSION

The reorganization found in hippocampal representation between tasks A and B in the present study appears to be due to changes in search strategy and/or trajectory planning. These data support and extend previous reports that hippocampal units do not simply encode for location, but rather for location within a given reference frame or context.[13] Consequently, the hippocampus can represent many different environments, as well as provide multiple representations of a given environment. Each representation could therefore be encoding a significant event in a given environment—a mechanism well suited to underlie episodic memory.

In both the middle-aged and old animals, the hippocampus showed a reliable representation of a given situation/task. However, the hippocampus of the aged rats showed less of a distinction between two different tasks within the same environment. A number of studies have shown age-related differences in the manner with which a stable or changed environment is represented by the hippocampus.[14-16] In those studies the animals were taken out of the environment before subsequent reintroduction, and the aged animals may have been affected by this manipulation. The current findings indicate that even when the animal remains within the environment, and must only encode a change in task demands, aging effects are found. Failure of the aged hippocampal system to form distinct representations of significant events in a given environment may give rise to episodic memory impairments in the elderly.

ACKNOWLEDGMENTS

This work was supported by National Institute on Aging, NIH grant R29-A613941-01A1, and University of Connecticut Research Foundation grant 441713. Preliminary data from this research was presented in a Society for Neuroscience abstract, and a more detailed manuscript is in press.[17]

REFERENCES

1. SCOVILLE, W.B. & B. MILNER. 1957. Loss of recent memory after bilateral hippocampal lesions. J. Neurol. Neurosurg. Psychiatry **20:** 11–21.
2. OLTON, D.S. & R.J. SAMUELSON. 1976. Remembrance of places passed: spatial memory in rats. J. Exp. Psychol. Anim. Behav. Proc. **2:** 97–116.
3. MORRIS, R.G. et al. 1999. The hippocampus and spatial memory in humans. In The Hippocampal and Parietal Foundations of Spatial Cognition. N. Burgess, K.J. Jeffery & J. O'Keefe, Eds.: 259–289. Oxford University Press. Oxford, U.K.
4. UTTL, B. & P. GRAF. 1993. Episodic spatial memory in adulthood. Psychol. Aging **8:** 257–273.
5. BARNES, C.A. 1979. Memory deficits associated with senescence: a neurophysiological and behavioral study in the rat. J. Comp. Physiol. Psychol. **93:** 74–104.
6. OLER, J.A. & E.J. MARKUS. 1998. Age-related deficits on the radial maze and in fear conditioning: hippocampal processing and consolidation. Hippocampus **8:** 402–415.
7. O'KEEFE, J. & J. DOSTROVSKY. 1971. The hippocampus as a spatial map. Preliminary evidence from unit activity in the freely-moving rat. Brain Res. **34:** 171–175.
8. RANCK, J.B., JR. 1973. Studies on single neurons in dorsal hippocampal formation and septum in unrestrained rats. Part 1. Behavioral correlates and firing repertiores. Exp. Neurol. **41:** 461–531.
9. JUNG, M.W. & B.L. MCNAUGHTON. 1993. Spatial selectivity of unit activity in the hippocampal granular layer. Hippocampus **3:** 165–182.
10. O'KEEFE, J. & L. NADEL. 1978. The Hippocampus as a Cognitive Map. Clarendon Press. Oxford, U.K.
11. MARKUS, E.J. et al. 1995. Interactions between location and task affect the spatial and directional firing of hippocampal neurons. J. Neurosci. **15:** 7079–7094.
12. SKAGGS, W.E. & B.L. MCNAUGHTON. 1998. Spatial firing properties of hippocampal CA1 populations in an environment containing two visually identical regions. J. Neurosci. **18:** 8455–8466.
13. REDISH, A.D. & D.S. TOURETZKY. 1997. Cognitive maps beyond the hippocampus. Hippocampus **7:** 15–35.
14. BARNES, C.A. et al. 1997. Multistability of cognitive maps in the hippocampus of aged rats. Nature **388:** 272–275.
15. TANILA, H. et al. 1997. Brain aging: changes in the nature of information coding by the hippocampus. J. Neurosci. **17:** 5155–5166.

16. TANILA, H. *et al.* 1997. Brain aging: impaired coding of novel environmental cues. J. Neurosci. **17:** 5167–5174.
17. OLER, J.A. & E.J. MARKUS. Age related deficits in the ability to encode contextual change: a place cell analysis. Hippocampus. In press.

Presubicular Input to the Dendrites of Layer-V Entorhinal Neurons in the Rat

THEO VAN HAEFTEN,[a] FLORIS G. WOUTERLOOD, AND MENNO P. WITTER

Department of Anatomy, Research Institute Neurosciences Vrije Universiteit, Faculty of Medicine, Vrije Universiteit Amsterdam, NL-1081 BT Amsterdam, the Netherlands

INTRODUCTION

The presubiculum is an inconspicuous, but functionally important, region of the parahippocampal cortex. It receives afferents form the retrosplenial and visual cortices, the anterior and laterodorsal nucleus of the thalamus, from the claustrum, the septal complex, and various nuclei of the brainstem.[1–4] In turn, the presubiculum distributes projections to the thalamus, the mammillary nuclei, the retrosplenial cortex, and the entorhinal cortex.[4,5] This latter projection is very dense and distributes bilaterally to layers I and III of the medial subdivision of the entorhinal cortex (MEA).[4] This projection comprises both excitatory and inhibitory fibers,[6] which have been shown to appose dendrites of entorhinal neurons, whose somata are located in layers I and III.[7] It is known that these target neurons give rise to the perforant pathway. The superficial layers of MEA, however, also contain the dendrites of neurons whose somata are located in deep layers V and VI.[8] Our intracellular tracing studies have shown that the apical dendrites of specific types of layer-V neurons arborize in layer I and to a lesser extent in layer III. Hence, we speculated that these neurons may be targeted by presubicular projections as well. In the present study, we have investigated this hypothesis by means of anterograde tracing in combination with selective labeling of putative target neurons in layer V of the MEA.

MATERIALS AND METHODS

Anesthetized rats ($n = 5$) were iontophoretically injected with the anterograde tracer phaseolus vulgaris-leucoagglutinin (Pha-L; Vector, Burlingame, CA) into the presubiculum. After a recovery period of one week, the animals underwent surgery again to iontophoretically inject minute amounts of the tracer Neurobiotin™ (Vector) around somata of neurons in layer V of the MEA. Two days later, the rats were transcardially perfused with an aldehyde-based fixative, their brains removed from the skull and subsequently cut on a freezing microtome. Sections were subjected to a standard double-staining protocol for light microscopy or a double-staining protocol with fluorescent-tagged compounds for two-laser confocal laser scanning microscopy and computer reconstruction.[9]

[a]Address for correspondence: Research Institute Neurosciences Vrije Universiteit, Department of Anatomy, Faculty of Medicine, Vrije Universiteit Amsterdam, 7 van der Boechorststraat, NL-1081 BT Amsterdam, The Netherlands. Tel.: (31)-20-4448049; fax: (31)-20-4448054.
e-mail: T.van_Haeften.anat@med.vu.nl

RESULTS

Unilateral injections of Pha-L in the presubiculum resulted in a massive fiber labeling in layers I and III of the ipsi- and contralateral MEA. In layers II and V, only a few labeled fibers were present. In all cases, the pattern of labeling in the contralateral MEA was the mirror image of that seen in the ipsilateral MEA. Injections of neurobiotin in layer V resulted in a very selective and complete labeling of a few somata in close vicinity of the injection site. The processes and axons of these labeled neurons could be followed into layer I. In those cases, where injections were made with both tracers, labeled layer-V neurons, whose spine-bearing dendrites ascended into the presubicular plexus, were observed. Close examination of these dendrites revealed many putative contacts of presubicular fibers with spines. Occasionally, appositions on dendritic shafts were observed. Because it is impossible to distinguish in the light microscope between true synaptic appositions and false positive appositions, sections containing both tracers were examined in a confocal laser scanning microscope. Possible appositions were studied at high magnification and 3D reconstructions were prepared. We have so far studied material from two animals and noted that presubicular fibers in many instances indeed formed presumed synaptic contacts with the dendrites of layer-V neurons.

CONCLUSION

Our findings confirmed earlier studies demonstrating that the presubiculum gives rise to strong projections to layers I and III of MEA.[4–7] Neurobiotin filling of layer-V neurons has revealed many spine-bearing dendritic processes traversing the lamina dissecans up into the superficial layers to arborize profusely in layer I. Close examination with the use of the confocal laser scanning microscope has demonstrated the presence in layers III and I of many close appositions between presubicular axons and layer-V dendritic spines, indicating the presence of synaptic contacts. We have thus obtained evidence supporting the hypothesis that neurons located in layer V of the EC have direct access to information delivered to the superficial layers by presubicular projections. Our findings demonstrate that the general conception of a functional separation between superficial neocortical input layers and deep hippocampal output layers of the entorhinal cortex is no longer tenable. We speculate that presubicular input to layer-V neurons may either be directly mediated to the neocortex and/or may influence the functioning of these neurons in the entorhinal–hippocampal network. Further detailed studies using high-power confocal 3D analysis are currently in progress.

ACKNOWLEDGMENTS

This work was supported by grant NWO:903-47-051 awarded to T.v.H. by the Netherlands Organization for Scientific Research.

REFERENCES

1. SWANSON, L.W. & W.M. COWAN. 1977. An autoradiographic study of the organization of the efferent connections of the hippocampal formation in the rat. J. Comp. Neurol. **172:** 49–84.
2. VOGT, B.A. & M.W. MILLER. 1983. Cortical connections between rat cingulate cortex and visual, motor, and postsubicular cortices. J. Comp. Neurol. **216:** 192–210.
3. WITTER, M.P. *et al.* 1989. Functional organization of the extrinsic and intrinsic circuitry of the parahippocampal region. Prog. Neurobiol. **33:** 161–253.
4. VAN GROEN, T. & J.M. WYSS. 1990. The connections of presubiculum and parasubiculum in the rat. Brain Res. **518:** 227–243.
5. SWANSON, L.W. *et al.* 1987. The limbic region. I. The septohippocampal system. Elsevier. Amsterdam.
6. VAN HAEFTEN, T. *et al.* 1997. GABAergic presubicular projections to the medial entorhinal cortex of the rat. J. Neurosci. **17:** 862–874.
7. CABELLERO-BLEDA, M. & M.P. WITTER. 1994. Projections from the presubiculum and parasubiculum to morphologically characterized entorhinal–hippocampal neurons in the rat. Exp. Brain Res. **101:** 93–108.
8. LORENTE DE NÓ, R. 1933. Studies on the structure of the cerebral cortex. J. Psychol. Neurol. **45:** 381–438.
9. WOUTERLOOD, F.G. *et al.* 1998. Two laser dual immunofluorescence confocal laser scanning microscopy using CY2- and CY5-conjugated secondary antibodies: unequivocal detection of co-localization of neuronal markers. Brain Res. Prot. **2:** 149–159.

Perirhinal Cortex and Thalamic Stimulation Induces LTP in Different Areas of the Amygdala

DAN YANIV,[a] GLENN E. SCHAFE,[b] JOSEPH E. LeDOUX,[b] AND
GAL RICHTER-LEVIN[a,c]

[a]*Department of Psychology, University of Haifa, Haifa 31905, Israel*

[b]*Center for Neural Science, New York University, New York, New York 10003, USA*

The parahippocampal region consists of the cortical areas that surround the hippocampus, including the perirhinal, the postrhinal, and entorhinal cortices. To a large degree, research into parahippocampal function is guided by the view that this area mediates interactions between cerebral cortex and hippocampus and thus contributes to object memory (association of objects with events) (see, for example, Suzuki et al.[1] and Murray[2]). Yet in recent years the amygdala and the perirhinal cortex (PRC) have been increasingly implicated in several aspects of cognitive and emotional learning, that is, associating objects/contexts with affective valences (for reviews, see Refs. 3–5). In fact, the rat PRC is regarded as a "gateway" for cortical sensory input to the amygdala,[6] before the input is further transferred to diencephalic motivational systems that regulate behavior.

A recent anatomical account of the PRC–amygdala system has distinguished between efferents arising from dorsal and ventral PRC.[7] The evidence indicated that the lateral nucleus of the amygdala (LA) receives input from the dorsal bank of the PRC (Brodmann's area 36), whereas both the fundus and ventral bank of the rhinal sulcus (Brodmann's area 35; vPRC) project heavily to the amygdaloid basal nucleus (B). In line with these data, we have recently characterized evoked-field potentials (EPs) in the vPRC-B pathway, and showed that these EPs are amenable to long-term potentiation (LTP) *in vivo*.[8] Given the essential role of the amygdala in the formation of emotional memories and that the PRC is involved in processing of complex, polymodal stimuli in both humans (e.g., Bohbot et al.[9]) and laboratory animals (reviewed by Suzuki,[4] but see Bussey et al.[10]), we suggested that higher order stimulus representations may gain their affective associations via cortical pathways to B which, presumably, functions as a highly integrative site within the amygdaloid processing circuitry.[8,11] This suggestion is consistent with a previous study showing that LTP can be induced in vivo by stimulation of hippocampal inputs to B[12] and seems complementary to an extensive body of research implicating the LA as an essential component of the circuitry through which (unimodal) auditory stimuli are endowed with

[c]Corresponding author: Gal Richter-Levin, Ph.D., Laboratory for Behavioral Neuroscience, Department of Psychology, University of Haifa, Haifa 31905, Israel. Tel.: +972-4-8240962; fax: +972-4-8249654.

e-mail: gal.r-l@psy.haifa.ac.il

emotional significance through Pavlovian fear conditioning.[13] For example, Rogan *et al.*[14] showed that sound processing in the LA is amplified following fear conditioning of the behaving rat, much as is the case after electrically induced LTP in the auditory thalamo-LA pathway.[15]

To further evaluate the hypothesis that the B is important for higher order aspects of plasticity within the amygdala just as LA is involved in simple stimuli-related plasticity, we have compared, in the present study, LTP evoked in the LA versus B by stimulation of the auditory thalamus (medial geniculate nucleus) versus vPRC. Consistent with our hypothesis, the results indicate that thalamic stimulation induced LTP in the LA but not the B, whereas cortical stimulation induced LTP in the B but not in the LA. Yet, due to its mutual connections with the LA, the B may also modify early information processing within the LA as well as control its own input from the LA.[11,16] The relatively new conception that information flow within the amygdala is reciprocal rather than unidirectional,[11] together with the present physiological evidence of plasticity in vPRC-B pathway, suggests that the basolateral amygdala complex, which includes LA and B, functions as a site of plasticity crucial for the formation of aversive emotional memories. (See Fanselow and Ledoux.[17])

REFERENCES

1. SUZUKI, W.A., S. ZOLA-MORGAN, L.R. SQUIRE & D.G. AMARAL. 1993. Lesions of the perirhinal and parahippocampal cortices in the monkey produce long-lasting memory impairments in the visual and tactual modalities. J. Neurosci. **13:** 2430–2451.
2. MURRAY, E.A. 1996. What have ablation studies told us about the neural substrates of stimulus memory? Semin. Neurosci. **8:** 13–22.
3. LEDOUX, J. E. 1995. Emotion: clues from the brain. Annu. Rev. Psychol. **46:** 209–235.
4. SUZUKI, W.A. 1996. The anatomy, physiology and functions of the perirhinal cortex. Curr. Opin. Neurobiol. **6:** 179–186.
5. TULVING, E. & H.J. MARKOWITSCH. 1997. Memory beyond the hippocampus. Curr. Opin. Neurobiol. **7:** 209–216.
6. KOLB, B. 1990. Association cortex. *In* The Cerebral Cortex of the Rat. B. Kolb & R.C. Tees, Eds.: 431–471. MIT Press. Cambridge. MA.
7. SHI, C.-J. & M.D. CASSELL. 1999. Perirhinal cortex projections to the amygdaloid complex and hippocampal formation in the rat. J. Comp. Neurol. **406:** 299–328.
8. YANIV, D. & G. RICHTER-LEVIN. 2000. LTP in the rat basal amygdala induced by perirhinal cortex stimulation *in vivo.* Neuroreport **11:** 525–530.
9. BOHBOT, V.D., M. KALINA, K. STEPANKOVA, *et al.* 1998. Spatial memory deficits in patients with lesions to the right hippocampus and to the right parahippocampal cortex. Neuropsychologia **36:** 1217–1238.
10. BUSSEY, T.J., J.L. MUIR & J.P. AGGLETON. 1999. Functionally dissociating aspects of event memory: the effects of combined perirhinal and postrhinal cortex lesions on object and place memory in the rat. J. Neurosci. **19:** 495–502.
11. PITKANEN, A., V. SAVANDER & J.E. LEDOUX. 1997. Organization of intraamygdaloid circuitries in the rat: An emerging framework for understanding functions of the amygdala. TINS **20:** 517–523.
12. MAREN, S. & M.S. FANSELOW. 1995. Synaptic plasticity in the basolateral amygdala induced by hippocampal fromation stimulation, in vivo. J. Neurosci. **15:** 7548–7564.
13. LEDOUX, J.E. 2000. Emotion circuits in the brain. Annu. Rev. Neurosci. **23:** 155–184.
14. ROGAN, M.T., U.V. STAUBLI & J.E. LEDOUX. 1997. Fear conditioning induces associative long-term potentiation in the amygdala. Nature **390:** 604–607.

15. ROGAN, M. & J.E. LEDOUX. 1995. LTP is accompanied by commensurate enhancement of auditory-evoked responses in a fear conditioning circuit. Neuron **15:** 127–136.
16. SAVANDER, V., R. MIETTINEN, J.E. LEDOUX & A. PITKANEN. 1997. Lateral nucleus of the rat amygdala is reciprocally connected with basal and accessory basal nuclei: a light and electron microscopic study. Neuroscience **77:** 767–781.
17. FANSELOW, M.S. & J.E. LEDOUX. 1999. Why we think plasticity underlying Pavlovian fear conditioning occurs in the basolateral amygdala. Neuron **23:** 229–232.

The Parahippocampal Region and Auditory-Mnemonic Processing

A. ENGELIEN,[a,b] E. STERN,[b] N. ISENBERG,[b,d] W. ENGELIEN,[b] C. FRITH,[c] AND D. SILBERSWEIG[b]

[b]Functional Neuroimaging Laboratory, Weill Medical College of Cornell University, 525 East 68th Street, New York, New York 10021, USA

[c]Wellcome Department of Cognitive Neurology, Institute of Neurology, University College London, 12 Queen Square, London WC1N 3BG, UK

[d]New Jersey Neuroscience Institute, JFK Medical Center, 65 James Street, Edison, New Jersey 08818, USA

The immediate recognition of environmental sounds is a phylogenetically old and important biological function and requires high levels of complex auditory feature integration. It is also closely linked to the process of matching incoming sounds to stored representations and encoding such events when salient. Neuroanatomically, the auditory cortices extend in parallel and serial organization through the temporal lobes from the primary auditory cortices towards the temporal pole and mesial temporal lobe, where highly processed, integrated information passes through the parahippocampal region. The latter is therefore well situated to play a role in automatic recognition and encoding of meaningful events in the environment.

The posterior parahippocampal cortices may constitute the main node of entry for auditory information to the medial temporal lobe memory system, where salient information is encoded into long-term memory. Sound stimulation has very rarely been examined in primate studies of the parahippocampal region. In the few studies reported, activity was elicited by complex sounds rather than simple tones. However, responses to such stimuli have not been directly compared, and the influence of salience versus mere acoustical complexity has not yet been addressed. We have shown that in man the left parahippocampal region is specifically activated during passive listening to meaningful real-world sounds compared to acoustically matched, degenerated meaningless sounds. We argue that such passive, yet carefully controlled, stimulation conditions may therefore prove a powerful tool for investigation of the importance of the parahippocampal region for the auditory domain. This paradigm can be applied in other species.

INTRODUCTION

The immediate recognition of environmental sounds is a phylogenetically old and important biological function. However, the neural correlates of this important function are not well understood, either in humans or in regard to primates or lower mam-

[a]Address for correspondence: Almut Engelien, M.D., Functional Neuroimaging Laboratory, Cornell University Medical College, 525 E. 68th St., Box 140, New York, NY 10021, USA. Tel.: (212) 746-3868; fax: (212) 746-5818.

e-mail: almut@hanazono.med.cornell.edu

malian species. In humans, two lines of research on auditory processing and its implementation in the brain seem prominent. The first line of studies has focused on the representation of simple acoustic parameters, such as pitch or intensity.[1–8] The second line of research, more concerned with higher order processing and meaningful sound events in humans, has virtually exclusively dealt with auditory–linguistic functions, that is, comprehension of spoken speech.[9–14] These lines of research are very important. Only the first one, however, which examines representations of basic physical parameters, allows one to draw direct comparisons across species. Many studies have successfully addressed the issues of tonotopic and amplitopic organization of primary auditory cortices in animal models.[15–18] The role of primary auditory cortices for sound localization[19–23] and preference for more acoustically more complex events[24,25] have also been examined. Only very few and recent studies, however, have systematically and comparatively addressed the role of auditory associational cortices for the processing of more complex tones.[26–29]

None of these studies has been specifically tailored to address the role of the parahippocampal region in auditory–mnemonic processing. As we will review below, the auditory cortices are highly connected to the parahippocampal region. In general, preprocessed information from higher order unimodal and heteromodal association studies is funneled into this region, although the possibility of an additional "shortcut" from auditory unimodal association cortex needs to be considered based on primate anatomical data. Physiological data on the parahippocampal region from primate models are extremely scarce and have never addressed neuronal responses to complex auditory stimuli that would be meaningful to the species examined.

Together with its efferent connectivity to the hippocampus, the parahippocampal region is crucially involved in long-term memory encoding.[30–34] Therefore, we predicted a specific role for the parahippocampal region in processing only salient, meaningful sound events that occur in the real world, which may automatically be encoded into long-term memory. A few studies in healthy human subjects have now addressed the neural correlates of processing and encoding complex, meaningful sounds using modern, noninvasive functional neuroimaging techniques. These studies support our hypothesis of the importance of the parahippocampal regions for processing meaningful, salient sounds. Here we review this work in the context of the existing auditory anatomical and physiological literature on the parahippocampal region, relying on the rhesus monkey in the absence of human data. We will also discuss possible future directions for studies on the parahippocampal region, specifically on its role for audition.

ANATOMY OF AUDITORY CORTICAL CONNECTIONS TO THE PARAHIPPOCAMPAL REGION

Before discussing anatomical connections of auditory cortices in the lateral temporal neocortex to the parahippocampal region, we want to give a brief definition of how the term is used in this article. We exclude the hippocampal formation (including the subiculum and dentate gyrus) from the parahippocampal region. The latter comprises the entorhinal and perirhinal cortices, as well as the posterior parahippocampal cortex, which has also been referred to as the parahippocampal area. We prefer and use the term posterior parahippocampal cortex, since this term is better defined and known in the primate anatomical literature, upon which our concept of the human parahippocampal regions still relies to a large degree.

In general, the parahippocampal region has been called the "gatekeeper to the hippocampus."[32,35] The classical doctrine holds that all information is conveyed to the hippocampal formation, particularly the hippocampus proper, through the entorhinal cortex, which in turn receives its information from the perirhinal and posterior parahippocampal cortices (for some recent challenge of this rule, see Lopes da Silva, this volume). Streaming of information from neocortices to other mesial temporal lobe structures such as the amygdalae is more variable in its connectivity pattern. In the following, we will briefly review anatomical studies on auditory afferents to posterior parahippocampal and perirhinal cortex. To date, the most detailed information pertinent to humans relies on primates, particularly the rhesus monkey.

In these animals, the parahippocampal cortex receives more input from second-order sensory association areas, whereas perirhinal cortex receives inputs from third-order sensory association cortices.[36] The auditory input to the posterior parahippocampal cortex stems mainly from auditory association areas in the superior temporal gyrus (Brodmann's area, in the following, BA 22), and inferior parietal lobule. It has been argued that some of these projections, which tend to be reciprocal, might be anatomically homologous to human "temporoparietal speech cortex."[37–40] Recently, the connectivity of auditory cortex projections specifically to the posterior part of parahippocampal cortices has been confirmed and refined by Suzuki,[41] who also now studies the connectivity between and within parahippocampal cortices.[42]

As an exception to the rule of nonprimary sensory cortex projecting to entorhinal cortex through posterior parahippocampal and/or perirhinal cortices, a direct projection from the superior temporal gyrus to entorhinal cortex has also been demonstrated.[43] Specifically, opercular lip and dorsal convexity of superior temporal gyrus project to medial entorhinal cortex, cortex bounding the depth of the superior temporal sulcus to perirhinal cortex (BA 35). Fundus and ventral bank of the superior temporal sulcus project to that portion of the parahippocampal gyrus that is caudally adjacent to the perirhinal cortex. Part of these projection lines come from an auditory association area, whereas the superior temporal sulcus areas in the monkey may be more polymodal. The projections from parahippocampal back to auditory association cortex have been studied by Tranel *et al.* and support the notion of largely reciprocal connections overall between these cortical areas.[40] In addition to these direct projections between the parahippocampal region and auditory cortices, auditory information may also reach the parahippocampal region through multisynaptic connections via frontal[44,45] and (para)insular regions.[45]

Little information is available on the human brain directly, especially for the posterior parahippocampal cortex, which is of greatest relevance to this paper. However, it seems that there is good analogy between rhesus monkey and human anatomy at least as regards the entorhinal cortex.[46] For reviews of the anatomy in macaques with discussion of homology with humans, see the work of Salzmann and Gloor.[35,47] Also in lower mammals, for example, the rat, the basic connectivity patterns of the parahippocampal regions seem to be like the one demonstrated in monkeys: projections from entorhinal to neocortices pass through the perirhinal and parahippocampal cortices. Regarding the details of the connectivity of the auditory cortices to the parahippocampal regions, however, it is notable that there may be some differences in lower mammalian species such as the rat and mouse: in these species, the perirhinal cortices seem to receive more unimodal auditory input than the posteror parahippocampal cortices (often labeled "postrhinal cortex" in this literature).[15,48]

AUDITORY PHYSIOLOGICAL STUDIES ON THE PARAHIPPOCAMPAL REGION IN PRIMATES AND HUMANS

Single-cell recording data on the processing of auditory stimuli in the parahippocampal regions in the macaque are extremely rare. First, this region poses a technical challenge for recording from awake animals. Second, responses from parahippocampal neurons were most often recorded in the context of hypotheses on the role of mesial temporal lobe structures for memory, and therefore sometimes not even reported separately from the hippocampal neurons' responses obtained in the same studies. Furthermore, the majority of these studies used visual stimulation in delayed matching to sample, that is, an active, trained task with an explicit memory component. During pure passive stimulation, MacLean et al. observed no responses to auditory stimuli in parahippocampal cortex; however, only pure sinusoidal tones were tested.[49] Desimone and Gross found 35% of cells in posterior parahippocampal cortex responding to complex auditory stimuli (as well as to visual), and an additional 2% specifically to auditory stimuli only.[50] An auditory correlate of the visual delayed-matching-to-sample, or modified Konorski, paradigm has only recently been studied in a careful combined behavioral and staged lesion approach, which will be further discussed below.[51] However, the auditory stimuli used in this experiment were not controlled for their genuine salience (rather than the trained familiarity) for the monkey, and single-cell recordings were not obtained.

In humans, we performed the first investigations of processing of meaningful environmental sound events in a series of functional neuroimaging experiments with positron emission tomography (PET). We were particularly interested in testing the participation of mesial temporal cortex in addition to auditory cortices for automatic matching of recognizable, meaningful sound events to stored representations, as well as automatic encoding of such salient events. In a new experimental approach to test this hypothesis, we altered the inherent semantic properties of complex sound stimuli rather than cognitive task instruction. Six healthy, right-handed men were examined while listening to meaningful versus meaningless acoustically matched nonverbal sounds in order to dissociate automatic semantic recognition from perceptual analysis. The crucial sound stimuli contrasts were generated by digital processing and analysis of the sounds, which are described in detail elsewhere. We established in an additional behavioral experiment that original sounds were correctly identified and degenerated sounds were not. Our PET activation results show that brain activity specifically associated with processing of meaningful versus meaningless sounds was lateralized to the left hemisphere and was specifically located in the parahippocampal region.

We also examined more active cognitive components of the processing of meaningful nonverbal sounds such as semantic categorization of sounds. Monitoring environmental sounds for a semantic target category is also mediated by the left hemisphere, by a distinct, distributed neocortical network comprising (pre)frontal, inferior parietal, and lateral middle temporal regions.[52] During performance of this task compared to passive listening to the same meaningful, identifiable sounds, parahippocampal cortices were not active. When encoding of such meaningful nonverbal sounds was explicitly required in the task instruction, however, other groups have demonstrated bilateral parahippocampal cortex activity (see Gabrieli, this volume).

DISCUSSION

We discuss here a functional neuroimaging study demonstrating the role of the left parahippocampal region in humans for the automatic processing of complex nonverbal, meaningful versus meaningless sounds in the context of anatomical and physiological knowledge from rhesus monkeys. Although our paradigm has no active cognitive task or motor output requirement, it does entail a number of processing components that were dissociated from the (bottom-up) acoustics, for which the two sound conditions were carefully matched. The meaningful sounds in contrast to the meaningless sounds are recognizable, that is, they have an identifiable semantic content, and in addition may be inherently more salient or "interesting," so that they may be more likely to be remembered. The latter means that during the one time presentation during the experiment, memory encoding may also be automatically engaged.

It may not be possible to disentangle these components completely based on this study alone. A central question here may be whether the functions of semantic recognition and long-term memory encoding can be dissociated, and if so, what their differential neural correlates are. Because the meaningful versus meaningless distinction, to our best knowledge, has not been made in the animal model literature, the macaque studies may only help for interpretation of the memory component. Regarding the well-studied, delayed-matching tasks in other sensory modalities, it has become increasingly clear in recent years that the parahippocampal regions play a very important role for retention of higher order, object-related sensory information, possibly even more so than the hippocampus proper.[53–55] Recent functional neuroimaging studies in humans also demonstrated parahippocampal activity associated with several mnemonic tasks.[30–34,56–58]

Functional neuroimaging methods have also been widely employed for studying the functional architecture of semantic processing in humans. With regard to semantic processing of nonverbal sounds, we demonstrated that this is a left hemisphere function,[52] as are semantic judgements on words and pictures[11,59,60] and the recognition of unique semantic items.[61] The laterality of finding is well in accord with these previous studies in man. Typically, in the *active* semantic tasks, associated activity was distributed in neural networks across the neocortical lobes. One study aimed to examine semantic networks when active spontaneously (during conscious "resting") and during a semantic decision/retrieval task, compared to other auditory perceptual tasks. The semantic network, which was noted to be downregulated from rest relative to the active tone perception task, and upregulated during the semantic retrieval task, comprised the left posterior parahippocampal cortex in addition to the above-mentioned dorsolateral (pre)frontal, inferior parietal, and temporal neocortical network in the left hemisphere.[60]

To summarize these lines of evidence on semantic and memory processing, the parahippocampal region in general may play an important role in memory formation for highly processed sensory information, and more specifically the left parahippocampal region for semantic information processing (as one node in a distributed neural network). To delineate which regions are necessary for a task, the consideration of behavioral studies after circumscribed brain lesions in both humans and monkeys may be equally important. Semantic recognition of meaningful sounds is disturbed in the neuropsychological syndrome of auditory agnosia. This disorder occurs after bilateral lateral auditory association cortex lesions.[52,62–64] With parahippocampal cortex lesions, auditory recognition, to the best of our knowledge, has not been specifically studied.

With regard to auditory (recognition) memory, some of the older lesion literature both in human neuropsychology and monkey models is currently revisited: the lesions associated with memory deficits often encompassed parahippocampal cortices as well as the hippocampus, so that the observed memory deficits may well depend on the parahippocampal region. Again, the information on deficits in the auditory verbal domain is scarcer than for the visual[65,66]; for nonverbal sound material, it is even more rare. The famous amnesic patient H.M., whose medial temporal lobe lesions extend from parts of the hippocampi into parts of the parahippocampal regions,[67] could not perform delayed paired comparison of simple acoustic stimuli. His discrimination of the same pairs of stimuli with 0 sec delay was intact.[68–70] The recent studies of auditory recognition memory in macaque monkeys[51] demonstrate that the auditory association cortices, or their undisturbed information output to the mesial temporal lobe, may be more crucial for auditory delayed matching to sample than the mesial temporal structures per se.

In sum, it therefore seems that the reciprocal connectivity in this temporal lobe system of the auditory association and parahippocampal cortices may be relevant for and engaged in both auditory recognition and encoding across species. We suggest that the left parahippocampal region may be important in automatically assessing the relevance of complex incoming sensory information to enable encoding of salient environmental events. It is possible that semantic content is a prerequisite for the left hemisphere laterality of this finding.

FUTURE DIRECTIONS

The functional neuroimaging studies discussed in this volume by us and Gabrieli *et al.* may in sum suggest that the posterior parahippocampal cortex in humans has an important role for encoding salient, meaningful sound events. In our paradigm, this function can be stimulated passively by presenting complex, meaningful sound events and acoustically matched, nonsalient control sounds. The strength of the functional neuroimaging approach is that it allows one to evaluate the contribution of the whole brain in action and can help to generate hypotheses on specific brain regions on a data-driven basis in addition to theoretical and modeling approaches. When paradigms are constructed in a passive, yet carefully controlled manner that is amenable to animal model studies, future studies with direct recordings from these cortical regions may help to delineate the precise type and timing of this neuronal activity.

REFERENCES

1. PANTEV, C. *et al.* 1988. Tonotopic organization of the human auditory cortex revealed by transient auditory evoked magnetic fields. Electroencephalogr. Clin. Neurophysiol. **69:** 160–170.
2. PANTEV, C. *et al.* 1989. Tonotopic organization of the auditory cortex: pitch versus frequency representation. Science **246:** 486–488.
3. PANTEV, C. *et al.* 1989. Neuromagnetic evidence of an amplitopic organization of the human auditory cortex. Electroencephalogr. Clin. Neurophysiol. **72:** 225–231.
4. PANTEV, C. *et al.* 1995. Specific tonotopic organizations of different areas of the human auditory cortex revealed by simultaneous magnetic and electric recordings. Electroencephalogr. Clin. Neurophysiol. **94:** 26–40.
5. WESSINGER, C.M. *et al.* 1997. Tonotopy in human auditory cortex examined with functional magnetic resonance imaging. Human Brain Mapping **5:** 18–25.
6. BELIN, P. *et al.* 1998. The functional anatomy of sound intensity discrimination. J. Neurosci. **18:** 6388–6394.
7. PANTEV, C. *et al.* 1998. Increased auditory cortical representation in musicians. Nature **392:** 811–814.
8. ENGELIEN, A. *et al.* 1999. Detailed tonotopic mapping with silent, event-related fMRI. Neuroimage **9:** S784.
9. BINDER, J.R. *et al.* 1996. Function of the left planum temporale in auditory and linguistic processing. Brain **119:** 1239–1247.
10. BINDER, J.R. *et al.* 1995. Lateralized human brain language systems demonstrated by task subtraction functional magnetic resonance imaging. Arch. Neurol. **52:** 59–601.
11. DEMONET, J.F. *et al.* 1992. The anatomy of phonological and semantic processing in normal subjects. Brain **115:** 1753–1768.
12. EULITZ, C. *et al.* 1994. Comparison of magnetic and metabolic brain activity during a verb generation task. Neuroreport **6:** 97–100.
13. PRICE, C. *et al.* 1992. Regional response differences within the human auditory cortex when listening to words. Neurosci. Lett. **146:** 179–182.
14. HIRANO, S. *et al.* 1997. Cortical activation by monaural speech sound stimulation demonstrated by positron emission tomography. Exp. Brain Res. **113:** 75–80.
15. BURWELL, R.D. & D.G. AMARAL. 1998. Cortical afferents of the perirhinal, postrhinal, and entorhinal cortices of the rat. J. Comp. Neurol. **398:** 179–205.
16. MERZENICH, M.M., J.H. KAAS & G.L. ROTH. 1976. Auditory cortex in the grey squirrel: tonotopic organization and architectonic fields. J. Comp. Neurol. **166:** 387–401.
17. MOREL, A., P.E. GARRAGHTY & J.H. KAAS. 1993. Tonotopic organization, architectonic fields, and connections of auditory cortex in macaque monkeys. J. Comp. Neurol. **335:** 437–459.
18. SCHREINER, C.E. & J.V. URBAS. 1986. Representation of amplitude modulation in the auditory cortex of the cat. I. The anterior auditory field (AAF). Hear. Res. **21:** 227–241.
19. HEFFNER, H.E. & R.S. HEFFNER. 1990. Effect of bilateral auditory cortex lesions on sound localization in Japanese macaques. J. Neurophysiol. **64:** 915–931.
20. MASTERTON, R.B. & T.J. IMIG. 1984. Neural mechanisms for sound localization. Annu. Rev. Physiol. **46:** 275–287.
21. JENKINS, W.M. & M.M. MERZENICH. 1984. Role of cat primary auditory cortex for sound-localization behavior. J. Neurophysiol. **52:** 819–847.
22. RAJAN, R., L.M. AITKIN & D.R. IRVINE. 1990. Azimuthal sensitivity of neurons in primary auditory cortex of cats. II. Organization along frequency-band strips. J. Neurophysiol. **64:** 888–902.
23. RAJAN, R. *et al.* 1990. Azimuthal sensitivity of neurons in primary auditory cortex of cats. I. Types of sensitivity and the effects of variations in stimulus parameters. J. Neurophysiol. **64:** 872–887.
24. DE CHARMS, R.C., D.T. BLAKE & M.M. MERZENICH. 1998. Optimizing sound features for cortical neurons. Science **280:** 1439–1443.
25. NELKEN, I., Y. ROTMAN & O. BAR YOSEF. 1999. Responses of auditory-cortex neurons to structural features of natural sounds. Nature **397:** 154–157.

26. RAUSCHECKER, J.P., B. TIAN & M. HAUSER. 1995. Processing of complex sounds in the macaque nonprimary auditory cortex. Science **268:** 111–114.
27. RAUSCHECKER, J.P. *et al.* 1997. Serial and parallel processing in rhesus monkey auditory cortex. J. Comp. Neurol. **382:** 89–103.
28. RAUSCHECKER, J.P. 1997. Processing of complex sounds in the auditory cortex of cat, monkey, and man. Acta Otolaryngol. Suppl. **532:** 34–38.
29. RAUSCHECKER, J.P. 1998. Cortical processing of complex sounds. Curr. Opin. Neurobiol. **8:** 516–521.
30. STERN, C.E. *et al.* 1996. The hippocampal formation participates in novel picture encoding: evidence from functional magnetic resonance imaging. Proc. Natl. Acad. Sci. USA **93:** 8660–8665.
31. ROMBOUTS, S.A. *et al.* 1997. Visual association encoding activates the medial temporal lobe: a functional magnetic resonance imaging study. Hippocampus **7:** 594–601.
32. TULVING, E. & H.J. MARKOWITSCH. 1997. Memory beyond the hippocampus. Curr. Opin. Neurobiol. **7:** 209–216.
33. BELLGOWAN, P.S. *et al.* 1998. Side of seizure focus predicts left medial temporal lobe activation during verbal encoding. Neurology **51:** 479–484.
34. EPSTEIN, R. *et al.* 1999. The parahippocampal place area: recognition, navigation, or encoding? Neuron **23:** 115–125.
35. GLOOR, P. 1997. The Temporal Lobe and Limbic System. Oxford University Press. New York.
36. PANDYA, D.N. & E.H. YETERIAN. 1985. *In* Association and Auditory Cortices. A. Peters & E.G. Jones, Eds.: 3–61. Plenum Press. New York.
37. JONES, E.G. & T.P. POWELL. 1970. An anatomical study of converging sensory pathways within the cerebral cortex of the monkey. Brain **93:** 793–820.
38. SELTZER, B. & D.N. PANDYA. 1976. Some cortical projections to the parahippocampal area in the rhesus monkey. Exp. Neurol. **50:** 146–160.
39. MESULAM, M.M. *et al.* 1977. Limbic and sensory connections of the inferior parietal lobule (area PG) in the rhesus monkey: a study with a new method for horseradish peroxidase histochemistry. Brain Res. **136:** 393–414.
40. TRANEL, D. *et al.* 1988. Parahippocampal projections to posterior auditory association cortex (area Tpt) in Old-World monkeys. Exp. Brain Res. **70:** 406–416.
41. SUZUKI, W.A. & D.G. AMARAL. 1994. Perirhinal and parahippocampal cortices of the macaque monkey: cortical afferents. J. Comp. Neurol. **350:** 497–533.
42. SUZUKI, W.A., T. YOON & D.L. FORSHAW. 1999. *In* Proceedings of the Society for Neuroscience 29th Annual Meeting. Miami Beach, FL.: 1901.
43. AMARAL, D.G., R. INSAUSTI & W.M. COWAN. 1983. Evidence for a direct projection from the superior temporal gyrus to the entorhinal cortex in the monkey. Brain Res. **275:** 263–277.
44. VAN HOESEN, G., D.N. PANDYA & N. BUTTERS. 1975. Some connections of the entorhinal (area 28) and perirhinal (area 35) cortices of the rhesus monkey. II. Frontal lobe afferents. Brain Res. **95:** 25–38.
45. INSAUSTI, R., D.G. AMARAL & W.M. COWAN. 1987. The entorhinal cortex of the monkey: II. Cortical afferents. J. Comp. Neurol. **264:** 356–395.
46. INSAUSTI, R. *et al.* 1995. The human entorhinal cortex: a cytoarchitectonic analysis. J. Comp. Neurol. **355:** 171–198.
47. SALZMANN, E. 1992. Importance of the hippocampus and parahippocampus with reference to normal and disordered memory function. Fortschr. Neurol. Psychiatr. **60:** 163–176.
48. BURWELL, R.D., M.P. WITTER & D.G. AMARAL. 1995. Perirhinal and postrhinal cortices of the rat: a review of the neuroanatomical literature and comparison with findings from the monkey brain. Hippocampus **5:** 390–408.
49. MACLEAN, P.D., T. YOKOTA & M.A. KINNARD. 1968. Photically sustained on-responses of units in posterior hippocampal gyrus of awake monkey. J. Neurophysiol. **31:** 870–883.
50. DESIMONE, R. & C.G. GROSS. 1979. Visual areas in the temporal cortex of the macaque. Brain Res. **178:** 363–380.
51. FRITZ, J.B. *et al.* 1999. *In* Proceedings of the Society for Neuroscience 29th Annual Meeting. Miami Beach, FL.: 147.

52. ENGELIEN, A. *et al.* 1995. The functional anatomy of recovery from auditory agnosia. A PET study of sound categorization in a neurological patient and normal controls. Brain **118:** 1395–1409.
53. ZOLA-MORGAN, S. *et al.* 1989. Lesions of perirhinal and parahippocampal cortex that spare the amygdala and hippocampal formation produce severe memory impairment. J. Neurosci. **9:** 4355–4370.
54. YOUNG, B.J. *et al.* 1997. Memory representation within the parahippocampal region. J. Neurosci. **17:** 5183–5195.
55. MURRAY, E.A., M.G. BAXTER & D. GAFFAN. 1998. Monkeys with rhinal cortex damage or neurotoxic hippocampal lesions are impaired on spatial scene learning and object reversals. Behav. Neurosci. **112:** 1291–303.
56. MAGUIRE, E.A., R.S. FRACKOWIAK & C.D. FRITH. 1996. Learning to find your way: a role for the human hippocampal formation. Proc. R. Soc. London B Biol. Sci. **263:** 1745–1750.
57. GUR, R.C. *et al.* 1997. Lateralized changes in regional cerebral blood flow during performance of verbal and facial recognition tasks: correlations with performance and "effort." Brain Cogn. **33:** 388–414.
58. GABRIELI, J.D. 1998. Cognitive neuroscience of human memory. Annu. Rev. Psychol. **49:** 87–115.
59. VANDENBERGHE, R. *et al.* 1996. Functional anatomy of a common semantic system for words and pictures. Nature **383:** 254–256.
60. BINDER, J.R. *et al.* 1999. Conceptual processing during the conscious resting state. A functional MRI study. J. Cogn. Neurosci. **11:** 80–95.
61. GORNO-TEMPINI, M.L., C.J. PRICE & R.S.J. FRACKOWIAK. 1999. *In* Proceedings of the Society for Neuroscience 29th Annual Meeting: 100.
62. VIGNOLO, L.A. 1969. *In* Contributions to Clinical Neuropsychology. A.L. Benton, Ed.: 172–208. Aldine. Chicago.
63. VIGNOLO, L.A. 1982. Auditory agnosia. Philos. Trans. R. Soc. London B Biol. Sci. **298:** 49–57.
64. ENGELIEN, A. 2000. Central Auditory Deficits. Two Case Reports including PET Activation Studies on Recovery Phenomena. LIT. Münster. In press.
65. FRISK, V. & B. MILNER. 1990. The role of the left hippocampal region in the acquisition and retention of story content. Neuropsychologia **28:** 349–359.
66. JOHNSRUDE, I. & B. MILNER. 1994. The effect of presentation rate on the comprehension and recall of speech after anterior temporal-lobe resection. Neuropsychologia **32:** 77–84.
67. CORKIN, S. *et al.* 1997. H.M.'s medial temporal lobe lesion: findings from magnetic resonance imaging. J. Neurosci. **17:** 3964–3979.
68. PRISKO, L. 1963. PhD thesis. McGill University, Montreal.
69. MILNER, B. & L. TAYLOR. 1972. Right-hemisphere superiority in tactile pattern-recognition after cerebral commissurotomy: evidence for nonverbal memory. Neuropsychologia **10:** 1–15.
70. MILNER, B., L.R. SQUIRE & E.R. KANDEL. 1998. Cognitive neuroscience and the study of memory. Neuron **20:** 445–468.

Impaired Sensory Gating and Attention in Rats with Developmental Abnormalities of the Mesocortex

Implications for Schizophrenia

L.M. TALAMINI,[a,b] B. ELLENBROEK,[c] T. KOCH,[b] AND J. KORF[b]

[b]Department of Psychiatry, University Hospital of Groningen, P.O. Box 30.000, 9700 RB Groningen, The Netherlands

[c]Department of Psychoneuropharmacology, University of Nijmegen, Gerard Groteplein 21, 6321 EZ, Nijmegen, The Netherlands

Anatomical investigations of postmortem brain tissue[1,2] and population studies[3,4] have led to neurodevelopmental theories on the pathogenesis of schizophrenia.[5,6] Although various association areas of the brain have been implicated in these theories, structural abnormalities in schizophrenia appear to be most pronounced in certain mesocortical areas of the brain, particularly in the parahippocampal region.[7] These areas occupy a high position in the hierarchy of cerebral information processing and are thought to play an important role in human cognition.[8] Interestingly, the parts of the mesocortex implicated in schizophrenia, such as the parahippocampal region, but also the orbitofrontal, mediofrontal, and anterior cingulate cortex, all originate precociously, during the earliest phases of cortical development.[9,10] We have recently developed a preparation in rats, in which maldevelopment of these regions can be investigated.[11] The approach involves the intoxification of gestating rats, between embryonic day 9 (E9) and E12, with methylazoxymethanol acetate (MAM), a short-acting, alkylating agent that leads to the death of neurons that are actively replicating DNA. It was shown that these procedures induce maldevelopment of mesocortical association areas in the fetuses, including the parahippocampal, anterior cingulate and prefrontal cortex. The abnormalities include cortical shortening and thinning, abnormal asymmetry, disorganized cytoarchitecture, and alterations of cortical nerve growth factor levels.[11–13] At the behavioral level, impairments affect pain perception, response to novelty,[13] and social behavior.[12] As discussed previously, these morphological and behavioral findings present a number of parallels to observations in schizophrenic subjects.

A prominent feature of schizophrenia, not considered in our studies thus far, is impaired attention. The allocation of attention in schizophrenic subjects appears to be impaired at both involuntary (automatic) and controlled levels. This is suggested by recent studies showing poor performance and abnormal evoked potentials in patients with schizophrenia during tasks requiring selective, divided, or sustained attention.[14–17] It has been proposed that attention deficits in schizophrenia might be

[a]Address for correspondence: Lucia M. Talamini, University of Amsterdam, Psychonomics, Roeterstraat 15, 1018 WB Amsterdam, The Netherlands. Tel.: 20.5256807; fax: 20.6391656.
e-mail: Talamini@psy.uva.nl

related to defective gating mechanisms.[18] Sensorimotor gating studies, using the acoustic startle reflex, have indeed demonstrated deficits in a substantial proportion of schizophrenic subjects (50–85%), although the relationship of these deficits with abnormalities of attention is not yet clear. While schizophrenic patients do not differ from control subjects in basal startle amplitude, they appear to habituate slowly to the startle stimulus and to display decreased PPI.[19] Habituation, in this context, is the reduction of startle amplitude occurring after repeated presentation of an initially novel startle stimulus; PPI refers to attenuation of the startle reflex following the presentation of a preceding, low-intensity, acoustic cue. Both phenomena represent involuntary modulations of a brainstem reflex.

Using the aforementioned animal model, the present study investigates whether impairments in sensory gating and attention can result from a subtle disturbance in brain development. Importantly, habituation and PPI of the acoustic startle reflex can be elicited from rats and humans with virtually identical stimulus parameters, thus promoting cross-species extrapolation of experimental findings.[19] Attention in the MAM-treated rats was studied using a "sudden silence" paradigm. In this test situation, the behavioral response to a sudden reduction in background white noise is measured.

MATERIALS AND METHODS

Animals and Housing

Thirty-eight gestating Wistar WI rats (Charles River, Germany), mated over a four-hour period on E0, were injected intraperitoneally (i.p.) with MAM (20 mg/kg in NaCl 0.9%) or with saline 0,9% on E9, E10, E11, or E12. The reaction of MAM with nucleic acids of fetal brain lasts from 2 to 24 hours after injection and is maximal approximately 12 hours post injection.[20] The offspring was group-housed under standard conditions and, upon reaching adulthood, was subjected either to the acoustic startle experiment ($n = 25$) or to the sudden silence paradigm ($n = 37$). Rats were handled twice daily, during at least five days, previous to testing. Observations were made during the animals' light phase (light on 8.00 P.M., light off 8.00 A.M.). The experiments were approved by the local animal welfare committee (FDC1045).

Habituation and Prepulse Inhibition

The startle experiment (in an acoustic startle chamber of San Diego Instruments) was designed to measure PPI and habituation in one session (for detailed methodological description see Ellenbroek *et al.*[21]). The session consisted of three blocks: During the first and last block, only startle pulses (120-dB, 40-msec broad band bursts) were delivered. During the middle block, startle pulses, "no stimulus" trails, and different prepulse-startle pairings were administered pseudo-randomly to measure PPI. The prepulses (20-msec broad band bursts) were 2, 4, 8, or 16 dB above background and were followed by a startle pulse after 100 msec. Intertrial intervals were between 10 and 20 seconds. A background white noise of 70 dB was maintained.

PPI was expressed as the ratio of mean startle amplitude on the prepulse trials and on the startle trials of the middle block. Two measures of habituation were calculated, reflecting habituation after an increasing number of startle stimuli. They were defined as the ratio of mean startle amplitude on the startle trials in the middle or last block and basal startle amplitude. Basal startle amplitude was defined as the mean startle amplitude in the first block of the session. Habituation and PPI were statistically analyzed in two independent, repeated measure procedures, with the groups of rats as the between-subject factor and, either the part of the session (first, middle, last), or the different prepulse intensities as the within-subject factor. Significant effects were further analyzed in individual ANOVA procedures for each level of habituation and each prepulse intensity. Simple contrasts (with the control group as a reference category) were determined to identify significant differences between the control group and the various MAM-treated groups. Within-group statistical analysis consisted of one-way ANOVAs, supplemented with Tukey's honestly significant difference (HSD) multiple comparison procedure. Tests were performed with basal startle amplitude as a covariate.

Sudden Silence Paradigm

The sudden silence test was performed in a sound-attenuated test chamber. White noise (70 dB) could be generated by a speaker mounted in the roof of the chamber. Our setup involved a five-minute pre-exposure to the test box with the noise generator on, in order to reduce the novelty response during the actual attention test. Twenty-four hours later, rats were subjected to the sudden silence paradigm consisting of a five minutes "noise on"–five minutes "noise off" exposure. During the sudden silence test, various behavioral elements were registered using a standard event recorder, among others the element "alert." Here, the animal does not ambulate, keeps at least three limbs on the ground, and scans the environment with its head raised. The other recorded behavioral elements were ambulation (moving around the cage), exploring (sniffing the floor and walls of the test box), rearing (vertical posture of the body with both forepaws raised or placed against the walls), burying (digging in the sawdust bedding of the test box), grooming (placing the mouth and paws on the body or on the head), and immobility (absence of movements; the head does not move and is not raised). Duration of the various behavioral elements was summed over the first (noise on) and over the second (noise off) half of the experiment, and expressed as a percentage of registration time. The data were analyzed through ANOVA for each behavioral element, with the experimental groups as the between-subject factor, followed by simple contrast analysis with the control group as reference.

RESULTS

Habituation and Prepulse Inhibition

The amplitude of the basal startle response (i.e., initial startle amplitude) did not differ significantly between groups (data not shown). Repeated measures analysis of habituation data shows both a significant effect of prenatal treatment ($F = 7.9$, df 4.19, $p = 0.001$) and an interaction effect between prenatal treatment and the levels of habituation ($F = 3.4$, df 8.40, $p < 0.005$). Similarly, analysis of PPI reveals a significant treatment effect ($F = 5.2$, df 4.19, $p < 0.01$), whereas the interaction effect

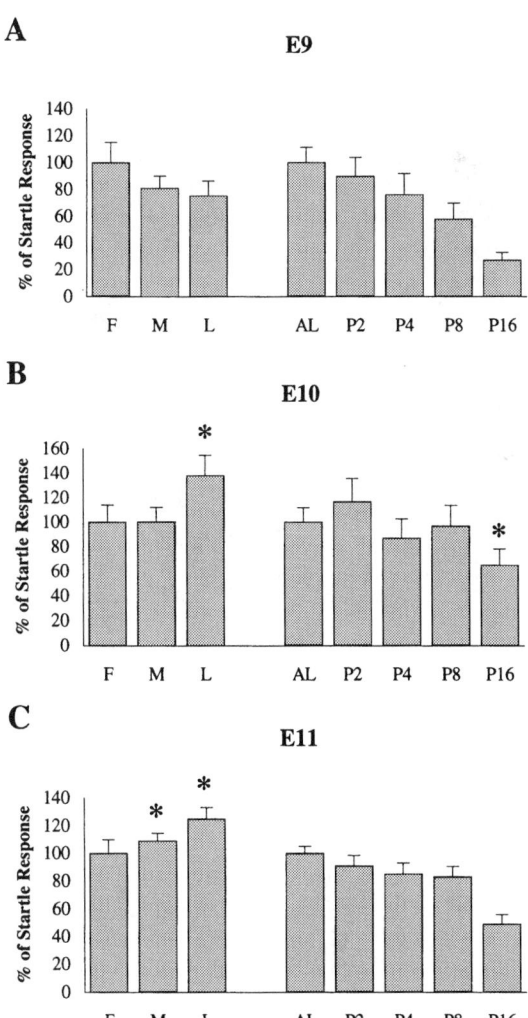

FIGURE 1. Mean scores for habituation and prepulse inhibition of the startle response, in each group. The *left side* of the graphs shows the startle response in the first (F), the middle (M), and the last part of the startle session (L), following a climbing number of startle stimulus presentations. The degree of habituation in the middle and last part of the session is expressed as a percentage of the basal startle response (F). The *right side* shows prepulse inhibition, following prepulses 2, 4, 8, and 16 dB above background (P2–P16). Startle amplitude on the prepulse trails is expressed as a percentage of startle amplitude on the startle stimulus alone (AL) trials. Habituation is severely impaired in the groups treated on E10 (**B**) and E11 (**C**). In addition, the E10-treated group displays a deficit in prepulse inhibition. * $p < 0.05$ in contrast analysis between groups, with the control group as reference category.

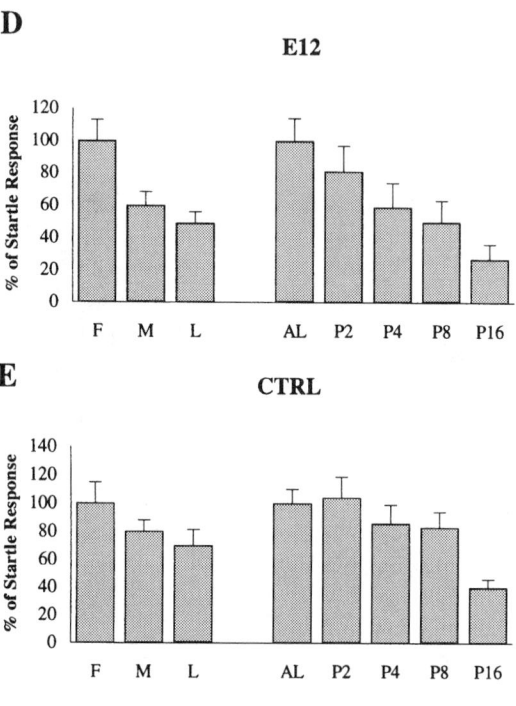

FIGURE 1. *Continued*

between treatment and prepulse intensity does not reach statistical significance (p <0.07). Further analysis, in general ANOVA procedures (FIG. 1), indicates statistically significant differences between the experimental groups for both measures of habituation (df 4.19; middle: $F = 4.17$, $p = 0.008$; late: $F = 7.8$, p <0.0001). The E10 and E11 group (FIG. 1B,C) displayed significantly less habituation than the control group, during the middle (E11: $t = 2.4$, p <0.03), and the last (E10: $t = 2.3$, p <0.03; E11: $t = 3.4$, $p = 0.003$) part of the habituation trial. In fact, during the late part of the startle experiment, mean startle response in groups E10 and E11 had increased to 130% and 140% of the initial response, respectively. Within groups, statistical analysis indicated absence of habituation in E10, while the E11-treated group displayed significant sensitization in the last part of the session ($F = 2.4$, df 2.97, Tukey's HSD: p <0.05). The experimental groups also differed significantly for all prepulse intensities (df 4.19; 2 dB: $F = 4.1$, p <0.02; 4 dB: $F = 3.3$, p <0.03; 8 dB: $F = 4.7$, $p = 0.008$; 16 dB: $F = 4.8$, $p = 0.007$). Here, the E10 group showed significantly less PPI than the control group in the condition with the highest prepulse intensity ($t = 2.4$, p <0.03; FIG. 1B). According to within-group analysis (df 4.145), E10 rats failed to show any statistically significant PPI.

A

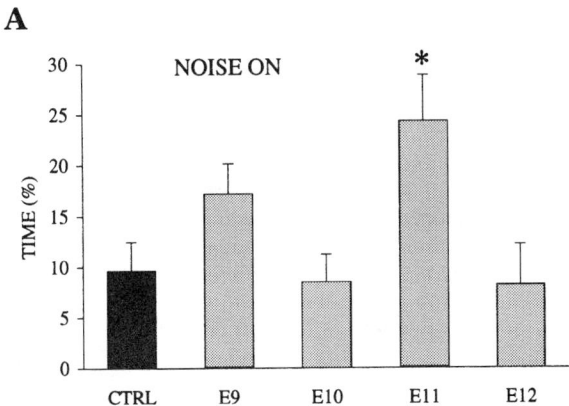

B

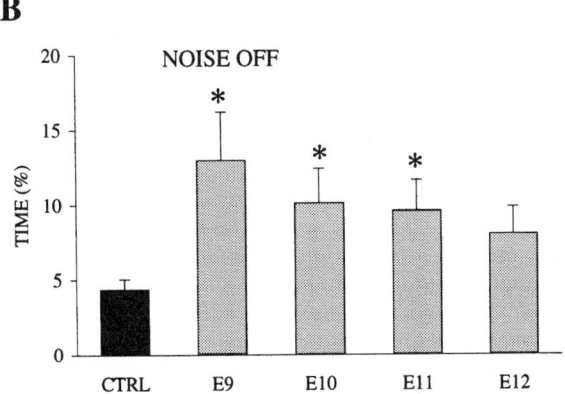

FIGURE 2. Mean percentage of time spent in the element "alert" is shown for the "noise-on" period (**A**) and the "noise-off" period of the sudden silence test. Duration of alert is significantly increased in E11 rats during the noise-on period. During the noise-off period, E9-, E10-, and E11-treated rats display increased durations of alert compared to the control group. * p <0.05 in post hoc comparisons.

Sudden Silence Paradigm

Analysis of variance indicated a difference between groups for the time spent in "alert" during both the "noise-on" (F = 3.4, df 4.31, p <0.02) and the "noise-off" period (F = 2.8, df 4.31, p <0.05). According to contrast analysis, E11 rats displayed a significantly increased percentage of alert behavior during the noise-on period (FIG. 2A) in comparison to controls (p <0.03). During the noise-off period (FIG. 2B) all MAM-treated groups, except the E12 group, displayed significantly increased amounts of alert behavior. The increase was largest in the E9 group (p <0.03) and somewhat smaller in the groups treated on E10 (p <0.04) and E11 (p <0.04).

DISCUSSION

These experiments show abnormalities in sensory gating and attention in rats prenatally exposed to MAM to induce schizophrenia-like abnormalities of neurodevelopment. The sensory gating deficits occur mainly in groups E10 and E11. Hereby, the E10 group displays reduced PPI of acoustic startle, while both groups show deficient habituation. The orientation–attention response, following a sudden change in the level of a background noise, is prolonged in groups E9, E10, and E11. In addition, the E11 group shows increased orienting to the sound stimulus during the "noise on" period. This latter effect may tentatively be interpreted as reflecting increased distractability.

As described in detail elsewhere,[11,13] the groups displaying impaired habituation and PPI (groups E10 and E11) suffered consequences of prenatal treatment in the lateral entorhinal region and, to a lesser extent, in the medial septal complex and the frontal area. The medial septum and prefrontal cortex are known to modulate acoustic startle.[22] Moreover, the entorhinal cortex represents a principal relay station between the hippocampus and the nucleus accumbens, which appears to be crucially involved in PPI.[22,23] It is, therefore, entirely possible that the MAM-induced abnormalities in this circuitry could affect PPI directly. Less is known about the central regulation of habituation to startle stimuli. Studies thus far show that short-term habituation is sustained in decerebrated animals and can be modulated by serotonergic drugs.[22]

With regard to the regulation of attention and the focusing of behavior on certain aspects of the environment, both the frontal and the (para)hippocampal cortex have been implicated. Specifically, the anterior cingulate and prefrontal cortex are activated during divided, selective and sustained attention,[24,25] while the hippocampal and parahippocampal regions appear to be necessary for novelty detection[26] and for the active focusing of behavior on novel environmental elements, respectively.[27] Again, it is not unlikely that the neurodevelopmental abnormalities in MAM-treated rats may directly underlie the impairments observed in the sudden silence paradigm, wherein various aspects of information filtering and attention may be expected to play a role. Notably, the sensory gating and attention deficits observed in the present experiments might be to some extent related. Interestingly in this context, the sensitizing to acoustic startle stimuli and the overall increased orientation–attention response in E11-treated rats suggest an exaggerated reaction to inconsequential auditive stimuli, which might extend to stimuli in general. Further research will be necessary to evaluate these possibilities.

Behavioral differences between the various MAM-treated groups presumably reflect differential morphological abnormalities, which shift with treatment day, following cerebral gradients of development. Notably, CNS hypoplasias are relatively mild in the earliest treated group; our studies thus far[11,13,13a] suggest that the E9-induced hypoplasias mostly concern the orbitofrontal region and the diagonal band area. With later treatment (groups E10 and E11), the lateral entorhinal cortex is additionally affected, and alterations in the septum shift upwards toward the medial septal nucleus. Finally, abnormalities in the E12 group encompass the entire entorhinal cortex (including the medial part), the subiculum, the perirhinal cortex, and the entire prefrontal cortex (also including the medial part), while tissue loss in the septum is most prominent in this group. In line with these more pronounced effects of MAM, there is an approximate 10% reduction of brain weight in the E12-treated group.

The present findings show that interruptions of cell proliferation during early corticogenesis in rats induce sensorimotor gating deficits analogous to those observed in schizophrenic subjects, as well as abnormalities of attention. As shown previously, similar prenatal insults induce various other impairments that may be related to schizophrenic symptoms, namely: social inadequacy and decreased social priming,[12] a reduced pain response,[13] impaired acquisition of passive avoidance,[13] delayed motor development, and subtle adult neurological impairment.[13a] Notably, morphological abnormalities induced at this stage of development, such as reductions of the entorhinal cortex and other mesocortical areas, disorganized cytoarchitecture, and abnormal temporal asymmetries, also present parallels with postmortem findings in schizophrenia.[1,6,7] We have herewith provided a model that combines pathogenic, neuropathological, and symptomatic aspects of schizophrenia into a single approach. The unique advantage of this approach is that it presents with a neuropathology that has similar characteristics to brain abnormalities in schizophrenia, and that it proposes a developmental mechanism by which this neuropathology might come about. As a consequence, the emergent behavioral and biochemical properties of the model are more likely to be based on neurobiological mechanisms similar to those acting in schizophrenia than is the case in other proposed models. The collective data from these experiments offers substantial support for a neurodevelopmental pathogenesis of schizophrenia and for the involvement of the mesocortex in this disorder.

REFERENCES

1. ARNOLD, S.E., B.T. HYMAN, G.V. VAN HOESEN, *et al.* 1991. Some cytoarchitectural abnormalities of the entorhinal cortex in schizophrenia. Arch. Gen. Psychiatry **48:** 625–632.
2. AKBARIAN, S., W.E. BUNNEY, S.G. POTKIN *et al.* 1993. Altered distribution of nicotinamide-adenine dinucleotide phosphate-diaphorase cells implies disturbances of cortical development. Arch. Gen. Psychiatry **50:** 169–177.
3. SHAM, P.C., E. O'CALLAGHAN, N. TAKEI, *et al.* 1992. Schizophrenia following pre-natal exposure to influenza epidemics between 1939 and 1960. Br. J. Psychiatry **160:** 461–466.
4. DAVIS, J.O., J.A. PHELPS & H.S. BRACHA. 1995. Prenatal development of monozygotic twins and concordance for schizophrenia. Schizophr. Bull. **21:** 357–366.
5. WOODS, B.T. 1998. Is schizophrenia a progressive neurodevelopmental disorder? Toward a unitary pathogenetic mechanism. Am. J. Psychiatry **155:** 661–670.
6. BRACHA, H.S. 1991. Etiology of structural asymmetry in schizophrenia: an alternative hypothesis. Schizophr. Bull. **17:** 551–553.
7. TALAMINI, L.M., J.W. LOUWERENS, C.J. SLOOF, *et al.* 1994. PET versus postmortem studies in schizophrenia research: significance for the pathogenesis and pharmacotherapy. *In* Advances in the Neurobiology of Schizophrenia. J.A. Den Boer, H.G.M. Westenberg & H.M. Van Praag, Eds.: 157–188. John Wiley & Sons. Chichester.
8. LOPEZ DA SILVA, F.H., M.P. WITTER, P.H. BOEIJINGA, *et al.* 1990. Anatomic organisation and physiology of the limbic cortex. Physiol. Rev. **70:** 453–511.
9. BAYER, S.A. 1990. Development of the lateral and medial limbic cortices in the rat in relation to cortical phylogeny. Exp. Neurol. **107:** 118–131.
10. KOSTOVIC, I., Z. PETANJEK & M. JUDAS. 1993. Early areal differentiation of the human cerebral cortex: entorhinal area. Hippocampus **3:** 447–458.

11. TALAMINI, L.M., T. KOCH, G. TER HORST, *et al.* 1998. Methylazoxymethanol acetate-induced abnormalities in the entorhinal cortex of the rat: parallels with morphological findings in schizophrenia. Brain Res. **789:** 293–306.
12. TALAMINI, L.M., T. KOCH, P.G.M. LUITEN, *et al.* 1999. Interruptions of early cortical development affect limbic association areas and social behaviour in rats: possible relevance for neurodevelopmental disorders. Brain Res. **847:** 105–120.
13. FIORE, M., L.M. TALAMINI, F. ANGELUCCI, *et al.* 1999. Pharmacologically induced damage in the entorhinal cortex alters behavior and brain NGF levels in young rats: a possible correlation with the development of schizophrenia–like deficits. Neuropharmacology **38:** 857–869.
13a. TALAMINI, L.M., 2000. Studies on the pathogenesis of schizophrenia in a neurodevelopmental animal model. Ph.D. Thesis, University of Groningen, Groningen, The Netherlands.
14. ALAIN, C., R. HARGRAVE & D.L. WOODS. 1998. Processing of auditory stimuli during visual attention in patients with schizophrenia. Biol. Psychiatry **44:** 1151–1159.
15. KASAI, K., K. OKAZAWA, K. NAKAGOME, *et al.* 1999. Mismatch negativity and N2b attenuation as an indicator for dysfunction of the preattentive and controlled processing for deviance detection in schizophrenia: a topographic event-related potential study. Schizophr. Res. **35:** 141–156.
16. LOBERG, E.M., K. HUGDAHL & M.F. GREEN. 1999. Hemispheric asymmetry in schizophrenia: a "dual deficits" model. Biol. Psychiatry **45:** 76–81.
17. STRANDBURG, R.J., J.T. MARSH & W.S. BROWN. 1999. Continuous processing related ERPS in adult schizophrenia: continuity with childhood onset schizophrenia. Biol. Psychiatry **45:** 1356–1369.
18. BRAFF, D.L. 1985. Attention, habituation and information processing in psychiatric disorders. *In* Psychiatry. Vol. 3. R. MICHELS *et al.*, Eds.: 1–12. Lippincott Company. Philadelphia.
19. SWERDLOW, N.R. & M.A. GEYER. 1998. Using an animal model of deficient sensorimotor gating to study the pathophysiology and new treatments of schizophrenia. Schizophr. Bull. **24:** 285–301.
20. MATSUMOTO, H., M. SPATZ & G.L. LAQUEUR. 1972. Quantitative changes with age in the DNA content of methylazoxymethanol-induced microencephalic rat brain. J. Neurochem. **19:** 297–306.
21. ELLENBROEK, B.A., M.A. GEYER & A.R. COOLS. 1995. The behavior of APO-SUS rats in animal models with construct validity for schizophrenia. J. Neurosci. **15:** 7604–7611.
22. KOCH, M. & H.U. SCHNITZLER. 1997. The acoustic startle response in rats—circuits mediating evocation, inhibition and potentiation. Behav. Brain Res. **89:** 35–49.
23. WITTER, M.P., H.J. GROENEWEGEN, F.H. LOPEZ DA SILVA, *et al.* 1989. Functional organization of the extrinsic and intrinsic circuitry of the parahippocampal region. Progr. Neurobiol. **33:** 161–253.
24. CORBETTA, M., F.M. MIEZIN, S. DOBMEYER, *et al.* 1991. Selective and divided attention during visual discriminations of shape, color, and speed: functional anatomy by positron emission tomography. J. Neurosci. **11:** 2383–2340.
25. VANDENBERGHE, R., J. DUNCAN, P. DUPONT, *et al.* 1997. Attention to one or two features in left or right visual field: a positron emission tomography study. J. Neurosci. **17:** 3739–3750.
26. DOLAN, R.J. & P.C. FLETCHER. 1997. Dissociating prefrontal and hippocampal function in episodic memory encoding. Nature **338:** 532–535.
27. SCHENK, F., F. INGLIN & M. GYGER. 1983. Activity and exploratory behavior after lesions of the medial entorhinal cortex in the woodmouse (*Apodemus sylvaticus*). Behav. Neural Biol. **37:** 89–107.

Morphometric MRI Analysis of the Parahippocampal Region in Temporal Lobe Epilepsy

NEDA BERNASCONI,[a] ANDREA BERNASCONI, ZOGRAFOS CARAMANOS, FREDERICK ANDERMANN, FRANÇOIS DUBEAU, AND DOUGLAS L. ARNOLD

Department of Neurology and Neurosurgery, McGill University and Montreal Neurological Institute and Hospital, Montreal, Quebec H3A 2B4, Canada

ABSTRACT: Despite neuropathological and electrophysiological evidence for the involvement of parahippocampal structures in temporal lobe epilepsy (TLE), little attention has been paid to morphometric changes in these structures, and the relation of these changes to TLE. We performed high-resolution MRI volumetric analysis to examine *in vivo* the morphology of the parahippocampal region in 20 healthy subjects and 6 TLE patients with MRI evidence of unilateral hippocampal atrophy. In normal controls the standardized volume of the left entorhinal cortex (EC) was 1305 ± 138 mm^3 and that of the right EC was 1376 ± 170 mm^3; the left perirhinal cortex (PC) was 2900 ± 554 mm^3 and the right PC was 2771 ± 486 mm^3; the left posterior parahippocampal cortex (PPC) was 2499 ± 583 mm^3 and the right PPC was 2234 ± 404 mm^3. Using a 2 standard deviation cutoff from the mean of normal controls, we found ipsilateral to the seizure focus: (*i*) a reduction in the volume of the EC in all patients; (*ii*) a reduction of the PC in 2/6 (33%) patients; (*iii*) no reduction in the volume of the PPC in any patient. In 3/6 (50%) of patients, the EC was also abnormally small contralateral to the seizure focus. In patients with unilateral TLE, the EC is the most affected structure within the parahippocampal region. Whether this is due to a primary role of the EC in the genesis of TLE or is the consequence of its pivotal position in the reciprocal flow of information between the hippocampus and the neo- and limbic cortices remains to be explored.

INTRODUCTION

The human mesial temporal region is composed of the hippocampus, the amygdala, and the parahippocampal region. The parahippocampal region itself is composed of the entorhinal cortex (EC), the perirhinal cortex (PC), and the posterior parahippocampal (areas TH and TF of von Bonin and Bailey[1]) cortex (PPC).

In early studies of surgically resected specimens of patients with temporal lobe epilepsy (TLE), the term "mesial temporal sclerosis" was introduced to describe widespread pathological changes of the hippocampus, the amygdala, and the sur-

[a]Address for correspondence: Dr. Neda Bernasconi, Brain Imaging Center, Montreal Neurological Hospital and Institute, 3801 University Street, Montreal, Quebec, Canada, H3A 2B4. Tel.: (514) 398-8185; fax: (514) 398-2975.
e-mail: neda@bic.mni.mcgill.ca

rounding cortical areas.[2] More recently, magnetic resonance imaging (MRI) studies in TLE have put the emphasis on the hippocampus. Hippocampal atrophy on MRI has been shown to correlate with the presence of hippocampal sclerosis.[3] We have recently shown a reduction in the volume of the EC ipsilateral to the seizure focus in patients with temporal lobe epilepsy[4] that is presumably an MRI correlate of neuronal loss and gliosis previously described.[5]

The purpose of this study was to examine if *in vivo* volume changes of different components of the parahippocampal region are apparent on MRI and to determine the distribution of atrophy within the parahippocampal region in patients with TLE.

METHODS

We selected six patients with medically intractable TLE (mean age, 37; range, 20–56) and unilateral hippocampal atrophy on volumetric MRI. Patients were compared to 20 neurologically normal controls (mean age, 27; range, 20–45).

Lateralization of Seizure Focus

Seizure type and the site of seizure onset were determined by a comprehensive evaluation including detailed history, neurological examination, review of medical and EEG records, and neuropsychological evaluation. The seizure focus was determined by predominantly ipsilateral interictal epileptic abnormalities (70% cutoff), by unequivocal unilateral seizure onset recorded during prolonged video-EEG monitoring using sphenoidal electrodes, and by response to surgical treatment in all six cases. All patients underwent a selective amygdalo-hippocampectomy. Qualitative histopathologic examination[6] of the resected tissue revealed hippocampal sclerosis in all patients. Because of subpial gyral aspiration, histopathology of the parahippocampal region structures was not available. All patients have been seizure-free since surgery with a mean postoperative follow-up of 20 months (range, 12 months to 2.5 years). On the basis of these criteria, TLE patients were divided into those with a left-sided (*n* = 3) or a right-sided (*n* = 3) seizure focus.

MRI Scanning

MRI volumetric images were acquired on a 1.5 T Gyroscan (Philips Medical System, Eindhoven, The Netherlands), using a T1 fast-field echo, TR = 18, TE = 10, one acquisition average pulse sequence, 30° flip angle, matrix size, 256 × 256, FOV = 256, thickness = 1 mm. Approximately 170 isotropic images with a voxel size of 1 mm × 1 mm × 1 mm were acquired.

Image Processing

Analysis was performed on a Silicon Graphics workstation (Mountain View, CA). Images were automatically registered into stereotaxic space[7] to adjust for differences in total brain volume and brain orientation and to facilitate the identification of boundaries by minimizing variability in slice orientation.[8] Each image underwent automated correction for intensity nonuniformity due to radiofrequency inhomogeneity of the MR scanner and intensity standardization.[9] This correction produces

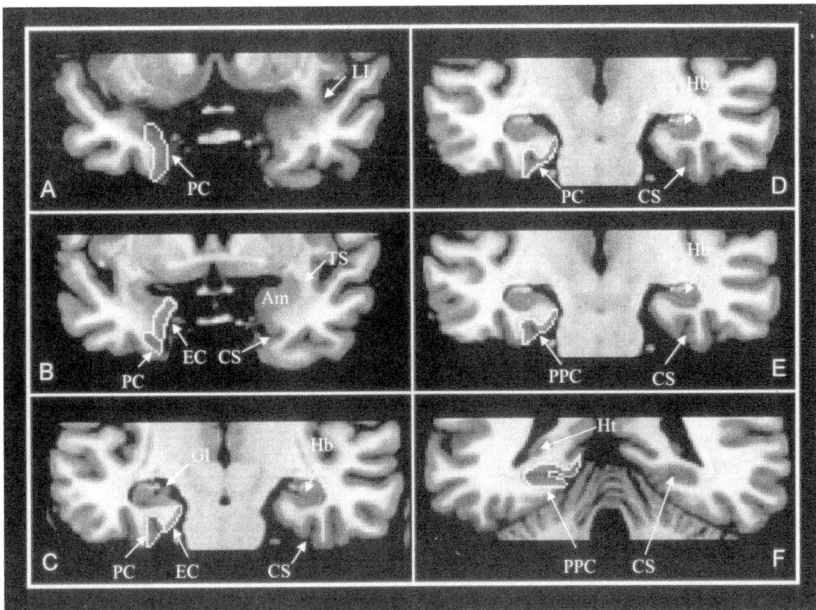

FIGURE 1. Major anatomical boundaries of parahippocampal region structures on coronal MR images. *A* is the most rostral, and *F* is the most caudal MR section. Only MR images displaying critical landmarks are shown. **(A)** Anterior border of the perirhinal cortex (PC) at the level of limen insulae (LI); **(B)** anterior border of the entorhinal cortex (EC) at the level of temporal stem (TS); **(C)** posterior border of the EC at the level of posterior limit of gyrus intralimbicus (GI); **(D)** posterior border of the PC, situated 2 mm caudal to the posterior end of the EC; **(E)** anterior border of the posterior parahippocampal cortex (PPC), situated 1 mm caudal to the posterior end of the PC; **(F)** posterior border of the PPC, situated at the level of the posterior end of the hippocampal tail (Ht). Am = amygdala; Hb = hippocampal body; CS = collateral sulcus.

consistent relative gray matter, white matter, and CSF intensities. The hippocampus,[10] the EC,[4,11] the PC,[11] and the PPC[12] were segmented manually using mouse-driven software according to previously described protocols (FIG. 1).

Statistical Analysis

The normality of the distribution of volume measurements for the entorhinal, perirhinal, and posterior parahippocampal cortices was assessed using normal probability plots. The statistical significance of differences in mean volumes between right and left sides was assessed using paired *t*-test. In the analysis of individual patients, values two standard deviations (SD) below the mean of normal controls were considered as abnormal.

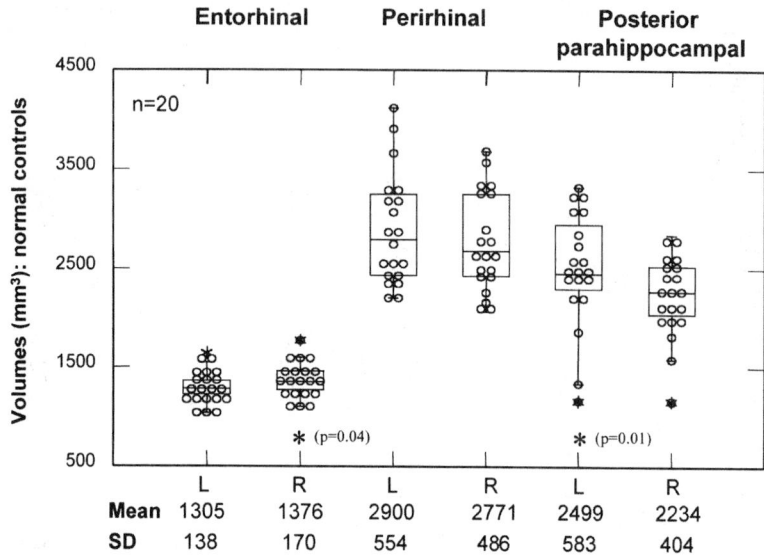

FIGURE 2. Box-and-whisker plots of the volumes of the entorhinal, perirhinal, and posterior parahippocampal cortices in normal controls. The center horizontal line marks the median of the sample; the upper and lower edges of the box (the hinges) mark the 25th and 75th percentiles (i.e., the central 50% of the values fall within the box)—the distance between these hinges being referred to as the Hspread, and the "whiskers" extend from the box and show the range of values that fall within 1.5 Hspread. The dots represent individual subjects. L and R refer to left and right. The mean and standard deviation (SD) is shown for each structure at the bottom of the figure.

RESULTS

In normal controls, the mean volume of the right EC (1376 ± 170 mm^3) was slightly greater than that of the left (1305 ± 138 mm^3; $p < 0.05$). The mean volume of the right PC was 2771 ± 486 mm^3 and that of the left was 2900 ± 554 mm^3 ($p > 0.05$). The mean volume of the left PPC (2499 ± 583 mm^3) was greater than that of the right (2234 ± 404 mm^3; $p < 0.01$) (Fig. 2).

Ipsilateral to the seizure focus, (i) the EC was abnormally small in all six patients; (ii) the PC was abnormally small in 2/6 patients; (iii) the PPC was normal in all six patients. Contralateral to the seizure focus, the EC was abnormally small in 3/6 patients. The PC and the PPC were normal in all patients (Fig. 3).

DISCUSSION

Our results show that in patients with intractable TLE and unilateral hippocampal atrophy, the EC is always abnormal, the PC is sometimes abnormal, and the PPC is

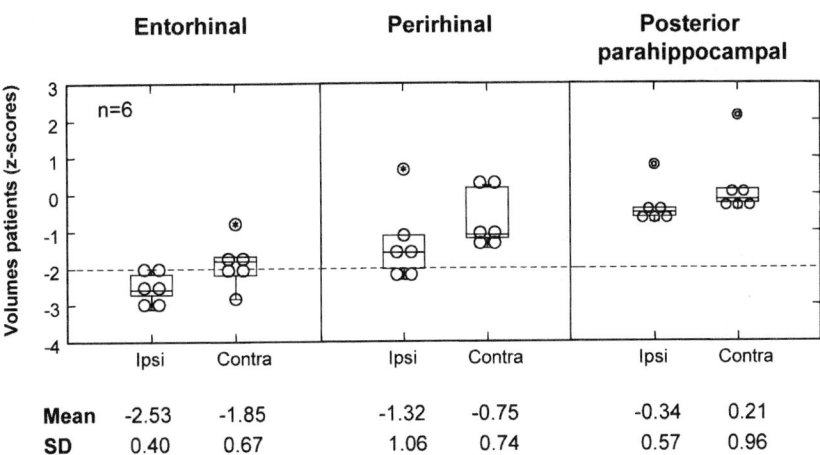

FIGURE 3. Box-and-whisker plots of the volumes of the entorhinal, perirhinal, and posterior parahippocampal cortices in TLE patients standardized relative to the normal controls. Scores are shown in units of standard deviations (SD) with 0 equaling the mean of normal controls. The dots represent individual subjects, and the filled squares represent the group means. The broken lines designate 2 SD below the mean of normal controls. Ipsi and contra refer to ipsilateral and contralateral to seizure focus.

always normal ipsilateral to the seizure focus. Within the parahippocampal region, the EC is the only structure that is bilaterally small in 50% of cases.

In an MRI volumetric analysis of the effect of long-lasting seizures in TLE patients, damage in the hippocampus, the amygdala, and the rostral portion of the parahippocampal gyrus has been described ipsilateral to the seizure focus.[13] In our study we divided the parahippocampal region into its three components. In doing so, we were able to show for the first time that atrophy is not equally distributed within the parahippocampal region. This information might be used in the planning of surgical treatment of pharmacologically intractable TLE.

Investigations with stereotactic electrodes have shown that seizure onset may be in the amygdala, the hippocampus, or the entorhinal cortex.[14] *In vitro* studies of focal epileptogenesis in combined hippocampal–entorhinal slices have demonstrated that the entorhinal cortex possesses an intrinsic capacity to generate epileptiform discharges.[15] After aminooxyacetic acid injection in the rat entorhinal cortex, there is extensive cell loss in layer III[16] of medial entorhinal cortex identical to the lesion found in human TLE.[5] The damage to the entorhinal cortex may contribute to long-lasting changes in excitability in the entorhinal cortex and the hippocampus and play a primary role in the genesis and spread of temporal lobe seizures.[17] However, the reason for a preferential damage to the entorhinal cortex in our patients remains unclear.

Our finding of a bilateral reduction in volume of the entorhinal cortex in 50% of cases concurs with the view that more widespread damage of mesial temporal lobe structures may occur even in patients with predominantly or strictly unilateral TLE. The fact that, within the parahippocampal region, only the entorhinal cortex is affected bilaterally may be due to its remarkable hyperexcitability.[17,18]

In this study we provide MRI corroboration of the pathological findings of neuronal loss and gliosis in the parahippocampal region, particularly in the entorhinal cortex. However, further studies are needed to define the roles of the different components of mesial temporal lobe in the genesis of temporal lobe epilepsy.

REFERENCES

1. BAILEY, P. & G. VON BONIN. 1951. The Isocortex of Man. University of Illinois Press. Urbana, IL.
2. FALCONER, M.A., E.A. SERAFETINIDES & J.A.N. CORSELLIS. 1964. Etiology and pathogenesis of temporal lobe epilepsy. Arch. Neurol. **10:** 233–248.
3. JACKSON, G.D., S.F. BERKOVIC, B.M. TRESS, et al. 1990. Hippocampal sclerosis can be reliably detected by magnetic resonance imaging. Neurology **40:** 1869–1875.
4. BERNASCONI, N., A. BERNASCONI, F. ANDERMANN, et al. 1999. Entorhinal cortex in temporal lobe epilepsy: a quantitative MRI study. Neurology **52:** 1870–1876.
5. DU, F., W.O. WHETSELL, B. ABOU-KHALIL & B. BLUMENKOPF. 1993. Preferential neuronal loss in layer III of the entorhinal cortex in patients with temporal lobe epilepsy. Epilepsy Res. **16:** 223–233.
6. MEENCKE, H.J. & G. VEITH. 1991. Hippocampal sclerosis in epilepsy. In Epilepsy Surgery. H. Lüders, Ed. Raven Press. New York.
7. TALAIRACH, J. & P. TOURNOUX. 1988. Co-planar stereotaxic atlas of the human brain. Thieme Medical Publishers. New York.
8. COLLINS, D.L., P. NEELIN, T.M. PETERS & A.C. EVANS. 1994. Automatic 3D intersubject registration of MR volumetric data in standardized Talairach space. J. Comput. Assist. Tomogr. **18:** 192–205.
9. SLED, J.G., A.P. ZIJDENBOS & A.C. EVANS. 1998. A nonparametric method for automatic correction of intensity non-uniformity in MRI data. IEEE Trans. Med. Imaging **17:** 87–97.
10. WATSON, C., F. ANDERMANN, P. GLOOR, et al. 1992. Anatomic basis of amygdaloid and hippocampal volume measurement by magnetic resonance imaging. Neurology **42:** 1743–1750.
11. INSAUSTI, R., K. JUOTTONEN, H. SOININEN, et al. 1998. MR volumetric analysis of the human entorhinal, perirhinal, and temporopolar cortices. AJNR Am. J. Neuroradiol. **19:** 659–671.
12. INSAUSTI, R., A.M. INSAUSTI, M.T. SOBREVIELA, et al. 1998. Human medial temporal lobe in aging: anatomical basis of memory preservation. Microsc. Res. Tech. **43:** 8–15.
13. SAUKKONEN, A., R. KÄLVIÄINEN, K. PARTANEN, et al. 1994. Do seizures cause neuronal damage? A MRI study in newly diagnosed and chronic epilepsy. Neuroreport **6:** 219–223.
14. SPENCER, S.S. & D.D. SPENCER. 1994. Entorhinal–hippocampal interactions in medial temporal lobe epilepsy. Epilepsia **35:** 721–727.
15. BEAR, J. & E.W. LOTHMAN. 1993. An in vitro study of focal epileptogenesis in combined hippocampal–parahippocampal slices. Epilepsy Res. **14:** 183–193.
16. DU, F. & R. SCHWARCZ. 1992. Aminooxyacetic acid causes selective neuronal loss in layer III of the rat medial entorhinal cortex. Neurosci. Lett. **147:** 185–188.
17. SCHARFMAN, H.E., J.H. GOODMAN, F. DU & R. SCHWARCZ. 1998. Chronic changes in synaptic responses of entorhinal and hippocampal neurons after amino-oxyacetic acid (AOAA)-induced entorhinal cortical neuron loss. J. Neurophysiol. **80:** 3031–3046.
18. BEAR, J., N.B. FOUNTAIN & E.W. LOTHMAN. 1996. Responses of the superficial entorhinal cortex in vitro in slices from naive and chronically epileptic rats. J. Neurophysiol. **76:** 2928–2940.

Index of Contributors